FIFTH EDITION

LANGE Q&A™

USMLE STEP 3

Donald A. Briscoe, MD
Program Director, Methodist Hospital (Houston) Family Medicine Residency
Medical Director, Denver Harbor Clinic
Clinical Assistant Professor of Family Medicine in Medicine
Weill Medical College of Cornell University
Houston, Texas

New York Chicago San Francisco Lisbon London Madrid Mexico City
Milan New Delhi San Juan Seoul Singapore Sydney Toronto

Lange Q&A™: USMLE Step 3, Fifth Edition

Copyright © 2008 by The McGraw-Hill Companies, Inc. All rights reserved. Printed in the United States of America. Except as permitted under the United States Copyright Act of 1976, no part of this publication may be reproduced or distributed in any form or by any means, or stored in a data base or retrieval system, without the prior written permission of the publisher.

Previous edition copyright © 2005 by The McGraw-Hill Companies, Inc.

Lange Q&A™ is a trademark of The McGraw-Hill Companies, Inc.

1 2 3 4 5 6 7 8 9 0   QPD/QPD   0 9 8

ISBN 978-0-07-149259-1
MHID 0-07-149259-3

Notice

Medicine is an ever-changing science. As new research and clinical experience broaden our knowledge, changes in treatment and drug therapy are required. The authors and the publisher of this work have checked with sources believed to be reliable in their efforts to provide information that is complete and generally in accord with the standards accepted at the time of publication. However, in view of the possibility of human error or changes in medical sciences, neither the authors nor the publisher nor any other party who has been involved in the preparation or publication of this work warrants that the information contained herein is in every respect accurate or complete, and they disclaim all responsibility for any errors or omissions or for the results obtained from use of the information contained in this work. Readers are encouraged to confirm the information contained herein with other sources. For example and in particular, readers are advised to check the product information sheet included in the package of each drug they plan to administer to be certain that the information contained in this work is accurate and that changes have not been made in the recommended dose or in the contraindications for administration. This recommendation is of particular importance in connection with new or infrequently used drugs.

This book was set in Palatino by International Typesetting and Composition.
The editor was Catherine A. Johnson.
The production supervisor was John Williams.
Project management was provided by Harleen Chopra, International Typesetting and Composition.
The cover design was by the Gazillion Group.
Quebecor World Dubuque was printer and binder.

This book is printed on acid-free paper.

Library of Congress Cataloging-in-Publication Data

Lange Q & A. USMLE Step 3 / [edited by] Donald A. Briscoe.—5th ed.
    p. ; cm.
   Includes index.
   ISBN-13: 978-0-07-149259-1 (pbk. : alk. paper)
   ISBN-10: 0-07-149259-3 (pbk. : alk. paper)
   1. Medicine—Examinations, questions, etc. 2. Physicians—Licenses—United
States—Examinations—Study guides. I. Briscoe, Donald A. II. Title: USMLE
Step 3. III. Title: Lange Q and A. USMLE Step 3.
   [DNLM: 1. Medicine—Examination Questions. W 18.2 L2742 2008]
  R834.5A662 2008
  610.76—dc22

                                      2007036055

Contents

47

Color insert appears between pages 94 and 95.

Contributors

Douglas G. Adler, MD, FACG, FASGE
Assistant Professor of Medicine
Director of Therapeutic Endoscopy
University of Utah, School of Medicine
Huntsman Cancer Center
Salt Lake City, Utah

Brian K. Bednarski, MD
Department of Surgery
University of North Carolina School of Medicine
Chapel Hill, North Carolina

Sean M. Blitzstein, MD
Director, Psychiatry Clerkship
Clinical Assistant Professor of Psychiatry
University of Illinois at Chicago
Chicago, Illinois

Edison Catalano, MD
Medical Director, Laboratory
Cooper University Hospital
Camden, New Jersey

Christian A. Chisholm, MD
Associate Professor
Department of Obstetrics and Gynecology
University of Virginia School of Medicine
Charlottesville, Virginia

Miguel A. Escobar, MD
Assistant Professor
Department of Pediatrics and Internal Medicine
University of Texas Health Science Center
at Houston
Houston, Texas

Christopher A. Greeley, MD, FAAP
Associate Professor of Pediatrics
Division of Community and General Pediatrics
University of Texas Health Science Center
at Houston
Houston, Texas

Vanessa H. Gregg, MD
Assistant Professor
Department of Obstetrics and Gynecology
University of Virginia Health System
Charlottesville, Virginia

Kathie L. Hullfish, MD
University of Virginia Health System
Charlottesville, Virginia

Philip C. Johnson, MD, FACP
Professor and Director
Division of General Medicine
University of Texas Medical School at Houston
Houston, Texas

Maureen C. Kelley, PhD
Assistant Professor
Department of Pediatrics
Treuman Katz Center for Pediatric Bioethics
University of Washington School of Medicine
Seattle, Washington

H. J. Kim, MD
Assistant Professor of Surgery
Division of Surgical Oncology
University of North Carolina School of Medicine
Lineberger Comprehensive Cancer Center
Chapel Hill, North Carolina

Terry L. McDermott, MD
Resident
Methodist Hospital (Houston) Family Medicine
Residency
Houston, Texas

Susan M. Miller, MD, MPH
Faculty, Methodist Hospital (Houston) Family
Medicine Residency
Associate Professor of Clinical Medicine
Weill Medical College of Cornell University
Houston, Texas

Seunghee Oh, MD
Resident, Methodist Hospital (Houston) Family
Medicine Residency
Houston, Texas

Philip R. Orlander, MD
Professor of Medicine
Director, Division of Endocrinology, Diabetes,
and Metabolism
Assistant Dean for Curricular Affairs
University of Texas Medical School at Houston
Houston, Texas

John T. Patlan, MD
Assistant Professor
Department of General Internal Medicine
The University of Texas—MD Anderson Cancer Center
Houston, Texas

Anush S. Pillai, DO
Faculty, Methodist Hospital (Houston) Family
Medicine Residency
Clinical Assistant Professor of Family Medicine in
Medicine
Weill Medical College of Cornell University
Houston, Texas

Richard A. Rubin, MD
Associate Clinical Professor of Medicine and
Rheumatology
Baylor College of Medicine
Clinical Chief of Rheumatology
The Methodist Hospital
Chief of Rheumatology
St. Lukes's Episcopal Hospital
Houston, Texas

Roland Schwarting, MD
Cooper University Hospital
Camden, New Jersey

Leora J. Tesche, MD
Department of Surgery
University of North Carolina School of Medicine
Chapel Hill, North Carolina

Introduction

This book is designed for those preparing for the United States Medical Licensing Examination (USMLE) Step 3. It provides a comprehensive review source with over 1000 "exam-type" multiple-choice questions covering the clinical sciences. Detailed explanations are provided for each question, with attempts to explain both why the correct answer is correct and, when appropriate, why the incorrect answers are incorrect. In addition, the last section of this book provides integrated, multispecialty practice tests, both to provide self-assessment and to simulate the multiple-choice parts of the Step 3 examination.

The United States Medical Licensing Examination, Step 3

Purpose of the Examination

The purpose of Step 3 is to determine if a physician possesses and can apply the medical knowledge and understanding of clinical science considered essential for the unsupervised practice of medicine, with emphasis placed on patient management in ambulatory care settings. The inclusion of Step 3 in the USMLE sequence of examinations ensures that attention is devoted to the importance of assessing the knowledge and skills of physicians who are assuming independent responsibility for providing general medical care to patients.

Examination Format

Step 3 consists of multiple-choice items and computer-based simulations, distributed according to the content blueprint. The examination material is prepared by committees broadly representing the medical profession. The committees comprise recognized experts in their fields, both academic and nonacademic practitioners, as well as members of state medical licensing boards.

Step 3 is a two-day examination. You must complete each day within 8 hours. The first day includes approximately 336 multiple-choice items divided into blocks of 48 items. Sixty minutes is allowed for completion of each block. There is a maximum of 7 hours of testing time and a minimum of 45 minutes of break time. There is also an optional 15-minute tutorial. The amount of break time may be increased by finishing the blocks or optional tutorial before the allowed time expires.

Day 2 of testing includes approximately 144 multiple-choice items divided into blocks of 36 items. Forty-five minutes is allotted for each of these blocks, with a total testing time of 3 hours for the completion of these blocks. The second day also includes a Primum tutorial, for which 15 minutes is allowed. This is followed by 9 case simulations, for which 4 hours is allotted. There is an optional survey at the end of the second day, which can be completed if time allows. A minimum of 45 minutes of break time is available on day 2.

The timing and structure of the testing days are subject to change without notice. Please refer to the USMLE web site (www.usmle.org) for the most up-to-date information.

The principal organizing dimension for Step 3 design is the clinical encounter frame. The concept of frames encompasses several elements that are critical to the definition of a physician-patient encounter. These elements include whether the problem is new or on-going, the urgency of the need for intervention relative to the underlying problem, the chronology of events and the degree of familiarity of the physician with the patient or the patient's history. In addition, each encounter occurs in a specific location. The primary encounter frames include initial workups, continuing care, and urgent interventions.

The second organizing dimension is the physician task, which includes six categories:

1. Obtaining history and performing physical examination;
2. Using laboratory and diagnostic studies;
3. Formulating the most likely diagnosis;
4. Evaluating the severity of the patient's problems;
5. Managing the patient (including health maintenance, interventions, therapeutics, applying legal and ethical principles); and
6. Applying basic science concepts (mechanisms).

Initial workup encounters are presentation of new, acutely occurring problems among patients seen for the first time. Tasks emphasized include extensive data gathering and initial therapeutic interventions. Continuing care encounters are characterized by management of previously diagnosed clinical problems among patients seen principally in ambulatory settings. Evaluating the severity of the problem(s) and prognosis, monitoring therapy and long-term management are emphasized. Urgent care encounters include life and/or organ-threatening emergencies, usually occurring in the emergency department or inpatient settings. Physician tasks emphasized include rapid assessment of complex presentations and prompt therapeutic decision making.

The 2007 USMLE Bulletin of Information specifies that the clinical encounter frames will be broken down as follows: 20–30% initial care; 50–60% continued care; 15–25% emergency care. The physician tasks will be broken down as follows: 8–12% obtaining history and performing physical examination; 8–12% using laboratory and diagnostic studies; 8–12% formulating most likely diagnosis; 8–12% prognosis; 8–12% applying scientific concepts and mechanisms of disease; 45–55% managing the patient, which is broken down into 5–9% health maintenance, 18–22% clinical intervention, 12–16% clinical therapeutics and 4–8% legal and ethical considerations. All of these percentages are subject to change. The most up-to-date information is available at the USMLE web site (www.usmle.org).

During the allowed time for an individual block, the questions may be answered in any order,

reviewed, and changed. After exiting a block, no further review of items or change of answers within that block is possible. Policies regarding review of test items may be changed without notice. The most current policies regarding review are posted on the USMLE web site at www.usmle.org. The computer interface includes, among other features, clickable icons for marking questions for review, automated review of marked and incomplete items, and a clock indicating the amount of time remaining. A tutorial on using the computer interface is available at the USMLE web site. A 15-minute optional tutorial will be available for your use on the day of your examination.

Step 3 cases are intended to reflect the diversity of health care populations with respect to age, cultural group, and occupation. The patient population mix is intended to be representative of data collected from various national databases that study health care in the United States.

Clinical Settings

The expected outcome of USMLE Step 3 is an unrestricted license to practice medicine without supervision. Although you may have already begun specialist training, for this examination you are to assume the role of a general physician. You are a member of an independent group practice associated with a number of managed care plans. Your office has regularly scheduled hours. You can admit patients to the 400-bed regional hospital, which provides care for both the urban and outlying rural communities. The hospital provides standard diagnostic, radiologic, and therapeutic options, including ICUs and cardiothoracic surgery. There is a labor and delivery suite. A fully equipped emergency department adjoins the hospital, and medical evacuation helicopter service is available for transfer to a regional trauma center. You do not have specialty-oriented hospital privileges but may request specialist consultation. The table of normal laboratory values provided represents the normal values for the hospital.

The multiple-choice items are organized into blocks that correspond to the clinical settings in which you will encounter the patients. Each setting is described at the beginning of its block. These descriptions are shown here as they would appear during the examination.

Setting I: Office/Health Center

You see patients in two locations: Your office suite, which is adjacent to a hospital, and at a community-based health center. Your office practice is a primary care generalist group. Most of the patients you see are from your own practice and are appearing for regularly scheduled return visits. Occasionally, you will encounter a patient whose primary care is managed by one of your associates. Reference may be made to the patient's medical records. Known patients may be managed by the telephone. You may have to respond to questions about information appearing in the public media, which will require interpretation of the medical literature. The laboratory and radiology departments have a full range of services available.

Setting II: Emergency Department and Inpatient Facilities

You encounter patients in the emergency department and inpatient facilities, including the hospital, the adjacent nursing home/extended-care facility, and detoxification unit. Most patients in the emergency department are new to you and are seeking urgent care, but occasionally, you arrange to meet there with a known patient who has telephoned you. You have general admitting privileges to the hospital, including to the children's and women's services. On occasion you see patients in the critical care unit. Postoperative patients are usually seen in their rooms unless the recovery room is specified. You may also be called to see patients in the psychiatric unit. There is a short–stay unit where you may see patients undergoing same–day operations or being held for observation. Also available to you are a full range of social services, including rape crisis intervention, family support, and security assistance backed up by local police.

Step 3 Test Item Formats

Multiple-Choice Items

Multiple-choice items are presented in several formats within each test block. Each of the formats requires selection of the one best choice. The general instructions for answering items are as follows:

Read each question carefully and in the order in which it is presented. Then select the one best response option of the choices offered. More than one option may be partially correct. You must select ONE BEST answer by clicking your mouse on the appropriate answer button or pressing the letter on the keyboard.

Single Items

This is the traditional, most frequently used multiple-choice format. It usually consists of a patient in a clinical setting and a reason for the visit. The item vignette is followed by four or five response options lettered A, B, C, D, and E. You are required to select the best answer to the question. Other options may be partially correct, but there is only ONE BEST answer.

Process for Single Items

- Read the patient description of each item carefully.
- Try to formulate an answer and then look for it in the list of options.
- Alternatively, read each option carefully and eliminate those that you think are incorrect.
- Of the remaining options, select the one that you believe is most correct.
- If unsure about an answer, it is better to guess, as unanswered questions are counted as incorrect.

The following is an example of a single item question.

Example item 1

1. A 45-year old African-American man comes to the office for the first time because he says, "I had blood in my urine this morning." He reports no other symptoms. On physical examination, his blood pressure is elevated and his kidneys are palpable bilaterally. The information in his history that is most pertinent to his current condition is:

    (A) chronic use of analgesics
    (B) cigarette smoking
    (C) a family history of renal disease
    (D) occupational exposure to carbon tetrachloride
    (E) recent sore throats

(Answer C)

Multiple Item Sets

A single patient-centered vignette may be associated with two or three consecutive questions about the information presented. Each question is linked to the vignette, but is testing a different point. Items are designed to be answered independently of each other. You are required to select the one best choice for each question. Other options may be partially correct, but there is only ONE BEST answer. The process of answering these items is the same as for single items.

Example Items 2–4

A 38-year-old white woman, who is a part-time teacher and mother of three children, comes to the office for evaluation of hypertension. You have been her physician since the birth of her first child 8 years ago. One week ago, an elevated blood pressure was detected during a regularly scheduled examination for entrance into graduate school. Vital signs today are:

Temp: 98.6° F
Pulse: 100 bpm
Resp: 22 per minute
BP: 164/100 mmHg (right arm, supine)

2. The most likely finding on physical examination is:

    (A) an abdominal bruit
    (B) cardiac enlargement
    (C) decreased femoral pulses
    (D) thyroid enlargement
    (E) normal retinas

(Answer E)

3. The most appropriate next step is to order:

    (A) complete blood count
    (B) serum electrolytes and creatinine
    (C) serum glucose
    (D) serum thyroxine
    (E) urine culture

(Answer B)

4. To assess this patient's risk factors for atherogenesis, the most appropriate test is determination of:

    (A) plasma renin activity
    (B) serum cholesterol
    (C) serum triglycerides
    (D) urinary aldosterone excretion
    (E) urinary metanephrine excretion

(Answer B)

Cases

A single-patient or family-centered vignette may ask as few as two and as many as three questions, each related to the initial opening vignette. Information is added as the case unfolds. **It is extremely important to answer the questions in the order presented.** Time often passes within a case and your orientation to an item early in a case may be altered by the additional information presented later in the case. If you do skip items, be sure to answer earlier questions with only the information presented to that point in the case. Each item is intended to be answered independently. You are required to select the ONE BEST choice to each question.

Example Items 5–7

A 24-year-old man comes to the office because of intermittent chest pain that began a few weeks ago. You have been his physician for the past 2 years and he has been in otherwise good health. He says that he is not having pain currently. A review of his medical record shows that his serum cholesterol concentration was normal at a preemployment physical examination 1 year ago. You have not seen him since that visit and he says that he has had no other complaints or problems in the interim. He reminds you that he smokes a pack of cigarettes a day. When you question him further, he says that he does not use any alcohol or illicit drugs. Although the details are vague, he describes the chest pain as a substernal tightness that is not related to exertion.

5. The finding on physical examination that would be most consistent with costochondritis as the cause of his chest pain is:

(A) crepitance over the second and third ribs anteriorly

(B) deep tenderness to hand pressure on the sternum

(C) localized point tenderness in the parasternal area

(D) pain on deep inspiration

(E) normal physical examination

(Answer C)

6. In light of the patient's original denial of drug use, the most appropriate next step to confirm a diagnosis of cocaine use is to:

(A) Ask the lab if serum is available for a toxicologic screening on his previous blood sample.

(B) Call his family to obtain corroborative history.

(C) Obtain a plasma catecholamine concentration.

(D) Obtain a urine sample for a routine urinalysis but also request a toxicologic screen.

(E) Present your findings to the patient and confront him with the suspected diagnosis.

(Answer E)

Cocaine use is confirmed. The patient admits a possible temporal relationship between his cocaine use and his chest pain. He expresses concern about long-term health risks.

7. He should be advised that:

(A) Cocaine-induced myocardial ischemia can be treated with beta-blockers.

(B) Death can occur from cocaine-induced myocardial infarction or arrhythmia.

(C) The presence of neuropsychiatric sequelae from drug use indicates those at risk for sudden death associated with cocaine use.

(D) Q wave myocardial infarction occurs only with smoked "crack" or intravenous cocaine use.

(E) Underlying coronary artery disease is the principal risk for sudden death associated with cocaine use.

(Answer B)

Primum Computer-based Case Simulations (CCS)

Primum CCS allows you to provide care for a simulated patient. You decide which diagnostic information to obtain and how to treat and monitor the patient's progress. In Primum CCS, you may request information from the history and physical examination; order labs, diagnostic studies, procedures or consultations; and start medications or other therapies. As time passes, the patient's condition changes based on the underlying problem and the interventions that you order. You must monitor the results of the tests that you order and the interventions that you make. When you confirm that there is nothing further that you want to do, you may advance simulated time in order to re-evaluate the patient's condition. You cannot go back in time but you can change your orders to reflect your updated management plan. The patient's chart contains an order sheet and reports resulting from your orders. You can review the vital signs, progress notes, patient updates, and test results. You may care for and move the patient among the office, home, emergency department, intensive care unit, and hospital ward.

In the simulation, you should function as the primary care physician who is responsible for managing each simulated patient. Management involves addressing a patient's problem(s) and/or concern(s) by obtaining diagnostic information, providing treatment, monitoring patient status and response to interventions, scheduling appointments and, when appropriate, attending to health maintenance screenings and patient education. You will manage one patient at a time and should continue to manage each patient until the "End of Case" message is displayed.

In your role as primary care physician, you must manage your patient in both inpatient and outpatient settings. This may involve management in multiple settings in a single case—initial care in the emergency department, admission to the inpatient unit, and follow-up in the outpatient setting. You should not assume that other members of the health care team (nurses, consultants, and so forth) will write orders for you. Some routine orders, such as vital signs at the beginning of the case or upon change of location, may be done automatically, but orders usually requested to monitor a patient's condition, such as cardiac monitors or pulse oximetry, are not automatically done. You are responsible for making all management decisions and determining needs, whether or not you would be expected to do so in real life.

As in real life, consultants should be called on when you deem appropriate. Typically, consultants are not helpful, as the exam is designed to assess your management skills. However, you will be evaluated on whether you request an appropriate consultation when it is indicated. For example, if a surgical procedure is indicated, it may be appropriate to request a surgical consultation. In some cases, it may be necessary to implement a course of action without the advice of a consultant or before a consultant is able to see the patient.

The CCS scoring process compares your patient management strategy with policies obtained from experts. Actions resembling a range of optimal strategies will produce a higher score. Dangerous and unnecessary actions will detract from your score. You must balance thoroughness, efficiency, avoidance of risk and timeliness in responding to the clinical situation.

Practice time with the CCS software is not available on the day of the test. You **must** review the CCS orientation material and practice the sample cases well in advance of your testing day in order to have an understanding of how the CCS system works. Sample cases are provided to Step 3 applicants on the USMLE CD and are available at the USMLE web site.

Specific Information of the Step 3 Examination

The USMLE is sponsored by the Federation of State Medical Boards (FSMB) and the National Board of Medical Examiners (NBME). Rules for the USMLE program are established by a composite committee that includes representatives of the FSMB, NBME, Educational Commission for Foreign Medical Graduates (ECFMG), and the American public. Information is published in an annual Bulletin of Information, which is available for download at the USMLE web site (www.usmle.org). You must be familiar with and will be subject to the policies and procedures of the Bulletin of Information for the year in which you take your examination. Changes in the USMLE program may occur after the release of the bulletin. If changes occur, information will be posted on the USMLE web site.

The registration entity for the Step 3 examination is the FSMB. You must contact the FSMB for information on how to apply for the USMLE, application materials, information on the status of your application or scheduling permit or information on obtaining a replacement scheduling permit (in the event that it is lost). The FSMB may be contacted at:

FSMB
Department of Examination Services
P.O. Box 619850
Dallas, TX 75261-9850
Website: www.fsmb.org
Email: usmle@fsmb.org

To be eligible for Step 3, the USMLE requires the following to be completed **prior** to submitting an application:

- Meet the Step 3 requirements set by the medical licensing authority to which you are applying.
- Obtain the MD degree (or its equivalent) or the DO degree (or its equivalent).
- Pass Step 1 and Step 2 (CK and CS).
- Obtain certification by the ECFMG or successfully complete a "Fifth Pathway" program if you are a graduate of a medical school outside of the United States or Canada.
- If you have taken Step 3 previously, you may not reapply prior to 60 days from the date of the prior Step 3 examination.
- The USMLE program limits all individuals to 3 attempts at Step 3 in a 12-month period.

Application procedures for Step 3 vary among jurisdictions. You should begin inquiries at least 3 months in advance of the dates on which you expect to take the test.

The Step 3 examination is given at Prometric Test Centers in the United States and its territories. Once your application has been approved, an eligibility period is assigned. A scheduling permit will be issued to you with instructions for making an appointment at a Prometric Test Center. The eligibility period starts immediately and extends for approximately 90 calendar days, so you should contact Prometric immediately after receiving your scheduling permit to schedule your test dates. If you are unable to take the test during your eligibility period, contact the FSMB to inquire about a 3-month eligibility period extension (a fee is charged for this and restrictions may apply). If you fail to take your examination within your eligibility period and wish to take it in the future, you will need to submit a new application and fee(s).

Physical Conditions

On the day(s) of your test, you should arrive at the Prometric center 30 minutes before your scheduled testing time. If you arrive late, you may not be admitted. If you arrive more than 30 minutes after your scheduled time, you will not be admitted.

When you arrive at the test center, you must present your scheduling permit and an acceptable form of identification. These include: passport, driver's license with photograph, national identity card, other government-issued identification, ECFMG-issued identification card. If you do not have your scheduling permit and identification, you will not be admitted to the test.

Test center staff monitor all testing sessions. You must follow their instructions throughout the examination. They are not authorized to answer questions regarding examination content, software, or scoring.

On the day of the examination, you are not allowed to bring any personal belongings into the testing area. If you bring any personal belongings to the test center, you must store them in a designated locker or cubicle outside of the testing room. You will be provided with laminated writing surfaces, dry erase markers, and an eraser, which must be returned after the test. Making notes of

any kind, except on the materials provided, is not permitted. You may not leave your testing station for breaks unless the break screen is visible on your computer monitor. During testing breaks, you may use a telephone or other communication device, but only for purposes not related to test content. You may not remove any materials (written, printed, recorded, and so forth) from the test center. Complete rules of conduct are available in the Bulletin of Information.

Organization of this Book

This book is organized to cover each of the clinical science areas that you will encounter on the Step 3 examination. Each chapter lists questions first, followed by the answers and explanations and a bibliography for further study. The question formats here have been chosen to conform to the style that you will encounter on the examination. This is done to familiarize you before you sit for the examination.

As is done for the actual examination, the sample test items are arranged in blocks of 48, for which 1 hour should be allotted, and organized by the clinical settings described above. The amount of time allowed is proportional to the amount of time that will be available for each block of questions during the actual examination.

Answers, Explanations, and Bibliography

In each of the sections of the book, the question sections are followed by a section containing the answers, explanations, and bibliography to the questions. This section tells you the answer to each question, provides an explanation and review of both why the answer is correct and why the other answers are incorrect and tells you where you can find more information on the subject. We encourage you to use this section as a basis for further study and understanding.

If you choose the correct answer to a question, you can then read the explanation for reinforcement and to add to your knowledge of the subject matter. If you choose the wrong answer to a question, you can read the explanation for a discussion of the material in question. You can also look up the reference cited for a more in-depth discussion.

How to Use this Book

There are two logical ways to get the most value from this book. We will call them Plan A and Plan B.

In Plan A, you go straight to the practice tests and complete them according to the instructions. After taking the tests and checking your answers, the number of questions that you answered incorrectly will be a good indicator of your initial knowledge state and the types of questions that you answered incorrectly will help point you in the right direction for further preparation and review. At this point, you can use the individual specialty chapters of the book to help you improve any areas of relative weakness.

In Plan B, you go through the clinical chapters first. Once you've completed this process, then you take the practice tests, check your answers and see how well prepared you are at this point. If you still have an area of significant weakness, it should be apparent in time for you to take remedial action.

In Plan A, by taking the practice test first, you get quick feedback regarding your initial areas of strength and weakness. You may find that you know all of the material very well, indicating that perhaps only a cursory review is necessary. This may be good to know early on in your exam preparation. On the other hand, you may find that you have some specific areas of weakness (such as pediatrics and psychiatry) and could then focus on these areas in your preparation—not only with this book but also with textbooks of pediatrics and psychiatry.

However, it is unlikely that you will not do some preparation prior to taking the USMLE Step 3 (especially since you have this book). Therefore, it may be more realistic to take the practice test after you have reviewed the specialty sections—as in Plan B. This will probably give you a more realistic test-type situation, as few of us may sit down for a test without studying first. In this case, you will have done some reviewing (from superficial to in-depth) and your practice test will reflect this studying time. If, after reviewing the specialty sections and taking the practice test, your scores indicate some weaknesses, you can then go back for further review of the subject sections and supplement your preparations with appropriate texts.

Now take a deep breath, relax, and good luck!

Acknowledgments

While one name may go on the cover of this book, this was far from a one-person job. I would first like to thank all of the contributors to this book, especially those who have now worked on multiple editions of this book. It has been a pleasure to work with all of you. I also need to thank Catherine Johnson, Laura Wenham, and the professional staff at McGraw-Hill publishing for trusting me to work on this again.

Since the last edition of the book was published, many professional changes have occurred in my "real job" and I need to acknowledge those with whom I work who have allowed me to continue my participation with this project. Thanks to Daniel Montez, the board of directors and outstanding staff of the Denver Harbor Clinic, our new residency home; Judy Paukert, the GME Department and Administration of the Methodist Hospital; the faculty—Anush Pillai, Kent Lee, Susan Miller, Jeané Simmons, and Stefanie Binder—residents and program coordinator Erika Robinson of the Methodist Hospital (Houston) FMRP. A special note of thanks must go to Terry McDermott and Seunghee Oh, two of my residents who did an excellent job of reviewing and improving each chapter of this edition.

As always, thanks to Heather, Cal, and Casey for putting up with me as deadlines approach.

Finally, on behalf of everyone involved with this project, I dedicate this book to those for whom it is intended—residents in the midst of their medical training. Step 3 is just one more hurdle to clear as you go. We wish you the best of luck on your examinations and in your careers.

Donald A. Briscoe, MD

USMLE STEP 3 LABORATORY VALUES

	REFERENCE RANGE	SI REFERENCE INTERVALS
BLOOD, PLASMA, SERUM		
* Alanine aminotransferase (ALT), serum	10–40 U/L	10–40 U/L
* Alkaline phosphatase, serum	Male: 30–100 U/L	Male: 30–100 U/L
	Female: 45–115 U/L	Female: 45–115 U/L
Amylase, serum	25–125 U/L	25–125 U/L
* Aspartate aminotransferase (AST), serum	15–40 U/L	15–40 U/L
* Bilirubin, serum (adult), total // direct	0.1–1.0 mg/dL // 0.0–0.3 mg/dL	2–17 µmol/L // 0–5 µmol/L
Calcium, serum (total)	8.4–10.2 mg/dL	2.1–2.8 mmol/L
* Cholesterol, serum		
Total	150–240 mg/dL	3.9–6.2 mmol/L
HDL	30–70 mg/dL	0.8–1.8 mmol/L
LDL	<160 mg/dL	<4.2 mmol/L
Cortisol, serum	8:00 AM: 5–23 µg/dL // 4:00 PM: 3–15 µg/dL	138–635 nmol/L // 82–413 nmol/L
	8:00 PM: # 50% of 8:00 AM	Fraction of 8:00 AM: # 0.50
Creatine kinase, serum	Male: 25–90 U/L	25–90 U/L
	Female: 10–70 U/L	10–70 U/L
* Creatinine, serum	0.6–1.2 mg/dL	53–106 µmol/L
Electrolytes, serum		
* Sodium (Na⁺)	135–146 mEq/L	135–146 mmol/L
* Potassium (K⁺)	3.5–5.0 mEq/L	3.5–5.0 mmol/L
* Chloride (Cl⁻)	95–105 mEq/L	95–105 mmol/L
* Bicarbonate (HCO₃⁻)	22–28 mEq/L	22–28 mmol/L
Ferritin, serum	Male: 15–200 ng/mL	15–200 µg/L
	Female: 12–150 ng/mL	12–150 µg/L
Follicle-stimulating hormone, serum/plasma	Male: 4–25 mIU/mL	4–25 U/L
	Female: premenopause 4–30 mIU/mL	4–30 U/L
	midcycle peak 10–90 mIU/mL	10–90 U/L
	postmenopause 40–250 mIU/mL	40–250 U/L
Gases, arterial blood (room air)		
PO₂	75–100 mmHg	10.0–14.0 kPa
PCO₂	35–45 mmHg	4.4–5.9 kPa
pH	7.35–7.45	[H⁺] 36–44 nmol/L
* Glucose, serum	Fasting: 70–110 mg/dL	3.8–6.1 mmol/L
	2-h postprandial: <120 mg/dL	<6.6 mmol/L
Immunoglobulins, serum		
IgA	76–390 mg/dL	0.76–3.90 g/L
IgE	0–380 IU/mL	0–380 kIU/L
IgG	650–1500 mg/dL	6.5–15 g/L
IgM	40–345 mg/dL	0.4–3.45 g/L
Iron	50–170 µg/dL	9–30 µmol/L
Lactate dehydrogenase, serum	45–90 U/L	45–90 U/L
Luteinizing hormone, serum/plasma	Male: 6–23 mIU/mL	6–23 U/L
	Female: follicular phase 5–30 mIU/mL	5–30 U/L
	midcycle 75–150 mIU/mL	75–150 U/L
	postmenopause 30–200 mIU/mL	30–200 U/L
Osmolality, serum	275–295 mOsmol/kg H₂O	275–295 mOsmol/kg H₂O
Phosphorus (inorganic), serum	3.0–4.5 mg/dL	1.0–1.5 mmol/L
Proteins, serum		
Total (recumbent)	6.0–7.8 g/dL	60–78 g/L
Albumin	3.5–5.5 g/dL	35–55 g/L
Globulin	2.3–3.5 g/dL	23–35 g/L
Thyroid-stimulating hormone (TSH), serum	0.5–5.0 µU/mL	0.5–5.0 mU/L
Thyroxine (T₄), serum	5–12 µg/dL .	64–155 nmol/L
Triglycerides	35–160 mg/dL	0.4–1.81 mmol/L
Triiodothyronine (T₃) resin uptake	25–35%	0.25–0.35
* Urea nitrogen, serum (BUN)	7–18 mg/dL	1.2–3.0 mmol/L
Uric acid, serum	3.0–8.2 mg/dL	0.18–0.48 mmol/L
CEREBROSPINAL FLUID		
Cell count	0–5 cells/mm³	0–5 × 10⁶/L
Chloride	118–132 mEq/L	118–132 mmo
Gamma globulin	3–12% total proteins	0.03–0.12
Glucose	40–70 mg/dL	2.2–3.9 mmol/L

(Continued)

	REFERENCE RANGE	SI REFERENCE INTERVALS
Pressure	70–180 mm H_2O	70–180 mm H_2O
Proteins, total	<40 mg/dL	<0.40 g/L
HEMATOLOGIC		
Bleeding time (template)	2–7 minutes	2–7 minutes
CD4 cell count	>500/mm^3	
Erythrocyte count	Male: 4.3–5.9 million/mm^3	4.3–5.9 × 10^{12}/L
	Female: 3.5–5.5 million/mm^3	3.5–5.5 × 10^{12}/L
Erythrocyte sedimentation rate (Westergren)	Male: 0–15 mm/h	0–15 mm/h
	Female: 0–20 mm/h	0–20 mm/h
Hematocrit	Male: 41–53%	0.41–0.53
	Female: 36–46%	0.36–0.46
Hemoglobin blood	Male: 13.5–17.5 g/dL	2.09–2.71 mmol/L
	Female: 12.0–16.0 g/dL	1.86–2.48 mmol/L
Hemoglobin A$_{1c}$	≤6%	≤0.06%
Leukocyte count and differential		
Leukocyte count	4500–11,000/mm^3	4.5–11.0 × 10^9/L
Neutrophils, segmented	54–62%	0.54–0.62
Neutrophils, band	3–5%	0.03–0.05
Eosinophils	1–3%	0.01–0.03
Basophils	0–0.75%	0.0–00.75
Lymphocytes	25–33%	0.25–0.33
Monocytes	3–7%	0.03–0.07
Mean corpuscular hemoglobin (MCH)	25–35 pg/cell	0.39–0.54 fmol/cell
Mean corpuscular hemoglobin concentration (MCHC)	31–36% Hb/cell	4.81–5.58 mmol Hb/L
Mean corpuscular volume (MCV)	80–100 μm^3	80–100 fl
Partial thromboplastin time (activated)	<28 s	<28 s
Platelet count	150,000–400,000/mm^3	150–400 × 10^9/L
Prothrombin time	<12 seconds	<12 seconds
Reticulocyte count	0.5–1.5% of red cells	0.005–0.015
Volume		
Plasma	Male: 25–43 mL/kg	0.025–0.043 L/kg
	Female: 28–45 mL/kg	0.028–0.045 L/kg
Red cell	Male: 20–36 mL/kg	0.020–0.036 L/kg
	Female: 19–31 mL/kg	0.019–0.031 L/kg
URINE		
Calcium	100–300 mg/24 h	2.5–7.5 mmol/24 h
Creatinine clearance	Male: 97–137 mL/min	
	Female: 88–128 mL/min	
Osmolality	50–1400 mOsmol/kg H_2O	
Oxalate	8–40 μg/mL	90–445 μmol/L
Proteins, total	<150 mg/24 h	<0.15 g/24 h

An astrisk (*) indicates a laboratory value included in the biochemical profile.

CHAPTER 1

Internal Medicine
Questions

Questions 1 through 4

A 45-year-old male comes to your office for his first annual checkup in the last 10 years. On first impression, he appears overweight but is otherwise healthy and has no specific complaints. He has a brother with diabetes and a sister with high blood pressure. Both of his parents are deceased and his father died of a stroke at age 73. He is a long-standing heavy smoker and only drinks alcohol on special occasions. On physical examination, his blood pressure is 166/90 in the left arm and 164/88 in the right arm. The rest of the examination is unremarkable. He is concerned about his health and does not want to end up on medication, like his siblings.

1. Regarding your initial recommendations, which of the following would be most appropriate?

    (A) You should take no action and ask him to return to the clinic in 1 year for a repeat blood pressure check.
    (B) You should immediately start him on an oral antihypertensive medication and ask him to return to the clinic in 1 week.
    (C) You should advise him to stop smoking, start a strict diet and exercise routine with the goal of losing weight, and return to the clinic in 6 months.
    (D) You should consider starting a workup for potential causes of secondary hypertension.
    (E) You should screen him for diabetes and evaluate him for other cardiovascular risk factors before proceeding any further.

2. In the initial evaluation of a patient such as this, which of the following should be routinely recommended?

    (A) a urine microalbumin/creatinine ratio
    (B) an echocardiogram
    (C) thyroid function tests
    (D) renal function tests (serum creatinine and blood urea nitrogen [BUN])
    (E) an exercise stress test

3. Which of the following describes the patient's blood pressure status?

    (A) normal blood pressure
    (B) prehypertension
    (C) stage 1 hypertension
    (D) stage 2 hypertension
    (E) stage 3 hypertension

4. Your patient returns to clinic a few weeks later for a follow-up appointment. Despite having lost 3 lbs and increasing his activity to walking 2 mi three times per week, his blood pressure remains elevated at 162/92. His initial evaluation revealed a fasting blood sugar of 156 and a hemoglobin (Hgb) A1C of 7.5. Along with starting hypoglycemic medications to control his diabetes, you recommend that he take an antihypertensive medication. At this point, you decide to start the patient on hypoglycemic medications to control his diabetes. What other intervention is appropriate at this time?

    (A) allow more time for the patient to practice lifestyle modifications
    (B) start treatment with an angiotensin-converting enzyme (ACE) inhibitor only
    (C) start treatment with a thiazide diuretic only
    (D) start treatment with a beta-blocker only
    (E) start treatment with a two-drug combination

EDDB

Questions 5 and 6

A 52-year-old male construction worker is seen in the emergency department (ED) at a local hospital with complaints of persistent cough for the past 4 months. He has been relatively healthy until a few months ago, when he lost his mother and developed severe depression which left him socially and professionally paralyzed. He has stopped doing any exercise or outdoor activity and spends most of his time at home eating, sleeping, and watching TV. In addition, he has noticed a 20-lb weight gain over this period but attributes it to his lack of exercise and increased food intake. His cough is worse at night, or any time when he lies down to sleep, and he notices a burning sensation in his throat associated with it. It is not associated with fever or chills, and his wife complains that he is constantly clearing his throat after meals. He smoked a few cigarettes per day as a young man in the Navy but quit more than 30 years ago. He denies recent travel or incarceration and has no recollection of any sick contacts. On examination, he is afebrile and appears mildly obese. His lung examination is clear. His oropharynx is red and mucosal membranes are dry and not inflamed.

5. Which of the following statements describes the likely cause of his chronic cough?

   (A) The patient likely suffers from a common cold due to a viral infection and will improve with symptomatic medications.

   (B) The patient most likely suffers from chronic bronchitis exacerbated by a bacterial infection.

   (C) The patient has developed gastroesophageal reflux disease (GERD).

   (D) The patient has developed late-onset occult asthma.

   (E) The patient has a "nervous" cough due to severe depression.

6. Which of the following therapies would be most beneficial in alleviating this patient's symptoms?

   (A) an inhaled, short-acting beta-2 agonist

   (B) a proton pump inhibitor (PPI)

   (C) an antitussive-expectorant syrup

   (D) weight loss and exercise

   (E) prolonged course of antibiotics

7. You are asked to interview a young couple who wish to conceive a child. Their first and only son was born with a rare, autosomal recessive glycogen storage disorder known as Pompe disease. Both parents are healthy and unaffected by this disease, but the father believes that he has heard of a distant cousin who also has this disease. They are concerned about the possibility that their next child will also be born with the affliction. In giving them advice about their chances of having a healthy child, you should:

   (A) Tell them not to worry about it; their next child will surely be healthy.

   (B) Tell them that their next child has a 25% chance of being born with the disease.

   (C) Tell them that there is a 50:50 chance that their next child will be affected.

   (D) Tell them that it is impossible to predict the likelihood that their next child will have the disease.

   (E) Advise them not to have any more children because they all will certainly be affected.

Questions 8 and 9

A 53-year-old female has made an appointment to see you concerning the recent onset of menopause. Her last menstrual period was 8 months ago and, over the last year, she had noticed that her periods were becoming lighter and less frequent. In addition, she has developed frequent hot flashes, and her mood has become very labile. She wishes to know what your advice is regarding hormone replacement therapy (HRT). She has heard recent reports in the news concerning an increased risk of developing cardiovascular complications, especially heart attacks and strokes. Although she is in great health, her father died at age 50 of a massive heart attack. Her mother is alive and well, and there is no history of breast cancer among the females in her family.

8. Regarding postmenopausal HRT, which of the following statements would be correct?

(A) Known benefits from HRT in post-menopausal women include a reduction in the incidence of osteoporosis and bone fractures (particularly hip fractures).

(B) Known benefits from HRT in post-menopausal women include a cardio-protective effect, which reduces the incidence of coronary artery disease (CAD) and myocardial infarction (MI).

(C) HRT increases the incidence of endometrial cancer in all patients.

(D) Although HRT reduces vasomotor instability and hot flashes after menopause, this effect is short-lived and there is no effect in mood stability.

(E) Despite recent press reports, any woman at risk for osteoporosis should take HRT, regardless of cardiovascular risk factors.

9. Which of the following would be the strongest argument to avoid HRT in this patient?

(A) HRT is unlikely to relieve her hot flashes.

(B) She has a positive family history of CAD.

(C) She is at high risk for developing breast cancer.

(D) She is at high risk for developing venous thromboembolism.

(E) She probably would develop breast tenderness and bloating.

10. A young college student is brought to your office by his fiancé for evaluation of weight loss. He tells you that, over the past few months, he seems to be unable to gain any weight despite having a ferocious appetite and that he is steadily losing weight. He has also noticed increased thirst and urination. Over the past few nights, he has awakened several times to go to the bathroom. You suspect that he may have developed diabetes. Which of the following is a diagnostic criterion for diabetes mellitus (DM)?

(A) a single fasting plasma glucose level of 140 mg/dL in an asymptomatic person

(B) a plasma glucose level of >175 mg/dL measured at least 8 hours after a meal

(C) a plasma glucose level of >124 mg/dL measured at least 4 hours after a meal

(D) a blood glucose level of 200 mg/dL, 2 hours after completing a glucose tolerance test with a 75-g oral glucose load

(E) a serum glycosylated HgbA1C level higher than 7%

Questions 11 and 12

A 67-year-old male with a history of type II diabetes and hypertension is hospitalized with complaints of retrosternal chest pain that radiates to the left arm and jaw. In the ED, an electrocardiogram (ECG) showed S-T segment depressions in the inferior and lateral leads. He has been given the diagnosis of *acute coronary syndrome* and admitted to the coronary care unit for further evaluation and treatment. Admission laboratory values reveal a total cholesterol of 270, a low-density lipoprotein (LDL) of 190, and a high-density lipoprotein (HDL) of 28. He is currently smoking a pack of cigarettes per day and lives a sedentary life. He is clearly overweight and his blood pressure, despite medication, remains elevated at 150/88. His last HgbA1C less than a month ago was 9.8%.

11. After being discharged from the hospital, which of the following cholesterol lowering regimens should be recommended to this patient?

(A) Low fat diet and exercise four times per week should reduce his cholesterol profile to acceptable levels.

(B) Starting a statin (3-hydroxy-3-methyl-glutaryl coenzyme A [HMG-CoA] reductase inhibitor) in addition to smoking cessation, diet, and exercise may reduce his risk of developing further cardiovascular complications.

(C) Starting niacin and recommending smoking cessation classes should be the first-line therapy in order to increase his HDL and reduce his risk for further cardiovascular complications.

(D) There is no role for cholesterol-lowering medications in secondary prevention of cardiovascular disease.

(E) The role of cholesterol-lowering drugs in reducing the risk for CAD is not well established and routine recommendation of such therapy after acute coronary syndrome should be avoided.

12. In addition to diet, exercise, and smoking cessation, which of the following would have the largest impact in reducing his cholesterol?

    (A) controlling his blood pressure

    (B) increasing his consumption of alcoholic beverages to three to four glasses of wine per day

    (C) improving his sleeping habits

    (D) adding thyroid hormone to his medications

    (E) controlling his diabetes

Questions 13 through 15

A 48-year-old female with a history of mild congestive heart failure (CHF) treated with furosemide presents to the emergency room (ER) for evaluation of 24 hours of epigastric pain, nausea, and vomiting after eating a large meal in a restaurant. Previously, the patient had experienced intermittent right upper quadrant pain after eating. On examination, the patient has a temperature of 98.5°F and a pulse of 100. Her examination is remarkable for epigastric tenderness to palpation, normal bowel sounds, and no rebound tenderness or guarding.

Laboratory studies are as follows:

Leukocyte count	4800/mm³
Alanine aminotransferase (ALT)	258 U/L
Aspartate aminotransferase (AST)	287 U/L
Alkaline phosphatase, serum	350 U/L
Bilirubin (total)	2.0 mg/dL
Bilirubin (indirect)	0.4 mg/dL
Amylase	2865 U/L
Lipase	3453 U/L

13. Which of the following is the most likely diagnosis?

    (A) acute gastroenteritis

    (B) acute gallstone pancreatitis

    (C) drug-induced pancreatitis

    (D) acute cholecystitis

    (E) acute cholangitis

14. What would the most appropriate next test to order be?

    (A) abdominal x-ray

    (B) abdominal computed tomographic (CT) scan

    (C) abdominal ultrasound

    (D) magnetic resonance imaging (MRI) of the abdomen

    (E) stool cultures and assessment for ova and parasites

15. The patient is made NPO (nothing by mouth) and vigorously hydrated. After 3 days, the amylase and lipase normalize, but the bilirubin rises to 4.2 mg/dL. An endoscopic retrograde cholangiopancreatography (ERCP) is performed, and the following cholangiogram is obtained (see Figure 1-1). What is the best treatment option at this time?

FIG. 1-1 (*Courtesy of Douglas G. Adler, MD.*)

    (A) papillary dilation and stone extraction

    (B) papillotomy (aka sphincterotomy) and stone extraction

    (C) placement of a transpapillary stent in the biliary tree

    (D) placement of a transpapillary stent in the pancreatic duct

    (E) no further manipulations are required

16. Your patient who was recently prescribed an antibiotic returns to your clinic for a follow-up visit. Although she was feeling better, the instructions on the bottle were to take the medication for total of 10 days. She wants to know if she still has to take the medication three times daily as she has improved. You explain to her that the dosing regimen is based on the biological half-life of a drug, which is generally related to which of the following?

    (A) the time for a drug to be absorbed into the blood
    (B) the time for a drug to take effect following administration
    (C) the time for the body burden of a drug to be reduced by 50%
    (D) the serum concentration of a drug that is 50% of the toxic level
    (E) a value that is half the duration of action of a drug

Questions 17 through 19

A 35-year-old woman with a history of major depressive disorder is brought into the ED by her boyfriend. He believes she may have overdosed on pain medication in an effort to hurt herself. He gives you three medication bottles which he discovered empty and states that they were nearly full before leaving for work earlier that morning. However, the timing of the ingestion is unclear. All three of the bottles apparently held acetaminophen-containing medications. Examination of the patient reveals a tired-appearing woman complaining of nausea and right upper quadrant abdominal pain.

17. Depletion of which of the following is primarily responsible for the hepatotoxicity being experienced by the patient?

    (A) N-acetyl-p-benzoquinone-imine (NAPQI)
    (B) taurine
    (C) citrulline
    (D) glutathione
    (E) ornithine

18. Which of the following pharmacologic treatments is most appropriate at this time?

    (A) no pharmacologic treatment is necessary
    (B) naloxone
    (C) flumazenil
    (D) physostigmine
    (E) N-acetylcysteine

19. Which of the following is the worst prognostic indicator if present in this patient?

    (A) arterial pH greater than 7.3
    (B) arterial lactate greater than 3.5 mmol/L
    (C) initiation of therapy 8 hours after acetaminophen ingestion
    (D) "probable-risk" of hepatotoxicity by the Rumack-Matthew nomogram
    (E) a history of chronic acetaminophen abuse

20. A 72-year-old male with type II diabetes, hypertension, and a history of recurrent pneumonia is admitted to the Medical intensive care unit (ICU) with a diagnosis of septic shock. His vital signs are: BP 80/60 mmHg, RR 24 breaths per minute, pulse 120 beats per minute (bpm), temp. 102.4°F, O_2 saturation 99% on room air. Of the choices listed below, what would be your initial management?

    (A) start IV dopamine
    (B) start empiric IV broad-spectrum antibiotics
    (C) bolus IV fluids
    (D) intubate and start ventilator support
    (E) start IV norepinephrine

Questions 21 through 23

A 42-year-old man without prior significant medical history comes to your office for evaluation of chronic diarrhea of 12 months duration, although the patient states he has had loose stools for many years. During this time he has lost 25 lbs. The diarrhea is large volume, occasionally greasy, and non-bloody. In addition, the patient has mild abdominal pain for much of the day. He has been smoking a pack of cigarettes a day for 20 years and drinks approximately five beers per day. His physical examination reveals a thin male with temporal wasting and generalized muscle loss. He has glossitis and angular cheilosis. He has excoriations on his elbows and knees and scattered papulovesicular lesions in these regions as well.

/kī'lōsəs/

21. Which of the following is the most likely diagnosis for this patient?

    (A) chronic pancreatitis
    (B) Crohn's disease
    (C) celiac sprue
    (D) Whipple disease
    (E) ulcerative colitis

22. Which of the following is the best test to confirm the suspected diagnosis?

    (A) abdominal CT scan with contrast
    (B) small bowel x-ray
    (C) esophagogastroduodenoscopy with small bowel biopsy
    (D) colonoscopy with colonic biopsy
    (E) 72-hour fecal fat quantification

23. What is the most serious long-term complication this patient could face?

    (A) pancreatic cancer
    (B) small bowel cancer
    (C) gastric cancer
    (D) colon cancer
    (E) rectal cancer

Questions 24 through 26

A 24-year-old male medical student is admitted to the hospital for the evaluation of a 3-month history of bloody stools. The patient has approximately six blood stained or blood streaked stools per day, associated with relatively little, if any, pain. He has not had any weight loss, and he has been able to attend classes without interruption. He denies any fecal incontinence. He has no prior medical history. Review of systems is remarkable only for occasional fevers and the fact that the patient quit smoking approximately 8 months ago. A colonoscopy is performed and reveals a granular, friable colonic mucosal surface with loss of normal vascular pattern from the anal verge to the hepatic flexure of the colon. Biopsies reveal prominent neutrophils in the epithelium and cryptitis with focal crypt abscesses, and no dysplasia. The patient is diagnosed with ulcerative colitis.

24. Which of the following is the best initial treatment for this patient?

    (A) colectomy
    (B) oral prednisone
    (C) oral metronidazole
    (D) cortisone enemas
    (E) intravenous cyclosporine

25. While on the inpatient service, the patient is noted to have a serum alkaline phosphatase of 380 U/L and a bilirubin of 2.4 mg/dL. An ERCP is performed, and the following cholangiogram is obtained (see Figure 1-2). In addition to ulcerative colitis, the patient likely has what other illness?

FIG. 1-2 (*Courtesy of Douglas G. Adler, MD.*)

(A) primary biliary cirrhosis

(B) Wilson disease

(C) alpha-1 antitrypsin deficiency

(D) hereditary hemochromatosis

(E) primary sclerosing cholangitis (PSC)

26. In addition to an increased lifetime risk of colon cancer, the patient is also at increased risk for which of the following tumors?

(A) hepatocellular carcinoma

(B) hepatoblastoma

(C) desmoid tumors

(D) small bowel lymphoma

(E) cholangiocarcinoma

Questions 27 and 28

A 61-year-old man comes to your office for a checkup. He currently feels well and has no focal complaints. He has a past medical history significant for well-controlled hypertension, and his gallbladder was removed 3 years ago in the setting of acute chole-cystitis. He does not smoke and drinks one to two alcoholic beverages per day. Family history is remarkable for colon cancer in his mother at age 45 and a brother at age 49. He has a sister who developed endometrial cancer at age 53. He has never undergone colon cancer screening and is interested in pursuing this.

27. Which colorectal cancer screening test would be best for this patient?

(A) virtual colonoscopy (aka CT colography)

(B) barium enema alone

(C) barium enema with flexible sigmoidoscopy

(D) fecal occult blood testing three times

(E) colonoscopy

28. The patient's family history is strongly suggestive of which of the following?

(A) familial adenomatous polyposis (FAP) syndrome

(B) hereditary nonpolyposis colorectal cancer (HNPCC) syndrome

(C) Peutz-Jeghers syndrome

(D) Cronkhite-Canada syndrome

(E) Turcot syndrome

Questions 29 through 31

A 50-year-old female presents to your office for evaluation of solid food dysphagia without weight loss. Symptoms have been present for 6 months and are progressive. The patient has had two episodes of near impaction, but copious water ingestion and repeated swallows allowed the food bolus to pass. She has never had to present to the ER for disimpaction. She drinks five to six beers per day, loves spicy foods, and smokes a pack of cigarettes daily with a total lifetime history of 30 pack-years. She has had intermittent heartburn symptoms for years and has not sought treatment. She takes hydrochlorothiazide for hypertension. Review of symptoms reveals chronic cough. Physical examination is unremarkable. Upper endoscopy reveals a distal esophageal stricture with inflammatory changes. Esophageal biopsies reveal benign mucosa with chronic inflammation. Gastric biopsies are unremarkable. *Helicobacter pylori* testing is negative.

29. What is the most likely etiology of the patient's stricture?

(A) alcohol ingestion

(B) tobacco use

(C) gastroesophageal reflux

(D) hydrochlorothiazide

(E) spicy food ingestion

30. What is the next best step in therapy for this patient?

(A) esophageal dilation

(B) histamine receptor antagonist therapy

(C) PPI therapy

(D) esophageal dilation with histamine receptor antagonist therapy

(E) esophageal dilation with PPI inhibitor therapy

31. The patient is at increased risk for which of the following illnesses?

    (A) esophageal squamous cell cancer
    (B) esophageal adenocarcinoma
    (C) gastric cancer
    (D) gastric lymphoma
    (E) duodenal adenocarcinoma

Questions 32 through 36

A 65-year-old man presents to your office for evaluation of abdominal pain. The patient states that he has epigastric pain that radiates to his back. The pain is worse with eating and improves with fasting. The pain has been present for 6 months and is gradually worsening. The patient has lost 15 lbs but feels his oral intake has been adequate. He complains of greasy stools and frequent thirst and urination. Examination reveals a thin male with temporal wasting and moderate abdominal pain with palpation. The patient consumes approximately 10–15 beers per day and smokes a pack of cigarettes per day for the past 20 years.

32. What would be the best initial test to do in this patient?

    (A) spot fecal fat collection
    (B) 72-hour fecal fat collection
    (C) CT scan of the abdomen
    (D) ERCP
    (E) upper endoscopy

33. On further questioning, the patient reports that he recently had a motor vehicle accident at night because he felt he could not see clearly. The most likely cause of this symptom is which of the following?

    (A) vitamin B_{12} deficiency
    (B) vitamin C deficiency
    (C) vitamin D deficiency
    (D) vitamin A deficiency
    (E) vitamin K deficiency

34. On further evaluation, the patient is found to be diabetic. He has an elevated HgbA1C and fasting hyperglycemia. The patient is sent for diabetic teaching sessions and begun on insulin therapy, but is unable to achieve euglycemia.

He experiences frequent bouts of symptomatic hypoglycemia requiring ER visits. What is the most likely cause for these episodes?

    (A) insulin overdose
    (B) impaired glucagon production
    (C) inadequate oral intake
    (D) vitamin K deficiency
    (E) vitamin B_{12} deficiency

35. The patient's weight loss would be best treated by which of the following regimens?

    (A) pancreatic enzyme replacement therapy
    (B) liquid caloric supplementation by mouth
    (C) liquid caloric supplementation via gastrostomy tube
    (D) total parenteral nutrition (TPN)
    (E) partial parenteral nutrition (PPN)

36. The patient's abdominal pain worsens and his weight loss progresses despite therapy, and you suspect that he may have a malignancy. If a malignancy was present, which tumor marker would be most likely to be elevated in this patient?

    (A) carcinoembryonic antigen (CEA)
    (B) prostate-specific antigen (PSA)
    (C) cancer antigen (CA)-125
    (D) α-Fetoprotein (AFP)
    (E) CA-19-9

Questions 37 through 39

A 60-year-old woman arrives at your office for a routine physical examination. During the course of her examination she asks you about osteoporosis. She is concerned about her risk for osteoporosis, as her mother suffered from multiple vertebral compression fractures at the age of 60. Your patient reports that she still smokes cigarettes ("although I know they are bad for me") and has one alcoholic beverage a week. She reports having had menopause 5 years ago and experiencing a deep venous thrombosis approximately 20 years ago. She is proud of the fact that she regularly exercises at the local fitness center. She has been taking 1500 mg of calcium with 800 IU of vitamin D every day. You suspect that she is at risk for osteoporosis.

37. Which of the following tests is best to detect and monitor osteoporosis?

    (A) plain film radiography
    (B) dual photon absorptiometry
    (C) single photon absorptiometry
    (D) dual-energy x-ray absorptiometry (DEXA)
    (E) quantitative CT scan

38. After performing the appropriate imaging study, you determine that your patient has osteoporosis. Of the following choices, which is a risk factor most likely contributing to her osteoporosis?

    (A) active lifestyle
    (B) late menopause
    (C) cigarette smoking
    (D) frequency of alcohol intake
    (E) her intake of calcium and vitamin D

39. After a thorough discussion with your patient, you determine that pharmacologic intervention would be beneficial given the severity of her osteoporosis. Which of the following is most appropriate for your patient?

    (A) estrogen replacement therapy
    (B) combined HRT with estrogen and progestin
    (C) alendronate
    (D) calcitonin intranasal spray
    (E) raloxifene

Questions 40 through 42

A 28-year-old male, well known to your clinic, presents for management of swelling, pain, and tenderness that has developed in his left ankle and right knee. It has persisted for 1 month. Your patient reports that he developed severe diarrhea after a picnic 1 month prior to the onset of his arthritis. During the interval between the diarrhea and onset of arthritis, he developed a "pink eye" that lasted for 4 days. He denies any symptoms of back pain or stiffness. You remember that he was treated with ceftriaxone and doxycycline for gonorrhea 2 years ago, which he acquired from sexual activity with multiple partners. Since that time, he has been in a monogamous relationship with his wife and has not had any genitourinary symptoms. He promises that he has been faithful to his wife and has not engaged in unprotected sexual activity outside his marriage. His physical examination is notable for a swollen left ankle, swollen right knee, and the absence of penile discharge or any skin lesions.

40. Which of the following is the most likely diagnosis?

    (A) pseudogout
    (B) gout
    (C) reactive arthritis
    (D) resistant gonococcal arthritis
    (E) ankylosing spondylitis

41. What would be the appropriate management for this patient's arthritis?

    (A) Screen him for the suspected disease with HLA-B27 testing.
    (B) Treat with daily indomethacin (150–200 mg daily).
    (C) Start him on empiric antibiotics.
    (D) Start treatment with prednisone 10 mg daily.
    (E) Assume that the patient is not being honest and perform the appropriate urogenital testing to confirm gonorrhea.

42. The patient's symptoms do not respond to your initial therapeutic management. You suspect that his condition is refractory to treatment. Which of the following should you consider at this time?

    (A) He may have human immunodeficiency virus (HIV) infection and should be tested.
    (B) His condition will require high doses of prednisone (60 mg daily) for adequate control.
    (C) His joints are obviously not infected and should be directly injected with corticosteroids.
    (D) He must have a disseminated bacterial infection that will require IV antibiotics.
    (E) He is resistant to indomethacin, so the dose should be doubled to 400 mg daily.

Questions 43 through 47

A 42-year-old man presents to your clinic with a 1-week history of pain and inflammation involving his right first metatarsophalangeal (MTP) joint. He describes the pain as sudden in onset and worse at night. He denies experiencing any fever or traumatic injury to the joint and states that he has never had this type of pain before. He denies any chronic medical conditions, any prior surgery, and any current medication use. Besides an erythematous and exquisitely tender right first MTP joint, the remainder of his physical examination is unremarkable.

43. Aspiration of the patient's right first MTP joint space is likely to reveal which of the following?

    (A) negatively birefringent crystals
    (B) positively birefringent crystals
    (C) nonbirefringent crystals
    (D) acellular synovial fluid
    (E) gram-positive cocci in clusters

44. Which of the following is true of the patient's condition?

    (A) It commonly presents in premenopausal women.
    (B) It commonly presents as a monoarticular arthritis.
    (C) Episodes of pain and inflammation become more frequent but resolve more quickly as the disease progresses.
    (D) The presence of tophi is a common early finding.
    (E) A blood test is the diagnostic gold standard.

45. Which of the following interventions is most appropriate at this time for your patient's condition?

    (A) probenecid
    (B) allopurinol
    (C) indomethacin
    (D) sulfinpyrazone
    (E) aspirin

46. What is a potential long-term complication of this patient's condition?

    (A) CHF
    (B) nephrolithiasis
    (C) anemia of chronic disease
    (D) recurrent urinary tract infection (UTI)
    (E) rheumatoid arthritis (RA)

47. After 1 week of treatment, your patient states that his pain and inflammation have resolved. You measure a serum urate level and find it elevated. Urinary urate excretion is high. Which of the following interventions is now most appropriate?

    (A) no further treatment is necessary
    (B) daily oral allopurinol
    (C) daily oral probenecid
    (D) daily oral colchicine with allopurinol
    (E) daily oral colchicine with probenecid

48. Which of the following produces the greatest increase in bone mineral density (BMD) in patients with osteoporosis?

    (A) estrogen
    (B) calcitonin
    (C) alendronate
    (D) teriparatide
    (E) raloxifene

Questions 49 through 52

A 23-year-old female graduate student with acne and asthma presents to you with a chief complaint of headaches. She has noted a gradual increase in the intensity and frequency of the headaches to the point where they are interfering with her daily activities and studies. Your examination shows an obese young lady with papilledema. The remainder of your physical examination is normal.

49. Which of the following is the most appropriate management at this time?

    (A) order an erythrocyte sedimentation rate (ESR)
    (B) order a glucose tolerance test
    (C) urine pregnancy test

(D) obtain a lumbar puncture to measure opening pressure

(E) obtain an MRI of the brain and orbits, with and without contrast

50. The test ordered above was negative. Which of the following is your most appropriate next step?

(A) instruct the patient on a weight loss program and follow-up in 3 months

(B) begin diuretic therapy

(C) start the patient on sumatriptan for migraine headaches

(D) perform a lumbar puncture to measure opening pressure

(E) obtain an MRI of the brain and orbits, with and without contrast

51. Which of the following is most commonly associated with this condition?

(A) obesity

(B) steroid use during asthma attacks

(C) tetracycline treatment for acne

(D) oral contraceptives

(E) pregnancy

52. Which of the following interventions is most appropriate initially for the patient's suspected diagnosis?

(A) this condition is self-limited

(B) ventricular-peritoneal shunt placement

(C) optic nerve fenestration

(D) serial lumbar punctures

(E) acetazolamide therapy

Questions 53 and 54

A 64-year-old Hispanic female with type II DM and hypertension for 15 years comes to your office after not seeing a physician for 5 years. The HgbA1C is 9. She reports that her vision has been deteriorating but new glasses from the optometrist have helped.

53. Which of the following findings during your examination would represent the highest risk for blindness in this patient?

(A) microaneurysms

(B) neovascularization at the optic nerve

(C) arteriovenous nicking

(D) cotton wool spots or focal infarcts

(E) hard exudates or lipid deposits

54. Your examination findings include all of the above. These form which of the following diagnoses?

(A) nonproliferative diabetic retinopathy

(B) proliferative retinopathy

(C) central serous chorioretinopathy

(D) microangiopathy of the retina

(E) hypertensive retinopathy

Questions 55 through 58

A 54-year-old Asian female with no significant medical history presents with frontal headache, eye pain, nausea, and vomiting. Her abdominal examination shows mild diffuse tenderness but no rebound or guarding. Her mucous membranes are dry. Her vision is blurry in both eyes, her eyes are injected but her extraocular muscles are intact. Her pupils are mid-dilated and fixed.

55. Which of the following is most likely to provide a diagnosis?

(A) abdominal ultrasound

(B) emergency exploratory laparoscopy

(C) MRI of the brain

(D) arterial blood gas

(E) ocular tonometry

56. What other finding is this patient most likely to have?

(A) cloudy corneas

(B) anemia

(C) anorexia

(D) dizziness or vertigo

(E) polyuria and polydipsia

57. Which of the following is the most likely diagnosis?

- (A) diabetic ketoacidosis (DKA)
- (B) appendicitis
- (C) angle closure glaucoma
- (D) perforated colon due to inflammatory bowel disease (IBD)
- (E) cerebellar malignancy

58. Which of the following is appropriate initial management of this patient?

- (A) urgent consultation of a general surgeon
- (B) urgent consultation of an ophthalmologist
- (C) prescription of an antiemetic with follow-up the next day in the office
- (D) bed rest with head of bed elevated to 45 degrees
- (E) performance of a dilated eye examination prior with referral if abnormalities seen

Questions 59 through 61

A 64-year-old male with a history of hypertension and tobacco abuse presents for follow-up after a routine physical during which he was found to have 4–5 red blood cells (RBCs) per high-power field (HPF) on a screening urinalysis. The urinalysis was negative for leukocytes, nitrites, epithelial cells, and ketones. The patient denies any complaints and the review of systems is essentially negative.

59. What would be your initial approach in the workup of this patient with asymptomatic microscopic hematuria?

- (A) check PSA and urine culture
- (B) CT scan with and without contrast of the abdomen and pelvis
- (C) intravenous pyelography (IVP)
- (D) observation and reassurance as patient is asymptomatic
- (E) repeat urinalysis

60. After your initial workup, what would the next course in management be?

- (A) change of antihypertensive agent and recommendation to patient to discontinue smoking
- (B) image the upper and lower urinary tracts
- (C) antibiotics for 1 month
- (D) expectant management with follow-up urinalysis in 6 months
- (E) nephrology consultation

61. In detecting microscopic hematuria, which of the following is true?

- (A) The office urine dipstick is 91–100% sensitive and 65–99% specific for detection of RBCs, Hgb, and myoglobin.
- (B) Urinalysis must reveal a minimum of 5 RBCs per HPF in order to continue the workup.
- (C) The presence of epithelial cells makes the urinalysis invalid.
- (D) The presence of "large blood" on a urine dipstick effectively distinguishes RBCs from myoglobinuria.
- (E) Any urinalysis with RBCs should be recollected via a catheterized specimen prior to initiating a workup for hematuria.

Questions 62 and 63

A 52-year-old man presents to the ED with a complaint of rectal bleeding and hematuria. He has a medical history significant for atrial fibrillation diagnosed 10 years ago and states that he takes metoprolol as well as warfarin for this condition. Upon examination, you find that his blood pressure is 122/78, his pulse is 84, his respiratory rate is 18, and his O_2 saturation is 98% on room air. He has an irregularly irregular heart rhythm, gingival bleeding, and some bruises on his extremities. He has a positive fecal occult blood test, and laboratory studies return showing an international normalized ratio (INR) of 16.5.

62. You order that the patient's warfarin be held. Which of the following is the most appropriate additional intervention at this time?

(A) repeat INR measurement as an outpatient in 5 days

(B) admit the patient to the hospital and conduct serial INR measurements

(C) administer vitamin K_1

(D) administer fresh frozen plasma

(E) administer vitamin K_1 and fresh frozen plasma

63. Reviewing the patient's medication list, you note that he mentions a "medication for depression" but does not recall the name. Which of the following is most concerning given the patient's current condition?

(A) amitriptyline
(B) trazodone
(C) fluoxetine
(D) venlafaxine
(E) imipramine

64. A 72-year-old African American male presents for a routine health examination. He states that he would like to have a "screening for cancer." In the United States, based on his sex, race, and age, what is the most likely malignancy for this patient?

(A) lung cancer
(B) prostate cancer
(C) colon cancer
(D) testicular cancer
(E) multiple myeloma

Questions 65 through 67

A 72-year-old man comes to your clinic for the first time, accompanied by his wife. His wife states that she is concerned because he has been growing increasingly forgetful over the past year. Within the past month, he has forgotten to turn off the stove and has got lost while walking to the post office one block away from their home. His past medical history is significant for well-controlled diabetes and chronic lower back pain. He has no history of falls or traumatic injury to the head. Examination of the patient is significant for a score of 18 on a Mini-Mental Status Examination (MMSE). During the administration of the MMSE, the patient blurts out

that his wife brought him to the doctor because she is having an extramarital relationship.

65. Which of the following accurately describes this patient's condition?

(A) There is no genetic basis for development of this disease.
(B) It is usually abrupt in onset.
(C) There is no correlation between age and prevalence of this disease.
(D) Environmental exposure is a proven risk factor for development of this disease.
(E) It is one of the most common terminal illnesses in developed nations.

66. Use of which of the following medications would be the most likely to lead to worsening of symptoms in this patient?

(A) risperidone
(B) amitriptyline
(C) olanzapine
(D) quetiapine
(E) trazodone

67. Despite appropriate treatment, the patient experiences a gradual decline in mental function. He develops erratic sleep habits, frequently awakening at night and wandering throughout his home. His wife states that she once found him sitting on the ground in their yard, unable to recall how he arrived there. During your latest examination of the patient, you note that he has lost the ability to sign his name, holding the pen as if he is unsure of what to do with it. Exasperated, his wife states that he is now dependent on her for performance of his activities of daily living. Which of the following is indicated in the treatment of the patient's condition at its current severity?

(A) tacrine (Cognex)
(B) gingko biloba
(C) rivastigmine (Exelon)
(D) memantine (Namenda)
(E) galantamine (Reminyl)

68. A 28-year-old woman presents to your clinic complaining of feeling "on edge." Upon further questioning, you discover that she has also noticed problems with irritability, insomnia, fatigue, and restlessness. She also has a history of worrying about things that seem to not bother those around her. She states these symptoms have been present for years but have recently become worse. When you try to gather more information, she interrupts to say that she cannot stay much longer because she is afraid that she will lose her new job as a machinist. Which of the following medications would be most appropriate in this patient?

   (A) diazepam
   (B) amitriptyline
   (C) doxepin
   (D) oxazepam
   (E) buspirone

69. A 54-year-old male with uncontrolled type II diabetes and well-controlled hypertension presents with complaints of erectile dysfunction. The patient requests Viagra (sildenafil), as his friends have used it with success. However, he is concerned as he was told by someone that Viagra can be fatal if used with some blood pressure medications. You would advise the patient that the use of which of the following is contraindicated in patients taking sildenafil?

   (A) isosorbide mononitrate
   (B) metoprolol
   (C) verapamil
   (D) captopril
   (E) clonidine

70. Bupivacaine is a local anesthetic agent that is much more potent and the duration of action of which is considerably longer than procaine. Possible reasons for this difference include which of the following?

   (A) higher partition coefficient for bupivacaine than for procaine
   (B) covalent binding to the receptor site
   (C) lower protein binding of bupivacaine than procaine

   (D) decreased rate of metabolism of procaine compared to bupivacaine
   (E) bupivacaine constricts blood vessels

Questions 71 through 74

A 68-year-old White male, with a history of hypertension, an 80 pack-year history of tobacco use and emphysema, is brought into the ER because of 4 days of progressive confusion and lethargy. His wife notes that he takes amlodipine for his hypertension. He does not use over-the-counter (OTC) medications, alcohol, or drugs. Furthermore, she indicates that he has unintentionally lost approximately 30 lbs in the last 6 months. His physical examination shows that he is afebrile with a blood pressure of 142/85, heart rate of 92 (no orthostatic changes), and a room-air O_2 saturation of 91%. He is 70 kg. The patient appears cachectic. He is arousable but lethargic and unable to follow any commands. His mucous membranes are moist, heart rate regular without murmurs or a S_3/S_4 gallop, and extremities without any edema. His pulmonary examination shows mildly diminished breath sounds in the right lower lobe with wheezing bilaterally. The patient is unable to follow commands during neurologic examination but moves all his extremities spontaneously. Laboratory results are as follows:

Blood
↓ Sodium: 109
Potassium: 3.8
Chloride: 103
CO_2: 33
BUN: 17
Creatinine: 1.1
Glucose: 95
Urine osmolality: 600
↓ Plasma osmolality: 229
White blood cell (WBC): 8000
Hgb: 15.8
Hematocrit (HCT): 45.3
Platelets: 410
Arterial blood gas: pH 7.36/pCO_2 60/pO_2 285
A chest x-ray (CXR) reveals a large right hilar mass.

---

71. What is the most likely cause of this patient's altered mental status?

   (A) sepsis syndrome with pneumonia
   (B) ischemic stroke
   (C) central pontine myelinolysis
   (D) cerebral edema
   (E) respiratory acidosis

72. Which of the following provides the best explanation for this patient's hyponatremia?
   (A) inappropriate high level of antidiuretic hormone
   (B) increased water intake (psychogenic polydipsia)
   (C) volume depletion due to decreased oral intake over the last week
   (D) the use of a thiazide for the treatment of hypertension
   (E) decreased expression of renal collecting duct "water channels"

73. Which of the following would be the optimal choice of solution to infuse in order to adequately correct this patient's hyponatremia?

   (A) D_5W with 20 meq/L KCl at 200 mL/h
   (B) 0.9% saline at 125 mL/h
   (C) 0.45% saline at 100 mL/h
   (D) 3% saline at 35 mL/h
   (E) 0.45% saline with 30 meq/L KCl at 100 mL/h

74. Which of the following is the correct statement regarding the treatment of hyponatremia?

   (A) Desmopressin acetate (DDAVP), used in conjunction with intravenous saline, will help correct the serum sodium.
   (B) Correction of sodium slowly by 3 meq/day will prevent any subsequent neurologic injury.
   (C) Correction of serum sodium by 15 meq over 24 hours could lead to permanent neurologic injury.
   (D) Diuretics should be avoided in the treatment of hyponatremia.
   (E) Potassium should always be added to IV saline solutions when treating both hyponatremia and hypokalemia.

Questions 75 through 79

A 53-year-old Black male, with a history of hypertension, hepatitis C, and newly diagnosed nonsmall cell lung cancer, undergoes his first round of chemotherapy, which includes cisplatin. You are called to see this patient 5 days into his hospitalization for oliguria and laboratory abnormalities. Other than the chemotherapy, he is receiving lansoprazole, acetaminophen, and an infusion of D5—0.9% normal saline at 50 mL/h. On examination, his BP is 98/60 and heart rate is irregular, between 40 and 50 bpm. His physical examination shows a middle-aged male in no acute distress. His cardiac examination is unremarkable, his lungs show bibasilar crackles, and the abdominal examination is positive for a palpable spleen tip without any hepatomegaly or abdominal tenderness. He has trace bilateral ankle edema. His distal pulses are irregular. The neurologic examination was unremarkable. His laboratory (serum sample) results are as follows:

	Day 1	Day 5
Sodium	135	145
Potassium	4.4	6.8
Chloride	100	108
CO_2	24	20
BUN	15	35
Creatinine	1.5	3.4
Glucose	118	152
Uric acid	6.5	15.3
Phosphate	4.4	8.3
Calcium	9.0	7.5
Uric acid	6.5	15.3
Lactate dehydrogenase (LDH)	285	994

75. Which electrolyte/acid-base abnormality is most likely responsible for the findings on physical examination?

   (A) hypernatremia
   (B) hyperkalemia
   (C) metabolic acidosis
   (D) hyperphosphatemia
   (E) hyperuricemia

76. What is the mechanism that best explains this patient's hyperkalemia?

(A) DKA

(B) acute kidney failure leading to an inability to excrete potassium in the urine

(C) release of potassium from the destruction of neoplastic cells

(D) chemotherapy-induced hyperkalemia

(E) type 4 renal tubular acidosis

77. What is the most likely etiology of this patient's acute renal failure?

(A) renal tubular deposition of uric acid

(B) calcium oxalate kidney stones causing partial urinary tract obstruction

(C) renal tubular injury due to cisplatin

(D) ischemic acute tubular necrosis from a decreased cardiac output

(E) type II cryoglobulinemia due to hepatitis C

78. What would be the most likely finding on this patient's ECG?

(A) shortened P-R segment

(B) prominent U wave

(C) widened QRS complexes

(D) flattened T waves

(E) atrial fibrillation

79. Which of the following would be a part of the IMMEDIATE treatment strategy in this patient?

(A) atropine 1 mg IV

(B) calcium chloride, given IV

(C) 50 g of Kayexalate, given orally

(D) 10 units of regular insulin, given subcutaneously

(E) one ampule of glucagon, given IV

Questions 80 through 83

A 53-year-old White female, with a history of systemic lupus erythematosus (SLE), hypertension, and peripheral vascular disease, is admitted to the hospital for chest pain and dyspnea. Her cardiac enzymes were positive for acute MI. She subsequently undergoes a cardiac catheterization and stenting of the right coronary artery. Her postcardiac catheterization course is unremarkable, and she is discharged home 3 days later with adequate blood pressure control. Five days later, she is brought to the ER by her husband for abdominal pain and nausea. Her medications consist of aspirin, metoprolol, and prednisone. On physical examination, her blood pressure is 190/95 and her heart rate is 85 bpm. In general, she appears nauseated but is in no acute distress. Her cardiac examination reveals a regular rate and rhythm without murmur or rub. Her lung fields are clear bilaterally. The abdominal examination is positive for diffuse discomfort, without guarding or rebound, and normoactive bowel sounds; her stool is positive for occult blood. Her lower extremities have trace edema bilaterally with 2+ distal pulses; moreover, she has a reddish-blue discoloration on both her lower extremities. You retrieve her records from prior hospitalization. The patient's laboratory results are as follows:

Blood	5 Days prior	Now	Urine
Sodium	140	135	
Potassium	4.4	5.2	Na+: 35
Chloride	106	113	Creatinine: 45
CO$_2$	24	20	Specific gravity: 1.012
BUN	15	52	Protein: trace
Creatinine	1.6	3.5	RBCs: 1–3
Glucose	80	115	WBCs: 10–12
Uric acid	6.0	5.8	+ Eosinophils
Amylase	90	205	No cellular casts
WBC	8000	12,000	
Hgb	13.5	12.1	
Platelets (PLT)	400,000	370,000	
% Eosinophils	1%	15%	

80. What is the most likely cause of this patient's acute renal failure?

(A) contrast nephropathy from cardiac catheterization

(B) acute interstitial nephritis

(C) prerenal etiology from occult gastrointestinal (GI) bleeding

(D) atheroembolic disease

(E) lupus nephritis flare

81. Which of the following tests is helpful in distinguishing volume depletion as a possible cause of acute renal failure?

    (A) kidney ultrasound
    (B) calculation of the fractional excretion of sodium
    (C) estimation of the glomerular filtration rate
    (D) examination of the urine sediment under microscopy
    (E) calculation of the anion gap

82. Which of the following is the optimal therapeutic agent for this patient's pain management?

    (A) intravenous Demerol
    (B) intramuscular ketorolac
    (C) oral indomethacin
    (D) intravenous morphine sulfate
    (E) ibuprofen 400 mg orally three times daily as needed

83. Which of the following laboratory findings would be most suggestive of active lupus nephritis?

    (A) urinary RBC casts
    (B) urinary WBC casts
    (C) >3.5 g of proteinuria on 24-hour urine sample
    (D) normal serum complement levels
    (E) urinary eosinophils by Hansel stain

Questions 84 through 88

A 63-year-old Native American male, with a 6-year history of DM, hypertension, and hyperlipidemia, comes to your office as a new patient for a routine examination. He has been experiencing frequent lower back pain and headaches for which he is taking ibuprofen daily for the past 5 weeks. Moreover, he is complaining of mild fatigue. In addition, he is taking aspirin, atorvastatin, verapamil, and glipizide. His physical examination shows a blood pressure of 165/80 and heart rate of 90 bpm. In general, he was not in any distress. His funduscopic examination reveals no signs of diabetic retinopathy. Cardiac examination reveals a regular rate and rhythm with an S_4 gallop. His lungs are clear and

abdominal examination is unremarkable without any bruit auscultated. He also has 2+ lower extremity pitting edema. Rectal examination reveals brown stool, negative for occult blood. His laboratory results are as follows:

	Blood	Urine
Sodium	137	Specific gravity: 1.012
Potassium	5.0	Protein: trace
Chloride	115 ↑	RBCs: 1–3
CO2	20	WBCs: 0–3
BUN	30	No cellular casts
Creatinine	1.6	
Glucose	131	24-h specimen: 5.2 g protein
Total protein	8.5	
Albumin	3.0	
AST	15	
Total bilirubin	0.3	
LDL cholesterol	160	
WBC	8,700	
Hgb	8.5	
HCT	24	
PLT	245,000	

A kidney ultrasound shows 12 cm kidneys bilaterally (normal = 12 cm).

84. Which of the following is a typical finding in this patient's condition?

    (A) hypocalcemia
    (B) macrocytic anemia
    (C) elevated thyroxine levels
    (D) hypocomplementemia
    (E) hematuria

85. With regard the workup of this man's proteinuria, what diagnostic test would you perform next?

    (A) serum and urine protein electrophoresis
    (B) kidney biopsy
    (C) complement levels
    (D) antiglomerular basement membrane (anti-GBM) antibody titer
    (E) glycosylated Hgb level

86. Which additional of the following would best help in the determination of the etiology of this patient's nephrotic syndrome?

    (A) fractional excretion of sodium
    (B) anion gap
    (C) estimation of glomerular filtration rate
    (D) fractional excretion of urea
    (E) split 24-hour urine for protein

87. Which of the following antihypertensive medications would be best implemented in patients with diabetic nephropathy?

    (A) lisinopril 10 mg orally once daily
    (B) clonidine 0.2 mg orally twice daily
    (C) metoprolol 25 mg orally twice daily
    (D) amlodipine 5 mg orally once daily
    (E) hydralazine 25 mg orally three times daily

88. Which of the following microscopic findings on kidney biopsy is most usually associated with HIV infection?

    (A) pauci-immune crescentic glomerulonephritis
    (B) focal segmental glomerulosclerosis (collapsing variant)
    (C) membranous nephropathy
    (D) membranoproliferative glomerulonephritis
    (E) anti-GBM disease

Questions 89 through 91

A patient you see routinely in the clinic has elevated liver function tests. ALT is 89, AST is 75, and the total bilirubin and alkaline phosphatase are normal. The patient has no past history of hepatitis, taking medications, or excessive drinking. You order hepatitis serologies. The results are as follows:

Positive: HBsAg and anti-HBc.
Negative: anti-HBs, anti-HBc IgM, anti-HAV, and anti-HCV

89. What is your interpretation?

    (A) The patient has acute hepatitis B.
    (B) The patient needs a test for IgM antibody to hepatitis A virus to rule out acute hepatitis A.

    (C) The patient needs a test for hepatitis C antigen to exclude acute hepatitis C.
    (D) The patient has chronic hepatitis B.
    (E) If the patient had a negative test for HBsAg, they could be infected with hepatitis delta.

90. What is the most appropriate next step for this patient?

    (A) Verify the diagnosis with a qualitative hepatitis B viral load.
    (B) Vaccinate the patient with hepatitis A vaccine.
    (C) Vaccinate the patient with hepatitis B vaccine.
    (D) Investigate other causes of hepatitis, such as cytomegalovirus (CMV) and Epstein-Barr virus.
    (E) Recommend the patient's spouse receive hepatitis A vaccine.

91. Which statement best describes this clinical situation?

    (A) If the patient was found to be HBe antigen positive, he would be considered highly infectious to spread hepatitis B.
    (B) This patient is in the "window period" because the antibody to hepatitis BsAg is negative.
    (C) This patient is not at risk for delta hepatitis because the patient has antibody to hepatitis B core.
    (D) The low level of transaminase elevations indicates that this patient is not a candidate for hepatitis B antiviral treatment.
    (E) If this patient has antibody to hepatitis Be, he is a candidate for antiviral therapy.

Questions 92 and 93

A 72-year-old diabetic is transferred to your hospital for fever and altered mental status in the late summer. Symptoms started in this patient 1 week prior to admission. On physical examination, the patient was disoriented. There were no focal neurologic findings. There was a fine rash on the patient's trunk. On oral examination, there were tongue fasciculations. A lumbar puncture was performed which showed a glucose of 71 and a protein of 94;↑ microscopy of the cerebrospinal fluid (CSF) revealed 9 RBC and 14 WBC (21 P, 68 L, 11 H). The creatinine phosphokinase was 506. An electroencephalogram and MRI of the brain were normal.

92. What is the best interpretation of these findings?

   (A) The patient may have cryptococcal meningitis.
   (B) The patient may have disseminated candidiasis.
   (C) The patient may have West Nile virus.
   (D) The patient may have *Coccidioides immitis* infection.
   (E) The patient may have rhinocerebral mucormycosis.

93. What further diagnostic test is the most appropriate?

   (A) Perform a West Nile virus IgM on the CSF.
   (B) Perform a serum cryptococcal antigen.
   (C) Perform *C. immitis* complement fixation tests.
   (D) Perform a sinus series.
   (E) Perform a purified protein derivative (PPD) skin test.

Questions 94 and 95

A 24-year-old male presents with sore throat, subjective fever, abdominal pain, and bad breath. He says that a neighbor's child is currently being treated for strep throat. On examination, his temperature is 101.1°F and his other vital signs are normal. He appears well. His throat is erythematous and his tonsils are enlarged, but there are no pharyngeal or tonsillar exudates. He has no cervical adenopathy. He has an occasional cough but his lungs are clear. His abdominal examination is normal.

94. The presence of which of the following findings is a clinical predictor for the diagnosis of streptococcal pharyngitis?

   (A) erythematous tonsils
   (B) cough

   (C) tonsillar exudates
   (D) posterior cervical lymphadenopathy
   (E) halitosis

95. Which of the following is the recommended first-line agent for the treatment of group A streptococcal pharyngitis?

   (A) levofloxacin
   (B) amoxicillin
   (C) penicillin
   (D) amoxicillin-clavulinic acid
   (E) clindamycin

Questions 96 through 98

A 22-year-old male presents to an acute care clinic in order to have two genital lesions evaluated. He first noticed the lesions about 2 weeks ago, but delayed seeking medical care because he believed they were harmless due to the lack of any discomfort. He states that he does engage in unprotected sexual intercourse, with the most recent time being 1 month ago. On examination, the glans penis features two distinct nontender papules with elevated edges surrounding ulcerated craters. They each measure 1 cm in diameter. There is also nontender bilateral inguinal lymphadenopathy.

96. Which of the following is true about this patient's condition?

   (A) The causative agent is a virus.
   (B) Light microscopy of fluid from the lesions will reveal gram-negative rods in chains.
   (C) The presence of multiple distinct lesions is uncommon.
   (D) There is a latent phase in which patients are asymptomatic.
   (E) Although associated with persistent symptoms if left untreated, it does not carry a significant risk for mortality.

97. The drug of choice for treating this patient works by which of the following mechanisms?

    (A) interfering with protein synthesis at the ribosome
    (B) attaching to sterols in cell membranes
    (C) inhibiting bacterial cell wall synthesis
    (D) inhibiting the transport of amino acids into bacteria
    (E) inhibiting dihydrofolate reductase

98. Six hours after treating this patient, he calls your office with complaints of new-onset headache, myalgia, and malaise. He also states that he felt feverish immediately prior to calling and measured his temperature, which was 99.8°F. Which of the following is most appropriate at this time?

    (A) Advise transport to the nearest ED for immediate evaluation.
    (B) Advise use of acetaminophen and provide reassurance.
    (C) Advise immediate use of Benadryl and then have the patient go to the nearest ED.
    (D) Start treatment with levaquin.
    (E) Start treatment with oral corticosteroids.

99. A 26-year-old HIV-positive man is admitted to the hospital for treatment of a varicella-zoster infection. On the fourth day of treatment, he develops an acute renal insufficiency. What is the most likely treatment-related mechanism accounting for the patient's acute renal insufficiency?

    (A) the formation of toxic metabolites
    (B) decreased glomerular filtration rate
    (C) the precipitation of acyclovir in renal tubules
    (D) direct tubular cytotoxic injury
    (E) hypersensitivity interstitial nephritis

Questions 100 through 102

A 34-year-old amateur spelunker develops cough, dyspnea, and fever 2 weeks after a caving expedition to caves in Kentucky. On physical examination, the patient's temperature is 102°F and respiratory rate is 24. On pulmonary examination, there are diffuse crackles bilaterally. A CXR is shown in Figure 1-3.

FIG. 1-3 (*Courtesy of Philip C. Johnson, MD.*)

100. Which of the following is the most likely cause of disease in this patient?

    (A) The patient likely developed influenza from close contact with the other members of the caving expedition.
    (B) The patient likely has disseminated aspergillosis.
    (C) The patient likely has miliary tuberculosis.
    (D) The patient likely has acute pulmonary histoplasmosis.
    (E) The patient likely has *Pneumocystis jiroveci* pneumonia.

101. What diagnostic test would be most appropriate?

    (A) serum cryptococcal antigen
    (B) fungal serologies
    (C) a PPD skin test
    (D) an HIV enzyme-linked immunosorbent assay (ELISA) test
    (E) arterial blood gas determination

102. Which of these is the most appropriate statement about infection control of this patient if the patient is hospitalized?

    (A) The patient is not likely to need respiratory isolation.
    (B) The patient should be placed in respiratory isolation if histoplasmosis is suspected.
    (C) The patient should be placed in respiratory isolation if *P. jiroveci* is suspected.

(D) The patient should be placed in respiratory isolation if pulmonary aspergillosis is suspected.

(E) The patient should be placed in respiratory isolation if cryptococcal pneumonia is suspected.

Questions 103 and 104

A 53-year-old insulin-dependent diabetic, who underwent a cadaveric renal transplant 1 year prior to admission, presents with fever and cough of 3 weeks duration. He works as a long-haul trucker, carting fruit from McAllen, Texas (on the Texas-Mexico border) to Fresno, California. He does not smoke. His PPD skin test prior to admission was positive. On physical examination, his respiratory rate is 25, his oral temperature is 101°F, his lungs have rhonchi and decreased breath sounds on the left. His CXR is shown in Figure 1-4.

FIG. 1-4 (*Courtesy of Philip C. Johnson, MD.*)

103. What organism besides *Mycobacterium tuberculosis* leads your differential as a cause of pneumonia in this case?

(A) *Haemophilus influenzae*
(B) CMV
(C) *P. jiroveci*
(D) *C. immitis*
(E) *Histoplasma capsulatum*

104. What is the best diagnostic approach?

(A) PPD skin testing
(B) urine histoplasma antigen testing
(C) serum cryptococcal antigen testing
(D) sputum for silver staining for *P. jiroveci*
(E) fiberoptic bronchoscopy with bronchial alveolar lavage

105. A 76-year-old alcoholic male with hypertension, type II diabetes, and a history of congestive heart presented with cough, fever, malaise, and chills. His initial vitals were: HR 110, T: 102°F, RR: 25, BP 90/60, O_2 saturation 93% on 4L/NC. The patient decompensated in the ER and was intubated. Intubation was achieved after three attempts secondary to patient vomiting during the initial attempts. Patient was admitted to the ICU with a diagnosis of sepsis and respiratory failure secondary to suspected pneumonia. After obtaining blood and sputum cultures, the initial empiric antibiotic coverage should be which of the following?

(A) gatifloxacin alone
(B) vancomycin and metronidazole
(C) ceftriaxone and azithromycin
(D) ceftriaxone, gatifloxacin, and azithromycin
(E) ampicillin/sulbactam and gatifloxacin

106. A 31-year-old female health care worker presents to your clinic after a needlestick injury from a patient who subsequently left against medical advice prior to laboratory analysis for HIV or hepatitis. You advise your colleague that:

(A) If the patient had HIV, her risk of seroconversion is 20%.
(B) If the patient had Hepatitis B, her risk of seroconversion is 2%.
(C) If the patient had Hepatitis C, her risk of seroconversion is 5%.
(D) If the patient had HIV, her risk of seroconversion is 0.3%.
(E) If the patient had Hepatitis C, her risk of seroconversion is 50%.

Questions 107 and 108

A 35-year-old woman schedules an appointment in an outpatient clinic for evaluation and treatment of a "mouth problem." She says that she has white spots in her mouth that have been present for a few weeks. In response to your questioning, she states that she has been experiencing fatigue and a 20-lb weight loss over the past several months, although she attributes these symptoms to a dramatic increase in work hours at her job over the same period of time. She denies having any other chronic medical issues and does not use any prescription or OTC medications. As you examine her, you note the presence of white plaques on her buccal mucosa, palate, and tongue. Scraping of the plaques with a tongue depressor elicits pain as well as a small amount of bleeding. Nontender generalized cervical and submandibular lymphadenopathy is present.

107. Which of the following questions would potentially yield the most useful information in this patient's diagnosis and treatment?

    (A) "Do you have a family history of cancer?"
    (B) "Have you traveled outside of the country within the past 12 months?"
    (C) "Have you engaged in unprotected sexual intercourse?"
    (D) "Do you have any sick contacts?"
    (E) "How much do you smoke?"

108. Which of the following immunizations is safe to administer to this patient?

    (A) inactivated influenza vaccine
    (B) live attenuated influenza vaccine (FluMist)
    (C) varicella vaccine
    (D) oral polio vaccine (OPV)
    (E) measles mumps rubella (MMR) vaccine

109. A 45-year-old male with type II diabetes, hypertension, and hyperlipidemia presents to your clinic as a new patient. He has been out of his cholesterol medications and came to your office requesting a refill. The patient brought his most recent lipid profile (done after he was off his cholesterol medication for 3 months) which revealed:

> Cholesterol (total): 242 mg/dL
> HDL cholesterol: 38 mg/dL
> Triglycerides (TGs): 660 mg/dL
> LDL cholesterol = unable to calculate due to high TGs

He also had recent liver function tests that were normal. Based on Adult Treatment Panel (ATP) III guidelines, which of the following medications should be the initial pharmacologic treatment for this patient?

    (A) atorvostatin
    (B) gemfibrozil
    (C) cholestyramine
    (D) omega-3 fatty acids
    (E) nicotinic acid

Questions 110 through 112

A 48-year-old woman complaining of dysuria is diagnosed with a UTI by urinalysis. Urine culture and sensitivities reveal that the causative organism belongs to the genus *Klebsiella* and is resistant to multiple antibiotics. Based upon the results available, you decide to begin therapy with gentamicin.

110. Before doing so, you explain to the patient that antibiotics such as gentamicin are often associated with which of the following?

    (A) hepatotoxicity
    (B) nephrotoxicity
    (C) interstitial pulmonary fibrosis
    (D) pulmonary edema
    (E) splenomegaly

111. Which of the following irreversible complications is also associated with gentamicin use?

    (A) vestibular dysfunction
    (B) cardiomyopathy
    (C) optic nerve dysfunction
    (D) myelodysplastic disease
    (E) cerebellar degeneration

112. Which of the following would lead to the classification of this patient's infection as "complicated?"

(A) a history of recurrent UTIs

(B) a diagnosis of type II DM

(C) the patient's gender

(D) a history of undergoing a laparoscopic appendectomy 1 month ago

(E) a postvoid residual volume of 25 cc

Questions 113 and 114

113. A 53-year-old fisherman develops pain and swelling of the right hand 8 hours after suffering a fish hook injury to the finger. On physical examination, the patient's temperature is 102.8°F and the patient appears septic. The patient's hand and a Gram stain of material aspirated from a bulla are shown in Figures 1-5 and 1-6.

FIG. 1-5 *(Courtesy of Philip C. Johnson, MD.)*

FIG. 1-6 *(Courtesy of Philip C. Johnson, MD.)*

What is the most likely etiology of this bacteremia?

(A) *Staphylococcus aureus* cellulitis

(B) group A, beta-hemolytic *Streptococcus* sepsis

(C) *Pasteurella multocida* cellulitis

(D) *Vibrio vulnificus* sepsis

(E) *Eikenella corrodens* cellulitis

114. After appropriate wound care and debridement of necrotic tissue as necessary, which antibiotics should be started in this patient?

(A) levofloxacin

(B) vancomycin

(C) doxycycline and ceftazidime

(D) nafcillin and gentamicin

(E) trimethoprim-sulfamethoxazole (TMP-SMZ)

115. You receive a call from the nurse at a nursing home for a 70-year-old patient of yours who was febrile overnight and had blood cultures, CXR, and urinalysis ordered by the housestaff. The patient was started empirically on a fluoro-quinolone orally. The nurse informs you that the CXR and urinalysis were normal but the blood culture grew out *Enterococcus faecalis*. The patient has been on oral fluoroquinolone for 36 hours and patient is still febrile but appears stable. Which of the following is most appropriate?

   (A) Continue the oral quinolone and add an intravenous first-generation cephalosporin.
   (B) Discontinue the oral quinolone and start treatment with an intravenous second-generation cephalosporin.
   (C) Discontinue the quinolone and start treatment with an intravenous third-generation cephalosporin.
   (D) Discontinue the quinolone and start treatment with intravenous ampicillin and an aminoglycoside.
   (E) Continue the quinolone, but change from oral to IV route of administration.

Questions 116 and 117

A 30-year-old female presents to your office for the evaluation of a rash on her back. It has been present and growing for about a week. Along with this rash, she has had a fever, headache, myalgias, and fatigue. Her symptoms started about a week after returning from a camping trip to New England. She denies having any bites from ticks or other insects and exposure to poison ivy and has had no wounds to her skin. On examination, her temperature is 99.5°F and her vital signs are otherwise normal. Her rash is shown in Figure 1-7. Her examination is otherwise unremarkable.

116. What is the most likely cause of her rash?

   (A) contact dermatitis secondary to plant exposure
   (B) infection transmitted by tick bite
   (C) infection transmitted by mosquito bite
   (D) group A *Streptococcus* suprainfection of small puncture wound
   (E) allergic reaction to ingested (i.e., food) allergen

FIG. 1-7 (Also see color insert.)

117. You order IgM and IgG ELISA testing for *Borrelia burgdorferi* and the results return as negative. Which of the following management options would be most appropriate?

   (A) Treat the patient with a topical steroid for presumed contact dermatitis.
   (B) Treat the patient with oral steroids for a presumed systemic allergic reaction.
   (C) Treat the patient with oral cephalexin for streptococcal cellulitis.
   (D) Treat the patient with doxycycline for Lyme disease.
   (E) No medication at present, but have the patient return in 6–8 weeks for repeat serologic testing and treat for Lyme disease if positive at that time.

Questions 118 through 120

A 39-year-old HIV-positive male presents for routine follow-up. He is on highly active antiretroviral therapy. A CD4 count is 250/µL. His vital signs are within normal limits and his examination is normal.

118. Which of the following management options is most appropriate at this time?

    (A) Continue with current regiment without change.
    (B) Add azithromycin for *Mycobacterium avium* complex prophylaxis.
    (C) Add TMP-SMZ (Bactrim DS) for *Pneumocystis carinii* prophylaxis.
    (D) Test the patient for IgG antibody to *Toxoplasma gondii* if such a test has not yet been done.
    (E) Start ganciclovir for CMV prophylaxis.

119. He has a PPD placed and follows up in 48 hours. At the site of the injection you find 6 mm of induration. A CXR is normal. He has never been treated for tuberculosis or a positive PPD before. Which management option is most appropriate?

    (A) Collect sputum samples for 3 days to send for AFB (acid fast bacilli) staining.
    (B) Empirically start four-drug therapy for active tuberculosis.
    (C) Empirically start isoniazid daily for 9 months.
    (D) Have the patient return in 1 week for a second PPD to assess for the presence of a "booster" phenomenon; treat with isoniazid if ≥10 mm induration.
    (E) No intervention at this time but repeat the test in 6 months.

120. One month later, a repeat measurement of the patient's CD4 count is 225/µL. Which of the following interventions would be the most appropriate at this time?

    (A) Continue the current regimen without change.
    (B) Modify the patient's antiretroviral therapy to prevent development of resistance.

    (C) Discontinue any prophylactic medications that the patient is taking.
    (D) Begin azithromycin for *M. avium* complex prophylaxis.
    (E) Recheck CD4 count due to suspected laboratory error.

121. While visiting a neighbor, a 14-year-old girl is bitten on the left hand by the neighbor's pet cat. The cat is an indoor pet and has had all of the required routine vaccinations. You see the girl in the office approximately 1 hour after the injury. On the dorsum of the left hand you see two shallow puncture wounds that are not actively bleeding. She has full range of motion of her hand, normal capillary refill, and sensation. You see in the chart that the patient had a diphtheria/tetanus (dT) booster vaccine last year. What is the most appropriate management at this time?

    (A) Recommend local care at home with hydrogen peroxide and topical antibiotics.
    (B) Give a booster dT and start oral cephalexin.
    (C) Give an intramuscular (IM) dose of penicillin and emergently refer to a hand surgeon for debridement.
    (D) Irrigate the wounds and prescribe oral amoxicillin/clavulanic acid (Augmentin).
    (E) Start oral ciprofloxacin and refer to the health department for rabies prophylaxis.

Questions 122 through 125

A 29-year-old woman complains of fatigue and decreased exercise tolerance. She takes no medications and denies changes in the color of the stool. Physical examination is significant for pale skin and conjunctivae. Stool was negative for blood. Laboratory evaluation revealed Hgb of 7.8 g/dL, reticulocytopenia, microcytosis, and hypochromia.

122. Which of the following would most likely be found on further laboratory testing?

	Mean corpuscular volume (MCV)	Ferritin	Erythrocyte protoporphyrin	Folate	B₁₂
A	N or D	N or I	I	N or D	N
B	D	D	I	N	N or D
C	I	N	N	D	N or I
D	I	N	N	N or I	D
E	D	N	N	N	N

N = normal, I = increased, D = decreased.

/'farənhīt/

123. The U.S. Preventive Services Task Force (USPSTF) recommends screening for iron deficiency in which of the following?

    (A) asymptomatic persons over the age of 65 at risk for gastric cancer

    (B) immigrants from developing countries

    (C) asymptomatic infants at high risk

    (D) pregnant women

    (E) blood donors

124. In vitamin B₁₂ or folate deficiency, which of the following statements is correct? /ˌmethəlmələˈänˌik/

    (A) High serum levels of homocysteine and decreased levels of methylmalonic acid are reliable indicators of cobalamin deficiency.

    (B) The recommended amount of dietary folate is 800 µg/day.

    (C) The peripheral smear in patients with cobalamin deficiency is identical to that found in folate deficiency. /kōˈbaləmən/

    (D) The most common cause of cobalamin deficiency is hypersecretion of gastric acid (i.e., Zollinger-Ellison syndrome).

    (E) Because body folate stores are high, individuals with low consumption of folate will take several years to become anemic.

125. Which of the following is the most appropriate next step in the management of the anemia in this woman?

    (A) Start iron therapy as soon as possible.

    (B) Transfuse RBCs and start iron therapy.

    (C) Start B₁₂ and folate replacement.

    (D) Identify the cause of the anemia with a thorough history and physical examination.

    (E) Start iron therapy and B₁₂ replacement.

Questions 126 and 127

A 23-year-old woman presents to your acute care clinic with a complaint of fever, sore throat, and malaise of sudden onset. Her prior medical history is significant for schizophrenia. Her vitals signs are: BP 116/80, HR 112, RR 26, Temp 100.6 degrees Fahrenheit. On physical examination, her oral cavity features painful aphthous ulcers as well as swollen gums. Initial laboratory testing includes a CBC which returns with the following results:

- Leukocyte count 800/mm³
- Hgb 12.1 g/dL
- HCT 37.0%
- Platelet count 212 × 10⁹/L
- Differential:
  - Neutrophils, segmented 52%
  - Neutrophils, bands 3%
  - Lymphocytes 35%
  - Monocytes 7%
  - Eosinophils 3%
  - Basophils 0%

126. Use of which of the following must be considered when formulating a differential diagnosis to explain this patient's symptoms?

    (A) haloperidol

    (B) chlorpromazine

    (C) risperidone

    (D) thioridazine

    (E) clozapine

127. Which of the following best describes the expected course of the patient's condition?

    (A) The condition is usually self-limiting and requires no intervention.

    (B) Use of G-CSF has been shown to speed recovery.

    (C) Dose reduction of the offending agent often leads to resolution of symptoms.

(D) If discovered earlier, discontinuation of the offending agent would have prevented progression of the condition to its current severity.

(E) Tardive dyskinesia usually develops as a late finding.

128. A 62-year-old female with a history of a recent pulmonary embolus presents to your office for follow-up on anticoagulation treatment. She takes warfarin on a daily basis. She reports that for the last week she has noticed mild rectal bleeding and multiple bruises over the extremities with minimal trauma. She is comfortable appearing with normal vital signs and is not orthostatic. You ordered a stat CBC and PT/INR which revealed a mildly decreased Hgb at 11 g/dL and an elevated INR of 7. Which of the following would be the most appropriate intervention?

(A) subcutaneous injections of heparin
(B) oral allopurinol
(C) intravenous protamine sulfate
(D) oral vitamin E
(E) oral vitamin K

129. A 42 year old male admitted for pulmonary embolus was placed on heparin, dosed by a weight based protocol. However, later in the day, you receive a call from the floor nurse stating that the patient had spontaneous epistaxis and a very high aPTT. Use of which of the following would be best at this time?

(A) cimetidine
(B) heparinase
(C) clofibrate
(D) protamine sulfate
(E) vitamin K

130. A 64 year old woman presents with bilateral symmetric arthralgias and morning stiffness for several years. She says that she has been worked up for RA in the past. On review of her records as well as the examination you note subcutaneous nodules, positive rheumatoid factor, and radiographs of the hands that revealed joint erosions. Which of her findings has the highest positive likelihood ratio (LR) for the diagnosis of RA?

(A) morning stiffness
(B) rheumatoid nodules on examination
(C) symmetric arthralgias
(D) joint erosions of the hand on xray
(E) positive rheumatoid factor.

131. A 58-year-old woman is concerned about her risk for osteoporosis and is seen by her general internist. Her mother was diagnosed with osteoporosis and had a hip fracture at age 84. She has no personal or family history of kidney stones or ulcer disease, and she has never had a fracture. She had a hysterectomy at age 48 and took estradiol for 2 years, but discontinued because of a fear of adverse effects. She does not have any vasomotor symptoms. She takes 1500 mg of calcium carbonate and 400 IU vitamin D daily. She is not on any other medications. On examination, she appears well developed and there is no evidence of kyphosis. A BMD test is performed that demonstrates a T score in the spine of —3.5 and in the hip of —2.8. CXR and mammogram are normal. Further evaluation demonstrates the following:

Serum calcium	11.4 mg/dL	(9.5–10.5)
Phosphate	2.1 mg/dL	(2.5–4.5)
24-h urine calcium	405 mg	(100–250)
Serum magnesium	1.8 meq/L	(1.3–2.1)
Serum creatinine	0.7 mg/dL	(0.5–1.4)
Hgb	14 g/L	(12–16)

Which of the following is the most likely diagnosis?

(A) milk-alkali syndrome
(B) primary hyperparathyroidism
(C) sarcoidosis
(D) secondary hyperparathyroidism
(E) osteomalacia

132. Vitamin D supplementation can be helpful in treating which disease?

    (A) hyperparathyroidism
    (B) hypoparathyroidism
    (C) alcoholic neuritis
    (D) pernicious anemia
    (E) scurvy

133. A 34-year-old woman was found to have a 2-cm right thyroid nodule at the time of a well woman examination. The remainder of the thyroid was palpably normal and there were no lymph nodes palpable. There was no history of thyroid disease or radiation therapy to her head or neck. She was clinically euthyroid. Thyroid-stimulating hormone (TSH) was normal. Which of the following tests would be the most useful in establishing a specific diagnosis?

    (A) ultrasound of the thyroid
    (B) nuclear scan of the thyroid
    (C) thyroid antibody studies
    (D) fine needle aspiration of the nodule
    (E) CT of the neck

Questions 134 through 136

A 32-year-old woman presents with complaints of irritability, heat intolerance, hyperdefecation, and frequent palpitations. She has lost 20 lb over the past six months. She has always been in good health and does not take any prescription or OTC medications. She denies any prior history of thyroid disease or exposure to head/neck irradiation, but she states that one of her relatives was diagnosed with a thyroid disorder at roughly the same age. Vital signs are as follows: BP 138/78, HR 112, RR 22, temp. 98.8°F. On examination, her thyroid is diffusely enlarged and smooth. Auscultation of the thyroid reveals a bruit. Her hair is fine in texture, and she has warm velvety skin. She has hyperactive deep tendon reflexes. There is a fine tremor in her outstretched hands.

134. Which of the following is a common finding in this condition?

    (A) macroglossia
    (B) hyperkeratosis

    (C) infiltrative ophthalmopathy
    (D) cerebellar ataxia
    (E) pericardial effusion

135. Which of the following sets of laboratory results would be consistent with this patient's presentation?

	TSH	free T3	free T4
(A)	low	low	high
(B)	low	normal	normal
(C)	low	high	high
(D)	high	low	low
(E)	high	high	high

136. Which of the following interventions is most appropriate at this time?

    (A) propylthiouracil
    (B) thyroidectomy
    (C) radioactive iodine therapy
    (D) propranolol
    (E) potassium iodide

137. A 40-year-old woman presents with nausea, vomiting, and weakness. She has been amenorrheic since the birth of her last child 1 year ago and has not felt well since that time. On examination, she appears chronically ill, her thyroid is not palpable, and there is no galactorrhea. Laboratory studies on admission include:

Sodium	120 meq/L	
Glucose	55 mg/dL	
Total T$_4$	2.0 µg/mL	(normal 4.5–12)
TSH	1.0 µU/mL	(normal 0.4–5.0)

The most appropriate next step is to start treatment with which of the following?

    (A) hydrocortisone
    (B) fluid restriction
    (C) desmopressin
    (D) glucagon
    (E) fludrocortisone

138. A 32-year-old woman complains of episodic confusion in the morning for the past 6 months. During one of these episodes, she was brought to the ER and her serum glucose was found to be 40 mg/dL. She was given intravenous dextrose and her symptoms resolved within 15 minutes. She has gained approximately 25 lbs during the past year. Which of the following would be the most appropriate next step?

   (A) measure serum insulin and proinsulin 2 hours after a mixed meal
   (B) MRI of the pancreas
   (C) measure insulin, C-peptide, and sulfonylurea level on the initial blood sample in ER
   (D) octreotide scan
   (E) advise a high protein diet with frequent feedings

Questions 139 and 140

A 74-year-old male with a history of hypertension, type II diabetes, myopia, and cataract surgery 2 weeks ago presents with the sudden onset of severe flashes of light and multiple new floaters in his right eye. He denies photophobia, ocular trauma, or diplopia. He also states that he feels as if there is a curtain lowering over his right eye.

139. What is the most likely cause of his symptoms?

   (A) central retinal artery occlusion
   (B) acute lens displacement
   (C) iritis
   (D) retinal detachment
   (E) staphylococcal endophthalmitis

140. Your examination and a stat ophthalmology consultation confirm your clinical diagnosis. Of the choices listed below, what would be the most appropriate next step to provide definite treatment for this patient?

   (A) lens removal and surgical replacement
   (B) corneal transplant
   (C) removal of vitreous humor (posterior vitrectomy)
   (D) intraocular antibiotics
   (E) stat angiogram and thrombolytics if needed

141. A 23-year-old pregnant woman with type 1 diabetes was admitted to the Obstetrics service for DKA. The DKA was appropriately treated and has resolved. You were consulted for medical management of the diabetes, as her sugars have been labile throughout the hospital stay. Your history and review of records reveals that the patient has a long-standing history of noncompliance with diet and medication regimens. She currently uses any insulin she can get and does not eat regular meals. She has fluctuating blood sugars with episodes of hypoglycemia. You counsel the patient extensively, order nutrition and diabetic teaching consults, and discuss keeping home glucose logs. Assuming the patient will follow your advice, which regimen would you recommend to minimize fluctuating glucose readings?

   (A) NPH insulin twice daily
   (B) insulin glargine once daily and insulin lispro before meals
   (C) Humulin 70/30 twice daily
   (D) NPH twice daily and regular insulin three times daily with meals
   (E) insulin glargine twice daily

142. A 54-year-old man presents with a 3-cm right thyroid nodule that was found incidentally by the patient while shaving. He denies any pain or discomfort. He denies any history of thyroid disease, any family history of thyroid disease, and any history of head/neck irradiation. He notes a 10-lb weight loss over the past 6 months. His examination is only remarkable for the firm right thyroid nodule. The remainder of the thyroid is not palpable. There is no adenopathy. Heart rate is 90/minute and regular. The skin is warm and moist, and a fine tremor is present when he holds his hands out. TSH level is <.02 μU/mL. Which of the following is the most appropriate next step?

   (A) thyroid ultrasound
   (B) antithyroid peroxidase antibodies
   (C) thyroid-stimulating immunoglobulins
   (D) fine needle aspiration of the nodule
   (E) thyroid nuclear scan

143. A 19-year-old woman who is 2 months postpartum complains of palpitations, heat intolerance, tremulousness, weight loss, and fatigue. Her thyroid is prominent and firm but nontender. Serum TSH level was undetectable. A nuclear medicine radioactive iodine uptake is performed and shows no uptake of iodine in the neck. Which of the following is the most appropriate next step?

(A) administer radioactive iodine
(B) initiate glucocorticoid therapy
(C) initiate levothyroxine therapy
(D) initiate propranolol therapy
(E) initiate methimazole therapy

144. A 60-year-old man with a history of severe chronic obstructive pulmonary disease (COPD), which is steroid dependent, is admitted to the ICU with pulmonary infiltrates and a sepsis syndrome. His hospital course is complicated by acute renal insufficiency and respiratory failure. Therapy includes glucocorticoids and dopamine. He has no history of thyroid disease. Several weeks into his hospital course, the following laboratory studies are performed:

Total T4	2.2	(5–12 µg/dL)
T3 resin uptake	55%	(25–35%)
Free thyroid index	1.2	(1.2–4.2)
TSH	0.20	(0.45 µU/mL)
Total T3	<30	(80–220 ng/dL)
Reverse T3	500	(80–250 ng/L)

Based on these laboratory studies, which of the following is the most appropriate next step?

(A) initiate levothyroxine therapy
(B) discontinue glucocorticoid therapy
(C) initiate methimazole therapy
(D) order MRI of the pituitary
(E) supportive treatment only

Questions 145 through 147

A 28-year-old woman presents for evaluation of primary infertility. She has had fewer than four periods per year since menarche at age 14, facial hirsutism, acne, and weight gain. On examination, she has a BP 150/100. Her body mass index (BMI) is 40. *Acanthosis nigricans* is noted along the posterior surface of her neck.

145. Which of the following laboratory studies is most likely to be abnormal in this patient?

(A) TSH
(B) prolactin
(C) glucose tolerance test
(D) growth hormone
(E) cosyntropin (Cortrosyn) stimulation test

146. Which of the following would be her most likely fasting lipid profile?

(A) high TGs, high HDL
(B) low TGs, low HDL
(C) high TGs, low HDL
(D) high LDL cholesterol
(E) normal lipid profile

147. How would you counsel this patient?

(A) The primary treatment for this problem is with medications.
(B) Weight loss is key to her management.
(C) Her hypertension would be best treated with a thiazide diuretic.
(D) Regardless of her lipid panel result, she should be on a statin.
(E) Her infertility is due to lack of estrogen production.

Questions 148 and 149

A 34-year-old female sex worker presents with a several week history of fatigue, malaise, fever, and a 10-lb weight loss. Over the last 2 weeks, the patient noted a rash on her face, torso, arms, legs, palms, and soles (Figures 1-8 and 1-9). The patient is HIV negative on a test 2 months ago, has had hepatitis B, gonorrhea, and chlamydia. The patient has an oral temperature of 100.6°F, and generalized lymphadenopathy. The patient does not have any lesions in the mucous membranes.

FIG. 1-8 *(Courtesy of Philip C. Johnson, MD.)* (Also see color insert.)

FIG. 1-9 *(Courtesy of Philip C. Johnson, MD.)* (Also see color insert.)

148. What is the diagnostic test most likely to explain this clinical presentation?

(A) a hepatitis B surface antigen test

(B) cervical smear for rapid tests for gonorrhea and chlamydiae

(C) a skin biopsy

(D) a rapid plasma reagin (RPR) and micro-hemagglutination assay for *Treponema pallidum* (MHA-TP) test

(E) an HIV viral load by polymerase chain reaction (PCR)

149. What is the appropriate treatment?

(A) benzathine penicillin 2.4 million units IM weekly for 3 weeks

(B) azithromycin 1 g orally

(C) aqueous penicillin 4 million units intravenously every 4 hours for 14 days

(D) doxycycline 100 mg twice a day for 2 weeks

(E) oral corticosteroids over 5 days

Questions 150 through 152

A 58-year-old male presents to your office for a well-male examination. It has been several years since he last visited a doctor, but he states that he has been in "excellent health." He denies any history of drinking, smoking, or using illegal drugs. He maintains a diet low in sodium and fat. An avid sports enthusiast, he also spends at least 2 hours per day engaged in some type of outdoor physical activity. On physical examination, you discover a translucent waxy papule with raised borders on the posterior aspect of his left shoulder.

150. Which of the following is true of this patient's skin condition?

(A) It is the most common malignancy in the United States.

(B) Total body skin examination reduces the morbidity and mortality associated with this condition.

(C) Metastasis is common.

(D) The cure rate is approximately 50%.

(E) If appropriately treated, the rate of recurrence (development of a second lesion) is equal to that found in the general population.

151. Which of the following is the most important risk factor for development of this skin condition?

    (A) immunosuppression
    (B) presence of a chronic inflammatory skin condition
    (C) chronic arsenic exposure
    (D) exposure to long-wavelength ultraviolet radiation
    (E) exposure to short-wavelength ultraviolet radiation

152. The treatment modality associated with the lowest recurrence rate is which of these?

    (A) radiation therapy
    (B) Mohs micrographic surgery
    (C) surgical excision
    (D) electrodesiccation with curettage
    (E) cryotherapy

Questions 153 and 154

An 18-year-old female presents for evaluation of facial acne. On examination, she has multiple comedones, papules, and pustules on her forehead, nose, cheeks, and chin. She also has several distinct nodules, each greater than 5 mm in diameter.

153. Which of the following is most appropriate for initial inclusion in a regimen to treat this patient's acne?

    (A) erythromycin gel
    (B) tretinoin 0.025% cream
    (C) clindamycin lotion
    (D) oral tetracycline
    (E) oral isotretinoin

154. After 6 months of appropriate treatment, the severity of your patient's acne remains essentially unchanged. You rule out several potential causes for the patient's recalcitrant acne and decide that more aggressive therapy is warranted. As you discuss this option with your patient, which of the following side effects of the proposed treatment necessitates extensive counseling prior to initiation of therapy?

    (A) pseudotumor cerebri
    (B) teratogenicity
    (C) hepatotoxicity
    (D) nephrotoxicity
    (E) cardiotoxicity

Questions 155 and 156

A 23-year-old presents with the history of a suspected spider bite to the left groin (Figure 1-10). On questioning, no one saw a spider. The patient has been healthy except occasional boils under his arms and in the groin. The patient is afebrile. No family members are sick.

FIG. 1-10 (Also see color insert.)

155. Appropriate treatment would include which of the following?

    (A) Benadryl and topical steroids
    (B) surgical debridement
    (C) incision and drainage
    (D) treatment with TMP-SMZ
    (E) observation and instructions to the patient to pop any pustules to help it drain

156. The patient is sent home and a day later develops chills, fever, and the lesion is spreading. Appropriate treatment would include which of the following?

    (A) hospital admission, blood cultures, and vancomycin
    (B) systemic corticosteroids

(C) surgical excision of any necrotic tissue

(D) observation and monitoring at home with oral clindamycin

(E) hospital admission, blood cultures, and ceftriaxone

Questions 157 and 158

157. A 45-year-old male has received intravenous contrast dye prior to CT scan of the abdomen. Twenty minutes later the patient reports severe pruritus. He denies respiratory distress, syncope, or palpitations. His blood pressure is 98/54, pulse is 90, and respiratory rate is 22. On physical examination, he has widespread urticaria. His lungs are clear to auscultation. The next appropriate step would be which of the following?

(A) administration of 0.5 mL of 1:1000 epinephrine subcutaneously

(B) administration of 0.5 mL of 1:100,000 epinephrine subcutaneously

(C) administration of 25 mg of diphenhydramine subcutaneously

(D) administration of intravenous glucocorticoids

(E) careful observation but no medications

158. This intervention works well in cases such as this due to activity directed toward which of these receptors?

(A) dopaminergic receptors

(B) muscarinic receptors

(C) nicotinic receptors

(D) adrenergic receptors

(E) *N*-methyl D-aspartate (NMDA) receptors

Questions 159 through 162

159. A 20-year-old male has had a recent wide local excision of a 1.5 mm melanoma from the right ankle. There is no evidence of metastatic disease. The most important prognostic factor for this patient is which of the following?

(A) the Breslow depth of the tumor

(B) the Clark level of the tumor

(C) the location of the tumor

(D) the age of the patient

(E) the number of prior severe blistering sunburns

160. Which of the following interventions is most appropriate in addition to wide local excision of the patient's melanoma?

(A) sentinel lymph node biopsy

(B) no further intervention is warranted

(C) adjuvant therapy with interferon alpha-2 for 1 year

(D) single-agent chemotherapy

(E) complete lymph node dissection

161. One year after his initial diagnosis and treatment, the patient develops a palpable right inguinal lymph node. Inguinal lymph node dissection reveals one node positive for metastatic melanoma; the remaining nodes are negative. A complete restaging workup shows no evidence of any additional metastatic disease. What is the correct stage for this patient?

(A) stage I

(B) stage IIa

(C) stage IIb

(D) stage III

(E) stage IV

162. Which of the following is true regarding melanoma?

(A) Chest radiographs are not recommended as a part of a patient's follow-up surveillance.

(B) Timely treatment of metastatic melanoma has been shown to have an effect on mean survival.

(C) Elevated serum LDH suggests metastatic melanoma.

(D) Patients without clinical lymphadenopathy are not at risk for metastatic involvement.

(E) High mitotic rate and a lower Clark level are poor prognostic signs.

163. A 43-year-old patient presents with his fourth episode of culture-proven shingles in a T7 distribution. What is the most likely associated underlying condition?

(A) leukemia

(B) lymphoma

(C) acquired immunodeficiency syndrome (AIDS)

(D) chronic prednisone therapy

(E) DM

164. A 24-year-old female presents to your office for excision of a nevus. After obtaining consent and prepping the site, you anesthetize the area with 1% lidocaine. However, as you start the procedure, you note that the patient is not sufficiently anesthetized. Your partner suggests the use of lidocaine with epinephrine. The addition of epinephrine with local anesthetics is useful because of which of the following properties?

(A) It prolongs and increases the depth of local anesthesia.

(B) It neutralizes the irritant action of the local anesthetic agent.

(C) It increases the rate of systemic absorption and therefore hastens the onset of action of the anesthetic agent.

(D) It increases the pH of the anesthetic so that less anesthetic is required to produce nerve block.

(E) It blocks neurotransmitter release (thus decreasing pain perception) via stimulation of presynaptic alpha-adrenergic receptors.

165. A 64-year-old man with hypertension presents for routine follow-up of his blood pressure. His home blood pressure log reveals readings in the 150/70 range. His home monitor had previously been verified by clinic BP readings. He denies any complaints. His current medications include HCTZ 25 mg daily, metoprolol 100 mg twice daily, enalapril 20 mg twice daily, and amlodipine 10 mg daily. He states he is adherent to his medication, drug, and exercise regimen as you recommended. At this time, how would you advise the patient?

(A) You need to take another blood pressure medication.

(B) I need to order some tests to look for secondary causes of high blood pressure.

(C) In spite of your efforts, you need to exercise more and lose more weight.

(D) Your blood pressure is acceptable where it is. Continue your current regimen.

(E) I need to refer you to a cardiologist.

166. C1 deficiency has three subcomponents, of which the most common is deficiency of C1q. Most of those patients will have clinical and serologic findings typical of which of these?

(A) polymyositis

(B) RA

(C) SLE

(D) recurrent *Streptococcus pneumoniae* infections

(E) recurrent *H. influenzae* type B infections.

Questions 167 and 168

A 21-year-old Asian female, with past medical history of exertional asthma, comes to your office complaining of mild low back pain. It started after her working out in the gym 3 days ago. The pain is 2–4 out of 10 in intensity, has no radiation, increases with bending or lying down for a long time, and improves with warm showers. You examine the patient, diagnose her with paravertebral muscle spasm, and give her prescriptions for cyclobenzaprine and naproxen to use as needed for pain and stiffness.

You receive a call from your patient 2 hours later. She is having generalized itching, dizziness, and swelling of the tongue and lips. She is having difficulty breathing. She tells you that she took the first dose of the medication you prescribed about 30 minutes ago.

167. What should you do at this time?

(A) Advise patient to use her albuterol inhaler as she is having an asthma attack.

(B) Advise her to take another dose of naproxen and stop cyclobenzaprine for now.

(C) Assure her that this is a common side effect to cyclobenzaprine; she will get used to it as she takes the next dose.

(D) Ask her to return to your clinic for evaluation.

(E) Ask her to call 911 immediately.

168. The most beneficial immediate intervention for this patient would be which of the following?

(A) oxygen

(B) albuterol nebulizer treatment

(C) IV fluids

(D) epinephrine

(E) diphenhydramine

169. A 34-year-old male presents with a penile lesion. Your history, physical examination, and serology confirm a diagnosis of syphilis. The patient reports that his mother told him he was "allergic" to penicillin. He does not recall any personal history of anaphylaxis or rash to antibiotics however he has never been "sick." How would you manage this patient?

(A) Admit to the ICU for penicillin desensitization as you don't want to risk anaphylaxis especially with the uncertain history.

(B) Do skin testing for penicillin allergy.

(C) Avoid penicillin or cephalosporins in future.

(D) Treat with erythromycin.

(E) Treat with penicillin as he is not likely to have a true allergy.

170. A 57-year-old male presents for annual examination. On history, you note a history of colon cancer that was successfully surgically resected 2 years ago. He had a negative postoperative colonoscopy 6 months later and another negative colonoscopy last year. Which of the following would be the most appropriate colon cancer screening regimen for this patient?

(A) colonoscopy or virtual colonoscopy in 1 year

(B) colonoscopy in 3 years

(C) colonoscopy or double contrast barium enema in 5 years

(D) colonoscopy annually

(E) digital examination and fecal occult blood test (FOBT) annually with colonoscopy in 10 years

Questions 171 through 174

A 19-year-old male who moved to your city 3 months ago comes to your office complaining of dry cough for the past 2–3 months. Along with the cough, he has had some shortness of breath with exertion. He denies fever, chills, nausea, vomiting, wheezing, and sneezing. The cough occurs mostly in the morning and improves as the day goes on. He denies similar complaints in the past and has no history of allergies. He says that his father had eczema and an allergy to eggs.

171. You order a CXR. Which of the following are you most likely to find?

(A) normal

(B) diffuse pulmonary congestion

(C) increased bronchial wall markings

(D) cardiomegaly

(E) flattening of the diaphragms

172. The pulmonary function test that is most likely to be diagnostic in this patient is which of these?

(A) increased total lung capacity

(B) increased functional residual capacity

(C) increased residual volume

(D) decreased forced expiratory volume in 1 second (FEV_1)

(E) decreased forced inspiratory volume

173. What is the single best treatment for preventing symptoms in this patient?

(A) long-acting beta-2 agonists

(B) an inhaled steroid

(C) an inhaled anticholinergic

(D) leukotriene modifiers

(E) long-acting oral bronchodilators

174. Which of the following properties of albuterol makes it a more appropriate choice than epinephrine for relief of acute episodes of bronchoconstriction?

    (A) rapid onset of action
    (B) longer duration of action
    (C) specificity for beta-1 receptors
    (D) specificity for beta-2 receptors
    (E) direct activation of both alpha- and beta-receptors

Questions 175 through 177

A 63-year-old male presents to your office with palpitations for the past 3 weeks. He has had no chest pains or dyspnea. He has no significant medical history and takes no medications. He does not smoke cigarettes and a recent lipid panel was normal. On examination, he is in no apparent distress. His pulse is 115 bpm and irregular. His BP is 125/77. His lungs are clear and his cardiac examination reveals an irregularly irregular rhythm with no murmurs, rubs, or gallops.

175. Which of the following is most likely to be found on an ECG?

    (A) saw-tooth P waves
    (B) wide QRS complexes
    (C) absent P waves
    (D) Q waves in leads II, III, and aVF
    (E) peaked T waves

176. An abnormal result of which of the following laboratory tests would be most likely to explain the cause of this condition?

    (A) TSH
    (B) troponin T
    (C) BUN and creatinine
    (D) serum glucose
    (E) arterial blood gas

177. Which of the following studies would be most appropriate to order at this time?

    (A) radionuclide ventriculography
    (B) exercise stress test
    (C) echocardiogram

    (D) cardiac catheterization
    (E) electrophysiologic studies

178. A 74-year-old male with gout, osteoporosis, and type II diabetes presents for routine follow-up. As you review his medication list you note that he is on insulin, vitamin D, glypizide, quinidine, and allopurinol. You now diagnose him with hypertension that requires pharmacologic management. Which of the following medications would be contraindicated in this patient?

    (A) enalapril
    (B) hydrochlorothiazide
    (C) diltiazem
    (D) losartan
    (E) atenolol

Questions 179 through 181

A 60-year-old male with a history of hypertension and hyperlipidemia undergoes an evaluation for angina. He states that he routinely experiences dyspnea, fatigue, and retrosternal chest discomfort when performing activities such as walking around the block on which his house is located or climbing the flight of stairs within his home. Besides taking medications for his blood pressure and cholesterol, he uses nitroglycerin which successfully alleviates his symptoms.

179. Which of the following best describes the severity of this patient's angina?

    (A) class I
    (B) class II
    (C) class III
    (D) class IV
    (E) Prinzmetal angina

180. The patient states that shortly after self-administering nitroglycerin, his heart feels like it races. He does not notice this sensation at any other times. Which of the following interventions would be most appropriate for counteracting this phenomenon?

    (A) discontinue nitroglycerin
    (B) increase the dose of nitroglycerin used

(C) use nifedipine instead of nitroglycerin

(D) continue nitroglycerin and start isoproterenol

(E) continue nitroglycerin and start propranolol

181. The patient undergoes a cardiac catheterization and is found to have 70% narrowing of the left anterior descending and proximal left circumflex arteries. Which of the following would be the most appropriate management of this condition?

(A) percutaneous transluminal coronary angioplasty (PTCA)

(B) medical management with a beta-blocker, statin, and aspirin

(C) medical management with an ACE inhibitor, statin, and aspirin

(D) referral for coronary artery bypass grafting (CABG)

(E) placement of a cardiac defibrillator

Questions 182 and 183

182. A 64-year-old female with no significant medical history presents with vague complaints of progressive generalized muscle weakness and fatigue. She denies any history of trauma or drug use and does not take any prescription, OTC or herbal medications. This is a new complaint and she has not had any prior workup. There is no evidence of trauma and a recent TSH was normal. On examination, you find mild muscle tenderness and atrophy. She has difficulty standing from a chair unless she pushes up with her arms at the same time. Her neurologic examination is normal. Which of the following tests would be most helpful in confirming your clinical diagnosis?

(A) complete blood count (CBC)

(B) antinuclear antibody (ANA)

(C) ESR

(D) MRI of spine

(E) aldolase

183. Your patient's test result confirms your clinical suspicion. The patient's symptoms have become more severe. Which of the following treatment options would be most appropriate?

(A) vitamin B_{12} injections

(B) electromyography (EMG)

(C) trigger point injections

(D) prednisone

(E) cyclobenzaprine

184. A 67-year-old female with past medical history of rheumatoid arthritis on chronic steroid treatment and past surgical history (PSH) of complete hysterectomy secondary to fibroids presents for routine visit. Patient states that she has had multiple arthralgias worsening over the last 2 years. She had a DEXA scan done that showed a T score of −1.5. She has been taking calcium + vitamin D, and even started an exercise program at her local gym. She was started on bisphosphonates, which she has tolerated well. Prior to discharging the patient, how soon would you counsel her to repeat the DEXA scan?

(A) never: although she has risk for osteoporosis, she has already made all the lifestyle changes and is on pharmacotherapy

(B) repeat in 5 years, since she only has osteopenia

(C) 6 months

(D) repeat in 1 year

(E) repeat in 2 years

Questions 185 through 188

A 55-year-old male is brought to the ED, by ambulance, because of crushing chest pain radiating to his left shoulder and arm that started 1 hour ago. He has a history of hypertension, high cholesterol, and has smoked a pack of cigarettes a day for 30 years. He has never had symptoms like this before.

185. Which of the following would be most likely to be seen on an ECG?

(A) Q waves

(B) P-R interval depression diffusely

(C) S-T segment elevation in anterior and inferior leads

(D) S-T segment elevation in anterior leads with reciprocal S-T segment depression in inferior leads

(E) normal ECG

186. While monitored in the ER, the patient's rhythm suddenly converts to ventricular tachycardia, and he becomes pulseless and unresponsive. Which of the following would be the most appropriate initial management of this situation?

(A) defibrillation
(B) synchronized cardioversion
(C) IV amiodarone
(D) IV lidocaine
(E) IV epinephrine

187. The patient's rhythm converts to asystole. What is the most appropriate first action to take?

(A) IV epinephrine
(B) IV atropine
(C) discontinuation of resuscitation
(D) direct current (DC) cardioversion
(E) check a second monitor lead

188. Fortunately, the patient survives this episode. As part of his long-term treatment, which of the following would be an appropriate therapeutic intervention to initiate due to its proven effect on survival rate?

(A) flecainide
(B) captopril
(C) quinidine
(D) digoxin
(E) nitroglycerin

Questions 189 through 191

An 18-year-old female presents for follow-up of a rash. She states that she has been using OTC antifungal preparations without success. She used OTC cortisone cream with mild improvement, but the lesions never disappeared. Her condition also recurred with full severity once the cortisone cream was discontinued. Her family history reveals a first degree relative with similar rash. The rash is over the elbows, trunk, and scalp (see Figure 1-11).

FIG. 1-11 *(Courtesy of Philip C. Johnson, MD.)* (Also see color insert.)

189. Which other physical finding would be consistent with your presumptive diagnosis?

(A) velvety, hyperpigmented patches over the axilla and neck
(B) pitting of the nails
(C) oily scalp
(D) subcutaneous nodules
(E) multiple tender and tense vesicles and bullae

190. Which of the following tests is most likely to confirm your clinical suspicion?

(A) ESR and ANA
(B) KOH prep and microscopic analysis of scraping from rash
(C) biopsy of the involved area
(D) capillary microscopy
(E) Lyme titers

191. Which of the following would be the appropriate initial treatment?

(A) methotrexate
(B) systemic steroids
(C) phototherapy
(D) topical steroids
(E) systemic biologicals

Questions 192 through 195

A 60-year-old morbidly obese man presents with complaints of fatigue, worsening exertional dyspnea, three-pillow orthopnea, lower extremity edema, and cough occasionally productive of frothy sputum. He has a long-standing history of type II diabetes and hypertension. On examination, you note the presence of bibasilar rales, an S_3 gallop, jugular venous distention, and 2+ pitting edema in both legs up to the knees. There does not appear to be an arrhythmia present.

192. Which test would be most sensitive for diagnosis of this condition?

    (A) troponin I
    (B) LDH
    (C) creatine kinase-MB isoenzyme (CK-MB)
    (D) brain natriuretic peptide (BNP)
    (E) CXR

193. Which of the following medications should be given initially?

    (A) metoprolol
    (B) diltiazem
    (C) furosemide
    (D) carvedilol
    (E) lisinopril

194. Which of the following has been shown to prolong survival in patients with this condition?

    (A) digoxin
    (B) nonsteroidal anti-inflammatory drugs (NSAIDs)
    (C) warfarin
    (D) carvedilol
    (E) diltiazem

195. A transesophageal echocardiogram (TEE) is performed which reveals a left ventricular ejection fraction (LVEF) of 30%. Which of the following accurately describes this patient and his condition?

    (A) A transthoracic echocardiogram (TTE) would give a more accurate estimation of the patient's true LVEF.
    (B) He has diastolic heart failure.

    (C) Digoxin would be an appropriate choice in attempting to control symptoms.
    (D) He has class I heart failure according to the New York Heart Association (NYHA) classification.
    (E) Hypertension is the most common cause.

Questions 196 through 198

A 70-year-old male is seen in the office for chest pain. He reports that he is getting substernal chest pain, without radiation, when he mows his lawn. The pain resolves with 10–15 minutes of rest. He has never had pain at rest. He has no other cardiac complaints and his review of systems is otherwise negative. He has an unremarkable medical history and takes only a baby aspirin a day. On examination, his blood pressure is 160/70, pulse 85, and respiratory rate 16. His cardiac examination is notable for a harsh, 3/6 systolic ejection murmur along the sternal border that radiates to the carotid arteries. His carotid pulsation is noted to rise slowly and is small and sustained. His lungs are clear. The remainder of his examination is normal.

196. Which of the following would be most likely to be seen on an ECG?

    (A) S-T segment elevations in the precordial leads
    (B) Q waves in the precordial leads
    (C) low-voltage QRS complexes
    (D) left ventricular hypertrophy pattern
    (E) normal ECG

197. Which of the following would be the most appropriate test to order next?

    (A) echocardiogram
    (B) exercise stress test
    (C) cardiac catheterization
    (D) 24-hour Holter monitor
    (E) electrophysiologic studies

198. Subsequent workup confirms the diagnosis of critical aortic stenosis. Which of the following treatments would be most appropriate at this time?

(A) a beta-blocker

(B) an ACE inhibitor

(C) a long-acting nitrate with as-needed sublingual nitroglycerin

(D) balloon valvuloplasty

(E) aortic valve replacement

199. A 42-year-old woman with hyperlipidemia, hypertension, and hypothyroidism presents to your office for a routine follow-up visit. Her blood pressure is well controlled with hydrochlorothiazide. She has been on a stable dose of levothyroxine for 8 years and measurement of her TSH today is within normal limits. However, her LDL cholesterol level remains elevated despite taking a statin for the past 9 months and complying with lifestyle modifications. You decide that the addition of a low dose of cholestyramine would provide her with additional benefit. How would you advise the patient before beginning this therapy?

(A) She should take other medications at least 1 hour before or 4 hours after cholestyramine.

(B) She should take a multivitamin tablet daily.

(C) She should ingest the cholestyramine in its dry form.

(D) She may mix the cholestyramine with water, juices, or carbonated beverages.

(E) She should discontinue the cholestyramine immediately if she experiences steatorrhea.

Questions 200 and 201

A 64-year-old male has been suffering from lower back pain for over 10 years. You have been following him for this period. You have prescribed stretching exercises and, occasionally, an anti-inflammatory medication to alleviate his pain. Although he has had no neurologic deficits in the past, today he has shown up in your office unexpectedly, complaining of bilateral lower back pain with numbness and tingling over the dorsal aspect of both feet. His symptoms have become progressively worse over the past 2 weeks and he is now unable to stand for more than 5 minutes without developing extreme pain and numbness. His symptoms are much improved by sitting down or kneeling over a chair. Climbing stairs seems to be tolerated well, but walking greatly exacerbates the pain. He denies bladder or bowel incontinence or retention, point tenderness or anesthesia in the lower back along the spinal cord or in the saddle area.

200. What is the likely diagnosis?

(A) spondyloarthropathy of the sacroilliac joint

(B) age-related early degenerative joint disease (DJD) of the hips

(C) spinal stenosis of the lumbosacral area

(D) muscle spasm of the lower back

(E) cauda equina syndrome

201. Which of the following imaging studies would be most helpful to confirm the diagnosis?

(A) an MRI of the lumbosacral spine

(B) an x-ray of the lumbosacral spine

(C) an indium-tagged WBC scan

(D) a bone scan of the sacrum

(E) nerve conduction study of the legs bilaterally

Questions 202 through 204

A 17-year-old male presents for evaluation of shortness of breath. He has episodes where he will audibly wheeze and have chest tightness. His symptoms worsen if he tries to exercise, especially when it is cold. He has used an OTC inhaler with good relief of his symptoms, but he finds that his symptoms are worsening. He now has episodes of wheezing on a daily basis and will have nighttime wheezing and coughing, on average, five or six times a month. You suspect a diagnosis of asthma.

202. Which of the following would confirm your suspicion of the diagnosis of asthma?

(A) presence of expiratory wheezing on examination

(B) increase in FEV_1 of 15% after giving inhaled albuterol

(C) a decreased serum IgE level

(D) presence of eosinophils on a sputum sample

(E) a peak expiratory flow measurement 30% below the predicted normal value for the patient

203. Your diagnostic workup confirms the diagnosis of asthma. What clinical classification of asthma does this patient have?

(A) exercise-induced asthma

(B) mild asthma

(C) mild persistent asthma

(D) moderate persistent asthma

(E) severe persistent asthma

204. Which of the following is the most appropriate pharmacologic regimen for this patient?

(A) a systemic antihistamine as needed

(B) a short-acting inhaled bronchodilator as needed

(C) a scheduled inhaled steroid and a short-acting inhaled bronchodilator as needed

(D) a scheduled long-acting beta agonist, a scheduled inhaled steroid, and a short-acting inhaled bronchodilator as needed

(E) a systemic corticosteroid, a scheduled inhaled steroid, and a scheduled long-acting beta agonist

Questions 205 and 206

205. A 74-year-old male with a history of hypertension, CAD, and a 50 pack-year history of smoking presents with complaints of pain and cramping sensation of the thigh and buttock areas for the past 2 months. On detailed history, patient reports that the pain is usually during ambulation and relieves with sitting down. The pain does not change with respect to sitting or supine position. He denies any recent trauma, weakness of the legs, or paresthesias. He takes his prescription medications regularly and denies using alcohol, drugs, or any herbs/supplements. Which of the following should be performed as an initial test to help confirm your clinical impression?

(A) ankle-brachial index (ABI)

(B) x-ray of the lumbar spine

(C) electromyelography and nerve conduction studies of the lower extremities

(D) lower extremity venous ultrasound with Dopplers

(E) angiography of the aorta and lower extremities

206. Which of the following measures should be implemented for the management of this patient's condition?

(A) referral to vascular surgeon

(B) glucosamine and chondroitin sulfate

(C) subcutaneous injections of low molecular weight heparin

(D) smoking cessation and walking program

(E) pentoxyfylline

Questions 207 through 209

A 48-year-old woman presents for evaluation of progressively worsening dyspnea. She relates the onset of symptoms to a "walking pneumonia" that she had a year ago. Her breathing has worsened progressively since that time. She has a "smoker's cough" productive of some clear or white phlegm, for which she frequently sucks on cough drops. She started smoking regularly at the age of 18. She currently smokes about a pack of cigarettes a day, down from as much as two packs per day. She is not on any medications regularly. She has no history of heart disease and has always had normal blood pressure.

207. Which of the following physical examination findings are you most likely to find in this patient?

(A) prolonged expiratory phase of respiration

(B) supraclavicular adenopathy

(C) rales one-quarter of the way up in both lungs

(D) clubbing of fingers

(E) prominent first heart sound

208. Which of the following is most likely to be found on a CXR?

(A) cardiomegaly

(B) residual infiltrate from inadequately treated pneumonia

(C) a pulmonary mass with hilar adenopathy

(D) hyperinflation of the lungs

(E) Kerley B lines

209. You recommend smoking cessation to your patient. She asks why, at this point, she should quit. Which of the following statements is true?

(A) Her pulmonary function will improve 50% or more if she quits.

(B) Quitting will not affect her pulmonary status but may reduce her risk of having a heart attack.

(C) At this point, quitting will not improve her survival.

(D) She is going to require supplemental oxygen and smoking will represent a significant fire hazard.

(E) If she is able to stay off of cigarettes, the rate of worsening of her lung function will slow.

Questions 210 and 211

A 19-year-old woman begins chemotherapy for an acute leukemia. Although you determine that her renal function is unimpaired prior to the initiation of treatment, you feel that she may be at high risk for development of tumor lysis syndrome given her condition's typically good response to chemotherapy.

210. Which of the following is an appropriate medication to use as a preventative measure prior to and during her treatment for leukemia?

(A) indomethacin

(B) colchicine

(C) allopurinol

(D) probenecid

(E) sulfinpyrazone

211. Which of the following is typically seen as a feature of tumor lysis syndrome?

(A) hypokalemia

(B) hypocalcemia

(C) hypophosphatemia

(D) acute necrosis of renal tubules

(E) urine alkalinization

Questions 212 and 213

212. A 37-year-old White executive secretary comes to you after she found a lump in her right breast while she was showering. She describes a lesion beneath her right nipple. You question her about her personal and family history. She began menarche at age 12, and she is still having regular menstrual periods. She has had two children; the first was born when she was 25 years old. She has no family history of breast, ovarian, or colon cancer on either her maternal or paternal side. You perform a physical examination including a careful examination of her breasts. You note that her breasts contain many small cysts bilaterally. However, you also palpate a localized, firm, nontender mass below the right areola. You also describe a peau d'orange appearance of the areola. What should you advise her?

(A) She appears to have fibrocystic disease and that she should return for a repeat physical examination in 6 months.

(B) Ask her to make another appointment to see you in 2 months.

(C) Order a mammogram.

(D) Obtain serum markers CA-27/29 and CEA.

(E) Order a breast ultrasound.

213. A mammogram is performed; however, the mammogram demonstrates no abnormality involving either breast. What next should be done?

(A) Tell your patient to feel reassured and return if the mass enlarges.

(B) Tell her to stop drinking caffeine, not to eat chocolate, and to reduce the stress in her life.

(C) Return for another physical examination and mammogram in 6 months.

(D) Order an ultrasound of the right breast and lymph node basin.

(E) Order a CT scan of the breast, chest, and axilla.

Questions 214 and 215

A 56-year-old Black male construction worker comes for evaluation of a worsening, nonproductive cough that he first noticed 2 months before. During the last week the cough has worsened and has become productive of yellow, blood-tinged sputum. He reports his appetite is poor, and he has lost approximately 15 lbs over the past 2 months. You take a social history and find out he has smoked two packs of cigarettes a day since he was 16 years old. He states that he drinks approximately 10 beers per week. You perform a physical examination. He appears chronically ill; however, his vital signs are normal. The head and neck examination is within normal limits. There are decreased breath sounds in the left upper chest. Breath sounds are distant in the other lung fields. The diaphragms are low. There is no palpable hepatosplenomegaly. You order a posterior-to-anterior (PA) and lateral CXR. The chest radiogram shows opacity of the left upper lobe. There are no pleural effusions. The cardiac silhouette is not enlarged. The mediastinum does not appear enlarged.

214.   What next should be ordered?

(A)   Culture sputum, blood, and urine; administer a broad-spectrum antibiotic; order apical lordotic x-ray views.

(B)   Culture sputum, blood, and urine; order a spiral CT scan of the chest.

(C)   Culture sputum, blood, and urine; order an MRI of the chest.

(D)   Treat with broad-spectrum antibiotics for pneumonia, and tell him to come back in 3 months to repeat the chest radiography.

(E)   Culture sputum, blood, and urine; order a positron emission tomographic (PET) scan.

215.   The patient has the follow-up test that you recommend. It shows a 5-cm mass compressing the left upper lobe bronchus with consolidation of the left upper lobe. Two 1 cm peribronchial lymph nodes near the left main stem bronchus and several 1.5–2.0 cm mediastinal lymph nodes are seen. The hilar nodes do not appear enlarged. There are no enlarged lymph nodes visualized in the right chest. There are no lesions seen in the right lung. There are emphysematous changes involving both lungs.

A biopsy of the lung mass shows a small cell carcinoma. What should be done next?

(A)   MRI of the brain with and without gadolinium contrast

(B)   complete pulmonary function studies followed by a left pneumonectomy

(C)   left upper lobectomy

(D)   radiation of the left upper lobe mass and the mediastinal lymph nodes

(E)   chemotherapy

216.   A 45-year-old female develops fever, dysuria, and back pain and is admitted to the hospital after evaluation in the ER discloses pyelonephritis. The patient is placed on broad-spectrum antibiotics and has a good improvement in her symptoms. On hospital day 4, the patient develops a new fever, leukocytosis, and profuse watery diarrhea. A colonoscopy is performed and the following finding is seen (Figure 1-12):

FIG. 1-12 (Also see color insert.)

What is the first-line therapy for treating this disorder?

(A)   metronidazole

(B)   vancomycin

(C)   oral corticosteroids

(D)   rectal administration of topical corticosteroids

(E)   sulfasalazine

217. A 45-year-old male presents to the hospital for acute abdominal pain and is found to have acute pancreatitis. He has no past medical history but recently has noticed urinary frequency and muscle weakness. He takes no medications. He denies alcohol use. His liver function tests during the episode are normal and magnetic resonance cholangiopancreatography study (MRCP) demonstrates an absence of stones in the biliary tree as well as a normal pancreatic duct. His serum calcium is found to be markedly elevated during this episode. The patient recovers clinically, and repeat serum calcium is also found to be elevated 1 month after hospital discharge. What is the most likely cause of his hypercalcemia?

  (A) metastatic bone disease
  (B) sarcoidosis
  (C) vitamin D overdose
  (D) hyperparathyroidism
  (E) laboratory error

Questions 218 through 220

A 25-year-old woman presents to your office complaining of cold hands. She describes them turning white as she reaches for orange juice in the frozen food section of the supermarket. It seems to be getting worse lately. She has no other symptoms but does note that she and her husband are contemplating pregnancy. Her examination today is unremarkable.

218. What condition is she describing?

  (A) Carpal Tunnel syndrome
  (B) Raynaud phenomenon
  (C) subacute bacterial endocarditis with emboli
  (D) SLE
  (E) RA

219. In this patient, which of the following studies would be most likely to describe an increased risk of future systemic disease?

  (A) echocardiogram
  (B) nerve conduction study

  (C) ANA
  (D) joint aspiration
  (E) arterial Doppler of the upper limbs with cold stimulation

220. Which of the following antibodies can cross the placenta and cause the syndrome of neonatal lupus?

  (A) anti-double-stranded DNA antibodies
  (B) antiscleroderma antibodies
  (C) anticardiolipin antibodies
  (D) Sjögren syndrome antibodies (SSA/SSB)
  (E) anticentromere antibody

Questions 221 through 223

A 55-year-old woman presents to your office with painful hands, causing difficulty opening jars and turning the key in the ignition of her car. She is fatigued and she notices joint stiffness, but limbers up by lunch. She has trouble getting her rings off because of enlarging knuckles. About a year ago, she tried some OTC ibuprofen, which seemed to help, but led to the development of a bleeding ulcer severe enough to require transfusion and ICU care. Otherwise, her health is good, and her review of systems is negative.

Your physical examination reveals tenderness and swelling at the index proximal interphalangeal and metacarpophalangeal joints bilaterally. There are small effusions on both knees. She has tenderness to lateral compression of the forefoot area bilaterally.

221. Which of the following tests is most likely to result in a diagnosis?

  (A) joint aspiration
  (B) ESR
  (C) serum uric acid
  (D) rheumatoid factor
  (E) ACE level

222. The following data are obtained: normal CBC; normal basic metabolic panel; ESR 40 mm/h; ALT 90 U/L; AST 110 U/L; alkaline phosphatase 70 U/L; bilirubin 0.2 mg/dL; uric acid 5.1 mg/dL; urinalysis is normal. ACE level is normal. Rheumatoid factor is 60 and ANA is positive 1:40 speckled pattern. The next most important test would be which of the following?

(A) hepatitis C antibody
(B) anti-double-stranded DNA antibodies
(C) serum protein electrophoresis
(D) C-reactive protein
(E) RPR

223. The test ordered above is negative and an anti-cyclic citrullinated peptide (anti-CCP) antibody is strongly positive (600). Which of the following is the probable source of her symptoms?

(A) cryoglobulinemia
(B) osteoarthritis
(C) polymyalgia rheumatica
(D) SLE
(E) RA

Questions 224 and 225

A 50-year-old man presents to your office with fatigue and weakness. He first noticed it a few weeks ago while trying to hang pictures with his wife. His legs have begun to ache as he walks up stairs. He has lost about 20 lbs in the last 3 months. Most recently, he has found that he is more constipated and has trouble rising from the commode. Your physical examination reveals modest proximal weakness, no articular swelling, rash, or any other pertinent findings.

Blood work from a recent insurance examination revealed:

Sodium 142 meq/L; potassium 3.8 meq/L; chloride 107 meq/L; bicarbonate 29 meq/L; BUN 30 mg/dL; Cr 1.6 mg/dL; WBC 6.8; Hgb 13.6 g/dL; HCT 40%; MCV 88.0 μm^3; platelets 240,000/mm^3; AST 200 U/L; ALT 250 U/L; alkaline phosphatase 70 U/L; bilirubin 0.3 mg/dL; ESR 40 mm/h.

224. Along with a creatine phosphokinase (CPK), which of the following tests should be ordered first?

(A) muscle biopsy
(B) gamma glutamyl transferase (GGT)
(C) MRI of the lumbar spine
(D) ultrasound of the liver and gallbladder
(E) kidney ultrasound with renal artery Doppler

225. His CPK is 2400 and an EMG shows fibrillation potentials, positive sleep waves, and myotonic discharges. In addition to addressing his myositis, diagnostic testing should be performed to evaluate for the possibility of which of these?

(A) Hodgkin lymphoma
(B) testicular cancer
(C) multiple myeloma
(D) lung cancer
(E) prostate cancer

Questions 226 and 227

A 35-year-old woman presents to your office complaining of fatigue and global achiness. She states that she has "not been myself" since she developed a bad whiplash after a motor vehicle accident. Her health has otherwise been good. About 3 years ago, she saw a cardiologist for chest pain. A full evaluation ensued including heart catheterization that showed no coronary disease, although her cholesterol levels were elevated and a statin was prescribed. She sleeps poorly and notes that she has gained a considerable amount of weight. She has seen a gastroenterologist who has told her that her abdominal pain and alternating constipation and diarrhea are because of irritable bowel syndrome.

Physical examination shows that her height is 5 ft 2 in. and her weight is 240 lb. Blood pressure is 126/78. Pulse is 86 and regular. Heart and lung examinations are completely normal. Her pharynx is normal and she has no lymphadenopathy. Abdominal examination shows diffuse mild tenderness, but no masses, rebound, guarding, or organomegaly. Rectal and pelvic examinations are normal. Muscular strength is 4/5 distally and proximally, but there is a considerable give way secondary to pain. She is tender bilaterally at the occiput across the trapezius, iliac crest at the greater trochanteric, anserine bursae bilaterally, and at the second intercostal space bilaterally.

226. Reasonable initial evaluations would include which of the following?

(A) electromyogram with nerve conduction studies
(B) muscle biopsy
(C) TSH
(D) Epstein-Barr virus titers
(E) cortisol level

227. In this patient, which of the following conditions may also be exacerbating her symptoms?

(A) sleep apnea
(B) hyperthyroidism
(C) RA
(D) celiac sprue
(E) medication side effect

Questions 228 and 229

An 82-year-old woman schedules an appointment to see you for neck and back pain. At age 50, she had an L4-L5 diskectomy and laminectomy. She also has long-standing hypothyroidism for which she takes levothyroxine 0.1 mg daily. Over the past few months, she has become more fatigued and describes pain in both of her arms, her low back, and the front of her thighs. She notes that the tops of her shoulders are also achy. She decided to call for an appointment because of worsening headache. She tells you that she has an appointment later this afternoon with her ophthalmologist, because she noticed some flickering of the vision in her left eye. Upon further questioning, she does acknowledge that she has cut her telephone conversation short with her daughter because her jaw begins to ache if she talks too long.

Physical examination shows that she has normal vital signs. She has diffuse scalp tenderness. The oral mucosa is normal without aphthous ulcers and the salivary pool is normal. Her pupils are equal, round, and reactive to light and accommodation, and extraocular muscles are intact. The funduscopic examination appears normal for her age. Neck motion is slightly reduced to lateral flexion and rotation. Her trapezii are tender to palpation, but there is no significant loss of range of motion in her shoulders. Her supraspinatus and infraspinatus tendons appear intact. Her quadriceps are mildly tender, but her gastrocnemius muscles are normal. Her strength is normal for age. Her reflexes are normal and symmetrical.

228. The most likely diagnosis is which of the following?

(A) polymyalgia rheumatica
(B) osteoarthritis of the cervical spine
(C) osteoarthritis of the lumbar spine
(D) bilateral rotator cuff tears
(E) temporal arteritis

229. Which of the following should be done next?

(A) start 80 mg prednisone daily
(B) start ibuprofen and refer for a temporal artery biopsy
(C) trigger point injections of triamcinolone in the trapezius muscles
(D) stat MRI/MRA of the head
(E) no treatment until after she is evaluated by the ophthalmologist and a rheumatologist

230. A 32-year-old man comes to the office for his annual checkup. He is asymptomatic and his physical exam is normal. He reports that his father died of colon cancer at age 46 and his older brother was recently diagnosed with colon cancer at age 37. His paternal aunt was previously diagnosed and treated for endometrial cancer. He is concerned about his family history of malignancy and wants to discuss cancer screening. What would be the most appropriate recommendation at this time?

(A) flexible sigmoidoscopy
(B) fecal occult blood testing, with referral for endoscopy if positive
(C) screening colonoscopy
(D) screening colonoscopy starting at age 50
(E) prophylactic colectomy

231. Which of the following risk factors has the strongest association with the development of malignant melanoma?

(A) dark skin and hair color with tendency to tan easily and not to burn easily
(B) personal history of sunburn, especially early in life

(C) pigmented lesion with asymmetric irregular borders, color variegation, and diameter 8 mm

(D) family history of non-melanoma skin cancer

(E) development of actinic keratosis

232. A 54-year-old man without significant past medical history presents to his primary care physician complaining of epigastric discomfort and early satiety. He subsequently undergoes an endoscopic procedure revealing an ulcerated mucosal lesion. The biopsy of this lesion is interpreted as a well-differentiated lymphoma. Which of the following statements regarding his treatment and prognosis is most accurate?

(A) His prognosis is poorer than if he were diagnosed with a gastric adenocarcinoma.

(B) This lymphoma is not associated with *Helicobacter pylori* infection.

(C) Antibiotic therapy may induce regression of the lesion in the majority of cases.

(D) Treatment will not offer curative potential, so he should be referred for hospice care.

(E) Gastric resection is recommended for well-differentiated, but not higher grade, lymphomas.

Questions 233 through 235

233. A 72-year-old man with a diagnosis of prostate cancer was recently seen in the clinic for restaging and re-evaluation. His bone scan showed development of widespread osseous metastases and his PSA was rising. He was started on leuprolide acetate, a gonadotropin releasing-hormone (GnRH) agonist. He now returns to the clinic complaining of new severe mid-thoracic back pain, which is worse with recumbency and worse with Valsalva maneuver. He also reports that he has a brief but intense electric shock sensation in his lower extremities when he bends over to tie his shoes. On physical exam, he had localized tenderness over the mid-thoracic spine, but his motor strength, sensation, and deep tendon reflexes are all intact. What is the most appropriate next step?

(A) Obtain an MRI of the thoracic spine.

(B) Refer for neurosurgical evaluation.

(C) Initiate radiation therapy to the affected thoracic spine.

(D) Start the patient on scheduled narcotics for relief of the back pain and follow up in 1 week.

(E) Stop the leuprolide and schedule the patient to return to clinic in 1 week for re-evaluation.

234. What is the most important prognostic factor regarding this patient's ultimate neurological outcome?

(A) patient's age and co-morbid conditions at time of diagnosis

(B) degree of neurological impairment at time of diagnosis and initiation of therapy

(C) number of vertebral bodies affected by metastatic disease

(D) tumor sensitivity to androgen stimulation or inhibition

(E) patient's overall functional status before the development of the spinal cord injury

235. What is the most likely explanation for the rapid onset of back pain and neurological difficulty after the initiation of leuprolide?

(A) The patient's tumor was likely androgen-independent and so did not respond to hormonal therapy, with rapid progression of his cancer.

(B) The patient likely experienced vasomotor symptoms such as hot flashes and discontinued the therapy, leading to the tumor progression.

(C) The GnRH agonist produced a transient rise in serum testosterone, causing a "tumor flare."

(D) The patient's response was an unpredictable idiopathic drug reaction.

(E) There is no plausible mechanism by which the medication could cause the development of spinal cord compression, and so it is likely unrelated to the patient's symptoms.

Questions 236 and 237

236. A 48-year-old woman with metastatic breast cancer presents to the Emergency Center complaining of a 4-day history of nausea, anorexia, and generalized weakness. Her husband reports that she has been more somnolent, sleeping 12–14 hours per day, and at times she seems confused. CT scan of the brain reveals no abnormalities. Initial laboratory evaluation reveals a normal CBC, but her BUN is elevated at 32 mg/dL with a slight elevation of serum creatinine above her baseline. Her serum calcium is elevated at 15 mg/dL. What is the most appropriate initial therapy for the patient's hypercalcemia?

(A) volume resuscitation with normal saline
(B) administration of furosemide every 6 hours
(C) subcutaneous calcitonin
(D) intravenous zoledronate
(E) treatment of the patient's underlying malignancy with chemotherapy

237. What is the most likely cause of her hypercalcemia?

(A) widespread osteolytic metastases
(B) ectopic production of a parathyroid hormone-related protein
(C) excessive administration of oral calcium and Vitamin D supplementation to prevent osteoporosis
(D) undiagnosed primary hyperparathyroidism
(E) side effect of medications such as thiazide diuretics

Questions 238 and 239

238. A 64-year-old man with a long history of smoking but no significant past medical history presents to his physician's office complaining of a 1–2 week history of worsening dyspnea, facial swelling, and discoloration. He has also had swelling and discomfort of his right arm. Physical examination reveals edema with plethora of the face and right arm, with prominent collateral veins over the chest wall. What

test is most likely to establish the cause of the patient's symptoms?

(A) PA and lateral chest radiograph
(B) echocardiogram
(C) CT of the chest with intravenous contrast
(D) ultrasound with Doppler flow studies of the right arm
(E) arteriogram of the carotid and axillary arteries

239. Following the establishment of a diagnosis, what is the most appropriate initial therapy?

(A) elevation of the head and monitoring for airway obstruction
(B) urgent radiation therapy
(C) administration of glucocorticoids
(D) empiric chemotherapy for suspected lung cancer
(E) surgical evaluation for resection of the obstructing mass

240. A 25-year-old woman with acute myelocytic leukemia is undergoing induction chemotherapy and presents to the Emergency Center complaining of a 1-day history of fever to 102° F with no other symptoms. Other than having a fever, her vital signs and physical examination are normal. Laboratory evaluation reveals pancytopenia, with a WBC count of 0.3 k/μL, hemoglobin concentration of 9.2 mg/dL, and platelet count of 23,000/μL. What is the most appropriate initial management?

(A) Obtain blood cultures, urine culture, a chest x-ray, and discharge patient to home with follow-up in 1–2 days to review culture results.
(B) Obtain blood cultures, urine culture, a chest x-ray, and admit the patient to the hospital for observation with plan to institute antibiotics if any culture becomes positive.
(C) Obtain blood culture, urine culture, a chest x-ray, and admit the patient to the hospital for empiric broad-spectrum antibiotics with Gram-negative coverage.

(D) Obtain blood culture, urine culture, a chest x-ray, and admit the patient to the hospital for empiric antibiotics with Gram-positive coverage.

(E) Forego cultures and admit the patient to the hospital for empiric antibiotics with both Gram-positive and Gram-negative coverage.

241. A 32-year-old man who is HIV-positive was found to have Burkitt's lymphoma with diffuse bulky abdominal disease. He now reports to the hospital and is scheduled to begin chemotherapy. Admission laboratory studies show elevations of his uric acid at 15 mg/dL, serum phosphorus at 8.5 mg/dL, creatinine at 2.9 mg/dL, and potassium at 6.1 mEq/L. What therapy is most likely to reverse the patient's metabolic abnormalities?

(A) administration of intravenous saline with mannitol to try to keep urine output >2.5 L/day

(B) allopurinol 300 mg/day

(C) administration of intravenous sodium bicarbonate to keep urinary pH >7.0

(D) hemodialysis

(E) administration of the recombinant uricase enzyme rasburicase to lower uric acid levels

242. A 72-year-old previously healthy woman was diagnosed with Stage II breast cancer and was initiated on FAC chemotherapy (5-fluorouracil, doxorubicin, cyclophosphamide) 3 months ago. She now presents to the emergency room complaining of exertional dyspnea, orthopnea, and lower extremity edema. Her vital signs are normal, her EKG is normal, and her chest x-ray shows cardiomegaly and pulmonary vascular congestion. What is the most likely cause of the patient's new symptoms?

(A) malignant pericardial effusion with cardiac tamponade

(B) acute pericarditis due to viral infection

(C) anthracycline-induced cardiomyopathy

(D) valvular aortic stenosis

(E) acute myocardial infarction

243. A previously healthy 34-year-old man, a lifelong nonsmoker, sought medical care at an Urgent Care Center for an upper respiratory infection. A chest x-ray was obtained, which revealed a peripherally located right lower lobe lung nodule. A follow-up CT of the chest showed the 1.8 cm nodule with multiple nonspecific calcifications, and no associated hilar or mediastinal adenopathy. What is the most appropriate next step?

(A) Refer the patient to a thoracic surgeon to evaluate for wedge resection for suspected malignancy.

(B) Repeat the CT chest in 3 months to assess for stability of the nodule.

(C) Refer the patient for a percutaneous needle biopsy of the lesion to rule out malignancy.

(D) Refer the patient to a pulmonologist to evaluate for possible bronchoscopy with transbronchial biopsy.

(E) Treat with empiric antibiotics for possible pneumonia and repeat the chest x-ray in 6 weeks to see if the nodular opacity has resolved.

Questions 244 through 246

244. A 32-year-old female presents for her first pap smear in more than 10 years. She has a history of heavy alcohol use and IV drug use and has performed sexual acts for drugs on numerous occasions. Testing performed today reveals her to have chlamydia cervicitis and trichomonas vaginalis and to be seropositive for hepatitis B and hepatitis C. HIV testing is negative. Her pap smear subsequently returns with carcinoma in-situ of the cervix. Infection with which of the following agents is most likely to have resulted in her cancer?

(A) human papillomavirus type 16

(B) hepatitis C virus

(C) hepatitis B virus

(D) *Chlamydia trachomatis*

(E) human papillomavirus type 11

245. What should be the next step in her work-up?

(A) human papillomavirus testing virus typing

(B) CT scan of the pelvis

(C) ultrasound of the uterus and ovaries

(D) cone biopsy of the cervix

(E) colposcopy and directed cervical biopsy

246. Subsequent work-up confirms the presence of micro-invasive cervical carcinoma [Stage Ia]. What would be the most appropriate treatment?

(A) simple hysterectomy

(B) radical hysterectomy with pelvic lymph node dissection

(C) cervical radiation therapy

(D) cervical radiation followed by chemotherapy

(E) hysterectomy followed by chemotherapy

247. Numerous types of cancers are associated with infectious diseases. For which of the following cancers is there a vaccine currently available against the infectious agent which leads to the tumor?

(A) Burkitt's lymphoma

(B) gastric carcinoma

(C) hepatocellular carcinoma

(D) nasopharyngeal carcinoma

(E) Kaposi's sarcoma

248. A 24-year-old male presents to the office for evaluation of a nodule on his left testicle. He noticed the mass while washing in the shower. He has had no pain, no weight loss, no change in sexual functioning, and no blood in his semen. Examination reveals the presence of a firm, nontender, 1 cm nodule on the testicle. No other masses and no inguinal adenopathy are noted. Ultrasound of the scrotum confirms that the mass is on the testicle. What would be the next step in management?

(A) 30-days of antibiotic for possible epididymitis followed by repeat examination

(B) radical inguinal orchiectomy

(C) needle biopsy of the mass

(D) trans-scrotal orchiectomy

(E) semen analysis and cytology for malignant cells

249. A 25-year-old man presents to the ER with a 3-month history of intermittent pounding headaches, sweating, and palpitations. He denies any symptoms of depression or anxiety. On examination, he is a thin gentleman, BP 240/120, heart rate 110/minute, thyroid not enlarged. There is no prior history of hypertension. The most likely diagnosis is which of the following?

(A) carcinoid syndrome

(B) thyroid cancer

(C) pheochromocytoma

(D) aldosteronoma

(E) renal artery stenosis

250. A 40-year-old woman presents with headaches and visual disturbances for the past 6 months. She suddenly developed amenorrhea 2 years ago. One year ago, she noticed milky discharge from her left breast. The most likely diagnosis is which of the following?

(A) prolactinoma

(B) premature ovarian failure

(C) Kallman syndrome

(D) Sheehan syndrome

(E) polycystic ovarian syndrome (PCOS)

251. A 28-year-old woman was noted to have a 3 cm thyroid nodule at the time of a well-woman examination. Her mother and maternal aunt died of thyroid cancer. On examination, her BP was 160/105, heart rate 90/minute. Laboratory studies:

Total T4	8	(5–12 µg/dL)
T3 resin uptake	30%	(25–35%)
Free thyroid index	2.4	(1.2–4.2)
TSH	2.0	(0.4–5 µU/mL)
Calcium	10.9	(9.5–10.5 mg/dL)
Calcitonin	8000	(<50 ng/mL)

Which of the following is the most likely diagnosis?

(A) papillary thyroid cancer
(B) follicular carcinoma with T3 toxicosis
(C) medullary thyroid carcinoma
(D) hyperfunctioning thyroid adenoma
(E) Hashimoto thyroiditis

252. An 18-year-old man with a history of type I diabetes since age 14 presents to the clinic for further management. He notes several episodes of hypoglycemia at around 2 a.m. that awaken him from sleep since starting on his school's tennis team. He practices in the afternoon. His 8 a.m. glucose readings prior to breakfast are all greater than 200 mg/dL. His current insulin regimen is as follows:

Breakfast: NPH 20 units with 5 units of regular insulin
Supper: NPH 15 units with 5 units of regular insulin

His average fingerstick glucose readings over the past week are as follows:

8 a.m.	240 mg/dL	breakfast
10 a.m.	110 mg/dL	
noon	90 mg/dL	lunch
2 p.m.	120 mg/dL	
5 p.m.	70 mg/dL	supper
8 p.m.	150 mg/dL	

Which of the following recommendations would most likely improve his glucose control?

(A) Discontinue insulin and start metformin.
(B) Schedule NPH at bedtime instead of before supper.
(C) Discontinue regular insulin at supper.
(D) Advise the coach that he cannot play tennis.
(E) Increase the regular insulin at breakfast.

253. A 32-year-old male is seen in the ER with a nondisplaced fracture of the ulna after a fall. Incidentally, the intern noticed that the patient is jaundiced and has a palpable spleen. He orders a CBC which shows a Hgb of 10.2 g/dL. The patient reveals that he has chronic anemia and intermittently has been prescribed iron. On further questioning, he says that he had a cholecystectomy at age 23 and that he has family members with similar symptoms. The intern reviews the peripheral smear and finds spherocytes. What would be the best way to confirm this man's diagnosis?

(A) splenectomy
(B) Hgb electrophoresis
(C) osmotic fragility
(D) G6PD level
(E) indirect Coombs test

254. A 74-year-old female with a history of hypertension and hypothyroidism is admitted with easy bruising, guaiac positive stools, and anemia (Hgb 8.1 g/dL). Screening coagulation tests reveal a prolonged activated partial thromboplastin time (aPTT) with a normal prothrombin time (PT) and platelet count. What is the next step in the diagnosis of this woman's problem?

(A) Perform upper and lower endoscopy with biopsies.
(B) Check factors II, VII, IX, and X levels.
(C) Check factor VII level.
(D) Check factors XI, VII, IX, and VIII levels
(E) Check an aPTT 1:1 mix with normal plasma and 1-hour incubation.

Questions 255 through 258

A 23-year-old African-American presents with acute-onset pain in the abdomen, back, and legs. On physical examination, his pulse is 115 bpm, respiratory rate is 20, blood pressure is 100/70 mmHg, and temperature is 101°F. There is scleral icterus, a systolic ejection murmur at the right upper sternal border, bilateral rhonchi, a right upper quadrant abdominal scar from a cholecystectomy, and a diffusely tender abdomen without rebound. A neurologic examination is normal. A peripheral blood smear is shown in Figure 1-13.

FIG. 1-13 *Photo of sickle cell blood smear. (Courtesy of Ethan Natelson, MD.) (Also see color insert.)*

255. Among the initial orders for this patient should be which of the following?

   (A) broad-spectrum antibiotics for community-acquired pneumonia
   (B) type and hold for 2 units packed RBCs
   (C) an arterial blood gas
   (D) a CT scan of the abdomen
   (E) analgesics

256. A CBC with differential and platelets later shows the Hgb to be 6.4, white blood count is 2100 with 85% polymorphonuclear forms, platelet count is 100, and the reticulocyte count is 0.5. Which of the following would be an appropriate next test?

   (A) serum antibody to parvovirus B19
   (B) broad-spectrum antibiotics for sepsis

   (C) consideration for splenectomy
   (D) a bone marrow biopsy
   (E) administration of granulocyte colony-stimulating factor (GnCSF)

257. Oxygen and IV fluids are given. A urine specific gravity is 1.010. Which of the following is the best explanation for this?

   (A) The patient is volume overloaded and fluid should be stopped.
   (B) The patient has developed diabetes insipidus.
   (C) The patient has developed a UTI leading to frequent urination.
   (D) This finding is secondary to repeated infarction of the renal papillae.
   (E) This complication is due to zinc wasting.

258. The patient develops pain in both hips and an MRI shows avascular necrosis. This is likely due to which of the following?

   (A) osteomyelitis due to *Salmonella* infection
   (B) HIV infection
   (C) a pituitary tumor causing Cushing syndrome
   (D) associated arthritis
   (E) chronic ischemia to the head of the femur

Answers and Explanations

1. **(E)**

2. **(D)**

3. **(D)**

4. **(E)**

Explanations 1 through 4

Although this is the first time that your patient has been noted to have an elevated blood pressure reading, given his family history and obesity, it is important to consider the coexistence of other cardiovascular risk factors. His evaluation should include, among other things, screening for DM and dyslipidemia along with an ECG. It is reasonable to ask the patient to submit himself to a strict diet (low in fat and salt) and to increase his exercise and activity, since these lifestyle modifications will likely result in weight loss, decreased blood pressure, and improve his risk profile for cardiovascular disease. Nonetheless, it is rarely enough to normalize blood pressure in all but the earliest stages of hypertension. Provided that no other comorbidities exist, the patient should return to clinic in no more than 2 months for a repeat blood pressure check. There is no need to consider secondary causes of hypertension, given his age and presentation. You should not start antihypertensive medications until further evaluation is completed, and a second elevated reading confirms your diagnosis of hypertension.

In the initial evaluation of hypertension (as per the Seventh Report of the Joint National Committee on Prevention, Detection, Evaluation, and Treatment of High Blood Pressure [JNC-7], 2003), it is important to evaluate the patient for end-organ damage. This should include the heart, kidneys, eyes, and nervous system. It is recommended to obtain a urinalysis to assess for proteinuria, glucosuria, or hematuria; to obtain an ECG to evaluate the heart for potential hypertrophy or early signs of cardiovascular disease; to obtain a fasting lipid profile, particularly after the age of 35, to assess the cardiovascular risk profile; and to check the patient's renal function to assess for damage or dysfunction. Thyroid function tests are only indicated in the workup of secondary causes of hypertension.

According to the JNC-7, this patient's blood pressure falls into the stage 2 hypertension classification in which either systolic blood pressure (SBP) is at least 160 mmHg or diastolic blood pressure (DBP) is at least 100 mmHg. Stage 1 hypertension is characterized by a SBP of 140–159 mmHg and a DBP of 90–99 mmHg. Prehypertension is characterized by a SBP of 120–139 mmHg and a DBP of 80–89 mmHg. Normal blood pressure is characterized by a SBP of less than 120 mmHg and a DBP of less than 80 mmHg. In classifying a patient's blood pressure and determining appropriate therapy, the higher of the two categories corresponding to the SBP and DBP is the one that is used.

Per JNC-7 guidelines, treatment of stage 2 hypertension should involve the consideration of a two-drug regimen initially. The goal blood pressure in patients with diabetes is a SBP less than 130 mmHg and a DBP less than 80 mmHg. An ACE inhibitor should be used as the drug class has been shown to slow the progression of diabetic nephropathy and reduce albuminuria. Thiazide diuretics, beta-blockers, and calcium channel blockers are appropriate choices to consider in this patient in addition to an ACE inhibitor. *(NIH Publication No. 03-5233, May 2003)*

5. **(C)**

6. **(B)**

Explanations 5 and 6

Although the most common cause of chronic cough in adults is the postnasal drip syndrome (not a choice in this question), the patient's cough is present only in the recumbent position and at night. This sign, as well as the fact that he has recently gained considerable amount of weight, point toward the correct diagnosis of GERD. All of the other answers are also potential causes of chronic cough among adults. The history and examination give some clues that point toward GERD (constant clearing of the throat, worse during recumbence, normal nasal mucosa, and worse after meals) and give some others that would make the alternative diagnoses less likely. While 4 months period is too long for a common cold, other infectious agents (including TB) are not likely given the lack of risk factors. It would be unusual for a patient to develop asthma at this age without other symptoms, and chronic bronchitis is even less likely given the remote history of smoking only a few cigarettes per day. Although nervous cough is also possible, this occurs more often as an escape from socially awkward situations or as a stress relieving method.

Because the symptoms are due to GERD, they should be treated with a PPI as initial therapy. Although weight loss and exercise may be beneficial in relieving GERD symptoms, they should be considered additional therapies and not curative. Antibiotics are not necessary since the patient does not show signs or symptoms of bacterial or fungal infection. The use of cough suppressants and expectorants would temporarily improve the cough but would do nothing to address the underlying disorder. Inhaled bronchodilators such as beta-2 agonist play no role in the treatment of GERD, unless the patient was to develop pneumonitis and dyspnea. *(Kaspar et al., 2005, pp. 203–205)*

7. **(B)** We are dealing here with a rare disease and certainly one that you most likely will not encounter in clinical medicine. However, to answer the question correctly you must only recognize that we are dealing with an autosomal recessive disease (a positive family history in either side of the family and the mandatory unaffected parents are normally hints). In order to be unaffected by the disease and to have a child who is affected, both parents must be carriers of one copy of the autosomal recessive gene. If we call the recessive gene for this disorder "p" and the normal, dominant gene "P," then we can create a 2×2 table demonstrating the likelihood of having a child with the two recessive genes necessary to develop the disease.

		Maternal	
		P	p
Paternal	P	PP	Pp
	p	pP	pp

We can see that there is a one-in-four chance of a child acquiring the two recessive genes necessary to develop the disease. All other answers are incorrect since they represent either an autosomal dominant disease (a 50:50 chance) or are inaccurate for recessive diseases (there is no chance that the child will be affected).

8. **(A)**

9. **(B)**

Explanations 8 and 9

Despite recent findings from the Women's Health Initiative (WHI) study, which show that HRT may not be cardioprotective and may increase the risk for cardiovascular events (MI and stroke) in postmenopausal women with a known history of cardiovascular disease, HRT remains an effective way to treat and alleviate vasomotor instability and reduce the risk of osteoporosis and bone fractures (particularly hip fractures). In addition, there is evidence to support that this effect, along with improvement in affect and mood stability, is long lived and persists during the course of therapy. The incidence of endometrial cancer appears to be reduced in those taking HRT. The use of HRT in those with risk factors for cardiovascular disease must be made on an individual case base, with carefully considering the risks versus the potential benefits of the intervention.

The WHI study has demonstrated an added risk for developing cardiovascular events, such as MI and stroke, among those with known coronary disease or populations at high risk for CAD. A significant family history of CAD (father died at early age of an MI) would place this patient in the category of higher risk. Although patients taking HRT are at an increase risk for developing venous thromboembolism, this would not preclude its use unless the patient had a known history of the disease. The incidence of breast cancer in women on HRT remains controversial and, in our patient's case, we are told that there is a negative family history, hence making it less of a concern. Bloating and breast tenderness may develop in patients taking HRT, but its occurrence would not be a reason not to start therapy on our patient. *(JAMA 2002;288:321–333)*

10. **(D)** The symptoms of polydipsia, polyuria, and weight loss are suggestive of new-onset diabetes in this young man. A diagnosis of DM can be made in any of the following ways: (1) A fasting plasma glucose level of at least 126 mg/dL; (2) a nonfasting plasma glucose level of at least 200 mg/dL in the presence of symptoms; or (3) an oral glucose tolerance test (OGTT) that yields a plasma glucose level of at least 200 mg/dL after 2 hours. Fasting is considered adequate at 8 hours. If unequivocal hyperglycemia is absent, testing should be repeated on a different day for confirmatory purposes before a diagnosis is made. Even though a glycosylated Hgb (A1C) of greater than 6% is suggestive of diabetes, the American Diabetes Association does not recommend the routine use of A1C in the diagnosis of diabetes. *(Diabetes Care 2004;27:S5–S10.)*

11. **(B)**

11. **(E)**

Explanations 11 and 12

The history of acute coronary syndrome and diabetes places this patient at high risk for cardiovascular complications (MI or stroke). His diabetes, as well as all other risk factors, must

be better controlled in order to decrease this risk. Statins (HMG-CoA reductase inhibitors) have been shown to lower cardiovascular morbidity and mortality in the primary and secondary prevention of cardiovascular complications. While niacin would indeed likely raise his HDL, data are still insufficient to recommend this as the main goal in reduction of cardiovascular events in patients with known CAD. The main goal at this point should be to lower LDL levels and total cholesterol to at least the recommended levels for patients at the highest risk for cardiovascular complication, with an emphasis on lowering the LDL to <100 mg/dL and total cholesterol to <200 mg/dL.

Although both hypothyroidism and diabetes are well-known causes of secondary hyperlipidemia, the case makes no mention of depressed thyroid function in this patient. It would be unreasonable to start hormone supplementation without evidence of hypothyroid state. Although beneficial in cardiovascular disease and stroke, controlling blood pressure has no known direct effect on lipid profile. Controlling diabetes would therefore be the only choice that would directly contribute to positively affecting his lipid profile, by lowering LDL and TG levels and, therefore, decreasing total cholesterol. Sleeping, although healthy and beneficial to general well being, has no direct effect on lipid metabolism. *(NIH Publication No. 01-3670, May 2001)*

13. **(B)**

14. **(C)**

15. **(B)**

Explanations 13 through 15

The patient has clinical and biochemical evidence of gallstone pancreatitis including epigastric pain, a history suggestive of prior biliary colic, elevated transaminases and bilirubin (suggestive of an obstructing common bile duct stone), and an elevated amylase and lipase. Gastroenteritis would not be expected to alter liver chemistries. Drug-induced pancreatitis is possible as furosemide has been shown to cause pancreatitis, but would not result in the abnormal liver chemistries. Acute cholecystitis and cholangitis would likely be associated with an elevated leukocyte count, right upper quadrant abdominal pain, and fever.

An abdominal ultrasound could assess the gallbladder for the presence of stones and signs of cholecystitis, such as gallbladder wall thickening or pericholecystic fluid. It could also look for a dilated biliary tree or an obstructing stone in the common bile duct. An abdominal x-ray could reveal a localized ileus ("sentinel loop") or calcifications suggestive of chronic pancreatitis, but would be of significantly lesser yield. A CT or MRI of the abdomen would provide images of the pancreas and liver, but are often clinically unhelpful early in the course of acute pancreatitis. An ERCP is not indicated at this point, as only one set of liver chemistries is available. Should the bilirubin rise or fail to fall, an ERCP might be warranted to decompress the biliary tree.

The patient has a common bile duct stone causing biliary obstruction. This stone likely caused the patient's acute pancreatitis as well. Papillotomy (also known as sphincterotomy) will allow endoscopic removal of the stone. The stone cannot be removed through the native papilla, as the sphincter of Oddi musculature would not allow such a large stone to pass. Thus, sphincterotomy must be performed to disrupt the sphincter musculature. Papillary balloon dilation is possible but is associated with an increased risk of pancreatitis. A biliary stent is a viable option to provide drainage, but is inferior to sphincterotomy and stone extraction. No manipulation of the pancreatic duct is warranted. The stone should not be left in place as it could lead to recurrent pancreatitis or cholangitis. (*Kaspar et al., 2005, pp. 1639, 1792–1797*)

16. **(C)** The biological half-life of a drug is the time required for 50% of the dose to be eliminated. This value is useful in determining the duration of a drug's effect and therefore proper drug dose regimes. (*Hardman et al., 2001, p. 18*)

17. **(D)**

18. **(E)**

19. **(B)**

Explanations 17 through 19

When acetaminophen is taken in normal doses, it is conjugated in the liver to harmless glucuronide and sulfate metabolites. These metabolic pathways become easily overwhelmed in the setting of a large overdose, however. If this occurs, the cytochrome P450 system directs conversion of the excess acetaminophen to a compound called NAPQI, which is conjugated with glutathione to form a nontoxic mercapturate metabolite. Once glutathione stores are exhausted in the liver, however, the excess NAPQI combines with proteins within hepatic cells causing hepatic cell death. Taurine is a mercaptan-containing amino acid involved in bile acid biochemistry. Citrulline aids in the detoxification and elimination of ammonia. Ornithine plays an important role in the urea cycle. (*Katzung, 2004, p. 36*)

N-acetylcysteine should be administered as promptly as possible for treatment of acetaminophen overdose. It works by helping restore hepatic glutathione stores and by providing sulfhydryl groups that bind toxic metabolites. *N*-acetylcysteine is administered orally in the form of an initial loading dose (140 mg/kg) followed by 17 doses (70 mg/kg each) given every 4 hours. In addition to this oral therapy, the Food and Drug Administration (FDA) approved 21-hour and 48-hour long intravenous treatment regimens in 2004. Left untreated, acetaminophen overdose carries a significant risk for hepatic failure and subsequent death depending on the amount of acetaminophen ingested, the presence of any preexisting liver disease, and interactions with any other medications that induce cytochrome P450 enzyme activity. Naloxone, flumazenil, and physostigmine are given as antidotes for toxicity related to opioid analgesics, benzodiazepines, and muscarinic receptor blockers, respectively. *(Harrison's Internal Medicine online, Chap. 286 "Toxic and Drug-induced Hepatitis"; Katzung, 2004, pp. 36, 521)*

Poor prognosis is associated with elevated serum lactate levels (above 3.5 mmol/L), acidemia (arterial pH less than 7.3), renal failure, and coagulopathy. The Rumack-Matthew nomogram provides a means of determining whether an individual falls into the possible-, probable-, or high-risk categories for developing hepatotoxicity based on serum acetaminophen levels and the number of hours since ingestion. Therapy with *N*-acetylcysteine is most effective if begun within 8 hours of the toxic ingestion but still has proven benefit if started within 24 hours. *(Harrison's Internal Medicine online, Chap. 286 "Toxic and Drug-induced Hepatitis.")*

20. **(C)** Septic shock results from inflammatory effects secondary to infection that ultimately leads to hemodynamic decompensation. The treatment encompasses three primary goals. The initial priority is to maintain a reasonable mean arterial pressure and cardiac output to keep the patient alive. Then the nidus of infection must be treated and the pathogenic sequence leading to septic shock should be interrupted. While these latter goals are being pursued, adequate organ system perfusion and function must be maintained, guided by cardiovascular monitoring.

Large fluid deficits exist in patients with septic shock. Up to 6–10 L of crystalloid solutions or 2–4 L of colloid solutions may be required for initial resuscitation in the first 24 hours. Volume repletion in patients with septic shock produces significant improvement in cardiac function and systemic oxygen delivery, thereby enhancing tissue perfusion and reversing anaerobic metabolism. Cardiac index will usually improve by 25–40% during fluid resuscitation. In approximately 50% of septic patients who initially present with hypotension, fluids alone will reverse hypotension and restore hemodynamic stability. Fluid resuscitation with isotonic crystalloids, such as normal saline or lactated Ringers solution, should be the initial therapy in shock. When fluid resuscitation fails to maintain adequate arterial pressure and organ perfusion, vasopressor therapy should be initiated.

In this patient, the initial therapy should be fluid resuscitation. If fluid resuscitation fails, then vasopressor therapy should be initiated with dopamine. If this alone fails, then adding another vasopressor/inotropic agent, such as norepinephrine, may be warranted. Although patients with septic shock should receive broad antibiotic coverage after being pan-cultured, this should not precede fluid resuscitation. As this patient is able to breathe independently while maintaining good O_2 saturation, intubation may be held off for now. If the patient starts to deteriorate (increased respiratory rate, low O_2 saturation, poor excursion, hypercapnia, hypoxia), intubation could be considered. *(Crit Care Med 2004;32(9): 1928–1948)*

21. **(C)**

22. **(C)**

23. **(B)**

Explanations 21 through 23

The patient has chronic diarrhea superimposed on a long history of loose stools, steatorrhea, and significant weight loss. While these features could be seen in several diseases, the presence of the pruritic vesiculopapular lesions on his extensor surfaces makes the diagnosis highly likely to be celiac sprue, with its frequently accompanying skin manifestation *dermatitis herpetiformis*. Crohn's disease is not usually associated with steatorrhea, and ulcerative colitis is often associated with bloody stools. Chronic pancreatitis and Whipple disease could cause a similar clinical picture but would not have the associated skin findings.

A small bowel biopsy would confirm histopathologic features consistent with celiac sprue, such as villous atrophy and crypt hyperplasia. A small bowel biopsy could also diagnose or rule out Whipple disease by looking for the pathognomonic PAS (periodic acid-Schiff) positive organism *Tropheryma whippelii*. Colonic biopsies would be unhelpful

/ˌhɔrpɛtəˈfɔrmɪs/

in celiac sprue. A fecal fat quantification would likely confirm and assess the degree of steatorrhea, but would offer little other diagnostic information. A small bowel x-ray is too nonspecific to confirm the diagnosis and an abdominal CT scan would likely be normal unless the patient had developed a complication of advanced sprue, such as intestinal lymphoma.

Patients with celiac sprue are at increased risk for malignancies of the small bowel with adenocarcinoma and lymphoma being the two most commonly encountered. Patients with celiac sprue are not at greatly increased risk of the other malignancies listed. Limited data suggest that strict adherence to a gluten-free diet may decrease the incidence of malignancy in these patients. *(Kaspar et al., 2005, pp. 1673–1675)*

24. (B)

25. (E)

26. (E)

Explanations 24 through 26

Oral corticosteroids are a mainstay of first-line treatment for moderate-to-severe ulcerative colitis. Starting doses of 40 mg PO daily of prednisone, with a slow taper, are often effective in reducing colonic inflammation, although some patients are unable to wean steroids or maintain remission once achieved. The patient does not have dysplasia in any biopsy specimens, nor does he have signs of systemic toxicity, so a colectomy would be premature. Oral metronidazole is ineffective in ulcerative colitis. Cortisone enemas would be helpful if the patient had isolated left-sided disease, but it is doubtful that enema therapy would reach his hepatic flexure. Intravenous cyclosporine would be used in severe colitis as a last measure before colectomy but this patient is not yet sick enough to warrant such therapy.

PSC occurs in approximately 3% of patients with ulcerative colitis and is its major liver complication. It is a chronic inflammatory condition of the biliary tree. It can typically manifest with

elevated alkaline phosphatase and bilirubin levels, and results in diffuse stricturing and pruning of the biliary tree. Wilson disease, hereditary hemochromatosis and alpha-1 antitrypsin deficiency are not associated with ulcerative colitis and are not cholestatic liver diseases. Primary biliary cirrhosis could account for these laboratory findings, but is rare in both males and patients with ulcerative colitis.

Patients with PSC are at increased risk of developing cholangiocarcinoma but not the other liver tumors mentioned. Patients with celiac sprue are at increased risk for small bowel cancers (adenocarcinoma, lymphoma). Patients with FAP are at increased risk to develop desmoid tumors. *(Kaspar et al., 2005, pp. 1682–1688)*

27. (E)

28. (B)

Explanations 27 and 28

The patient should undergo screening colonoscopy, especially with his strongly positive family history of first-degree relatives developing colon cancer before age 50. Colonoscopy is the only test that can directly evaluate the entire colon and rectum. Most polyps can be removed completely at colonoscopy, and large lesions or masses can be directly biopsied. Virtual colonoscopy and barium enema combined with flexible sigmoidoscopy are good tests, but any positive findings on either of these tests would warrant further examination with colonoscopy. Barium enema alone is insufficient for screening. Fecal occult blood testing is helpful as a screening tool, but would be inadequate alone in this patient given his family history.

The patient satisfies criteria for HNPCC, a syndrome seen in patients with germline mutations in DNA mismatch repair (MMR) genes. He has three first-degree relatives with cancer of the colorectum, endometrium, small bowel, ureter, or renal pelvis (all of whom are first-degree relatives of each other). The colorectal cancers involve at least two generations and at least one case was diagnosed before age 50. FAP involves a mutation of the APC gene and results in dense colonic polyposis, mandibular osteomas, and universal colon cancer at a young age unless colectomy is performed. Peutz-Jeghers syndrome results in hamartomatous polyps of the gut as well as mucocutaneous pigmentation changes. Cronkhite-Canada syndrome manifests as GI polyposis, alopecia, cutaneous hyperpigmentation, malnutrition, and dystrophic fingernails. Turcot syndrome is a variant of FAP in which patients can also develop medulloblastoma, glioblastoma multiforme, and hypertrophy of retinal pigmented epithelium. *(Kaspar et al., 2005, pp. 582–583)*

29. **(C)**

30. **(E)**

31. **(B)**

Explanations 29 through 31

The patient has a peptic stricture, seen in the setting of long-standing untreated gastroesophageal reflux with esophagitis. The history of progressive solid food dysphagia without weight loss is typical. Tobacco, alcohol, thiazide diuretics, and spicy foods do not predispose to benign esophageal strictures.

The patient has developed a peptic stricture, a serious complication of GERD. The patient needs esophageal dilation (either with mechanical or pneumatic dilators) and maximal acid suppression. PPI therapy is superior to histamine receptor antagonist therapy in terms of healing erosive esophagitis.

Patients with long-standing GERD are at increased risk of developing Barrett esophagus, a risk factor for esophageal adenocarcinoma. GERD is not a risk factor for esophageal squamous cell cancer, gastric cancer, or duodenal cancer. Patients with chronic *H. pylori* infection (which this patient did not have) are at increased risk for a form of gastric lymphoma known as a MALT-oma. *(Kaspar et al., 2005, pp. 1645–1647)*

32. **(C)**

33. **(D)**

34. **(B)**

35. **(A)**

36. **(E)**

Explanations 32 through 36

The patient's history and examination are worrisome for pancreatic disease, and he has strong signs of pancreatic insufficiency. His long history of alcohol use suggests the possibility of chronic pancreatitis or pancreatic cancer. Fecal fat studies would only confirm or quantify his steatorrhea. A CT scan would image the pancreas for changes consistent with chronic pancreatitis (duct dilation, calcifications, pseudocysts) and could look for a neoplasm of the pancreas as well. ERCP is not indicated as a first-line test in patients with abdominal pain given its risk of causing acute pancreatitis. Upper endoscopy would be helpful to rule out peptic ulcer disease and other gastric complaints, but would not provide more global information about the abdomen.

The patient has greasy stools and weight loss, findings seen in patients with steatorrhea due to chronic pancreatitis. Patients with steatorrhea malabsorb fat-soluble vitamins (vitamins A, D, E, and K). "Night blindness" (poor night vision) due to vitamin A deficiency is common among patients with advanced chronic pancreatitis and likely led to this patient's motor vehicle accident.

The patient has DM as a consequence of pancreatic endocrine insufficiency, another feature of chronic pancreatitis. Diabetes develops when greater than 80–90% of the gland has been destroyed. Patients with chronic pancreatitis have a coexisting loss of glucagon from islet cells and, thus, often become brittle diabetics, with hypoglycemia seen after insulin administration. Vitamin K and B_{12} deficiency, which the patient may have, do not cause hypoglycemia. The patient was previously noted to eat well, so inadequate oral intake is unlikely. Diabetic education should decrease the rate of chronic insulin overdosage.

The patient has pancreatic exocrine insufficiency and thus cannot produce enough pancreatic enzymes to digest his food. Pancreatic enzyme replacement therapy in tablet form is a mainstay of therapy for chronic pancreatitis. It can rapidly reverse this problem by providing exogenously produced pancreatic enzymes to break down fats, carbohydrates, and proteins for absorption in the small bowel. The patient would not benefit from additional oral feedings without enzyme supplementation and would only worsen his steatorrhea by doing so. He can take food orally, so feeding via gastrostomy, TPN, or PPN are not indicated.

The patient's worsening pain and weight loss despite therapy is worrisome for the development of pancreatic cancer. CA-19-9 is frequently (but not universally) elevated in pancreatic cancers, although it can be elevated in cholangiocarcinoma as well. PSA is associated with prostate cancer. CEA is associated with colon cancer. CA-125 is associated with ovarian cancer. AFP is associated with hepatocellular carcinoma. *(Kaspar et al., 2005, pp. 1799–1803)*

37. (D)

38. (C)

39. (C)

Explanations 37 through 39

DEXA is the newest, least expensive, and quickest method of assessing BMD. The precision of DEXA is approximately 1–2%. Standard radiography is inadequate for accurate bone mass assessment. Single photon absorptiometry is used to scan bone, which is in a superficial location with little adjacent soft tissue (e.g., radius). It may not be an accurate reflector of the density in the spine or hip, which are the sites of greatest potential risk for fracture. The quantitative CT scan and dual photon absorptiometry take more time, expose the patient to more radiation, and, in the case of quantitative CT scanning, significantly increase costs, when compared to DEXA.

The major risk factors for osteoporosis are family history, slender body build, fair skin, early menopause, sedentary lifestyle, cigarette smoking, medications (corticosteroids or L-thyroxine), more than two drinks a day of alcohol or caffeine, and low calcium intake. The current recommendation for oral calcium in men and premenopausal women is 1000 mg/day. Postmenopausal women and patients with osteoporosis should have 1500 mg calcium a day and 400–800 IU of vitamin D, which promotes intestinal calcium absorption. This patient's intake of calcium and vitamin D is not a risk factor for osteoporosis. *(Ruddy, pp. 1635–1637)*

Alendronate is a bisphosphonate, which is approved for the prevention and treatment of postmenopausal osteoporosis. Among the many results of the WHI, it was found that combined estrogen plus progestin therapy was associated with an increased risk of non-fatal MI or death from coronary heart disease (CHD). Consequently, while it is recognized that postmenopausal women who are taking estrogen to alleviate postmenopausal symptoms may also experience skeletal benefits, the prevention of osteoporosis should not be a reason in itself to start estrogen therapy. Calcitonin inhibits osteoclastic bone resorption, but is not sufficiently potent to prevent bone loss in early postmenopausal women (within 5 years of menopause). It is best reserved for use in patients with osteoporosis unresponsive to other therapies. Raloxifene is a selective estrogen receptor modulator (SERM), which is effective for prevention of bone loss in early postmenopausal women and treatment of established osteoporosis, but it also increases the risk of venous thromboembolic disease which makes it an inappropriate choice for this patient. *(Cecil Textbook of Medicine, pp. 1551–1554; Harrison's Internal Medicine online, Chap. 333 "Osteoporosis")*

40. (C)

41. (B)

42. (A)

Explanations 40 through 42

Reactive arthritis (previously called Reiter syndrome) consists of a triad of nonspecific urethritis, conjunctivitis, and asymmetric arthritis, usually involving the large joints of the lower extremities. Genitourinary causes of reactive arthritis include *Chlamydia* or *Ureaplasma*. GI infections due to *Salmonella*, *Shigella*, *Yersinia*, *Klebsiella*, and *Campylobacter* can also cause reactive arthritis. Gout attacks are typically monoarticular and begin abruptly (often during the night or early morning) with the affected joint being exquisitely painful, warm, red, and swollen. These attacks often spontaneously resolve in 3–10 days. While the symptoms from pseudogout may mimic those of gout, they tend to be less painful and take longer to reach peak intensity. Gonococcal arthritis is seen more often in females, is associated with migratory arthralgia, tends to favor the upper limbs and knees and may be associated with cutaneous lesions (pustules). The absence of attacks and joint distribution makes gout and pseudogout less likely. The history of conjunctivitis and association with diarrhea makes the diagnosis of reactive arthritis more likely than resistant gonococcal arthritis. His clinical symptoms do not suggest ankylosing spondylitis, although if he was HLA-B27 positive he would be at increased risk of developing spondylitis.

This patient has the classic symptoms and exposure risk (GI infection) to suggest reactive arthritis. For the articular symptoms, reduction of inflammation and restoration of function can be achieved with nonsteroidal anti-inflammatories alone. A sufficient number of patients with reactive arthritis will not be HLA-B27 positive, thus rendering this test useless as a screening test. However, it may be useful when the clinical picture is incomplete (such as absence of antecedent infection or lack of extraarticular features). Once an antecedent infection has triggered reactive arthritis, it is unlikely that antibiotics will affect the course of the illness (except in the case of chlamydia-associated urogenital disease where a trial of prolonged antibiotic therapy may be reasonable). Systemic corticosteroids are usually ineffective in reactive arthritis, but may be tried for resistant disease or conditions such as AIDS in which cytotoxic therapy is contraindicated. Given the absence of skin lesions, penile discharge, or urogenital symptoms, one would be hard-pressed to challenge the patient's statement that he has not engaged in unprotected sex at the risk of jeopardizing the physician-patient relationship.

Reactive arthritis may be the first manifestation of HIV infection. Therefore, HIV antibody status should be determined when the appropriate risk factors and/or clinical features are present. As mentioned previously, systemic steroids are usually ineffective for reactive arthritis and, with the possibility of joint infection, would necessitate ruling out infection by arthrocentesis of the affected joints. Joint infection cannot be ruled out based on his presentation, and joint sepsis must be excluded prior to corticosteroid injection. The clinical presentation is classic for reactive arthritis, and the absence of systemic symptoms makes the likelihood of disseminated bacterial infection low. Indomethacin, at a dose of 150–200 mg/day, is the prototypic NSAID medication for treatment of reactive arthritis. Doses higher than this are associated with significant GI complications and do not improve efficacy in a patient resistant to the standard dose. In the event that the patient does not respond to 200 mg of indomethacin or alternative NSAIDs, disease-modifying antirheumatic drugs (DMARD) such as methotrexate, azathioprine, or sulfasalazine may be used, provided that HIV test results are negative, as these immunosuppressants have been reported to precipitate the onset of AIDS in HIV-positive patients. (*Ruddy, pp. 1055–1062*)

43. **(A)**

44. **(B)**

45. **(C)**

46. **(B)**

47. **(D)**

Explanations 43 through 47

This patient's presentation is consistent with gout. Aspiration of his first MTP joint is likely to reveal the presence of needle-shaped, negatively birefringent crystals. Rhomboid-shaped, positively birefringent crystals are characteristic of calcium pyrophosphate deposition disease, or pseudogout, with the knee being the joint most commonly affected. Nonbirefringent crystals are found in hydroxyapatite crystal deposition disease. The synovial fluid from joints affected by gout typically show evidence of inflammation in the form of leukocytosis with a predominance of polymorphonuclear neutrophils. The presence of bacteria in synovial fluid is characteristic of infection rather than gout, although gout and infectious arthritis may coexist. (*Cecil Textbook of Medicine, pp. 1703–1708*)

Acute gouty arthritis usually presents in a monoarticular or oligoarticular distribution, with the first MTP joint most commonly affected. The diagnostic gold standard is detection of urate crystals within the synovial fluid of affected joints. It most commonly affects adult men with a peak incidence in the fifth decade of life. While patients with gout typically also have hyperuricemia, only a small fraction of the people with hyperuricemia actually have or will develop gout. Tophi are primarily seen in patients with long-standing hyperuricemia and is considered a finding of chronic gouty arthritis. As the disease progresses, acute attacks become more frequent and last longer if left untreated. (*Cecil Textbook of Medicine, pp. 1703–1708*)

Indomethacin inhibits the prostaglandin synthesis that facilitates the inflammation of acute gout and inhibits the phagocytosis of urate crystals by leukocytes. This inhibits the cell lysis and release of cytotoxic factors that initiate the inflammatory cascade. Allopurinol (an inhibitor of urate synthesis) and probenecid and sulfinpyrazone (promoters of urate excretion) are useful for preventing gout but are not effective during an acute gout attack. Aspirin is inappropriate in the treatment of gout since it can inhibit urate elimination and, therefore, increase hyperuricemia. (*Katzung, 2004, pp. 596–599*)

Because severe hyperuricemia can lead to the precipitation of urate within the renal tubules, nephrolithiasis is a common complication seen in gout. UTIs may or may not result in the setting of gout-induced nephrolithiasis. CHF, anemia, and RA are not related to gout. (*Cecil Textbook of Medicine, p. 1708*)

Allopurinol is the first-line drug for long-term use in patients with excessive urate excretion. It functions by irreversibly inhibiting xanthine oxidase, which is necessary for urate formation. However, allopurinol can precipitate acute gout attacks during the period immediately after initiation of therapy. So, colchicine is typically used in addition to allopurinol for its anti-inflammatory effects. Probenecid is a first-line drug in patients who have normal-to-low urate excretion. Lack of long-term pharmacologic therapy is inappropriate. (*Cecil Textbook of Medicine, pp. 1706–1708; Katzung, 2004, pp. 326–327*)

48. **(D)** Teriparatide is a recently approved recombinant form of parathyroid hormone that stimulates bone formation, rather than inhibiting resorption, and which is associated with a marked reduction in the incidence of bone fractures. Estrogen and the estrogen receptor modulator raloxifene, alendronate, and calcitonin all inhibit bone resorption and increase BMD, but the percent increase in bone density is less than occurs with teriparatide.

49. **(E)**

50. **(D)**

51. **(A)**

52. **(E)**

Explanations 49 through 52

Papilledema is optic disc swelling and implies raised intracranial pressure. Headache is a common associated symptom. The initial evaluation of papilledema should involve imaging, either by MRI or CT scan with and without contrast, to exclude mass lesions. If these studies are negative, then the subarachnoid opening pressure should be measured by lumbar puncture.

An ESR is unlikely to be diagnostic in this case. It would be more important in the evaluation of vision loss or headache in a person over the age of 50. Neither a pregnancy test nor a glucose tolerance test would provide information on the cause of increased intracranial pressure.

Pseudotumor cerebri is a condition of idiopathic intracranial hypertension. It is a diagnosis of exclusion that would be made in the presence of papilledema, normal imaging studies, and elevated opening pressure on lumbar puncture with normal CSF studies. The majority of patients with pseudotumor cerbri are young, female, and obese. This condition is treated with a carbonic anhydrase inhibitor, such as acetazolamide, which lowers intracranial pressure by reducing the production of CSF. Weight reduction, while important, is often unsuccessful in improving the condition by itself. Steroids, tetracycline, pregnancy, and oral contraceptives are not associated with the development of pseudotumor cerbri. *(Kaspar et al., 2005, pp. 171–172)*

Pseudotumor cerebri may ultimately resolve spontaneously, but there is a significant risk for development of impaired vision or even blindness if left untreated. The goal of treatment is the reduction of intracranial pressure. This may be accomplished in a number of ways. Use of medications such as acetazolamide or furosemide is considered a first-line therapy, with the aim of reducing CSF production. If pharmacologic treatment proves unsuccessful, alternative treatment options include surgical options such as optic nerve fenestration or creation of a ventricular-peritoneal shunt. Performing serial lumbar punctures is also possible but carries a number of associated risks including development of infections or headaches. *(Cecil Textbook of Medicine, p. 2229)*

53. (B)

54. (B)

Explanations 53 and 54

Persons with DM are 25 times more likely to become legally blind than persons without diabetes. Blindness is primarily the result of

progressive diabetic retinopathy and clinically significant macular edema. The presence of retinal vascular microaneurysms, blot hemorrhages, and cotton wool spots mark the presence of nonproliferative diabetic retinopathy. Increased retinal vascular permeability, alterations in blood flow, and abnormal microvasculature lead to retinal ischemia. In response to the ischemia, new blood vessels may form at the optic nerve and/or macula (neovascularization). This marks the presence of proliferative diabetic retinopathy. These new vessels rupture easily and may lead to vitreous hemorrhage, fibrosis, and retinal detachment. *(Kaspar et al., 2005, p. 2121)*

55. (E)

56. (A)

57. (C)

58. (B)

Explanations 55 through 58

The presence of headache, eye pain, nausea, and vomiting should prompt the consideration of the diagnosis of acute angle closure glaucoma. This is a rare but serious condition in which the aqueous outflow is obstructed, and the intraocular pressure abruptly rises. Susceptible eyes have a narrow anterior chamber and when the pupil becomes dilated, the peripheral iris blocks the outflow via the anterior chamber angle. Edema of the cornea occurs, resulting in cloudiness on examination. Diagnosis is made by measuring the intraocular pressure during an acute attack. Treatment includes medications to induce miosis in an effort to relieve the blockage or, if that fails, surgical intervention.

In some patients, the headache or GI symptoms can overshadow the ocular symptoms, resulting in a delay in diagnosis and unnecessary workup for other conditions. In this case, the lack of findings on abdominal examination makes appendicitis or perforated bowel unlikely. DKA can present with primarily GI symptoms, but would not explain the ocular symptoms. Similarly, cerebellar or other brain tumors may cause headache, nausea, and vomiting, but would not be causes of a painful, red eye. *(Kaspar et al., 2005, p. 170)*

Since acute angle-closure glaucoma is considered an emergency requiring specialized treatment, an ophthalmologist should always be consulted immediately upon diagnosis. Definitive treatment for acute angle-closure glaucoma involves peripheral iridotomy. The goal of medical treatment is to reduce intraocular pressure in preparation for surgery. Pharmacologic treatments which are commonly used to decrease intraocular pressure include oral or intravenous acetazolamide, topical beta-blockers, topical pilocarpine, and topical alpha-adrenergic agonists. Patients may also be placed in a supine position to relieve some of the increased intraocular pressure. Since acute angle-closure glaucoma involves a problem with the pupil being fixed in a dilated position, induction of further pupillary dilation for the purpose of ophthalmoscopic evaluation carries with it a risk for exacerbation of symptoms. *(Harrison's Internal Medicine online, Chap. 25, Sect. 4 "Disorders of the Eye")*

59. (E)

60. (B)

61. (A)

Explanations 59 through 61

Asymptomatic microscopic hematuria is defined by the American Urological Association as three or more RBCs per high power field on urinary sediment from two out of three properly collected urinalyses. A proper sample can be a midstream clean-catch specimen. The urine dipstick is roughly 91–100% sensitive and 65–99% specific for detection of RBCs, Hgb, and myoglobin. Urine dipstick is not reliable in distinguishing myoglobin from Hgb or RBCs. Therefore, urinalysis with microscopy should be ordered to assess the number of RBCs per high power field. Microscopic hematuria is usually an incidental finding but deserves a

thorough workup, as 10% can be due to malignancy. The initial approach is to repeat the urinalysis to rule out infection. If the urinalysis suggests infection by the presence of WBCs or nitrites, a culture should be ordered and the patient treated appropriately. If RBCs are present without any leukocytes, nitrites, or epithelial cells on the repeated urinalysis, a proper workup should ensue. After history and physical are done to rule out risk factors, comorbidities, or other etiologies to account for the hematuria, one must look to diagnostic tests. A serum creatinine is useful to assess for renal insufficiency. During the course of the workup, if the urinalysis and serum creatinine suggest a glomerular etiology (casts, elevated creatinine, dysmorphic RBCs) a renal consultation and possible renal biopsy may be warranted. Evaluation of the upper tract with either an IVP or CT scan of the abdomen/pelvis with and without contrast should be ordered to rule out renal cell carcinoma, nephrolithiasis, or aneurysms. Next, the lower tract should be visualized by cystoscopy and washings sent for cytology. If all the above workup is negative, the patient can be reassured and followed with a repeat urinalysis in 6 months. *(Am Fam Physician 2006;73(10):1748–1754)*

62. (E)

63. (C)

Explanations 62 and 63

This patient has a markedly supratherapeutic INR and clinical evidence of bleeding. Discontinuation or dosage reduction of warfarin is an appropriate intervention by itself in patients with an INR less than 5.0 or in patients without signs of bleeding. In patients with bleeding or with an INR greater than 5.0, however, further interventions are indicated. Vitamin K_1 administration provides a more rapid reversal of the anticoagulation caused by warfarin, but it takes 6–8 hours to begin having an effect and up to 24 hours to achieve its maximal effect. Immediate reversal may be obtained by the administration of fresh frozen plasma intravenously in addition to vitamin K_1. *(Cecil Textbook of Medicine, p. 163)*

Elimination of warfarin from the body depends on the activity of cytochrome P450 in the liver. Therefore, drugs which inhibit cytochrome P450 will lead to a reduction in warfarin clearance and will consequently lead to an increase in the anticoagulation effect obtained from a specific dose of warfarin. Examples of drugs which inhibit cytochrome P450 include selective serotonin reuptake inhibitors (SSRIs), cimetidine, fluoroquinolones, metronidazole, isoniazid, amiodarone, quinidine, erythromycin, cyclosporine, HIV protease inhibitors, and azole antifungals. Amitriptyline, trazodone, venlafaxine, and imipramine neither inhibit nor induce cytochrome P450 activity. *(Katzung, 2004, p. 35, 307)*

64. **(B)** Prostate cancer is the leading cancer in African American males in the United States. The cancer with the highest rate of mortality for the same subpopulation is lung cancer. Of African-American men diagnosed with a new cancer, approximately 42% will have prostate cancer, 14.6% lung cancer, and 10% colorectal cancer. The leading causes of cancer deaths in the same population are lung (28.4%), prostate (15.6%), and colorectal cancer (10.5%). *(American Cancer Society. 2005-2006, available at: www.cancer.org/downloads/STT/CAFF2005 AACorr PWSecured.pdf)*

65. **(E)**

66. **(B)**

67. **(D)**

Explanations 65 through 67

This patient's symptoms are most consistent with Alzheimer disease. Alzheimer disease is a prominent condition in developed nations, ranking as the third most common terminal illness behind heart disease and cancer. It is the most common form of dementia, with over 4 million Americans having the condition in the United States alone. There is a direct correlation between advanced age and increasing prevalence of Alzheimer disease. While there is an early-onset form of familial Alzheimer disease

that may appear as early as the third decade of life, this accounts for only a small percentage of total Alzheimer cases. There does appear to be a genetic component to the development of Alzheimer disease, as it has been demonstrated that first-degree relatives of Alzheimer patients possess an increased risk for development of the condition. Genes on chromosomes 1, 14, and 21 have been implicated in this association. While age and family history are important risk factors, there is no evidence proving that environmental factors lead to an increased chance for development of the disease. Progression of Alzheimer dementia is typically insidious, spanning as many as several years. *(Cecil Textbook of Medicine, pp. 2253–2255; Harrison's Internal Medicine online, Chap. 350 "Alzheimer's Disease and Other Dementias")*

Anticholinergic agents and any other medication with anticholinergic effects are contraindicated in the setting of Alzheimer dementia. Their use may lead to worsening of cognition and may contribute to decreased efficacy of medications used in the treatment of Alzheimer dementia. Tricyclic antidepressants such as amitriptyline should be avoided for this reason. Risperidone, olanzapine, and quetiapine are atypical antipsychotic medications which are useful in the treatment of emotional withdrawal and delusions which may arise in Alzheimer patients. Trazodone, carbamazepine, and divalproex are mood-stabilizing medications which are useful in patients who display marked agitation. While trazodone does display some anticholinergic side effects, they are far less pronounced than those seen with amitriptyline. *(Cecil Textbook of Medicine, p. 2255; Katzung, 2004, pp. 270–272)*

Memantine, the only drug listed as an option that is approved for the treatment of moderate-to-severe Alzheimer disease, is an NMDA receptor antagonist and the first Alzheimer drug of this type approved in the United States. It blocks the activity of glutamate, a neurotransmitter involved in information processing, storage, and retrieval. NMDA receptors facilitate calcium influx into neurons. Too much calcium, though, can result in cell death. All of the other drugs are acetylcholinesterase inhibitors that increase the concentration of acetylcholine in the brain. *(Katzung, 2004, pp. 1010–1011)*

68. **(E)** This patient's symptoms are consistent with an anxiety disorder. Given her occupation, an anxiolytic medication with no sedative properties would be most preferable. Buspirone is a nonsedating anxiolytic agent that is a partial agonist at 5-HT$_{1A}$ receptors. Unlike benzodiazepines, such as diazepam and oxazepam (Serax), it has no hypnotic, anticonvulsant, or muscle relaxant properties. Amitriptyline and doxepin have also been used to treat anxiety, especially when associated with depression; however, these drugs are also sedating. *(Katzung, 2004, p. 360)*

69. **(A)** Sildenafil is a phosphodiesterase inhibitor effective in the treatment of erectile dysfunction the mechanism of action of which is related to an increase in intracellular cyclic guanosine monophosphate (GMP). Nitrates increase cyclic GMP via the activation of guanylyl cyclase. When the two drugs interact, there can be a dramatic fall in blood pressure related to extreme vasodilation. The other selections can reduce blood pressure; however, since their mechanisms of action are not associated with the intracellular concentration of cyclic GMP, there is no synergistic interaction with sildenafil. *(Hardin et al., pp. 850–851)*

70. **(A)** Local anesthetics exist in solution in both uncharged base and charged cationic forms. The base diffuses across the nerve sheath and membrane and then re-equilibrates within the axoplasm. It is intracellular penetration of the cation into, and attachment to a receptor at a site within the sodium channel, that leads to inhibition of sodium conductance and ultimate conduction blockade. Bupivacaine is typical of amide-linked local anesthetics with high anesthetic potency and long duration of action (class III). Procaine is typical of class I agents that are ester linked and have low anesthetic potency and short duration of action. Important features of group III compounds include: (1) high degree of lipid solubility or high partition coefficient that aid in penetration

of the drug, (2) high degree of protein binding that aids in attachment of the drug once it has penetrated the cell, and (3) pK_a closer to pH = 7.4 so that more of the drug is in the unionized form and is free to penetrate the membrane. Ester-linked anesthetics, such as procaine, are rapidly metabolized by pseudocholinesterases, whereas bupivacaine is slowly degraded by hepatic enzymes. *(Hardman et al., 2001, pp. 331–339)*

71. **(D)**

72. **(A)**

73. **(D)**

74. **(C)**

Explanations 71 through 74

The patient has hypotonic hyponatremia, which can lead to increased water shifting into the brain, resulting in cerebral edema. This patient has nothing in history or physical examination to suggest a stroke or the presence of sepsis as the etiology of his altered mental status. Central pontine myelinolysis is a potentially devastating neurologic complication that can result from the treatment of hyponatremia, not hyponatremia itself. While respiratory acidosis could potentially contribute to this patient's change in mental status, cerebral edema due to hypotonicity is the most likely etiology.

The patient's laboratory studies indicate a low plasma osmolality with an inappropriately increased urine osmolality. With this degree of hypotonicity, the urine should be maximally dilute (osmolality of <100 mOsmol/kg H$_2$O). The high urine osmolality suggests the presence of antidiuretic hormone. In psychogenic polydipsia, the urine would be maximally dilute. Choice C is unlikely since his physical examination does not suggest volume depletion; furthermore, the patient is taking a calcium channel blocker, not a diuretic, for the treatment of his hypertension. Decreased expression of renal collecting duct water channels would lead to water wasting and, thus, the development of diabetes insipidus and hypernatremia.

The patient has symptomatic hypotonic hyponatremia with signs of cerebral edema. This requires immediate attention. Choices A, C, and E are essentially hypotonic solutions which should be withheld in patients with hyponatremia. The serum sodium in this case should be increased by at least 5% for the treatment of cerebral edema. The use of 0.9% saline would require nearly 5 L of infusate to address this cerebral edema. This could lead to pulmonary edema and volume overload. The use of hypertonic saline (3% saline) is the ideal solution to use in this scenario, as the infusion of 3% saline will correct the symptoms while avoiding volume overload. As in all cases of hyponatremia management, frequent serum sodium assays are necessary in order to avoid too rapid of a correction, which could result in neurologic injury—pontine myelinolysis.

The optimal rate of correction to avoid pontine myelinolysis is controversial; however, correction should not exceed 8–12 meq/L in the first 24 hours or 25 meq/L in the first 48 hours. DDAVP is of no clinical use in the management of hyponatremia. Loop diuretics can be of use in the treatment of hyponatremia, especially in hypervolemic hyponatremia, as they result in a hypotonic diuresis and aid in the removal of excess water. Choice B is not accurate, as too slow of a correction in symptomatic hyponatremia can result in neurologic injury through the persistence of cerebral edema. Choice E is incorrect, as hypokalemia can usually be corrected by oral intake of potassium, making IV supplementation not always necessary. *(Brenner & Rector, pp. 896–903)*

75. **(B)**

76. **(C)**

77. **(A)**

78. **(C)**

79. **(B)**

Explanations 75 through 79

The patient has tumor lysis syndrome. The destruction of malignant cells by chemotherapeutic agents will lead to the release of intracellular contents, including potassium, phosphorus, and uric acid (from nucleic acids). This can result in hyperkalemia, hyperuricemia, and hyperphosphatemia.

Hyperkalemia will produce significant ECG abnormalities, including peaked T waves and widened QRS complexes. The presence of bradycardia and irregular heart rate on physical examination are suggestive of the cardiac effects of hyperkalemia, which can lead to life-threatening arrhythmias if not addressed.

Patients with tumor lysis syndrome can develop a severe hyperuricemia. The kidneys are responsible for the excretion of uric acid. In acidic urine, the uric acid can crystallize in collecting tubules, resulting in intratubular obstruction and acute kidney failure. Calcium oxalate stones are not a part of this entity. Cisplatin can cause renal potassium and magnesium losses, which is not the case in this patient. The laboratory data suggest the release of intracellular contents (high LDH, uric acid, potassium, and phosphate) and the diagnosis of urate nephropathy as the cause of his acute kidney failure.

As mentioned before, hyperkalemia will produce significant ECG abnormalities, including peaked T waves and widened QRS complexes. Prominent U waves are found in hypokalemia, not hyperkalemia. Atrial fibrillation is not typically seen in hyperkalemia.

This patient is having hemodynamic instability because of life-threatening hyperkalemia. Calcium chloride, in this case, is necessary to help stabilize the myocardium from the effects of hyperkalemia, although it will not have an effect on the serum potassium itself. Intravenous insulin, given in conjunction with dextrose (in order to prevent hypoglycemia), is the first-line treatment for hyperkalemia, as it will promote the movement of potassium intracellularly. Albuterol is also effective in the treatment of hyperkalemia, as a beta agonist will promote the cellular uptake of potassium. Kayexalate binds potassium in the large intestine and helps remove total body potassium; however, this is not immediately helpful in treating life-threatening hyperkalemia because of the increased time to onset of action. *(Brenner & Rector, pp. 1006–1007, 1022, 1635–1636)*

80. (D)

81. (B)

82. (D)

83. (A)

Explanations 80 through 83

This patient has atheroembolic disease, most likely from the dislodging of arterial plaque during or after the cardiac catheterization, with subsequent kidney embolization. The findings in her history and physical examination that would suggest this are the presence of significant hypertension, abdominal pain, the red-blue rash on her extremities (livedo reticularis), and eosinophilia with urinary eosinophils. Furthermore, the time course of the development of acute renal failure is suggestive of atheroembolic disease. The typical time course for contrast nephropathy is of an immediate onset, usually with subsequent recovery. However, in patients with atheroembolic disease, the kidney failure can occur much later after the procedure. Contrast nephropathy is not associated with the laboratory abnormalities and physical examination findings seen in this case. Interstitial nephritis is unlikely, as is a lupus nephritis flare, given her classic presentation for emboli.

Calculation of the fractional excretion of sodium (FeNa) is helpful in differentiating between "prerenal" causes (FeNa <1%) of acute renal failure versus intrinsic causes (FeNa >1%). A kidney ultrasound is helpful in determining the presence of urinary tract obstruction. Neither the anion gap nor calculation of glomerular filtration rate is helpful in determining if volume depletion is a possible etiology of acute renal failure. Examination of urine sediment would be helpful in determining the

presence of a glomerular etiology of acute renal failure, not a prerenal etiology.

Demerol and metabolites can accumulate in patients with depressed kidney function, leading to increased levels and, potentially, convulsions. NSAIDs should be avoided in patients with acute kidney failure, as these drugs are potential nephrotoxins and could prevent a recovery of kidney function. Ketorolac, indomethacin, and ibuprofen are all NSAIDs. Therefore, morphine is the best option of those given.

WBC casts are suggestive of pyelonephritis. High levels of proteinuria are significant for the diagnosis of nephrotic syndrome, but not lupus nephritis specifically. Urine eosinophils are usually seen in patients with acute interstitial nephritis or atheroembolic disease. Lupus nephritis is usually associated with depressed serum complement levels. Of these tests, RBC casts are the most suggestive of glomerulonephritis. *(Brenner & Rector, pp. 1079–1084, 1382–1388)*

84. (A)

85. (A)

86. (B)

87. (A)

88. (B)

Explanations 84 through 88

This patient's presentation and laboratory data are consistent with nephrotic syndrome. Nephrotic syndrome is typically associated with proteinuria of greater than 3.5 g/day, hypoalbuminemia, edema, and hyperlipidemia. Abnormalities commonly seen in nephrotic syndrome include hypocalcemia (due to vitamin D deficiency), low thyroxine levels (due to loss of thyroxine-binding globulin [TBG]), and microcytic, hypochromic anemia (due to transferrin loss). Hypocomplementemia may be found in some forms of nephrotic syndrome, but this is not a typical finding. Hematuria is one of the components found in nephritic syndrome. *(Kaspar et al., 2005, pp. 1584–1585)*

This patient has history, physical, and laboratory findings that suggest possible multiple myeloma. For example, his history is pertinent for lower back pain and headaches. Moreover, Bence-Jones protein is not usually detected by urine dipstick but will be detected during a 24-hour urine collection. This would explain why there is relatively little urine protein detected on dipstick but over 5 g on the 24-hour urine. Lastly, multiple myeloma should be considered in an older patient with unexplained anemia. Given these findings, a serum and urine protein electrophoresis would be the best test to order next. A kidney biopsy would usually be diagnostic, but is unnecessary if the electrophoresis is positive. Complement levels and anti-GBM titer would not be of any use at the present time. Checking glycosylated Hgb will inform you of the adequacy of glucose control, but will be of little use with regard to the workup of the nephrotic syndrome.

This patient has a low anion gap due to the presence of unmeasured cations in the blood. In this case, they arise from circulating immunoglobulins. The fractional excretion of sodium and urea can be helpful in differentiating prerenal causes from other etiologies of acute renal failure. A split 24-hour urine for protein is helpful in determining the presence of orthostatic proteinuria.

Initiation of ACE inhibitors or angiotensin receptor blockers is the best option in patients with diabetic nephropathy, as these medications have been shown to slow the progression of kidney disease. The other medications listed may be used adjunctively, with an ACE inhibitor or angiotensin receptor blocker, if adequate blood pressure control could not be achieved with monotherapy.

HIV-associated nephropathy is typically associated with a collapsing glomerulopathy, a variant of focal segmental glomerulosclerosis. Membranous nephropathy is associated with a number of other infections, including syphilis, hepatitis B, and hepatitis C virus. Membranoproliferative glomerulonephritis has also been associated with hepatitis C virus. *(Brenner & Rector, p. 1441)*

89. (D)

90. (B)

91. (A)

Explanations 89 through 91

This patient has chronic hepatitis B. The different serologic studies for hepatitis B are shown in Figures 1-14 and 1-15. The patient does not have acute hepatitis B because the IgM antibody to hepatitis B core is negative, and the total antibody to hepatitis B core is positive. Antibody to hepatitis B core occurs prior to the development of antibody to hepatitis B surface. IgM is found in acute infections; primarily IgG is seen in chronic infections.

FIG. 1-14

FIG. 1-15

The presence of antibody to hepatitis B core with a positive hepatitis B surface antigen is indicative of chronic infection. Delta hepatitis infection requires the hepatitis B surface antigen. Delta hepatitis can occur concurrently with acute hepatitis B infection or later in the setting of chronic hepatitis B infection (Figures 1-16 and 1-17). There is no test for hepatitis C antigen. This is not a presentation of acute hepatitis A, which usually has very high transaminases. The antibody to hepatitis A virus occurs after 1 month and is associated with high transaminases (Figure 1-18).

Hepatitis A vaccine is indicated for patients with chronic liver disease. If this patient had hepatitis C, then hepatitis B vaccine would also

Hepatitis A Virus Infection

FIG. 1-18

HBV - HDV Coinfection

FIG. 1-16

HBV - HDV Superinfection
Typical Serologic Course

FIG. 1-17

be indicated. Hepatitis B vaccine is essentially hepatitis B surface antigen that causes the production of hepatitis B surface antibody. Since this patient has hepatitis B surface antigen already, choice C would be incorrect. Verifying the diagnosis with a qualitative hepatitis B viral load is not necessary. A quantitative hepatitis B viral load might be useful to evaluate for potential antiviral therapy. The only reason hepatitis A would be recommended for the patient's spouse would be if the patient had acute hepatitis A. Investigating for other causes of hepatitis is not necessary as the diagnosis of chronic hepatitis B is already established.

If the patient was found to be HBeAg positive, he would be considered highly infectious for the spread of hepatitis B. Hepatitis Be antigen is the DNA polymerase that shows active replication of the hepatitis B virion. These patients are 100 times more infectious than those lacking the hepatitis Be antigen. The window period is a situation where a patient is just recovering from hepatitis B. Hepatitis Bs antigen is negative and the antibody to hepatitis Bs has not been developed. The diagnosis is made by antibody to hepatitis B core. This is seen in Figure 1-6. Any patient who is hepatitis B surface antigen positive is at risk for delta hepatitis. This patient would be at risk for delta hepatitis by virtue of having a positive hepatitis B surface antigen. There is no level of transaminases, even normal transaminases, which would preclude antiviral therapy. The level of viral production indicated by the hepatitis B quantitative viral load, along with an assessment of the underlying liver pathology, is the best indication of need for treatment. As mentioned earlier, the antibody to hepatitis B would show the patient is less infectious and likely have a lower viral load. *(Mandell, pp. 300–305, 1671, 1934–1936)*

92. (C)

93. (A)

Explanations 92 and 93

This is a clinical presentation of West Nile virus infection. The tongue fasciculations go along with an inflammation at the base of the brain. The patient is at the right age for West Nile virus infection and he is immunocompromised due to diabetes. The diagnosis can be made by performing a West Nile virus IgM titer on the CSF. Diabetics can have cryptococcal meningitis. Lumbar puncture in this setting is usually normal with increased opening pressure, and rhabdomyolysis is not a feature of this disease. Diabetics are more at risk for candidiasis. However, the patient has no history of instrumentation, IV catheters, or other situations that would lead to disseminated candidiasis. Diabetics are at increased risk for *C. immitis* infection, but we have no history of the patient living in an area endemic for this organism. Diabetics are at increased risk for rhinocerebral mucormycosis. An MRI of the head might have shown involvement of the sinus. However, this patient's presentation is not consistent with rhinocerebral mucormycosis. *(Huhn GD, Am Fam Physician 2003;68:653–660, 671–672)*

94. (C)

95. (C)

Explanations 94 and 95

Pharyngitis is a commonly encountered problem in primary care. Patients with upper respiratory symptoms are often convinced that they need antibiotics. Often the etiology is viral, but ruling out bacterial etiology is crucial as the secondary complications can be severe. In terms of group A strep pharyngitis, it is often difficult to make a clinical diagnosis based on one or two factors. Many studies have been performed to guide the clinician in making an empiric diagnosis of group A strep pharyngitis. Fever, tonsillar exudates, tender anterior cervical lymphadenopathy, absence of cough and tonsillar hypertrophy are all positive predictors. A patient who has at least two of these criteria should have a rapid strep test or culture—with treatment initiated if the test is positive. When a patient meets three or more criteria and is ill appearing, empiric treatment may be justified. If the patient has a negative rapid strep test and the clinician is suspicious, empiric treatment may be started and throat culture should be obtained. A patient with a positive culture or rapid strep test should be treated, but a test of cure does not need to be performed. The throat culture has a sensitivity of 97% and specificity of 99%, while the rapid strep test has a sensitivity of 80–97% and a specificity of >95%. *(Am Fam Physician 2004;69(6): 1465–1470)*

The first-line medication for patients diagnosed with streptococcal pharyngitis is penicillin. If the patient is allergic to penicillin, erythromycin or first-generation cephalosporins may be used. *(Clin Infect Dis 2002;35(2):113–125)*

96. (D)

97. (C)

98. (B)

Explanations 96 through 98

This patient's presentation is consistent with primary syphilis. Primary syphilis manifests itself usually in the form of solitary or multiple raised, firm papules which eventually erode to form ulcerative craters with raised, indurated margins surrounding the centralized ulcer.

These lesions, called chancres, most commonly involve the glans penis in males and the vulva or cervix in females, although they may appear rarely in other areas. Syphilis is caused by the spirochete, *T. pallidum*, which can be visualized by darkfield microscopy, by silver stain, or by fluorescent antibody microscopy. There is an incubation period of approximately 3 weeks separating the time of initial exposure to *T. pallidum* and the time of chancre formation. Syphilis is characterized by the presence of latent stages in which there are no signs of clinical disease present.

Penicillin is the drug of choice for the treatment of syphilis. In addition to treating patients with diagnosed syphilis, it is recommended that treatment also be administered to all sexual contacts of the past 90 days. It has been demonstrated that up to 30% of asymptomatic sexual contacts of patients with infectious lesions within the past 30 days go on to develop syphilis if left untreated. If left untreated, patients may ultimately develop tertiary syphilis characterized by significant destructive neurologic and cardiovascular symptoms. The mortality rate for untreated tertiary syphilis is approximately 20%. (*Cecil Textbook of Medicine, pp. 1923–1932*)

Cephalosporins and penicillin antibiotics act by interfering with the late stages of bacterial cell wall synthesis, although the precise biochemical reactions are not entirely understood. Peptidoglycan provides mechanical stability to the cell wall because of its high degree of cross-linking with alternating amino pyranoside sugar residues (*N*-acetylglucosamine and *N*-acetylmuramic acid). The completion of the cross-linking occurs by the action of the enzyme transpeptidase. This transpeptidase reaction, in which the terminal glycine residue of the pentaglycine bridge is joined to the fourth residue of the pentapeptide (D-alanine) thereby releasing the fifth residue (D-alanine), is inhibited by beta-lactams. (*Hardman et al., 2001, pp. 1190–1191*)

The patient's symptoms immediately after initiation of treatment are consistent with the Jarisch-Herxheimer reaction. This reaction is characterized by low-grade fever, chills, myalgias, and headache all with an onset within 2–6 hours of initiation of treatment. Other possible symptoms may include tachycardia, tachypnea, and vasodilation with resultant mild hypotension although these are significantly rarer. The Jarisch-Herxheimer reaction is common (occurring in up to 50% of patients with primary syphilis) and is a self-limiting condition, usually resolving within 12–24 hours. Symptomatic treatment may be beneficial but no other interventions are necessary. (*Harrison's Internal Medicine online, Chap. 153, Sect. 9 "Syphilis"*)

99. **(C)** HIV-positive patients who develop a varicella-zoster infection require aggressive antibiotic therapy. Intravenous acyclovir should be adminstered for a period of 7 days, and oral maintenance therapy should be started for secondary prophylaxis. While acyclovir is usually well tolerated, it can be nephrotoxic when given intravenously. It may crystallize within renal tubules and cause subsequent acute tubular necrosis. Acyclovir is more likely to cause nephrotoxic effects if there is associated dehydration or a preexisting renal insufficiency. Individuals who have a preexisting renal insufficiency should have the dose and frequency of acyclovir administration adjusted according to their baseline creatinine clearance. (*Cecil Textbook of Medicine, pp. 1960–1961, 2340–2341*)

100. **(D)**

101. **(E)**

102. **(A)**

Explanations 100 through 102

The patient has diffuse interstitial infiltrates on CXR that correspond in time and presentation to acute inhalation histoplasmosis. This would be seen in a patient, such as an amateur spelunker, who has been in a cave with bats. It is the act of crawling through the cave that disturbs the spores of histoplasmosis that grow in the bat guano. The incubation period for influenza is 1–2 days. It is passed primarily by secretions from the nose spread by hands. The other members of the expedition were not sick, as they might be with influenza. Disseminated

/,aspərɪjil'ɔsɔs/

aspergillosis occurs in immunocompromised patients who have defects in both cell-mediated and humoral immunity. This patient does not have this. While the CXR could mimic miliary tuberculosis, the association with caving 14 days before would make tuberculosis less likely and histoplasmosis more likely. There is no history that the patient is immunocompromised with HIV and would be at risk for *P. jiroveci* pneumonia.

Fungal serologies would establish the diagnosis, but acute and convalescent serologies would take 3 weeks for results. These are only useful in outbreak investigations. The other choices do not fit due to the reasons above. Treatment of acute respiratory histoplasmosis is based on severe hypoxia and would require arterial blood gases to establish the need for therapy.

None of the fungal infections mentioned are transmissible person to person, therefore respiratory isolation would not be necessary. Histoplasmosis is a dimorphic fungus that grows as a yeast at body temperature and a mold at room temperature. The mold produces the spores that are infectious. A similar situation occurs for *Cryptococcus neoformans*. *C. immitis* and aspergillosis are not transmitted from person to person. (*Mandell, pp. 2720–2723*)

103. (D)

104. (E)

Explanations 103 and 104

The clinical picture is most consistent with disease caused by *C. immitis*. This is due both to the nature of the cavitary lesion on CXR and the endemic area. Figure 1-4 shows a peripheral, thin-walled cavitary lesion on CXR as well as a right lower lobe infiltrate. As a renal transplant recipient 1 year out, this patient is likely to have infections with tuberculosis and disseminated fungal infections. It is interesting that the route that he travels is through the lower Sonoran life zone where coccidiomycosis is endemic. CMV produces a diffuse interstitial infiltrate pattern on CXR, as does *Pneumocystis* and *H. capsulatum*.

/al'veələr/

Fiberoptic bronchoscopy with bronchial alveolar lavage should be performed in any patient with this clinical presentation who is immunocompromised because of the lack of ability to produce a good sputum specimen. We know that the patient is PPD positive, so skin testing is not useful. The patient is not mentioned to be in the endemic area for histoplasmosis. Serum cryptococcal antigen testing is a remote possibility. While *Cryptococcus* can produce a pulmonary disease with cavitary lesions, in immunocompromised hosts such as this, the patient more likely would present with meningitis. (*Mandell, pp. 2749–2752*)

105. **(E)** Patients with pneumonia who are admitted to the ICU should be given empiric antibiotic coverage once the cultures are sent. According to the guidelines set forth by the Infectious Disease Society of America, empiric antibiotic coverage could be initiated with any of the following:

- Generally preferred are: an extended-spectrum cephalosporin or beta-lactam with beta-lactamase inhibitor plus either fluoroquinolone or macrolide
- History of structural lung disease: antipseudomonal agents (piperacillin, piperacillin-tazobactam, carbapenem, or cefepime) plus a fluoroquinolone (including high-dose ciprofloxacin)
- Beta-lactam allergy: fluoroquinolone ± clindamycin
- Suspected aspiration: fluoroquinolone with or without clindamycin, metronidazole, or a beta-lactam with beta-lactamase inhibitor

This patient is at high risk for aspiration because of his vomiting and history of alcoholism. Thus, choice E would be the most appropriate initial regimen in order to cover gram-positive, gram-negative, atypical, and anaerobic pathogens. The ampicillin-sulbactam covers gram positive, negative, and anaerobes. The flouroquinolone adds the atypical coverage in addition to providing gram-positive/-negative coverage. (*Clin Infect Dis 2000;31(2): 347–382, Epub Sep 7, 2000*)

106. **(D)** The rate of HBV transmission to susceptible health care workers ranges from 6 to 30% after a single needlestick exposure to an HBV-positive patient. The average incidence of anti-HCV seroconversion after unintentional needle sticks or sharps exposure from an HCV-positive source is 1.8% (range, 07%). Average risk of HIV transmission after a percutaneous exposure to HIV-infected blood is approximately 0.3%. Postexposure prophylaxis may reduce the risk of transmission of HIV following a needlestick. *(Online Version: Emergency Medicine: A Comprehensive Study Guide, 6th ed., Sect. 13, 2004)*

107. **(C)**

108. **(A)**

Explanations 107 and 108

This patient's presenting symptoms are consistent with oropharyngeal candidiasis, or thrush. While risk factors for the development of thrush include recent antibiotic use, use of inhaled corticosteroids, and head or neck radiation, thrush is also commonly encountered in immunocompromised patients, such as those positive for HIV. Due to the patient's apparently benign prior medical history and the new onset of multiple complaints in addition to her oral candidal infection, an HIV infection should be considered. In order to assess a patient's risk for HIV exposure, a thorough history should be taken. Risk factors for HIV infection include unprotected sexual intercourse, multiple sexual partners, IV drug use, occupational exposure to blood or bodily fluids, blood transfusion prior to 1985, and use of nonsterile equipment in tattooing or body piercing. *(Cecil Textbook of Medicine, p. 2053)*

Generally, individuals positive for HIV should not receive live vaccines. Administration of inactivated influenza vaccine is recommended annually in all individuals positive for HIV. Live attenuated influenza vaccine was FDA approved in 2003 in an intranasal formulation but is contraindicated in individuals with immunocompromise. The varicella and MMR vaccines should not be administered to patients with severely symptomatic HIV infection. The OPV is no longer recommended for use in the United States despite its continued use in many other parts of the world. Instead, inactivated polio vaccine (IPV) is recommended and is safe for use in HIV-positive individuals. *(2006, available at: www.cdc.gov).*

109. **(B)** According to the Third Report of the National Cholesterol Education Program (NCEP) on the ATP III once the TG levels are in very high range (>500 mg/dL) the focus changes from LDL to reducing TGs, as such high levels can trigger acute pancreatitis. Once the LDL is lower than 500 mg/dL, the attention can be turned toward lowering LDL for CHD reduction. The results of various recent meta-analyses revealed that elevated TGs are also an independent risk factor for CHD. Some factors that may lead to elevated TG include obesity, physical inactivity, tobacco use, alcohol use, high carbohydrate diets, diabetes, chronic kidney disease, familial disorders, and certain drugs. ATP III adopts the following classification for serum TGs:

- Normal TGs: <150 mg/dL
- Borderline-high TGs: 150–199 mg/dL
- High TGs: 200–499 mg/dL
- Very high TGs: ≥500 mg/dL

Nicotinic acid and fibrates have the largest reduction in TG (25–30% and 35–50%, respectively) and are thus the first-line recommendations in addition to diet modification and exercise in cases of very high TG. Statins reduce TG by roughly 10–33%, while bile acid sequestrant can have no effect or even increase TG levels. Fish oils in high doses can be used in recalcitrant cases as they may reduce TG by up to 50%; however GI side effects are common. It is also important to note that active omega-3 fatty acids make up only 30–50% of many fish oil supplements, whereas Omacor has 90% omega-3 fatty acids. Although this class of agents can reduce TG effectively, they have the unwanted effect of elevating LDL-C levels. *(ATP III Guidelines. Executive Summary, p. 28)*

110. (B)

111. (A)

112. (B)

Explanations 110 through 112

Aminoglycosides such as gentamicin accumulate in the proximal tubular cells of the kidney, resulting in a defect in renal concentrating ability and reduced glomerular filtration after several days. This renal impairment is almost always reversible. Of all the aminoglycosides, gentamicin and tobramycin are the most nephrotoxic. Aminoglycosides may also cause ototoxicity in the form of irreversible auditory or vestibular damage. There is a direct relationship between aminoglycoside dosage and the risk for development of ototoxicity, so doses should be adjusted according to a patient's baseline renal function. *(Hardman et al., 2001, p. 1229; Katzung, 2004, p. 397)*

Complicated UTIs involve metabolic or hormonal abnormalities such as those seen in DM or during pregnancy; the presence of foreign bodies such as calculi, tumors, or catheters; the presence of strictures causing turbulent urine flow or vesicoureteral reflux; incomplete voiding such as that seen in neurogenic bladder, prostate hyperplasia or cancer; and, the presence of unusual infecting microorganisms. A history of recurrent UTI does not in itself lead to the classification of subsequent infections as complicated. Due to anatomic differences in urethral length between males and females, any UTI in a male is considered complicated. A history of recent surgery does not correlate with development of a complicated UTI unless the surgical procedure resulted in the creation of some anatomic abnormality which increased the risk of infection; examples of such abnormalities include adhesions or strictures. A postvoid residual volume greater than 50–100 mL suggests abnormal bladder emptying, which would predispose an individual to development of UTIs. *(Cecil Textbook of Medicine, p. 1909)*

113. (D)

114. (C)

Explanations 113 and 114

V. vulnificus is associated with sepsis in patients with liver disease who eat raw oysters or those with salt water contamination of wounds, like those caused by fish hooks. *P. multocida* is a cause of cellulitis caused by exposure to cat saliva as a result of a bite or a clawing injury. *E. corrodens* is associated with cellulitis caused by a human bite. *Staphylococcus* and *Streptococcus* are the most common causes of cellulitis. The Gram stain shows gram-negative, comma-shaped organisms typical for vibrios. *(Mandell, p. 2274)*

Close attention should be paid to the wound site in the setting of a *V. vulnificus* infection. The wound site must be thoroughly cleaned and any necrotic tissue debrided. If necessary, fasciotomy or limb amputation should be performed. Antibiotic therapy should begin immediately as well. Use of a combination of doxycycline and a third-generation cephalosporin such as ceftazidime is considered first-line. Quinolones may be considered as alternative therapy in the case of drug allergy or contraindication. A combination regimen using TMP-SMZ and an aminoglycoside is indicated for treatment in children since doxycycline and quinolones are contraindicated. *(Cecil Textbook of Medicine, pp. 1760–1761; CDC Disease Listing for V. vulnificus, available at: www.cdc.gov)*

115. (D) No cephalosporin is appropriate for the treatment of *E. faecalis*. This organism is occasionally sensitive to fluoroquinolones, but this choice is unreliable. The combination of ampicillin and an aminoglycoside is synergistic for susceptible *E. faecalis*. *(Mandell, p. 2151)*

116. (B)

117. (D)

Explanations 116 and 117

Lyme disease is the most common vector-borne disease in the United States. It is caused by infection with *B. burgdorferi*, a spirochete that is transmitted to humans through the bite of ticks of the Ixodes family. These ticks are very small, so frequently the victim is unaware of having been bitten. After an incubation of 3–30 days, a red macule or papule develops at the site of the bite, which expands to form a large annular lesion with partial central clearing or several red rings within an outside ring. The lesion, erythema migrans, is often said to resemble a "bull's-eye" target. Within a few days or weeks of this, the patient often complains of flu-like symptoms— fever, chills, myalgias, headache, fatigue— caused by the hematogenous spread of the spirochete. Lyme disease has been found in most of the United States, but is most common in the New England states, where over 20% of *Ixodes* ticks are infected with the spirochete. Left untreated, patients may progress to develop multiple complications, including neurologic, musculoskeletal, or cardiac involvement.

Lyme disease is usually diagnosed by recognition of the symptoms and signs, along with serologic testing. However, serologic tests may be negative for several weeks after infection. IgG and IgM should be tested in acute and convalescent samples. Only 20–30% of exposures will have positive acute antibody responses, whereas 70–80% will have positive convalescent titers. Samples that are positive by ELISA assay should be confirmed by Western blot testing. Empirical antibiotic therapy, preferably with doxycycline, is recommended for patients with a high probability of Lyme disease—such as those with erythema migrans. Doxycycline is the preferred antibiotic for treatment of early stage Lyme disease in adults because of its effectiveness against Lyme disease and other infections, such as human granulocytic ehrlichiosis, which is also transmitted by *Ixodes* ticks. Waiting to treat until convalescent titers become positive would not be recommended in this patient, who has a high likelihood of having Lyme disease, as it may result in more complications developing and the need for longer and more

/er,like'ōsis/

intensive treatment. For more advanced stages of disease, such as the presence of nervous system involvement or third-degree heart block, parenteral antibiotic treatment is necessary. Ceftriaxone is the treatment of choice in this setting. *(Kaspar et al., 2005, pp. 1061–1064)*

118. **(D)**

119. **(C)**

120. **(A)**

Explanations 118 through 120   /ka'rīnē,ē/

Guidelines for the prevention of opportunistic infections in persons with HIV recommend institution of TMP-SMZ for *P. carinii* pneumonia prophylaxis when the CD4 count falls below 200 cells/μL. Azithromycin or clarithromycin are recommended for *M. avium* complex when the CD4 count falls below 50 cells/μL. All HIV-infected individuals should be tested for IgG antibody against *T. gondii* as soon as possible after being diagnosed with HIV infection. Counselling should also be provided regarding avoidance of exposure to sources of *Toxoplasma*. Ganciclovir would be recommended for CMV prophylaxis if there were a history of prior end-organ disease. *(Kaspar et al., 2005, p. 1881; Centers for Disease Control, available at: www.cdc.gov)*

In a patient with HIV, a PPD is considered positive if there is 5 mm of induration. In a patient with a normal CXR, no symptoms of active disease and no history of treatment for a prior positive PPD, the recommended treatment would be isoniazid for 9 months. In the absence of a suspicious appearing CXR or symptoms, AFB testing would be unnecessary. A booster test would also be unnecessary, as the initial test is already positive. Multidrug therapy would be indicated only for confirmed or suspected active tuberculosis. *(Centers for Disease Control, available at: www.cdc.gov)*

PCP prophylaxis should be discontinued if a patient's CD4 count increases to at least 200 cells/μL for at least 3 consecutive months. Discontinuation at this point limits the risks for development of drug resistance, drug toxicities, and drug interactions while doing so at a point where the antibiotic would confer little benefit in terms of opportunistic disease prevention. Prophylaxis should be reinitiated as soon as the CD4 count drops below 200 cells/μL again. While drug resistance is always a concern, modification of the patient's antiretroviral therapy would be inappropriate at this point given the responsiveness shown in his CD4 cell count. *(Centers for Disease Control, available at: www.cdc.gov)*

121. **(D)** Animal bites, most commonly from pet dogs and cats, result in over 1 million wounds in the United States each year. Bites and scratches from cats are prone to infection with organisms that are normally found in the animal's oropharynx. These infections tend to be polymicrobic and include alpha-hemolytic streptococci, staphylococci, and *Pasteurella* species, among others. *Pasteurella* infections tend to spread rapidly, often within hours. Cat bites may also result in the transmission of rabies and tetanus. In the setting of a well cared for indoor house pet, rabies would be unlikely and rabies vaccine unnecessary, although reporting the injury to the health department may be required (depending on local statute). A dT booster would not be necessary, as she had one within a year. Surgical debridement would not be necessary for a shallow wound with normal hand function. If there were signs of tendon, nerve, or vascular injury, then surgical evaluation would be mandatory. Local care alone would not be appropriate because of the propensity for cat bite wounds to become infected. Antibiotic prophylaxis is recommended for most cat bite wounds, particularly those involving the hands. The recommended first-line agent is a combination of beta-lactam and beta-lactamase inhibitor, such as amoxicillin/clavulanic acid. An alternative regimen includes clindamycin with either TMP-SMZ (Bactrim DS) or a fluoroquinolone. *(Kaspar et al., 2005, pp. 817–819)*

122. **(B)**

123. **(D)**

124. **(C)**

125. **(D)**

Explanations 122 through 125

Iron-deficiency anemia (IDA) is characterized by a low MCV, low ferritin, and a high erythrocyte protoporphyrin in serum. Microcytosis and hypochromia are the hallmark in the peripheral smear. Elevated erythrocyte protoporphyrin in serum can also be seen in anemia of chronic disease and chronic lead poisoning.

The USPSTF recommends screening pregnant women for IDA, but found insufficient evidence to recommend for or against routine screening in other asymptomatic persons. However, the guidelines did recommend routine iron supplementation in asymptomatic infants 6–12 months of age who are at high risk of IDA. Infants are considered to be at high risk if they are living in poverty; are Black, Native American, or Alaskan Native; are immigrants from a developing country; are preterm or low birth weight; or if their primary dietary intake is unfortified cow's milk.

The most common cause of cobalamin deficiency is pernicious anemia. Rarely, hypersecretion of gastric acid (i.e., Zollinger-Ellison syndrome) results in cobalamin deficiency. The peripheral smears in folate and cobalamin deficiency are indistinguishable, showing macrocytosis and hypersegmented neutrophils. Both methylmalonic acid and homocysteine levels become elevated with cobalamin deficiency. Folate deficiency is caused by decreased intake, increased utilization, or impaired absorption. Because body stores of folate are low, persons who have an inadequate consumption will become anemic in several months. The recommended amount of dietary folate is 400 μg/day.

Anemia is not a diagnosis in itself; it is an objective sign of the presence of a disease. It is always secondary to an underlying condition. In most cases, a thorough history and physical examination can help elicit the pathogenesis of the anemia and direct appropriate treatment. *(Hoffman, pp. 397–406, 446–470)*

126. (E)

127. (B)

Explanations 126 and 127

This patient's presentation is consistent with agranulocytosis, which is defined by an absolute neutrophil count (ANC) of fewer than 500/mm^3. ANC is defined as the percentage of the WBC count that is accounted for by segmented neutrophils and bands. In the case of this patient, the ANC is 55% of the WBC count or 440/mm^3. Individuals with agranulocytosis commonly experience a sudden onset of malaise, fever, chills, and pharyngitis. They may also develop painful aphthous ulcers affecting the oropharyngeal mucosa. Suppression of the bone marrow, including agranulocytosis, is associated with the use of clozapine. The incidence approaches 1% within several months of treatment, independent of dose. Patients on clozapine should be monitored closely with weekly measurement of the CBC. Mild leukocytosis and other blood dyscrasias occur much less frequently with other antipsychotic drugs. *(Cecil Textbook of Medicine, p. 2221; Hardman et al., 2001, p. 503)*

Usually, there is a prodrome of several weeks duration in which the WBC count gradually declines. Decreasing the dose or discontinuing the offending agent does not always prevent progression to full blown agranulocytosis. Patients with drug-induced neutropenia recover more quickly with the assistance of granulocyte colony-stimulating factor (G-CSF). Additionally, individuals suffering from agranulocytosis frequently develop infections which require the use of antibiotic therapy. In these cases, further supportive and symptomatic care may be necessary depending on the severity of infection. Delaying or withholding intervention is inappropriate. Tardive dyskinesia is an adverse effect related to use of antipsychotic medications; it is not inherently related to agranulocytosis. *(Harrison's Internal Medicine online, Chap. 100 "Hematopoietic Cell Transplantation")*

128. (E) Warfarin acts as a vitamin K antagonist by blocking the regeneration of the reduced form of the vitamin. The result is a decrease in clotting factors II, VII, IX, and X leading to an increase in bleeding time. Warfarin toxicity can be alleviated by increasing the availability of vitamin K. *(Hardman et al., 2001, pp. 1526–1530)*

129. (D) Protamine sulfate is a strongly basic molecule that is thought to inhibit acidic heparin electrostatically. It may not, however, affect heparin-induced platelet aggregation. Cimetidine is an H$_2$-antagonist that increases the anticoagulant response by an as yet unknown mechanism. Clofibrate is an agent used to reduce plasma lipid levels. Vitamin K is used to reverse the effect of warfarin. Heparinase is not used clinically. *(Katzung, 2004, p. 548)*

130. (D) RA is primarily a clinical diagnosis. The history and physical examination are crucial to confirming the diagnosis and ruling out differential diagnosis. No one laboratory analysis can make the diagnosis, however using laboratory analysis in conjunction with a detailed history and examination can help to confirm the clinical suspicion. Some findings that may suggest RA include: morning stiffness (LR 1.9), symmetric arthralgias (LR 1.2), rheumatoid nodules (LR 3.0), positive serum rheumatoid factor (LR 8.4), and radiographic changes of hands/wrists that demonstrate erosions or hypodensity adjacent to the joints (LR 11). Rheumatoid factor is present in about 70% of patients with the diagnosis at some point in the course, however in less than 30% of patients with early RA. ANA may be positive in 20–40% of RA patients but may also be positive in many other disease states. Anti-CCP antibodies have been reported to have a sensitivity of 40–70% and specificity of 95%. The presence of both RF and anti-CCP is very highly specific for the diagnosis of RA. *(Am Fam Physician 2005;72(6):1037–1047)*

131. (B) Primary hyperparathyroidism is common in postmenopausal women and more than 80% present without any symptoms. The most common findings are bone loss, usually in association with estrogen deficiency. The elevated calcium, decreased phosphate, and increased urinary calcium are typical of this disorder. Milk-alkali syndrome is primarily historical disease occurring in patients receiving large quantities of calcium and alkali, and presenting with renal insufficiency, elevated phosphate, and alkalosis. Her normal renal function and relatively low dose of calcium exclude this entity. Familial hypocalciuric hypercalcemia is autosomal dominant and is diagnosed by a low urinary calcium clearance. The lack of renal insufficiency excludes secondary hyperparathyroidism. The normal CXR and Hgb make sarcoidosis and multiple myeloma unlikely. Postmenopausal osteoporosis and osteomalacia are excluded by the elevated calcium level. (Larsen, pp. 1323–1332)

132. **(B)** Vitamin D is actually a hormone that, along with parathyroid hormone and calcitonin, regulates plasma calcium concentration. One action of vitamin D is to increase plasma Ca^{2+}, which can be reduced in hypoparathyroidism. Scurvy is associated with vitamin C deficiency. Alcoholic neuritis is associated with thiamine deficiency. (Hardman et al., 2001, pp. 1731–1732)

133. **(D)** In evaluating a sporadic thyroid nodule in a patient who is euthyroid, it is critical to determine whether the nodule is malignant or benign. The most diagnostic test is the fine needle aspiration. Ultrasound will only distinguish between cystic and solid structures, and most nodules have some solid component. The nuclear scan will demonstrate a photopenic area in over 85% of patients. Neither these tests nor CT scan will reliably separate benign from malignant nodules. Thyroid antibody studies do not play a role in the evaluation of a thyroid nodule in a euthyroid patient. They are sometimes used in the evaluation of thyroiditis. (Kaspar et al., 2005, p. 2083)

134. **(C)**

135. **(C)**

136. **(A)**

Explanations 134 through 136

This patient's presentation is consistent with Graves' disease. Infiltrative ophthalmopathy is a common finding in this condition. Approximately 20–40% of patients with Graves' disease possess clinically evident eye disease. Complaints include photophobia, diplopia, reduced visual acuity, and easy tearing; and, signs of corneal or conjunctival irritation are oftentimes present. Periorbital edema, chemosis, lid retraction with restricted ocular movement, proptosis, and upward gaze impairment may also be found. Optic nerve compression may also arise, leading to decreased visual acuity, visual field defects, impaired color vision, and papilledema. Macroglossia, hyperkeratosis, cerebellar ataxia, and pericardial effusion are all findings in hypothyroidism. (Cecil Textbook of Medicine, pp. 1396–1400)

Free T3 levels are elevated in all patients with Graves' disease. Most patients also have elevated free T4 levels, but occasionally this level will remain within the normal reference range in a state known as T3 toxicosis. This generally occurs during the initial phases of Graves' disease or at the onset of a relapse. TSH levels are suppressed by the elevated thyroid hormone levels. (Cecil Textbook of Medicine, pp. 1396–1400)

Propylthiouracil is a preferred initial treatment option in the setting of Graves' disease. Thyroidectomy is contraindicated in patients who are severely hyperthyroid; it remains a viable option, however, in patients who achieve a euthyroid state with the aid of antithyroid medications. Radioactive iodine therapy may cause increased release of thyroid hormone, leading to a worsening of thyrotoxicity; it is generally used in older patients with moderate hyperthyroidism, in patients with allergies to antithyroid medications, and in cases where a course of antithyroid medication fails to send a patient into a long-term euthyroid state. Radioactive iodine therapy is contraindicated in pregnancy and in breastfeeding. The beta-adrenergic antagonist propranolol is useful in controlling symptoms of hyperthyroidism such as tachycardia, tremor, and anxiety; however, it does not treat the underlying problem of thyroid hormone excess and does not induce a euthyroid state. Potassium iodide is commonly used in conjunction with an antithyroid medication such as propylthiouracil for several weeks preceding a thyroidectomy, acting to decrease the vascularity of a hyperthyroid gland and to help induce a euthyroid state prior to surgery. *(Cecil Textbook of Medicine, pp. 1396–1400)*

Propylthiouracil inhibits the incorporation of iodine into tyrosyl residues of thyroglobulin and also inhibits the coupling of iodotyrosyl residues to form iodothyronines. These effects are the result of inactivation of the enzyme peroxidase, which occurs when the heme moiety is in the oxidized state. *(Hardman et al., 2001, pp. 1580–1582)*

137. (A) The patient has Sheehan syndrome, necrosis of the pituitary associated with childbirth. She has panhypopituitarism, but the most urgent hormone to replace is hydrocortisone. Thyroid hormone should not be replaced until after glucocorticoids are administered. The hyponatremia will correct with glucocorticoids and saline. The patient is not deficient in mineralocorticoids, as she does not have primary adrenal insufficiency; therefore, fludrocortisone is not indicated. *(Larsen, p. 258)*

138. (C) The patient appears to have significant hypoglycemia and neuroglycopenia. The differential diagnosis includes medications such as sulfonylureas; alcohol; endocrine deficiency syndromes such as adrenal insufficiency, hypopituitarism, and hypothyroidism; surreptitious insulin administration; and insulinoma. The best way to establish the diagnosis is to measure the levels of each of these levels on the critical sample demonstrating hypoglycemia. *(Larsen, pp. 1599–1604)*

139. (D)

140. (C)

Explanations 139 and 140

Retinal detachment is fairly uncommon but should be considered for any patient with visual loss. Risk factors for retinal detachment include advanced age, myopia, cataract surgery, focal retinal atrophy, congenital eye diseases, fibromuscular hyperplasia (FMH) retinal detachment, prematurity, uveitis, diabetic retinopathy, and hereditary vitreoretinopathy. Patients may be asymptomatic but usually present with sudden onset of flashes of light, new floaters, visual field defects, and a sensation of a "curtain" coming down over their visual field. Prompt ophthalmology evaluation, preferably by a retinal specialist, is warranted. Immediate care is paramount as often retinal tears can be managed so as to prevent retinal detachment. Symptomatic retinal tears can be managed with laser or cryo burns to create a chorioretinal scar that prevents fluid access to the subretinal space. This is effective 95% of the time to prevent progression to a retinal detachment. Retinal detachment can be surgically corrected with scleral buckling techniques (90% success rate) or posterior vitrectomy (75–90% success rate). *(Am Fam Physician 2004;69(7):1691–1698)*

141. (B) See Table 1-1 below for onset, peak, and duration of the various types of insulin.

TABLE 1-1   PHARMACOKINETICS OF INSULIN PREPARATIONS

Insulin type	Onset	Peak	Duration
NPH	1–3 h	4–9 h	12–16 h
Regular	30–45 min	2–4 h	5–7 h
Lente	1–2 h	6–8 h	12–18 h
Ultralente	2–4 h	8–14 h	18–24 h
Lispro or Aspart	2–10 min	1.5–2.5 h	4–5 h
Glargine	1–2 h	No peaks/valleys Usually steady basal levels	18–26 h

Multiple randomized-controlled trials have shown that tight blood sugar control type I diabetics will reduce the risk of micro- and macrovascular complications, such as retinopathy, neuropathy, and cardiovascular disease. The Diabetes Control and Complications Trial (DCCT) showed that, compared with conventional therapy, intensive therapy significantly reduced the risk of retinopathy progression and clinical neuropathy. Other studies have shown that intensive therapy prevented one cardiovascular event for every 25 patients treated over a 10-year period in a relatively young group of patients. Intensive therapy is not without risk, however. The risk of severe hypoglycemia and subsequent coma or seizure was significantly higher in the intensive therapy group. Control of type I diabetes is dependent on controlling diet with regular low fat meals, keeping blood sugar logs (fasting/preprandial and postprandial) and adherence to insulin. In type I diabetes, oral hypoglycemics are not useful, as patients have a lack of endogenous insulin production. Most oral hypoglycemic agents work either as insulin sensitizers, secretagogues, or a combination. Type I diabetics need insulin for glycemic control and for prevention of ketoacidosis. Patient acceptance and compliance is critical, for which education is key. Patients must be taught the implications of poor control, and the means to optimize control. Blood sugar testing techniques and nutrition counseling are essential features of success. Regular cardiovascular exercise is also of paramount importance. For patients with poor diet regimens, medication compliance, and blood sugar testing, a long-acting agent without peaks and valleys of insulin levels would be an ideal agent for basal insulin. For patients who have no regular mealtimes and history of hypoglycemia, rapid-acting insulin is taken at the time of meals is recommended. Patients should also be taught to count carbohydrates and adjust the insulin accordingly (1 g carbohydrate = 1 unit of lispro). Another option is to use a sliding scale for the lispro based on the premeal sugar levels (using 1 unit for every 30–50 mg/dL that the blood sugar is above target). Thus, based on these recommendations, the best option for this patient would be to use insulin glargine as the basal insulin and insulin lispro at the time of meals. However, regular follow-up and compliance with lifestyle measures are key to achieve optimal short- and long-term control and reduction of complications. (*Am Fam Physician 2006;74(6):971–978*)

142. **(E)** The very low TSH suggests that the patient is hyperthyroid, most likely because of an autonomously functioning thyroid adenoma or hot nodule. In general, these nodules are more than 3 cm in diameter in order to be associated with hyperthyroidism. They are associated with a very low rate of malignancy and do not require fine needle aspiration. The diagnosis would be confirmed by the finding of uptake in the area of the nodule on scan with suppression of uptake in the rest of the thyroid. (*Kaspar et al., 2005, p. 2083*)

143. **(D)** The patient has the clinical features of hyperthyroidism due to postpartum thyroiditis. This is caused by an autoimmune process with leakage of stored thyroid hormone from the gland. The hyperthyroidism is self-limited and is not associated with new synthesis of thyroid hormone. Therefore, methimazole is not indicated. The thyroid is not painful, as it is in subacute (de Quervain) thyroiditis, so glucocorticoids are not indicated. The radioactive iodine uptake is low, so radioactive iodine treatment is not indicated. Symptom control with propranolol is the only therapy needed during this phase of the illness. (*Kaspar et al., 2005, p. 2075*)

144. **(E)** The patient exhibits the typical features of the nonthyroidal illness syndrome. The total thyroxine level is low, but TBG is also low (based on the elevated T3 resin uptake), so that the free thyroid index is still in the normal range. The low TBG is related to the patient's nutritional deficiency. The low T3 and TSH levels are related to his illness and the use of both glucocorticoids and dopamine, which decrease TSH. The reverse T3 level is high because of the blockade of T4 to T3 conversion caused by the illness. This finding excludes hypopituitarism as an underlying cause. There is no specific therapy for this problem other than treating the underlying illness. (*Kaspar et al., 2005, p. 2075*)

145. **(C)**

146. **(C)**

147. **(B)**

Explanations 145 through 147

The patient has the typical features of PCOS associated with insulin resistance and the metabolic syndrome. The presence of hyperandrogenism and oligomenorrhea, without other known causes (such as congenital adrenal hyperplasia), makes the diagnosis of PCOS. The hirsutism and acne are the result of the hyperandrogenism associated with PCOS. Thyroid disorders and hyperprolactinemia can contribute to menstrual disturbances but would not be expected to cause the signs of androgen excess or *A. nigricans*. A cosyntropin stimulation test would be used for the diagnosis of adrenal insufficiency. Growth hormone levels may be elevated in acromegaly or in some pituitary tumors. Women with PCOS have a high risk of glucose intolerance, diabetes, dyslipidemia, and hypertension. Individuals with insulin resistance syndromes typically exhibit hypertriglyceridemia with low HDL levels. The key to management of PCOS is weight loss. Even modest weight loss (10–20 lbs) can result in significant improvement in metabolic and physiologic parameters, such as blood pressure and insulin resistance, and improved fertility. *(Larsen, pp. 627–633)*

148. (D)

149. (A)

Explanations 148 and 149

The skin lesions shown in Figures 1-8 and 1-9 show erythematous maculopapular lesions. There are only a few conditions that cause a rash on the palms and soles. These include syphilis, gonorrhea, and Stevens-Johnson syndrome. Disseminated gonnorhea does not cause lesions on the face. This is not a potential presentation of hepatitis B or chlamydia. A skin biopsy is not indicated. RPR and MHA-TP tests will be positive in syphilis in a high titer. All patients with syphilis need to have HIV testing. The rash of primary HIV infection is a faint erythematous rash on the trunk and is not always present. Early in primary HIV infection, a PCR determination can be negative. *(Mandell, 6th ed., Chap. 235).*

In the absence of neurosyphilis, benzthine penicillin 2.4 million units IM weekly for 3 weeks is the treatment of choice for patients with syphilis of unknown duration or greater than a year. While azithromycin 1 g orally will treat gonorrhea and chlamydia, it will not treat syphilis. Aqueous penicillin 4 million units intravenously every 4 hours for 14 days is the treatment of choice for neurosyphilis. An alternate treatment for latent syphilis in patients who are penicillin allergic is doxycycline 100 mg twice daily for 30 days. Oral corticosteroids are not indicated in this case. *(Sanford Guide to Antimicrobial therapy, 2006).*

150. (A)

151. (E)

152. (B)

Explanations 150 through 152

Nonmelanoma skin cancer is the most common cancer in the United States. Of this group of cancers, approximately 70–80% are basal cell carcinomas (BCC). The majority of the remaining 20–30% are squamous cell carcinomas (SCC). Metastasis is less common in BCC than SCC, with an estimated risk for metastasis of less than 0.1%. There is no evidence that total body skin examination reduces morbidity or mortality associated with BCC. The cure rate of BCC ranges anywhere from 80 to 99% depending on the treatment modality employed. Despite adequate treatment, individuals with a prior BCC lesion are at increased risk for development of a subsequent BCC (with a 40% risk of development 3–5 years after treatment). *(Cecil Textbook of Medicine, pp. 1252–1253; Harrison's Internal Medicine online, Chap. 73 "Cancer of the Skin")*

The most important risk factor for development of BCC is exposure to UVB (or short-wavelength ultraviolet) radiation. There is some evidence, however, that UVA (or long-wavelength ultraviolet) radiation also confers a risk. Sporadic, intense episodes of sun exposure, particularly during childhood, are associated with increased risk of BCC development later in life. Conversely, SCC is apparently associated with cumulative sun exposure, regardless of intensity. Other risk factors implicated in BCC development include arsenic exposure, immunosuppression, exposure to other forms of radiation, and the presence of other skin-affecting conditions such as xeroderma pigmentosum and basal cell nevus syndrome.

Several modalities exist for the treatment of BCC. The modality associated with the lowest recurrence rate is Mohs micrographic surgery, which is associated with a cure rate in excess of 98%. Because Mohs surgery utilizes the least amount of tissue possible while attempting to ensure complete tumor removal, it is a modality which should be used when treating BCC affecting cosmetically important body regions or regions where tissue preservation is important (such as the ears, eyelids, nose, and lips). Other treatment modalities used are radiation therapy, surgical excision, electrodesiccation with curettage, cryotherapy, topical 5-fluorouracil, and topical immuno-modulators. (*Cecil Textbook of Medicine, pp. 1252–1253; Harrison's Internal Medicine online, Chap. 73 "Cancer of the Skin"*)

153. (D)

154. (B)

Explanations 153 and 154

This patient has nodulocystic acne which is characterized by the presence of multiple comedones, inflammatory papules, pustules, and large nodules. Characteristically, the nodules measure greater than 5 mm in diameter. Initial therapy should include a systemic antibiotic such as tetracycline or erythromycin. Use of local therapy alone may be adequate in individuals with comedonal acne. In cases of acne which feature more of an inflammatory component (with papules and pustules), topical and oral antibiotics are useful. Oral isotretinoin is indicated for severe nodulocystic acne that is unresponsive to other therapies.

Use of isoretinoin is tightly regulated due to the severity of its primary adverse effect, teratogenicity. Health care providers prescribing isotretinoin must receive specialized education and training as well as certification from the manufacturer prior to being able to prescribe or administer the medication to their patients. Female patients must receive contraception counseling and must have two negative pregnancy tests prior to initiation of therapy. They must also have an additional negative pregnancy test prior to each subsequent refill. Recipients of oral isotretinoin should also be warned of the risk of mood changes and depression which have been anecdotally associated with therapy. Other side effects of oral isotretinoin therapy include hypertriglyceridemia and development of dry skin with cheilitis. (*Harrison's Internal Medicine online, Chap. 47 "Eczema, Psoriasis, Cutaneous Infections, Acne, and Other Common Skin Disorders"*)

155. (D)

156. (A)

Explanations 155 and 156

Figure 1-10 shows a pustule or furuncle with a necrotic center. With the patient having a history of boils under his arms and groin, a *S. aureus* infection should be suspected. Community-acquired methicillin-resistant *S. aureus* (MRSA) infection has been described to present as an appearance similar to a spider bite. Brown recluse spider bites have necrotic centers, but do not usually form pustules. TMP-SMZ is the best oral agent available for MRSA. Benadryl and topical steroids would not be indicated. Surgical debridement is not indicated. If there is a large pustule, incision and drainage of the wound may be useful. Alternatively, a needle aspirant of drainage could be sent for culture. Patients should be instructed not to press on these lesions to express puss. This causes bacterimia and can later lead to serious systemic infections due to *S. aureus*.

If a patient with *S. aureus* infection becomes febrile, he should be admitted to the hospital for systemic antibiotics. Blood cultures should be taken. *S. aureus* easily forms abscesses in the skin and in other tissues. Blood-borne infection causes endocarditis, renal furuncles, and osteomyelitis. These would appear within several weeks of the bacterimia. To prevent this, systemic antibiotics should be administered. Oral administration of static drugs such clindamycin would not be indicated for diseases that could potentially develop endocarditis later. *(Mandell, 6th ed., Chap. 192)*

157. (A)

158. (D)

Explanations 157 and 158

Anaphylaxis is an acute multisystem allergic reaction to a particular antigen in a sensitized patient. The reaction may be mild or severe. Clinical manifestations may include urticaria and angioedema; laryngeal edema with dyspnea; bronchospasm; tachycardia and hypotension; and vomiting and diarrhea. The correct initial step in the treatment of mild anaphylaxis is the administration of 0.3–0.5 mL of 1:1000 epinephrine subcutaneously. *(Kaspar et al., 2005, pp. 1949–1950)*

Epinephrine is the drug of choice for treating severe anaphylactic shock because it is active at both alpha- and beta-adrenergic receptors. The alpha-adrenergic effects constrict the smaller arterioles and precapillary sphincters, thereby markedly reducing cutaneous blood flow. Veins and large arteries also respond to epinephrine. The beta-adrenergic effects of epinephrine cause relaxation of the bronchial smooth muscle and induce a powerful bronchodilation, which is most evident when the bronchial muscle is contracted, as in anaphylactic shock. *(Hardman et al., 2001, pp. 223–225)*

159. (A)

160. (A)

161. (D)

162. (C)

Explanations 159 through 162

In patients who have melanoma that is confined to the skin (i.e., no evidence of metastatic

disease), the most important prognostic factor is the Breslow histologic depth of the tumor. The age of the patient and location of the tumor also play a role in prognosis, but to a lesser degree. The forearm and leg tend to have a better prognosis; scalp, hands, feet, and mucous membranes have a worse prognosis. Older persons tend to have poorer prognoses, as well. *(Harrison's Principles of Internal Medicine, 15th ed., p. 555)*

Standard treatment for melanoma involves surgical excision. Sentinel lymph node biopsy should also be performed in any patient who has a melanoma that is at least 1 mm thick. This aids in determining whether melanoma cells have metastasized to the local lymph node basin. If the sentinel lymph node biopsy is negative for melanoma cells, no further lymph node studies are necessary. However, a positive biopsy warrants complete lymph node dissection. In addition to this situation, complete lymph node dissection is indicated in the setting of clinical lymphadenopathy regardless of evident distant metastasis. High-dose interferon alpha-2 therapy is a viable option for use as adjuvant therapy in patients at high risk for disease recurrence, having been shown to prolong periods of remission and possibly improve mortality. Single-agent chemotherapy is generally used in patients with stage IV melanoma and is considered more for palliative purposes. *(Cecil Textbook of Medicine, pp. 1248–1252)*

Melanoma patients who have metastases confined to the regional lymph node basin are stage III. Patients who have metastases beyond the regional lymph node basin are stage IV. *(Harrison's Principles of Internal Medicine, 15th ed., p. 555)*

Elevated serum LDH is suggestive of metastatic melanoma. Treatment of metastatic melanoma (stage IV) is directed toward palliation as there is no evidence that treatment has an effect on survival. The lack of clinical lymphadenopathy does not exclude the possibility of occult micrometastases, which lends support to the practice of sentinel node biopsy. Besides metastasis, poor prognostic signs include high mitotic rate, a high Clark level of invasion, presence of ulceration, and the presence of microscopic satellites. Chest radiographs are indicated as a part of routine surveillance and follow-up after treatment of an initial melanoma. (*Cecil Textbook of Medicine, pp. 1248–1252*)

163. **(C)** The incidence and severity of shingles is increased in most immunosuppressed patients. This population includes patients with lymphoma, leukemia, or HIV; patients who have received bone marrow transplantation; and patients on chronic immunosuppressive therapy. However, HIV patients are notable for their tendency to suffer multiple recurrences of shingles. (*Fitzpatrick, p. 2077*)

164. **(A)** The duration of action of a local anesthetic is proportional to its contact time with the nerves. Therefore, if the drug can be localized at the nerve, the period of analgesia should be prolonged. Using a vasoconstrictor such as epinephrine decreases the systemic absorption of the local anesthetic. Once the absorption is decreased, the anesthetic remains longer at the desired site and is systemically absorbed at a slower rate, which allows destruction by enzymes and less systemic toxicity. (*Hardman et al., 2001, pp. 372–373*)

165. **(B)** Resistant hypertension is defined as blood pressure not at goal despite adequate doses of a three-drug regimen including a diuretic. One of the first considerations is medication compliance and white coat hypertension. White coat hypertension can be assessed by the use of ambulatory blood pressure monitoring. A patient's home monitor should be assessed for accuracy against the office monitor. The patient's technique should also be verified. One should also assess for other agents that may lead to resistant hypertension despite pharmacologic therapy (e.g., tobacco use, NSAIDs, steroids, recreational drugs, oral decongestants, herbal medications). If the above are ruled out, one should initiate a workup to assess for a secondary cause for the hypertension, which may include chronic kidney disease, coarctation of the aorta, Cushing syndrome, steroid treatment, drug-induced hypertension, pheochromocytoma, primary aldosteronism, renovascular

hypertension, sleep apnea, and thyroid/parathyroid disease.

This patient has been on four drugs and has no history of noncompliance. The patient also has no evidence of white coat hypertension as the home readings match the office readings. As there is no history of prior evaluation, the most appropriate step is to initiate a workup of secondary causes. If the workup identifies a cause, treat based on the findings. If the workup is negative, perhaps initiating a central agent or specialist consultation may be warranted. (*JNC-7 Full Report*)

166. **(C)** Deficiency of C1q, along with other C1, C2, and C4 deficiencies, results in immune complex syndromes that are clinically similar to lupus. Deficiencies of C5, C6, C7, and C8 often result in recurrent, invasive *Neisseria* (*meningitidis* or *gonorrhoea*) infections. (*Kaspar et al., 2005, p. 1826*)

/nī'sirēə/

167. **(E)**

168. **(D)**

Explanations 167 and 168

This patient is exhibiting signs and symptoms of an anaphylactic reaction, likely to one of the medications that she recently took. Angioedema is occurring (swelling of the lips and tongue). Her dyspnea may be a manifestation of laryngeal edema or of bronchospasm. She is at high risk for respiratory compromise and, therefore, of the options listed, having her activate the emergency medical system is the most appropriate. Calling 911 from your office would be another option.

Of the interventions listed, epinephrine would provide the most benefit in correcting the underlying problem. The alpha- and beta-adrenergic effects result in vasoconstriction, bronchial smooth-muscle relaxation, and reduction on vascular permeability. Oxygen may be required if the patient is hypoxic, IV fluids may be necessary for persistent hypotension and albuterol may benefit the treatment of bronchospasm, but epinephrine would most immediately address the multiple systemic effects of anaphylaxis. *(Kaspar et al., 2005, pp. 1915–1916)*

169. **(B)** A questionable history of penicillin allergy by a patient often incorrectly labels patients as penicillin allergic. Physicians are often afraid of a true anaphylactic reaction and turn to a second-line medication. Most patients who state they were penicillin allergic or were told by a parent they were allergic were confusing a complication of the illness, such as a rash from viral prodrome. In fact, 80–90% of patients who self-report a nonanaphylactic reaction or were informed by a parent of a penicillin allergy are not penicillin allergic when assessed with skin allergy testing. The frequency of all adverse reactions to penicillin in the general population ranges from 0.7 to 10%. Approximately 98% of patients with a reported history of penicillin allergy (except anaphylaxis) and a negative skin test can safely receive penicillin. In patients who have an unclear history of penicillin allergy (pretest likelihood greater than that of general population) and who would benefit from penicillin, skin testing should be performed and penicillin used for patients with negative results. If however, the pretest likelihood of allergy is similar to the prevalence in the general population, skin testing can be foregone, and treatment with penicillin offered. In patients with definite penicillin allergy or anaphylaxis in whom penicillin therapy is the only option, inpatient admission for penicillin desensitization is warranted. *(JAMA 2001;285:2498–2505)*

170. **(B)** As per the American Cancer Society, American College of Colorectal Surgery, and the American College of Gastroenterology, the colon cancer screening guidelines for persons with prior history of colon cancer are as follows:

- Initially, a "clearing" colonoscopy should be performed to evaluate for synchronous disease located elsewhere in the colon. If the cancer is not obstructing, this can be done with a preoperative colonoscopy. If it is obstructing, CT colonography (virtual colonoscopy) or barium enema can be used preoperatively and colonoscopy can be performed either intraoperatively or 3–6 months postoperatively.

- If curative resection is performed for colon or rectal cancer, a follow-up colonoscopy should be performed 1 year postoperatively. If this is normal, the next scope should be 3 years later. If all endoscopy is normal then a subsequent interval of 5 years is recommended. *(Rex, et al., CA Cancer J Clin 2006;56(3):160–167; quiz 185–186; Gastrointestinal Consortium Panel. Colorectal cancer screening and surveillance: clinical guidelines and rationale. Update based on new evidence. Gastroenterology 2003;124(2): 544–560)*

171. **(A)**

172. **(D)**

173. **(B)**

174. **(D)**

Explanations 171 through 174

This patient is manifesting symptoms consistent with asthma. With the history of recently moving to a new area, along with a family history of allergies and eczema, his asthma may be further classified as allergic asthma. Episodic symptoms of cough, dyspnea, and wheezing are likely to occur. The diagnosis of asthma is made by demonstrating reversible airway obstruction. Airway obstruction is likely to be manifested by a reduction in the FEV_1. An increase in the FEV_1 of 15% after the use of a bronchodilator is the definition of reversibility. A CXR is most likely to be normal. Numerous cardiac conditions, such as CHF, cardiomyopathies, or pericardial effusions, may result in cardiomegaly on a CXR. Diffuse infiltrates may be seen with infections, interstitial lung disease, or other conditions. Flattened diaphragms would be consistent with prolonged obstructive lung disease, such as emphysema.

The treatment of choice for the prevention of symptoms in all stages of asthma other than mild intermittent is inhaled steroid. All patients with asthma should also have a short-acting bronchodilator for acute symptomatic relief. A leukotriene modifier would be an alternative recommendation and might be a good addition to an inhaled steroid, as they also have FDA indications for patients with allergic rhinitis. *(Kaspar et al., 2005, pp. 1456–1463)*

Albuterol is a beta-adrenergic agonist that is selective for beta-2 receptors. Activity at these receptors leads to relaxation of respiratory, uterine, and vascular smooth muscle. In the setting of an asthma attack, albuterol is the drug of choice for reversing bronchoconstriction. In conditions such as acute heart failure and certain types of shock, it is desirable to increase cardiac output and overall blood flow to the tissues, so epinephrine (which functions as a direct nonselective alpha and beta agonist) is a more appropriate option. *(Katzung, 2004, pp. 80–83)*

175. (C)

176. (A)

177. (C)

Explanations 175 through 177

Atrial fibrillation is the most common sustained clinical arrhythmia. It occurs in approximately 4% of the population over the age of 60. It is diagnosed by the presence of irregularly irregular QRS complexes on an ECG with an absence of P waves. The QRS complex is most commonly narrow, as this is a supraventricular arrhythmia. Wide QRS complexes can occur if there is an underlying conduction abnormality, such as Wolff-Parkinson-White syndrome or a bundle branch block. Saw-tooth P waves occur in atrial flutter, another atrial arrhythmia that may present similarly to atrial fibrillation but which is less common. The saw-tooth P waves, or flutter waves, are representative of an atrial rate typically in the range of 300–350/minute.

Not infrequently, atrial flutter will lead to atrial fibrillation. Q waves in II, III, and aVF would be seen if there had been a previous inferior MI. Peaked T waves are seen in certain conditions, such as hyperkalemia, but are not routinely associated with atrial fibrillation.

Atrial fibrillation may be precipitated by both cardiac and noncardiac conditions. Among the noncardiac conditions are metabolic abnormalities, which include hyperthyroidism. Of the tests listed, a suppressed TSH level, consistent with hyperthyroidism, would be most likely to be causative of atrial fibrillation. Troponin may be elevated in acute myocardial ischemia. Atrial fibrillation can occur following a MI, particularly when complicated by CHF. This is not consistent with the clinical scenario presented. Renal disease and diabetes may contribute to some of the conditions that can predispose to the development of atrial fibrillation, such as metabolic derangements or CAD. Acute and chronic pulmonary disease may also precipitate atrial fibrillation. In the setting of a man who is otherwise healthy and without significant medical history, new-onset atrial fibrillation would be less likely to be the initial presentation of diabetes, renal failure, or pulmonary disease than hyperthyroidism. For this reason, choice A is the single best answer of those provided.

The initial evaluation of atrial fibrillation should generally include a detailed history and physical examination, ECG, CXR, thyroid function tests, and an echocardiogram. The echo would provide information on the overall ventricular function and evidence of valvular disease. It would also allow for the measurement of atrial size, which provides prognostic information on the ability to achieve and maintain a sinus rhythm. The presence of atrial thrombus could also be determined. An exercise stress test may be useful if the arrhythmia was precipitated by exercise. Electrophysiologic studies are usually reserved for the setting of disease that is refractory to medical management. Cardiac catheterization would be appropriate in the setting of confirmed or suspected ischemic heart disease as a cause of the condition.

Radionuclide ventriculography would provide significantly less overall information than an echocardiogram in this setting and would not be as useful as an initial test. (*Goldman and Braunwald, pp. 333–339*)

178. **(B)** Quinidine can prolong the Q-T interval resulting in the development of polymorphic ventricular tachycardia (torsade de pointes). Hypokalemia, a side effect of thiazide diuretics, increases the risk of torsade de pointes, which can then degenerate into fatal ventricular fibrillation. Thiazide diuretics may decrease the effectiveness of uricosuric agents, insulin, and sulfonylureas and may increase the effects of vitamin D. However, these effects tend not to be life threatening. (*Hardman et al., 2001, pp. 877, 965–966*)

179. **(C)**

180. **(E)**

181. **(D)**

Explanations 179 through 181

Two generally accepted conventions for grading the severity of angina pectoris are those of the Canadian Cardiovascular Society (CCS) and the NYHA. The NYHA classification attempts to quantify the functional limitations imposed on an individual by their symptoms. Class I angina is defined as angina which does not appear as a patient undertakes ordinary physical activity. Symptoms caused by ordinary physical activity characterize class II angina. In class III angina, there is a moderate limitation of activity such that a patient remains comfortable at rest but symptoms appear during less-than-ordinary activities. In class IV angina, symptoms are present at rest so a patient is unable to perform any physical activity without feeling discomfort. Prinzmetal angina describes a syndrome of ischemic pain occurring at rest but not necessarily with exertion; it is diagnosed with detection of transient ST-T elevation with rest pain. (*Harrison's Internal Medicine online, Chap. 227 "Unstable Angina and Non-ST-Elevation Myocardial Infarction"*)

The goal of treatment of angina is to relieve symptoms and prolong exercise capacity by improving the relationship of oxygen demand and supply. Nitroglycerin is a smooth muscle relaxant that produces both venodilation (reduced preload) and arteriolar dilation (reduced afterload). Although the combined effect is to reduce myocardial oxygen demands, the potential exists for reflex tachycardia and increased contractility. To avoid the potential for increased oxygen demand and decreased coronary blood flow, a beta-blocker such as propranolol may be used concurrently with nitroglycerin. Another option is the careful titration of the nitroglycerin dose used. Discontinuation of nitroglycerin without further intervention would inappropriately leave the patient's angina pain untreated. Replacing nitroglycerin with the calcium channel blocker nifedipine may not address the problem of reflex tachycardia as nifedipine can also lead to a rapid vasodilation and subsequent drop in blood pressure (which, in turn, leads to increased sympathetic outflow and an increase in heart rate). Addition of isoproterenol would be inappropriate since it increases myocardial oxygen demand. (*Katzung, 2004, pp. 83, 113–114*)

Major indications for CABG surgery include the presence of triple-vessel disease; severe left main stem artery stenosis (greater than 50%); and left main equivalent disease (greater than 70% stenosis of the left anterior descending and proximal left circumflex arteries), especially in the setting of impaired left ventricular function (decreased LVEF). The outcomes from bypass surgery in these situations are superior to any form of medical therapy. Left main stenosis and left main equivalent stenosis are contraindications for performance of PTCA. Defibrillator placement is indicated in situations where a prior cardiac arrest is known to have been due to an irreversible cause or due to an undetermined cause in the presence of persistent arrhythmia. (*Braunwald, pp. 1353–1361; 1999 Guidelines for CABG Surgery, American College of Cardiology, and the American Heart Association*)

Explanations 182 and 183

182. (E)

183. (D)

Polymyositis usually presents with patients complaining of gradual muscle weakness and myalgias. The peak incidence occurs in the fifth and sixth decades, with women being affected more commonly than men. Aside from the history and physical examination, laboratory analysis such as elevated muscle enzymes such as CPK and aldolase usually confirm the diagnosis. ESR levels may not be significantly elevated in over 50% of the patients. ANA may be positive in many patients, however this does not distinguish the condition. EMG may be helpful in making the diagnosis as certain features— such as polyphasic potentials, fibrillations, and high-frequency action potentials—are more consistent with polymyositis. Muscle biopsy is the most specific test, however the patchy distribution may lead to false negative tests on occasion. Muscle biopsy may reveal endomysial infiltration of the inflammatory infiltrate. Usually, the initial treatment of choice is high-dose steroids, that is, prednisone 60 mg with tapering down after clinical response to the lowest effective dose. If steroids fail, immunosuppressant such as methotrexate or azathioprine may be tried. *(Harrison's Principles of Internal Medicine, 15th ed., pp. 2524–2529)*

184. (D) Osteoporosis is generally defined as a T score of –2.5 SD or greater on assessment of BMD. Osteopenia is generally defined as a T score between 1 and 2.5 SD below the peak BMD for a healthy young person of the same gender. Osteoporosis screening with an assessment of BMD should be offered to the following groups:

- All women 65 years old or older
- All adult women with a history of a fracture (or fractures) not caused by severe trauma (such as a motor vehicle accident)
- Younger postmenopausal women who have clinical risk factors for fractures

- Modifiable risk factors: current cigarette smoking, low body weight (<127 lbs), estrogen deficiency, premature menopause, excessive thyroid hormone replacement, chronic corticosteroid therapy, low calcium intake (life-long), alcoholism, uncorrected visual impairment, inadequate physical activity, recurrent falls
- Nonmodifiable risk factors: personal or family history of fragility, family history of osteoporosis, White or Asian race, age, gender, poor health/frailty, dementia, hypogonadism in males, fracture without substantial trauma

Serial assessments for BMD may be useful but one must remember the precision error among the tests. Using DEXA, a BMD must have a 3–5% difference to be clinically significant. Patients who are on pharmacologic treatment with bisphosphonates may only show this much change in 1 year. Therefore, static BMD or slight reduction should not be regarded as treatment failure.

At present, there are no hard evidence-based guidelines for the most efficient use for BMD monitoring. However, the following guidelines are generally accepted:

- *For patients with "normal" baseline BMD* (T score more than –1.0), consider a follow-up measurement every 3–5 years. Patients whose bone density is well above the minimal acceptable level may not need further bone density testing.
- *For patients in an osteoporosis prevention program*, perform a follow-up measurement every 1–2 years until bone mass stability is documented. After BMD has stabilized, perform follow-up measurements every 2–3 years.
- *For patients on a therapeutic program*, perform a follow-up measurement yearly for 2 years. If bone mass has stabilized after 2 years, perform a follow-up measurement every 2 years. Otherwise, continue with annual follow-up measurements until stability of bone mass is achieved. *(Hodgson, al., 2001 edition, with selected updates for 2003. Endocr Pract 2003;9(6):544–564)*

185. (D)

186. (A)

187. (E)

188. (B)

Explanations 185 through 188

The clinical scenario described is classic for an acute MI. The patient has multiple risk factors, including smoking, hypertension, and elevated cholesterol. His symptoms of crushing chest pain radiating to the left arm is commonly seen in this setting. Often the first electrocardiographic sign of acute ischemia is the development of hyperacute T waves. The ECG will usually show S-T segment elevations in the area of the involved occluded vessel, with reciprocal S-T segment depressions in uninvolved areas. This can be followed by the eventual resolution of S-T segment abnormalities and the development of T wave inversions and Q waves. Diffuse P-R depressions are often the initial manifestation of pericarditis, a less common cause of acute chest pain. This often progresses to diffuse S-T segment elevations, the presence of which helps to distinguish pericarditis from the focal S-T elevations more classically associated with a thrombosed coronary artery. Q waves would be unlikely to occur within 1 hour of the onset of symptoms. In this clinical setting, a normal ECG, while possible, would be less likely to occur. (Goldman and Braunwald, pp. 262–263)

Ventricular arrhythmias, both tachycardia and fibrillation, are recognized complications of acute MI. The presence of ventricular fibrillation or pulseless ventricular tachycardia should lead to the primary "ABCD" survey, as outlined in the American Heart Association's ACLS protocols. The mnemonic stands for **ai**rway, **b**reathing, **c**irculation, and **d**efibrillation. Epinephrine, lidocaine, or amiodarone are reserved for the setting where defibrillation is ineffective. Synchronized cardioversion would be used in efforts to convert a patient's rhythm in the setting of a stable tachycardia.

(American Heart Association, ACLS provider manual, 2001, pp. 75–90)

According to ACLS protocols, the primary survey for asystole is "ABCCD"—**a**irway, **b**reathing, **c**irculation, **c**onfirmation of true asystole, and **d**efibrillation (or recognition that asystole is not a shockable rhythm). In a patient monitored in an emergency or telemetry setting, confirmation of true asystole would include checking a second lead, confirming that the leads are attached to the patient, and that cables are correctly attached. The use of epinephrine and atropine, or the consideration of discontinuation of resuscitation, would be appropriate after the confirmation of true asystole. (ACLS provider manual, pp. 109–122)

ACE inhibitors have been shown to improve remodeling after acute MI and to reduce the mortality rate in patients who survive MI. Beta-blockers have also been proven to reduce mortality by a mechanism believed to involve arrhythmia suppression. Flecainide and quinidine are antiarrhythmic drugs which may actually increase mortality. Digoxin and nitroglycerin, although effective in increasing cardiac output and decreasing workload on the heart, do not necessarily prolong survival. (Cecil Textbook of Medicine, p. 419; Katzung, 2004, pp. 154–156)

189. (B)

190. (C)

191. (D)

Explanations 189 through 191

Psoriasis is a benign chronic, inflammatory skin disorder with a genetic basis that affects approximately 2% of the population in the United States. The condition varies in its presentation from person to person, with some having only local involvement and others having a severe generalized involvement. The incidence occurs in a bimodal distribution, with peaks persons in their 20s and 50s. Those with earlier onset generally will have a more severe disease over the course of their lifetime.

Psoriasis has several variants, or sub types, including plaque type (most common), eruptive (guttate), generalized pustular, and erythrodermic psoriasis. Some patients may be asymptomatic or may have only minor itching. Others may have involvement of most of their body, with severe disfigurement and poor quality of life. Psoriasis may involve any skin area; however, areas such as the scalp, extensor surfaces, palms, soles, and nails should always be examined.

The typical lesions are described as erythematous, well-demarcated plaques with overlying scales. Fine stippling (pitting) of the nails is highly suggestive of psoriasis. In addition to the skin findings, patients may also have arthritis. The lesions can be reactivated with local injury or irritation of normal skin (Koebner phenomenon).

The diagnosis is predominantly clinical, based on the history and examination. There are no laboratory measures that will diagnose psoriasis. Skin biopsy, although not pathognomonic, would show features consistent with psoriasis and would help to rule out other similar appearing conditions.

The treatment options for psoriasis depend on the type, extent, area of involvement, and quality of impairment of the patient. Initial treatments especially for limited disease may be topical steroids, coal tar topical preparations, topical retinoids, and/or topical vitamin D analogs. If the involvement is more severe, other options such as ultraviolet light therapy, systemic immunomodulators, or systemic immunosuppressants may be used. Systemic steroids are not recommended, as withdrawal may lead to a flare-up or aggravation of the condition. However, some specialists may choose this option, with close follow-up, if other avenues have failed. *(Tierney, et al., pp. 94–121; Wolf, et al., pp. 54–57)*

192. (D)

193. (C)

194. (D)

195. (C)

Explanations 192 through 195

This patient's presentation is most consistent with pulmonary edema from decompensated CHF. The BNP test has been found to be both sensitive and specific for the diagnosis of CHF. It can be a very useful test to order when a patient is dyspneic to help to determine if CHF is the cause. Troponin, CK-MB, and LDH are markers of damage to cardiac muscle and can be diagnostic in a MI. While MI can be a cause of CHF, and most patients presenting with CHF will have cardiac enzymes drawn as part of their evaluation, cardiac enzymes are neither sensitive nor specific for CHF. Similarly, a CXR can determine the presence of pulmonary edema but not its cause.

Acute pulmonary edema secondary to CHF will require management with diuresis for acute symptomatic relief. ACE inhibitors and beta-blockers do decrease mortality and morbidity in CHF; however their use in acute decompensated heart failure is suspected as they may induce hypotension and further cardiogenic shock. Digoxin is used for symptomatic relief either when other modalities fail or when rate control from atrial fibrillation is an issue. In patients with CHF and atrial fibrillation, beta-blockers have shown better effect and reduced morbidity than digoxin. Nevertheless, in the acute setting of decompensated heart failure with pulmonary edema, diuresis is the optimal initial treatment, not digoxin. In chronic heart failure, digoxin is reserved for patients with systolic failure that are symptomatic despite adequate ACE inhibitor and beta-blocker use. Furosemide is effective in treating the acute pulmonary edema associated with CHF by virtue of its potent diuretic action, which rapidly eliminates excess body fluid volume. *(Peacock, 2003)*

ACE inhibitors and some beta-adrenergic antagonists (metoprolol, bisoprolol, and carvedilol) have been proven to reduce mortality in patients with CHF. Additionally, the Randomized Aldactone Evaluation Study

(RALES) trial showed that the addition of spironolactone to patients with class IV heart failure symptoms who were already receiving ACE inhibitors led to a further decrease in the risk of death by up to 25%. Digoxin has been shown to improve symptoms in patients with severe CHF; however, it has no effect on mortality due to its proarrhythmic effect. Warfarin should be considered in patients who have a previous history of thromboembolism or atrial fibrillation. Some calcium channel blockers such as diltiazem should be avoided in patients with impaired left ventricular function due to negative inotropic effects. Serious complications which may result from the use of calcium channel blockers include worsening heart failure, pulmonary edema, and cardiogenic shock. *(Harrison's Internal Medicine online, Chap. 216, Sect. 3 "Heart Failure and Cor Pulmonale")*

Furosemide is effective in treating the acute pulmonary edema associated with CHF by virtue of its potent diuretic action, which rapidly eliminates excess body fluid volume. Both propranolol and verapamil may decrease cardiac output and thus exacerbate congestion. Mannitol tends to increase vascular fluid volume, which can result in increased congestion. Spironolactone is not potent enough as a diuretic to be effective in treating this condition. *(Hardman et al., 2001, pp. 904, 924)*

The patient's LVEF is decreased, which is a finding consistent with systolic dysfunction. In this case, digoxin would be an appropriate choice for control of symptoms. Currently, digoxin is not considered appropriate for use in the setting of diastolic dysfunction. Diastolic dysfunction, which is most commonly caused by long-standing hypertension, is characterized by a normal or increased ejection fraction. The main advantage that a TEE has over a TTE is the easier visualization of certain anatomic structures which may be obscured or distorted by conditions such as morbid obesity. Consequently, a TTE would not give a more accurate estimation of LVEF than a TEE. By the NYHA classification of heart failure, class I heart failure involves no dyspnea or fatigue during normal physical activity; the

patient in this case is clearly beyond this stage. *(Cecil Textbook of Medicine, pp. 291–310)*

196. (D)

197. (A)

198. (E)

Explanations 196 through 198

Aortic stenosis is one of the most common valvular abnormalities found in adults. It can be congenital—such as a unicuspid or bicuspid valve—or acquired. In young adults, acquired aortic stenosis is often seen as a consequence of rheumatic fever. This is becoming less common in developed nations. In adults over the age of 65, the most common cause of aortic stenosis is age-related degenerative, calcific aortic stenosis. The valvular cusps are immobilized and the stenosis caused by calcium deposits along the flexion lines of the valves. Acquired aortic stenosis typically has a prolonged asymptomatic period. During this time the stenosis may be found incidentally by auscultation of the characteristic harsh, holosystolic murmur in the aortic valve area that radiates to the carotid arteries. There may also be a slow, small, and sustained arterial pulsation (pulsus parvus and tardus) due to the relative outflow obstruction. The cardinal symptoms of aortic stenosis that signal advancing disease, and increased risk of mortality, are angina, heart failure, and syncope. An ECG will show left ventricular hypertrophy in approximately 85% of symptomatic cases of aortic stenosis. A normal ECG is possible but would be more likely in early, asymptomatic stages. S-T segment elevation would be more consistent with acute cardiac ischemia and Q waves would be more consistent with a completed MI. Low-voltage QRS complexes can be seen in several conditions, including pericardial effusion, COPD, or obesity.

When considering the diagnosis of aortic stenosis, the initial diagnostic test of choice would be echocardiography. It would provide information on both the structure (bicuspid, tricuspid, and the like) and the function (valve area, pressures) of the valve. The size and function of the left ventricle can also be determined. If aortic stenosis is found on echocardiogram and the patient is symptomatic, the next test would be cardiac catheterization. This would allow for direct measurement of the pressure gradient across the valve. It would also allow for evaluation of the status of the coronary arteries in order to determine whether CABG would need to be performed along with valve replacement. Exercise stress testing is relatively contraindicated in the setting of symptomatic aortic stenosis. Holter monitoring would only be useful if there were a concomitant arrhythmia. Electrophysiologic studies would not play a role in the typical evaluation of aortic stenosis.

The management of symptomatic critical aortic stenosis is surgical. If the patient is a surgical candidate, the treatment of choice is aortic valve replacement. Balloon valvuloplasty would be an option either as a temporizing measure when surgery could not be immediately performed or when the patient is not a surgical candidate. A high percentage of patients develop recurrent stenosis within 6 months of this procedure. Antihypertensive and vasodilating medications must be used with extreme caution, and usually should be avoided, as they can impair the ability of the ventricle to create the pressure needed to pump blood across the narrowed aortic valve. (Braunwald, pp. 1671–1680)

199. **(A)** Cholestyramine is a bile acid sequestrant which binds bile acids and similar steroids in the intestine, thereby reducing concentrations of LDLs in the circulation. Orally administered drugs may also bind to cholestyramine, however, impairing their efficacy by impairing absorption in the gut. This problem can be alleviated by administering other oral medications at least 1 hour before or 4 hours after cholestyramine. Examples of compounds which may be bound by cholestyramine include warfarin, digoxin, glipizide, phenytoin, methyldopa, thiazide diuretics, niacin, and statins. Fat-soluble vitamins (A, D, E, and K) may also bind to cholestyramine. Cholestyramine powder should never be administered in its dry form due to the risk of aspiration. It should be combined with water, pureed-consistency food, or a noncarbonated beverage. Use of carbonated liquids as a solvent may exacerbate the common side effects of heartburn and indigestion. Fat-soluble vitamins (A, D, E, and K) may also bind to cholestyramine; if steatorrhea develops, with associated impairment of fat-soluble vitamins, vitamin supplementation is recommended. (Hardman et al., 2001, pp. 989–990; Katzung, 2004, p. 316)

200. **(C)**

201. **(A)**

Explanations 200 and 201

Although all of the given diagnoses could produce similar symptoms, there are distinct findings which suggest a diagnosis of spinal stenosis. Spinal stenosis is a degenerative disorder of the spine which normally presents after the age of 50. Neurologic symptoms, including dysesthesias and paraesthesias, and pain are often bilateral and not localized, since it commonly affects multiple vertebrae. The symptoms are improved with flexion of the spine (sitting or climbing stairs) and worsened by straightening the spine (standing). There is no localized pain in the sacrum and no bowel or bladder incontinence, so a diagnosis of cauda equina syndrome or spondyloarthopathy is less likely. Muscle spasms and early DJD should not produce such neurologic findings.

The most sensitive and specific imaging study in the diagnosis of spinal stenosis, among those given above, is an MRI of the spine at the affected area. Although x-rays of the spine have been frequently used in the past in the evaluation of lower back pain, they have been shown to be of limited value in diagnosing pathology. Bone scans may detect malignancy or infection before radiography does, but are of no value in spinal stenosis. Indium scans would be useful in occult inflammatory pathology and nerve conduction studies would suggest a neuropathic deficit, but would not help in localizing the defect. (Kaspar et al., 2005, p. 83)

202. (B)

203. (D)

204. (D)

Explanations 202 through 204

Asthma is a chronic lung disease characterized by inflammation of the airways, causing recurrent symptoms. The characteristic symptoms are wheezing, chest tightness, shortness of breath, or cough. Symptoms often worsen in the face of certain triggers, which include allergens, cold air, exercise, or other irritants. Physical examination may reveal hyperexpansion of the thorax, expiratory wheezing with a prolonged expiratory phase of respiration, and signs of allergies or atopic dermatitis.

Asthma can be diagnosed by a history of episodic symptoms of airway obstruction (wheeze, dyspnea, cough, chest tightness), establishing the presence of airflow obstruction that is at least partially reversible and ruling out other causes of these symptoms/signs. Airflow obstruction can be shown by spirometry revealing an FEV_1 of <80% predicted or an FEV_1/forced vital capacity of <65% of the lower limit of normal. Reversibility can be shown by an FEV_1 increase of ≥15% and at least 200 mL with the use of a short-acting beta agonist.

Expiratory wheezing on examination is commonly seen in asthma but is a nonspecific finding. Many patients with asthma have elevated serum IgE levels; it is unusual to find asthma in individuals who have a low level of serum IgE. The sputum of asthmatics may contain eosinophils, Charcot-Leyden crystals, Curschmann spirals, or Creola bodies. However, eosinophils may also be present in the sputum of patients with other conditions such as Churg-Strauss syndrome or eosinophilic pneumonia. Peak-flow monitoring is useful for the short- and long-term monitoring of asthma patients and for exacerbation management (by aiding in the determination of exacerbation severity which directs therapeutic decision making). (*Cecil Textbook of Medicine, pp. 502–509*)

Asthma is generally classified as mild, mild persistent, moderate persistent, or severe persistent based on the frequency of symptoms and the degree of airflow obstruction (see Table 1-2). Based on this patient's frequency of symptoms, he falls into the moderate persistent class. An often neglected diagnosis is exercise-induced asthma which is characterized by attacks immediately following exertion and by the lack of any long-term sequelae or increase in airway reactivity. (*Harrison's Internal Medicine online, Chap. 236 "Asthma"*)

The preferred treatment for severe persistent asthma includes a combination of a scheduled long-acting inhaled beta agonist and a scheduled inhaled steroid. Additionally, a short-acting inhaled beta agonist should be used for symptomatic relief on an as-needed basis. Beyond this regimen, glucocorticoid tablets or syrup may be used if needed in the event that additional control is necessary. It is standard practice to use a stepwise approach to the management of asthma. (*Harrison's Internal Medicine online, Chap. 236 "Asthma"*)

205. (A)

206. (D)

Explanations 205 and 206

Peripheral arterial disease (PAD) affects roughly 12% of the U.S. population with higher prevalence rates in persons over the age of 70. The classic symptoms of PAD are intermittent claudication which is usually described by patients as cramping pain in the calf, legs, thighs, or buttocks during any type of exercise that quickly relieves with rest. This scenario of worsening with activity and relief with rest is consistent with the disease process, as the pain results from ischemia. The ischemia is worse during periods of increased oxygen demand where the vascular insufficiency fails to meet the demand.

Not all patients with PAD are symptomatic, thus an assessment of risk factors and a thorough physical examination are usually key to making the diagnosis in asymptomatic patients. The ABI is an easy, inexpensive, noninvasive test with a high correlation to angiography that can be done in the office. ABI is the usual initial test to screen for PAD.

FIG. 1-7 (Question 116)

FIG. 1-8 *(Courtesy of Philip C. Johnson, MD.)* (Question 148)

FIG. 1-9 *(Courtesy of Philip C. Johnson, MD.)* (Question 148)

FIG. 1-10 (Question 155)

FIG. 1-11 *(Courtesy of Philip C. Johnson, MD.)* (Question 189)

FIG. 1-12 (Question 216)

FIG. 1-13 *Photo of sickle cell blood smear. (Courtesy of Ethan Natelson, MD.)* **(Question 255)**

FIG. 4-2 *(Courtesy of Kathy Hullfish, MD.)* **(Question 26)**

FIG. 2-9 *(Courtesy of H.J. Kim, MD.)* **(Question 87)**

FIG. 4-3 *(Courtesy of Kathy Hullfish, MD.)* **(Question 39)**

FIG. 3-2 *(Reproduced, with permission, from Wolff K, Johnson RA, Suurmond R. Color Atlas and Synopsis of Clinical Dermatology, 5th ed. New York, NY: McGraw-Hill, 2005, p. 589.)* **(Question 35)**

FIG. 7-9 *(Courtesy of Roland Schwarting, MD.)* **(Question 47)**

TABLE 1-2   CLASSIFICATION OF ASTHMA SEVERITY

Classification	Days with symptoms	Nights with symptoms	PEF or FEV$_1$ (PEF is % of personal best; FEV$_1$ is % of predicted)	PEF variability	Treatment
Severe persistent	Continual	Frequent	≤60%	>30%	Preferred: high dose inhaled steroid and long-acting beta agonist AND, if needed, corticosteroid tablets or syrup
Moderate persistent	Daily	≥5/month	>60–<80%	>30%	Preferred: low-to-medium dose inhaled steroid and long-acting beta agonist Alternative: increase inhaled steroid within medium dose range OR low-to-medium dose inhaled steroid and leukotriene modifier or theophylline if needed (particularly in patients with recurring severe exacerbations): Preferred: increase inhaled steroid within medium dose range and long-acting beta agonist Alternative: increase inhaled steroid within medium dose range and add leukotrienemodifier or theophylline
Mild persistent	3–6/ week	3–4/month	≥80%	20–30%	Preferred: low dose inhaled steroid Alternative: cromolyn, nedocromil, leukotriene modifier, or theophylline
Mild intermittent	≤2/week	≤2/month	≥80%	<20%	No daily medication needed severe exacerbations may occur, separated by long periods of normal function and no symptoms. A course of systemic corticosteroids is recommended

All patients: Short-acting bronchodilator as needed for symptoms
Source: (Reproduced from) Practical Guide for the Diagnosis and Management of Asthma, NIH: National Heart, Lung and Blood Institute, 1997; NAEPP Expert Panel Report; Guidelines for the Diagnosis and Management of Asthma–Update on Selected Topics, 2002; NIH: National Heart, Lung and Blood Institute, 2002.

A value of greater than 1.0 is considered normal, whereas values less than 0.9 are consistent with varying grades of PAD:

- 1.0 or greater: normal
- 0.81–0.9: mild PAD
- 0.51–0.8: moderate PAD
- <0.5: severe PAD

The sensitivity of the ABI can be increased if performed post exercise. The ABI, however, has its limitations in patients with noncompressible, calcified vessels such as the elderly or in patients with diabetes. An ABI of greater than 1.3 may suggest the above scenario and its utility would be suspect. In these cases, more detailed testing may be warranted. Other modalities to assess PAD include arterial Dopplers, magnetic resonance angiography, and conventional angiography.

The initial therapy for patients with PAD should be a trial of a structured walking program along with smoking cessation. Walking programs have been shown to increase walking distance without symptoms. In addition, walking also improves endothelial function, collateral vessel formation and function, and control of blood pressure, lipids, and blood sugars.

Pentoxyfylline has been traditionally recommended for PAD; however its efficacy is modest at best based on newer trial data. Antiplatelet agents may also be added for PAD as it will improve cardiovascular risk and perhaps modify the pathogenesis for PAD. Ultimately, risk factor modification is key for prevention and reduction of complications and comorbidities. Severe PAD or patients who require more specialized intervention may require vascular surgery consultation. *(Friedman, et al., Postgrad Med 2006;119(2):21–27. Available at: www.postgradmed. com/issues/2006/07/021)*

207. (A)

208. (D)

209. (E)

Explanations 207 through 209

COPD is a group of chronic and progressive pulmonary disorders that cause reduced expiratory flow. Most of the obstruction is fixed, although some reversibility can be found. COPD affects approximately 16 million Americans and smoking is, by far, the greatest risk factor. Onset is typically in the fifth decade and the typical presenting symptoms are dyspnea and cough. Patients often relate these to an acute illness (walking pneumonia in this case) but the decline in pulmonary function has been present for some time prior to the onset of symptoms. The physical examination has poor sensitivity and may, in early disease, only show wheezing on forced expiration and a prolonged expiratory phase of respiration. Clubbing is not typically a manifestation of COPD and its presence should lead to a search for another cause, such as lung cancer. In the setting of pulmonary hypertension, sometimes one can hear a pronounced pulmonic component to the second heart sound, although hyperinflation may obscure this finding. Bilateral pulmonary crackles would be more consistent with pulmonary edema. Supraclavicular adenopathy should lead to a workup to exclude cancer, especially of breast, lung, ovarian, or GI origin.

Hyperinflation of the lungs is the most likely CXR finding in this case. This would manifest as flattened diaphragms with elongated lungs and a long, narrow cardiac shadow. Kerley B lines would be more characteristic of pulmonary edema from left-sided heart failure, rather than COPD. A pulmonary mass with adenopathy would be more consistent with lung cancer—certainly a possibility in a long-time smoker, but much less common than COPD. A residual infiltrate from pneumonia a year ago would be highly unlikely.

Smoking cessation should always be recommended when COPD is diagnosed. It has been shown that the rate of decline of the FEV_1 can revert back to that of a nonsmoker. While pulmonary function may improve some, it likely will not improve dramatically. Quitting smoking can prolong survival and delay the onset of disability along with reducing the risk of malignancy and cardiovascular disease development. (*Harrison's Principles of Internal Medicine, 15th ed., pp. 1491–1499*)

210. (C)

211. (B)

Explanations 210 and 211

Tumor lysis syndrome refers to a series of metabolic disturbances resultant from cancer treatment. It generally occurs when a large number of cancer cells are killed rapidly, releasing the contents of those cells into the systemic circulation. These contents include various ions. Tumor lysis syndrome is typically characterized by a combination of hyperuricemia, hyperkalemia, hyperphosphatemia, hypocalcemia, and lactic acidosis. Besides treatment of electrolyte abnormalities, urine alkalinization and aggressive hydration are frequently included as a part of treatment. Patients with tumor lysis syndrome may also develop oliguric acute renal failure, which arises from the precipitation of uric acid, hypoxanthine, or calcium phosphate within the renal tubules. Acute tubular necrosis is generally not seen in the setting of tumor lysis syndrome. (*Harrison's Internal Medicine online, Chap. 88, Sect. 1 "Oncologic Emergencies"*)

Allopurinol reduces the synthesis of uric acid by blocking the metabolism of xanthine and hypoxanthine to uric acid via xanthine oxidase inhibition. This makes it useful in reducing the risk of hyperuricemia from tumor lysis. Urinary alkalinization and aggressive hydration are also components of treatment. Probenecid and sulfinpyrazone enhance urate excretion by blocking the reabsorption of urate from the proximal tubule. Colchicine is effective in treating acute gout attacks by inhibiting leukocyte migration and phagocytosis. Indomethacin, and other NSAIDs, can be effective in treating acute gout attacks by inhibiting urate crystal phagocytosis. However, low-dose aspirin may actually increase the risk of gout. (*Katzung, 2004, pp. 596–599*)

212. (C)

213. (D)

Explanations 212 and 213

Any new palpable breast lesion in females (or males) of any age necessitates a mammographic evaluation and biopsy. Delay is inadvisable. Serum tumor markers, such as CA-27/29 (or even less specifically CEA), are useful to follow tumor response to therapy; however tumor markers are not reliable as diagnostic tools in breast cancer because of a relatively low sensitivity. Lobular carcinomas are frequently not visualized on mammogram, particularly standard mammograms; ultrasound however detects these tumors and should be ordered when a palpable lesion is not detected on a mammogram. *(Berg WA, 2004; U.K. Trial of Early Detection of Breast Cancer Group, Lancet 1999;343:1909–1914; J Clin Oncol 2001;19(6):1865–1878. Erratum in: J Clin Oncol 2001;19(21):4185–4188. J Clin Oncol 2002;20(8):2213)*

214. (B)

215. (A)

Explanations 214 and 215

Because there is a smoking history, it is appropriate to order a spiral CT scan to better delineate whether the mass is a tumor, an infectious process, or both. Tumor blocking a bronchus can frequently be associated with a pneumonia involving lung behind the compressed bronchus; therefore, the evaluation should include collecting the appropriate cultures along with the further imaging. *(Petty T. Ann Intern Med 2004;141:649–650)*

The full staging of small cell lung cancer is very important both for prognosis to relate to the patient and his family and to define the most appropriate therapy. Therefore, it is appropriate to order the MRI studies of the head along with CT scans with contrast of the abdomen and pelvis, a bone scan and a bone marrow aspirate and biopsy to determine if the disease is limited to the thorax or has metastasized to other organs. Small cell lung cancer limited to the thorax is potentially a disease that can achieve complete, long-term remissions with appropriate therapy. Small cell lung cancer metastatic beyond the chest can be well palliated but, at this time, our current treatments are unable to induce a long-term disease-free remission. Surgery alone is not an appropriate treatment for small cell lung cancer. Even with a successful complete tumor resection, without systemic therapy (chemotherapy), the small cell lung cancer recurs in 100% of cases within months to several years. *(Devita VT, 2000, pp. 983–1018)*

216. (A) The colonoscopy image demonstrates the pseudomembranes classically seen in pseudomembranous colitis, also known as *Clostridium difficile* colitis. *C. difficile* colitis is commonly encountered in patients on broad-spectrum antibiotics, although almost any antibiotic can predispose a patient to this illness. The disease is toxin mediated, and is frequently seen when antibiotics disrupt the normal balance of gut flora, allowing *C. difficile* to more widely colonize the bowel than it would normally. Crohn colitis and ulcerative colitis would have different patterns of ulceration of the mucosa, which is not seen here. Ischemic colitis would appear as an area or areas of blanched, edematous, or frankly necrotic mucosa due to an interruption of vascular flow. Microscopic colitis, which can cause a chronic form of watery diarrhea, typically has a normal appearance at colonoscopy.

The first-line therapy for patients diagnosed with pseudomembranous colitis is typically a course of oral metronidazole. Patients can also receive oral vancomycin, although this is usually reserved for persistent or recurrent infection. Oral vancomycin also carries a much higher cost than metronidazole. Oral or topical steroids would be contraindicated in the setting of an infection, although these medications are frequently used in patients with IBD such as ulcerative colitis or Crohn colitis. Sulfasalazine is a topical anti-inflammatory agent that is also used for patients with IBD. *(Harrison's Principles of Internal Medicine, 15th ed., pp. 923–924, 926–927)*

217. (D) The patient likely has hyperparathyroidism. Hyperparathyroidism can lead to chronic hypercalcemia, a known cause of acute pancreatitis. A serum calcium level can be elevated in many patients during acute pancreatitis due to dehydration and should be checked after the event has resolved. Hyperparathyroidism would also explain his urinary frequency and muscle weakness. Laboratory error is unlikely given that the level is elevated on two occasions. Metastatic bone disease and sarcoidosis can also cause hypercalcemia but hyperparathyroidism is more commonly associated with pancreatitis. Vitamin D overdose is unlikely given his lack of medication use. *(Harrison's Principles of Internal Medicine, 15th ed., pp. 2209–2213)*

218. (B)

219. (C)

220. (D)

Explanations 218 through 220

Vasospasm severe enough to reduce flow and produce cyanosis after exposure to cold is called Raynaud phenomenon. Some make a further distinction between Raynaud syndrome when the phenomenon is associated with another systemic disorder and Raynaud disease when there is no established systemic process. Similarly, Raynaud phenomenon in the absence of a systemic illness may also be referred to as primary Raynaud phenomenon, and Raynaud in the presence of another systemic illness may be termed secondary Raynaud phenomenon.

In this case, there is no evidence of another systemic illness. Clinical features suggesting SLE or RA are absent. Subacute bacterial endocarditis likewise would be expected to be associated with fever, which is absent in this patient. In addition, one would expect to see areas of necrosis either in the soft tissue (Janeway spots) or under the fingernails (splinter hemorrhages) were any kind of embolic phenomenon is present. *(Harrison's Principles of Internal Medicine, 15th ed., pp. 1438–1439)*

Given the patient's age, it is reasonable to explore the possibility of an associated systemic illness. If one were present, basic laboratories such as blood count, urinalysis, and chemistries are important. ANA is a reasonable screening study in this case. It does have a

prognostic value increasing the likelihood of the development of a systemic process in the future. If positive, further serologic studies might then be helpful in establishing a more specific diagnosis. The arterial Doppler with cold stimulation can be a useful test in showing a marked drop in blood flow with cold exposure. Still, with such a classical description, it is hard to imagine how this test would be helpful either diagnostically or therapeutically.

Antidouble-stranded DNA antibodies would establish the diagnosis of SLE. Likewise, the antiscleroderma antibodies (anti-Scl-70) would be a very important prognostic marker once the ANA is positive and certainly would occasion a rheumatic disease consultation. Patients with hypercoagulable states, including those with positive cardiolipin antibodies, can often mimic Raynaud's. Given that the patient wants to become pregnant, this would be an important study to obtain. Sjögren antibodies, both SSA and SSB, are important in this case because of the contemplated pregnancy. Sjögren antibodies can cross the placenta and create the syndrome of neonatal lupus (complete heart block, thrombocytopenia, and rash). *(Harrison's Principles of Internal Medicine, 15th ed., pp. 1922–1928)*

221. (D)

222. (A)

223. (E)

Explanations 221 through 223

In all likelihood, this patient is presenting with a systemic inflammatory arthritis. Clearly, treatment will need to be initiated. In order to effectively and promptly treat her, you will need to understand the current state of her physiology. Therefore, basic laboratory studies including blood count, full chemistries, and urinalysis should be obtained. At this point, the most likely diagnosis is RA, and the rheumatoid factor and sedimentation rate may be helpful. Theoretically, sarcoidosis can present in this way but, epidemiologically, this is much less likely. Because of this and because the ACE level is fairly nonspecific, it should not be part of the

RF+ ANA- HCV

initial workup. Neither joint fluid aspiration nor uric acid levels are likely to be diagnostic. The elevation of serum transaminase in the face of elevated sedimentation rate, moderate or low positive ANA, and rheumatoid factors raise the question about hepatitis C. About 50% of patients with active hepatitis C will have cryoglobulinemia. Cryoglobulins can produce low moderate positive rheumatoid factors. Therefore, it is extremely important in this circumstance to be certain that hepatitis C is not present.

With such a low positive ANA, the likelihood that this is classical Lupus is low, and double-stranded DNA antibodies are not likely to be revealing. C-reactive protein may confirm the presence of inflammation, but it won't provide additional information over the sedimentation rate. Syphilis, "the great imitator," again may occasionally have arthritis as a manifestation—but rarely without other features. The remaining studies while they might be useful later but are unlikely to be helpful as the next most important test obtained.

The probable source of the patient's symptoms is RA. Osteoarthritis can produce articular swelling, but on physical examination, there is rarely bogginess in the synovium. Anti-CCP antibody is an antibody directed against the citrullinated portion of fillagen. It has the highest specificity for RA of any antibody known. It is usually present early and may predict more severe disease. (*Am Fam Physician 2005;72:1037–1047, 1049–1050*)

224. (B)

225. (D)

Explanations 224 and 225

The clinical features presented by the patient suggest a myopathy. It is often forgotten that serum transaminases are found in the muscle as well as the liver. Thus, a significant inflammatory myopathy may present with elevated serum transaminases in addition to symptoms. In this patient with normal alkaline phosphatase and bilirubin, initial measurement of the GGT would help rule out liver pathology and would be more appropriate initially than ultrasonography.

Rhabdomyolysis may lead to renal dysfunction or even renal failure and a kidney ultrasound may eventually be appropriate, but a urinalysis would be recommended first. An MRI of the lumbar spine is not needed for this evaluation.

It has long been established that there is an association between dermatomyositis, polymyositis, and malignancy. Although the malignancy risk is slightly higher in patients with dermatomyositis than with polymyositis, the malignancy association with both diseases is well established. The overall risk of cancer is highest in the first 3 years after the diagnosis of the myopathy, but it also continues over the individual's lifetime. Cancers most highly associated with inflammatory myopathy include lung, pancreatic, GI tract, non-Hodgkin lymphoma, and ovarian. (*Am Fam Physician 2001;64:1565–1572*)

226. (C)

227. (A)

Explanations 226 and 227

The most likely diagnosis in this case is fibromyalgia. Occasionally, hypothyroidism can present in this way, and a low-grade myopathy can create many of these symptoms. A reasonable workup would include chemistries, TSH, and CPK.

The usefulness of Epstein-Barr virus titers in this case is minimal. Epidemiologic studies reveal that about 90% of Americans over the age of 20 have been exposed to Epstein-Barr virus even if they never had a clinical scenario of mononucleosis. Your physical examination did not show any question of acute infectious mononucleosis. Findings of elevated IgG antibodies to Epstein-Barr virus would only reveal the fact that she has had the disease in the past. Absent titers might assure you that there was no evidence of a previous infection, but it is unclear how that would help you sort out the current situation. (*Cecil Textbook of Medicine, 22nd ed., pp. 1710–1712*)

228. (E)

229. (A)

Explanations 228 and 229

The diagnosis is almost certainly temporal arteritis. Age over 70, headache with scalp tenderness, jaw claudication, and visual disturbance would suggest the diagnosis even if the sedimentation rate came back within the normal range. Since the patient's supraspinatus and infraspinatus strength are normal, complete rotator cuff tear seems unlikely. Rotator cuff tears would also not explain the leg component. Osteoarthritis of the neck and back could explain many of her clinical features, particularly if spinal stenosis is present, but would not account for the jaw claudication or the headaches with scalp tenderness. Many patients with temporal arteritis have features of polymyalgia rheumatica, but in this case, temporal arteritis is the best working diagnosis.

Temporal arteritis is one of the few unequivocal rheumatic disease emergencies. The patient should be given large doses of prednisone immediately. An ESR should be obtained, but as noted above, even a normal study would not prevent the prednisone from being prescribed at this point. You should also contact the ophthalmologist because there can be retinal clues not picked up on standard office funduscopy. In addition, many ophthalmologists now will do the temporal artery biopsy in their patients. This is a very reasonable next step for the patient and will unequivocally establish the diagnosis. Temporal arteritis may have skip lesions, and thus, a fairly significant length of the temporal artery should be taken by the surgeon. MRI of the brain, even with MRA, will not help establish a diagnosis of temporal arteritis and will needlessly delay diagnosis, possibly causing the patient to lose vision. (*Cecil Textbook of Medicine, 22nd ed., pp. 1693–1695*)

230. (C) The patient appears to be at risk for hereditaty nonpolyposis colon cancer (HNPCC) or Lynch syndrome. This autosomally dominant inherited cancer predisposition is characterized by colorectal cancer involving at least two generations, with one or more cases being diagnosed before age 50, and patients may have multiple primary cancers (affected women often also have endometrial or ovarian

cancer). It is recommended that HNPCC family members undergo screening colonoscopy every two years beginning at age 25. The colon cancers in HNPCC often involve the proximal colon, so flexible sigmoidoscopy would be an insufficient tool for screening the at-risk bowel.

HNPCC should be differentiated from familial adenomatous polyposis (FAP), another inherited colon cancer predisposition. This well-studied and described autosomal dominant inherited condition is much less common than HNPCC. Affected patients develop thousands of adenomatous premalignant polyps, which are generally evenly distributed from cecum to anus and usually become evident between puberty and age 25. Because the polyps are so widespread and evenly distributed, proctosigmoidoscopy is usually a sufficient screening procedure for at-risk family members. When diagnosed with FAP, it is recommended that patients under prophylactic colectomy. If not treated surgically, almost all patients will develop colorectal cancer by age 40.

Colonoscopy beginning at age 50 would be recommended for persons at average risk for colon cancer. (*Harrison's Principles of Internal Medicine, 16th ed., pp. 527–528*)

231. (C) History of excess sun exposure and sunburn early in life is associated with increased incidence of skin cancers, including melanoma (2–4 times increased risk), but the highest risk would be the development of a suspicious pigmented lesion. Clinicians can be guided by the "ABCD" rules: asymmetry, irregular borders, color variegation within the same lesion, and diameter >6 mm. Other risk factors for melanoma would include fair skin and hair with tendency to burn easily and a family history of melanoma. Actinic keratoses are premalignant lesions, but can develop into cutaneous squamous cell malignancies, not melanoma. (*Harrison's Principles of Internal Medicine, 16th ed., pp. 498–503*)

232. (A) Although gastric lymphomas are less common than adenocarcinomas, they are much more treatable with a more favorable prognosis. Gastric lymphomas, especially well-differentiated mucosa-associated lymphoid tissue (MALT),

are associated with *Helicobacter pylori* infection, and antibiotic therapy to eradicate *H. pylori* has been associated with regression of 75% of such tumors. Higher-grade gastric lymphomas may require chemotherapy with a standard regimen, such as CHOP, and consideration for surgical resection with curative intent. *(Harrison's Principles of Internal Medicine, 16th ed., p. 526)*

233. (A)

234. (B)

235. (C)

Explanations 233 through 235

The patient has symptoms of spinal cord compression and needs an urgent MRI to establish the diagnosis. Spinal cord compression usually develops when patients have metastases to the vertebral body with epidural extension of the tumor, displacing the underlying thecal sac, and causing cord edema and injury. Patients with cord compression usually experience new or worsening pain symptoms days or weeks before the development of motor weakness below the level of compression. Loss of sensation and loss of bowel or bladder control occur even later. Clues that the pain symptoms may represent cord injury include pain that is worse with recumbency or Valsalva and the occurrence of Lhermitte's sign, an electric sensation down the back and into the extremities with extension or flexion of the neck or spine. Initiation of therapy, such as radiation therapy or neurosurgical intervention, might be necessary later but would be premature before the diagnosis is established with an imaging study. If the patient's history or physical exam suggests spinal cord compression, initiation of corticosteroids should be started immediately while diagnostic imaging is pending. Pain control with adequate narcotic analgesia is important and may be instituted while the appropriate diagnostic studies are being obtained. Delay of 1 week would be inappropriate due to the urgent nature of the problem and risk of neurological compromise.

The patient's neurological status at the time of diagnosis is the most important prognostic factor: 75–80% of patients who are ambulatory at the time of diagnosis will retain locomotion. But, if already paraplegic, only 10% will regain the ability to walk. While this patient appeared neurologically intact, the development of neurological deficits can progress over a period of days, making rapid diagnosis and institution of appropriate therapy such as corticosteroids and radiotherapy an urgent consideration. Other factors such as age, presence of co-morbid medical conditions, functional status, and tumor androgen-sensitivity are important to the patient's overall cancer prognosis. *(Harrison's Principls of Internal Medicine, 16th ed., pp. 577–579)*

Standard therapy for patients with metastatic prostate cancer is to block testosterone action or decrease its production to inhibit tumor stimulation. Surgical orchiectomy would be the most definitive anti-androgen therapy, but most patients favor medical therapy. Leuprolide is a gonadotropin-releasing hormone (GnRH) analogue, which produces a transient rise in luteinizing hormone (LH) and follicle-stimulating hormone (FSH), which is then followed by downregulation of pituitary receptors and subsequent "chemical castration." The transient LH and FSH rise causes an initial rise in serum testosterone concentration, and may produce a "tumor flare," with worsening of symptoms during the first 1–2 weeks of therapy, including bone pain and bladder outlet obstruction, and for patients with epidural tumor, can precipitate spinal cord compression. When the level of testosterone falls, patients may experience side effects such as testicular atrophy, loss of libido, and vasomotor symptoms. *(Harrison's Principles of Internal Medicine, 16th ed., p. 548)*

236. (A)

237. (B)

Explanations 236 and 237

The patient is hypercalcemic and has laboratory features suggesting dehydration, as do most patients with symptomatic hypercalcemia. Initial management would include saline rehydration, which replaces volume deficits, dilutes the elevated serum calcium, and promotes urinary calcium excretion. The addition of loop diuretics such as furosemide can also increase calciuresis, but should only be added after the patient has had adequate volume repletion. Administration of bisphosphanates, such as pamidronate or zoledronate, provide more powerful reduction of serum calcium by inhibiting bone resorption and liberation of calcium. Their effects may last for several weeks, but their onset of action does not occur for 1–2 days. Subcutaneous calcitonin can provide a faster onset of action to inhibit bone resorption within a few hours, but patients develop tachyphylaxis and become unresponsive to the drug effect within 24–48 hours.

Most cancer patients with hypercalcemia develop this problem as a paraneoplastic phenomenon, due to the production of a parathyroid hormone-related protein (PTHrP). This problem, called humoral hypercalcemia of malignancy (HHM), is very common, affecting 5–10% of all cancer patients. The diagnosis is usually straightforward, as there is a readily-available laboratory assay for PTHrP. Other cancer patients develop HHM due to the production of an enzyme that converts 25-hydroxyvitamin D to the more active 1,25-hydroxyvitamin D, similar to the hypercalcemia seen in patients with granulomatous diseases. Severe hypercalcemia solely due to the presence of osteolytic metastases is much less common. Hyperparathyroidism and medications such as thiazide diuretics can also cause elevations of serum calcium, but usually not to the severe levels seen in HHM. (*Harrison's Principles of Internal Medicine, 16th ed., pp. 566–567*)

238. (C)

239. (A)

Explanations 238 and 239

The patient's most likely diagnosis is superior vena cava syndrome (SVCS), which is usually due to external compression of the SVC by tumor or lymph nodes, sometimes associated with intraluminal thrombosis. The diagnosis is established by CT of the chest with intravenous contrast, which can demonstrate the level and extent of obstruction, as well as the presence of any caval thrombus.

Plain chest radiography may show some mediastinal widening, but yields much less information. Echocardiography would be appropriate if the patient had suspected pericardial effusion with tamponade, but that would not produce unilateral arm edema and discoloration. Doppler studies of the deep veins of the arm would be useful if the problem were isolated to the upper extremity. In this case, the cerebral venous drainage is also involved, so the obstruction is more proximal, i.e. at the level of the SVC. Arteriogram would not be indicated, since the issue in this case is venous obstruction, not arterial insufficiency.

Unless the patient has cerebral edema with mental status changes or upper airway compromise due to tracheal obstruction, the diagnosis of SVCS is not immediately life-threatening, and emergent therapy is not usually indicated. The majority of patients with SVCS present with this as the initial presentation of their malignancy, before a tissue diagnosis has been established. This is problematic, since therapy is guided by the underlying malignancy (radiation therapy for non-small cell lung cancers, chemotherapy +/− radiation for small cell lung cancers or lymphomas), but empiric initiation of radiation or glucorticoids (if the underlying diagnosis is lymphoma) may obscure the histologic diagnosis. The most important initial step is to try to obtain a biopsy to establish the cancer type before initiating therapy. If symptoms are severe, placement of intravascular stents may provide rapid symptomatic relief without compromising subsequent diagnostic or therapeutic efforts. Surgical intervention is rarely indicated, and usually only for benign causes of SVCS. (*Harrison's Principles of Internal Medicine, 16th ed., pp. 575–576*)

240. (C) This patient has neutropenia (neutrophil count <500/μL) with fever. For high-risk patients, such as patients with leukemia, the standard of care is to obtain cultures and a chest radiograph, perform any other studies as indicated by the patient's clinical presentation, and initiate empiric antibiotic therapy. Guidelines from the Infectious Disease Society of America recommend empiric broad-spectrum coverage for Gram-negative organisms, including anti-pseudomonal coverage. Antibiotics such as vancomycin, for Gram-positive infection, are added if there is hypotension, suspicion for a central venous catheter-related infection, or recent or current evidence for Gram-positive infection (such as MRSA colonization, or positive culture for Gram-positive cocci). (*Harrison's Principles of Internal Medicine, 16th ed., pp. 494–495; 2002 IDSA Guidelines for the use of antimicrobial agents in neutropenic patients with cancer. Clin Infect Dis 2002;34:730*)

241. (D) This patient has tumor lysis syndrome (TLS), a group of metabolic derangements due to rapid cell turnover with release of intracellular contents, such as phosphate and potassium, and increased purine metabolism, leading to hyperuricemia. It is usually seen after the initiation of cytotoxic chemotherapy, but occasionally occurs spontaneously in patients with bulky disease such as Burkitt's lymphoma. The uric acid crystallizes in the renal tubules and can cause oliguric renal failure. Once renal failure has occurred, patients usually require hemodialysis until renal function recovers. Each of the other choices may be employed to prevent the development of TLS in high-risk patients prior to beginning chemotherapy. (*Harrison's Principles of Internal Medicine, 16th ed., pp. 581–582*)

242. (C) This patient has clinical signs of congestive heart failure. Cardiomyopathy may be a complication of chemotherapy containing anthracyclines (doxorubicin, daunorubicin, idarubicin, epirubicin). The cumulative anthracycline dose is the most widely recognized risk factor for this problem, although it is more common in patients over 70, patients with any other history of heart disease, or those with a history of thoracic radiation treatment. Other reversible causes of heart failure such as ischemic cardiomyopathy should be investigated. Patients with anthracycline cardiomyopathy frequently have recovery of systolic function with standard medical heart failure therapy.

Lack of chest pain and a normal EKG make acute pericarditis or acute myocardial infarction unlikely. Pericardial effusion with tamponade might cause dyspnea and edema, but not pulmonary vascular congestion or pulmonary edema. (*Harrison's Principles of Internal Medicine, 16th ed., pp. 519–522*)

243. (B) This patient has a solitary pulmonary nodule. Overall, 35% of these lesions are malignant, usually primary lung cancers. In patients under 35 years of age without a smoking history, <1% of such lesions are malignant. Certain patterns of calcification within the nodule suggest a benign cause ("bulls-eye" pattern in granulomas, and "popcorn ball" in hamartomas), but these features alone cannot exclude malignancy. For low-risk patients such as this man, if the lesion remains stable on serial imaging studies (such as serial CT every 3–6 months) for 2 years, then no biopsy is deemed necessary to exclude malignancy. (*Harrison's Principles of Internal Medicine, 16th ed., pp. 512–513*)

244. (A)

245. (E)

246. (A)

Explanations 244 through 246

Human papillomavirus has been associated with the development of multiple squamous cell malignancies, including cervical cancer (HPV types 16, 18, 31, 45, and 51–53), as well as anal, penile, and vulvar cancers. Recent evidence has also linked some oropharyngeal squamous cell cancers to HPV infection as well. The risk for HPV-associated cancer is increased in patients with HIV co-infection. HPV type 11 may cause genital warts but is not a likely cause of cervical cancer. The presence of other sexually transmitted diseases, such as chlamydia or hepatitis B, may help to identify women at high risk for cervical cancer, but they are not direct causes of cervical cancer.

Following the abnormal pap smear findings, the next step in the diagnosis of this patient would be a colposcopy with biopsy of any visualized cervical abnormalities. At this point, HPV testing and typing would not add to or change the work-up, so they would not be necessary. HPV testing and typing can be helpful in the evaluation of women with lower grade cervical cytological abnormalities, such as ASCUS. The other tests noted may be performed later in the diagnostic work-up, after the results of the biopsies are known.

Stage Ia cervical cancer is usually treated with simple hysterectomy with good outcomes. Women who wish to preserve fertility may sometimes be treated with cervical conization with close follow-up. (*Harrison's Principles of Internal Medicine, 16th ed., pp. 557, 533; Cervical cancer. Am Fam Physician 2000;61:1369–1376*)

247. (C) Burkitt's lymphoma and nasopharyngeal carcinomas are associated with the Epstein-Barr virus. Gastric carcinoma is associated with *H. pylori* infection. Kaposi's sarcoma is associated with human herpesvirus 7. The rate of hepatocellular carcinoma is greatly increased in those with chronic hepatitis B and C. Hepatitis B virus infection is the leading cause of hepatocellular carcinoma worldwide, usually after congenital infection in Asia and Africa. Of these infections, only hepatitis B has a widely available, routinely recommended vaccine. (*Harrison's Principles of Internal Medicine, 16th ed., p. 534*)

248. (B) A painless, firm testicular mass is a classic presentation of testicular cancer, although some men have pain or scrotal swelling as well. When such a mass is found on examination, ultrasound is the next indicated study to confirm whether the mass is truly located on the testicle or if it is associated with another structure, most commonly the epididymis. Once the presence is confirmed, an inguinal orchiectomy is the procedure of choice for both diagnostic and therapeutic purposes, as the vascular and lymphatic drainage of the testis is through the inguinal canal. Antibiotic therapy may play a role if the enlarged area is in the epididymis and not the testicle. Semen cytology plays no role in the work-up of suspected testicular malignancy. (*Testicular cancer. Am Fam Physician. 1999 May 1;59(9):2539–2544, 2549–2550.*)

249. (C) The classic triad of pheochromocytoma is sweating, headache, and palpitations. When these are associated with hypertension, they have a sensitivity and specificity of >90% for the diagnosis. Paroxysms are not a component of aldosterone secreting tumors or renal artery stenosis. Hyperthyroidism and panic attacks would be in the differential diagnosis, but thyroid cancer is not associated with hypertension. (*Cecil Textbook of Medicine, 22nd ed., pp. 1420–1424*)

250. (A) Galactorrhea with amenorrhea is consistent with hyperprolactinemia. The additional history of headache and possible visual field changes or cranial nerve abnormalities is strongly suggestive of a pituitary tumor. In this setting, the most likely diagnosis is prolactinoma. Ovarian failure, Kallman syndrome, and Sheehan syndrome would not present with galactorrhea. Kallman syndrome is associated with primary amenorrhea and anosmia. PCOS presents with a long history of irregular cycles and hyperandrogenism. (*Cecil Textbook of Medicine, 22nd ed., pp. 1376–1377*)

251. (C) The patient has a strong family history of thyroid cancer and has a thyroid nodule, hypertension, tachycardia, and hypercalcemia. These are hallmarks of Multiple Endocrine Neoplasia Type 2 (MEN-2) syndrome, which is associated with medullary thyroid cancer, pheochromocytoma, and hyperparathyroidism. The very high calcitonin level is an excellent tumor marker for medullary thyroid cancer and a fine needle aspiration is not indicated. She will need to have an evaluation and treatment for pheochromocytoma prior to treatment of her thyroid cancer. (*Cecil Textbook of Medicine, 22nd ed., pp. 1458–1459*)

252. (B) The patient has type I diabetes, therefore oral agents are contraindicated. The glucose pattern he has is known as the Somogyi phenomenon. His increased activity has made him more insulin sensitive, especially at the time of the day that he is most at risk of hypoglycemic reactions. When NPH is given at supper time, the peak action will be ~2 a.m. Changing the timing of the NPH to bedtime, will advance the peak to ~4–6 a.m., a time when the patient is becoming increasingly insulin resistant (Dawn phenomenon). As his glucose is already increasing at supper, discontinuing the regular insulin at that time may avoid nocturnal hypoglycemia, but at the expense of higher

glucose values. Increasing the regular insulin at breakfast will likely cause hypoglycemia prior to lunch. *(Am Fam Physician 1999)*

253. **(C)** Hereditary spherocytosis (HS) is a familial hemolytic disorder with clinical features, ranging from an asymptomatic condition to a fulminant hemolytic anemia. The morphologic hallmark of HS is the microspherocyte, which result from membrane protein defects leading to cytoskeleton instability. Spectrin deficiency leads to loss of erythrocyte surface area, which produces spherical RBCs. Spherocytic RBCs are culled from the circulation by the spleen leading to the development of splenomegaly. Spectrin deficiency and the degree of deficiency correlate with the extent of spherocytosis, the degree of abnormality on osmotic fragility test results, and the severity of hemolysis. Hemolysis primarily is confined to the spleen and, therefore, is extravascular. Although four abnormalities in red cell membrane proteins have been identified, spectrin deficiency is the most common. Spectrin deficiency results from impaired synthesis, whereas in other instances, it is caused by quantitative or qualitative deficiencies of other proteins that integrate spectrin into the cell membrane. In the absence of these binding proteins, free spectrin is degraded, leading to spectrin deficiency. The major complications are aplastic or megaloblastic crisis, hemolytic crisis, cholecystitis and cholelithiasis, and severe neonatal hemolysis.

   The classic laboratory features of HS include minimal or no anemia, reticulocytosis, an increased mean corpuscular hemoglobin concentration (MCHC), spherocytes on the peripheral blood smear, hyperbilirubinemia, and abnormal results on the osmotic fragility test. The most sensitive test to help detect HS is the osmotic fragility test performed after incubating RBCs for 18–24 hours under sterile conditions at 37°C. Osmotic fragility measures RBC resistance to hemolysis when exposed to a series of increasingly dilute saline solutions. The sooner hemolysis occurs, the greater the osmotic fragility of the cells. *(Shah S, Vega R. Hereditary spherocytosis. Pediatr Rev 2004;25(5):168–172)*

254. **(E)** A 1:1 mixing study is done when the PT or PTT is prolonged. The patient's plasma is mixed with normal plasma and the abnormal test is repeated. If the mixing of normal plasma corrects the abnormal test (PT or PTT), then a factor deficiency is suggested; otherwise, an inhibitor is suspected. Similarly, an incubated mixing study is done 1 hour (and occasionally 2 hours) after mixing of the patient plasma with normal plasma. It is used to differentiate a lupus anticoagulant from factor inhibitors. *(Hematol Oncol Clin North Am 1994;8:809–853; Sallah & Kato, Postgrad Med 1998;103:209–210)*

255. **(E)**

256. **(A)**

257. **(D)**

258. **(E)**

Explanations 255 through 258

   This patient has sickle cell anemia. This is evident from sickle cells forms on the peripheral blood smear in Figure 1-13. Pain medication is an important initial concern. It is often difficult to determine whether a patient in sickle cell crisis has an ongoing infection. Infections can precipitate sickle cell crisis. With respect to community-acquired pneumonia, the diagnosis is difficult. A patient with sickle cell crisis can have fever as a result of the sickle crisis. They can have an increased respiratory rate, physical examination, and CXR findings which suggest pneumonia as a result of pulmonary infarctions. A white blood count can be elevated due to marrow stimulation. In the presence of the acute chest syndrome, characterized by chest pain, hypoxia, and CXR infiltrates, antibiotics would be indicated. Without further information, it is hard to decide to empirically start broad-spectrum antibiotics for community-acquired pneumonia. Transfusions should generally be avoided in patients with sickle cell anemia who are not symptomatic due to the anemia. Since patients in sickle cell crisis have intravascular hemolysis, their reticulocyte counts are usually high and they can replace their blood quickly. Repeated small transfusions will lead to autoantibodies that will make further transfusions difficult. Arterial blood gas determination should not be the first step, given the above information. A CT scan of the abdomen is not indicated given the nonspecific nature of the patient's abdominal findings.

Parvovirus B19 can cause aplastic crisis in patients with hemoglobinopathies, including sickle cell disease. A tip to this diagnosis is the decreased reticulocyte count in a patient who normally would have a high reticulocyte count. Given the information listed above, there is no indication for broad-spectrum antibiotics. Splenectomy is not a reasonable alternative at this point. Patients with sickle cell disease have autosplenectomy by the time they are adults. A bone marrow biopsy maybe indicated because of the low platelet count, but not initially. GnCSF is not indicated because the patient does not have neutropenia.

Patients with sickle cell disease typically have isosthenuria. This is due to repeated /pə'pilī/ infarction of the renal papilli. This causes destruction and interference with the counter current mechanism that causes urine concentration. As a result, patients with sickle cell anemia have the inability to concentrate their urine. This results in fluid and electrolyte abnormalities. Patients in sickle cell crisis are usually fluid depleted. This and the sickled blood cells cause hyperviscosity and microinfarctions. There is no evidence that the patient has diabetes insipidus, which usually has a urine specific gravity less than 1.005. Patients with UTIs do

/ī, säs thə'ncyūrēə/

not have isosthenuria due to RBCs and WBCs that increase the urine specific gravity. Sickle cell patients may have zinc deficiency, but this is not a cause of isosthenuria.

Patients with sickle cell anemia frequently have avascular necrosis of the hips and sometimes shoulders. This is not due to infection. While patients with HIV can have avascular necrosis of the hips, sickle cell anemia is a risk factor for this in and of itself. There is no evidence that the patient has Cushing syndrome. Patients taking chronic corticosteroids can have avascular necrosis of the hip. While patients with sickle cell anemia can develop arthritis, this is not a cause of avascular necrosis.

Patients with sickle cell disease undergo splenectomy in childhood due to repeated sickling and infarction. Patients with Hgb SC disease may have splenomegaly. Patients with sickle cell disease have a decreased susceptibility to malaria. Priapism occurs in men with sickle cell disease, rather than erectile dysfunction. Peripheral neuropathy is not a common complication of sickle cell disease, but strokes are frequently one of the causes of death in these patients. Pulmonary microinfarctions are common, and patients can also have pulmonary embolism, but there is no increase in deep venous thrombosis. *(Cecil Textbook of Medicine, 22nd ed., pp. 1030–1039, Chap. 171 "Sickle Cell Anemia and associated Hemoglobinopathies"; Mandell, 6th ed., Chap. 143 "Parvovirus B19")*

BIBLIOGRAPHY

American Diabetes Association. Diagnosis and classification of diabetes mellitus. *Diabetes Care* 2004;27:S5–S10.

American Cancer Society. Cancer Facts and Figures for African Americans 2005–2006. Available at: www.cancer.org/downloadsSTT/CAFF2005AACorrPWSecured.pdf.

Berg WA Diagnostic accuracy of mammography, clinical examination, US, and MR imaging in preoperative assessment of breast cancer. *Radiology* 2004.

Bisno AL, Gerber MA, Gwaltney JM, et al. Practice guidelines for the diagnosis and management of group A streptococcal pharyngitis. *Clin Infect Dis* 2002;35(2):113–125.

Braunwald E, Hauser SL, Jameson JL, et al. *Harrison's Principles of Internal Medicine*, 15th ed. New York, NY: McGraw-Hill, 2001.

Brenner BM. *Brenner & Rectors's The Kidney*, 7th ed. Philadelphia, PA: W.B. Saunders, 2004.

Canavan TP, Dashi NR. Cervical cancer. *Am Fam Physician* 2000;61:1369–1376.

Centers for Disease Control and Prevention Advisory Committee on Immunization Practices (ACIP) "General Recommendations on Immunization," 2006, available at: www.cdc.gov.

Devita VT. *Cancer Principles and Practice of Oncology*, 6th ed., 2000, pp. 983–1018.

Freedberg IM, Eisen AZ, Wolff K, et al., eds. *Fitzpatrick's Dermatology in General Medicine.* New York, NY: McGraw-Hill, 2003.

Friedman DG, Kravertz JD, Braveta DM, et al. *Peripheral arterial disease.* Postgrad Med 2006; 119(2):21–27. Available at: www.postgradmed.com/issues/2006/07/021.

Gastrointestinal Consortium Panel. Colorectal cancer screening and surveillance: clinical guidelines and rationale. Update based on new evidence. *Gastroenterology* 2003;124(2):544–560.

Goldman L, Ausiello D, eds. *Cecil Textbook of Medicine*, 22nd ed. Philadelphia, PA: W.B. Saunders, 2004.

Hardman JG, Limbird LE, Molinoff PB, et al., eds. *Goodman & Gilman's The Pharmacological Basis of Therapeutics*, 10th ed. New York, NY: McGraw-Hill, 2001.

Hirsch IB. Type 1 diabetes mellitus and the use of flexible insulin regimens. *Am Fam Physician* 1999;60:2343–2356.

Hodgson SF, Watts NB, Bilezikian JP, et al. American Association of Clinical Endocrinologists medical guidelines for clinical practice for the prevention and treatment of postmenopausal osteoporosis: 2001 edition, with selected updates for 2003. *Endocr Pract* 2003;9(6):544–564.

Hoffman R, Benz EJ, Shattil SJ, et al. *Hematology: Basic Principles and Practice*, 3rd ed. New York, NY: Churchill Livingstone, 2000.

Huhn GD. West Nile virus in the United States: update on an emerging infectious disease. *Am Fam Physician* 2003;68:653–660, 671–672.

IDSA guidelines for the use of antimicrobial agents in neutropenic patients with cancer. *Clin Infect Dis* 2002:34:730.

Kaspar DL, Braunwald E, Fauci AS, et al., eds. *Harrison's Principles of Internal Medicine, 16th ed.* New York, NY: McGraw-Hill, 2005.

Katzung BG, ed. *Basic & Clinical Pharmacology*, 9th ed. New York, NY: McGraw-Hill, 2004.

Kinkade S. Testicular cancer. *Am Fam Physician* 1999 May 1;59(9):2539–2544, 2549–2550.

Koler RA, Montemarano A. Dermatomyositis. *Am Fam Physician* 2001;64:1565–1572.

Kottke-Marchant K. Laboratory diagnosis of hemorrhagic and thrombotic disorders. *Hematol Oncol Clin North Am* 1994;8:809–853.

Kunimoto DY, Kanitkar KD, Makar MS, et al. *The Wills Eye Manual: Office and Emergency Room Diagnosis and Treatment of Eye Disease*, 4th ed. Philadelphia, PA: Lippincott Williams & Wilkins, 2004.

Larsen PR, Davies TF, Hay ID, et al. *Williams Textbook of Endocrinology*, 10th ed. Philadelphia, PA: W.B. Saunders, 2003.

Mandell GL, Bennett JE, Mandell DR. *Mandell, Douglas and Bennett's Principles and Practice of Infectious Diseases*, 5th ed. Philadelphia, PA: Churchill Livingstone, 2000.

National Institutes of Health. *The Third Report of the National Cholesterol Education Program Expert Panel on the Detection, Evaluation, and Treatment of High*

Blood Cholesterol in Adults. Bethesda, MD: National Institutes of Health, 2001.

National Institutes of Health. *The 7th Report of the Joint National Committee on the Prevention, Detection, Evaluation, and Treatment of High Blood Pressure.* Bethesda, MD: National Institutes of Health, 2003. NIH Publication No. 03-5233.

Peacock WF. Congestive heart failure and pulmonary edema. In: Tintinalli J, Kelen G, Stapczynski J, eds. *Emergency Medicine: A Comprehensive Study Guide,* 6th ed. New York, NY: McGraw-Hill, 2003.

Rex DK, Kahi CJ, Levin B, et al. Guidelines for colonoscopy surveillance after cancer resection: a consensus update by the American Cancer Society and US Multi-Society Task Force on Colorectal Cancer. *CA Cancer J Clin* 2006;56(3):160–167; quiz 185–186.

Rindfleisch JA, Muller D. Diagnosis and management of rheumatoid arthritis. *Am Fam Physician* 2005;72:1037–1047, 1049–1050.

Ruddy S, Harris J, Sledge CM, et al. *Kelley's Textbook of Rheumatology,* 6th ed. Philadelphia, PA: W.B. Saunders, 2001.

Salkind AR, Cuddy PG, Foxworth JW. Is this patient allergic to penicillin? An evidence-based analysis of the likelihood of penicillin allergy. *JAMA* 2001;285:2498–2505.

Sallah S, Kato G. Evaluation of bleeding disorders. A detailed history and laboratory tests provide clues. *Postgrad Med* 1998;103:209–210.

U.K. Trial of Early Detection of Breast Cancer Group. 16-Year mortality from breast cancer in the U.K. trial of early detection of breast cancer. *Lancet* 1999;343:1909–1914.

Women's Health Initiative Investigators. *Risks and benefits of estrogen plus progestin in healthy postmenopausal women. JAMA* 2002;288:321–333.

Woo SB, Hellstein JW, Kalmar JR. Systematic review: bisphosphonates and osteonecrosis of the jaws. *Ann Intern Med* 2006;144(10):753–761.

CHAPTER 2

Surgery
Questions

1. 1. A 22-year-old male presents to the emergency department (ED) with complaints of right-sided chest pain and dyspnea. He has no other significant medical history. There is no history of trauma. On examination, he has a pulse of 95, BP of 110/70, and SpO_2 of 95% on 2 L. A chest x-ray reveals a large right pneumothorax. Which of the following statements is true?

   (A) Since the patient is hemodynamically stable, he can be observed with oxygen supplementation, pain control, and serial chest x-rays.
   (B) The patient is likely to have a tall, thin habitus.
   (C) This condition is probably due to small lacerations in the apex of the right lung.
   (D) His risk of recurrence is 10%.
   (E) Recurrences are usually on the contralateral side since adhesions prevent recurrence on the ipsilateral side.

2. A 10-month-old male presents with a 12-hour history of episodes of crying, holding his stomach, and bending over in pain. The parents report one "reddish" stool. He has no past medical history or episodes of similar events. He did have 24 hours of viral symptoms, which resolved a few days ago. The following study was obtained. Which of the following statements is true? (See Figure 2-1.)

FIG. 2-1 (*Courtesy of H.J. Kim, MD.*)

   (A) The initial treatment for this child involves emergent laparotomy.
   (B) Air contrast enema can be diagnostic AND therapeutic.
   (C) Colonic mass is the usual source of this problem in a child.
   (D) "Dance's sign" is the appearance on x-ray of "telescoped" intestine.
   (E) Recurrence is likely after treatment.

3. A 4-week-old, previously healthy male presents with projectile emesis after feeds. His mother states that he has had 2 weeks of postprandial emesis, which became projectile in the past 2 days. She states that it looks like formula and has never been bilious. Which of the following statements is true?

(A) Physical examination is almost always normal in patients with this condition.

(B) Upper gastrointestinal (GI) contrast study is the best diagnostic option.

(C) This patient should be taken emergently to the operating room (OR) once the diagnosis is made.

(D) If uncorrected, these infants will progress to complete obstruction.

(E) Surgical therapy involves bypassing the site of obstruction.

4. A 1-month-old female presents after an episode of bilious emesis. She became irritable 12 hours ago, began vomiting 6 hours ago, and is now lethargic. She had one small stool that was somewhat bloody 2 hours ago. Which of the following statements is true?

(A) An upper GI contrast study should be obtained immediately.

(B) The most likely explanation is pyloric stenosis.

(C) The patient should be admitted for IV fluid resuscitation and observation. If she does not improve over the next 24 hours, a surgical consultation should be obtained.

(D) An air contrast enema is the most appropriate next step.

(E) A nasogastric tube should be inserted and IV antibiotics started to treat probable necrotizing enterocolitis.

5. Which of the following statements is true concerning Meckel's diverticulum?

(A) It is found within 2 in. of the ileocecal valve.

(B) It represents a remnant of the embryonic vitelline duct.

(C) Ectopic colonic epithelium is found in it.

(D) Diagnosis is best made by CT scan.

(E) The diverticulum is usually found on the mesenteric border of the bowel.

Questions 6 and 7

6. A 55-year-old man with hepatic cirrhosis from alcohol abuse presents with a massive hematemesis. This is his third admission for upper GI hemorrhage in the past 2 months. He is currently receiving appropriate therapy for liver failure, including a beta-blocker and diuretics. He is lethargic and confused. His pulse is 100 and blood pressure is 85/40. His initial hematocrit is 20. After fluid resuscitation, which of the following is the most appropriate management strategy?

(A) The transplant team should be called immediately.

(B) The bleeding is probably secondary to an uncontrolled duodenal ulcer related to his alcohol use.

(C) Red blood cells should be administered immediately, but fresh frozen plasma should be withheld if possible.

(D) Endoscopic control options include sclerotherapy and banding.

(E) Transjugular intrahepatic portal systemic shunt (TIPS) is not an option in the immediate period.

7. Endoscopic attempts to control the bleeding are initially successful, but the patient has a recurrent bleed 2 days later. The medicine team obtains a surgical consultation for placement of a shunt. Which of the following statements is true?

(A) The best shunts are nonselective, meaning that they divert all blood from the portal system.

(B) Synthetic graft materials should never be used because of the risk of infection.

(C) A mesocaval shunt involves connecting the superior mesenteric vein (SMV) to the inferior vena cava (IVC).

(D) Encephalopathy rarely worsens after the placement of the shunt. In fact, it often improves in these patients.

(E) Postoperative mortality for emergency shunts is related more to the type of shunt placed rather than the degree of hepatic failure in the patient.

8. Which of the following is a contraindication to sentinel lymph node biopsy in breast cancer?

(A) clinically negative axillary examination

(B) multicentric disease

(C) lesion under the nipple

(D) history of previous breast biopsy

(E) patient preference for breast conservation

9. A 45-year-old male was involved in a motor vehicle collision. He was a restrained passenger in a high speed, head-on collision with a death at the scene. He is brought to the ED unresponsive with a pulse of 140, a BP of 70/30, and a SpO_2 of 80%. He has multiple facial lacerations, a dilated right pupil, a contusion on his chest, and a distended abdomen. The medic team has placed two large-bore IVs and given him 2 L of lactated Ringer's solution. The initial step in the care of this patient is:

(A) Given the mechanism, low oxygen saturation, and the presence of a contusion on his chest, the patient likely has a pneumothorax. A chest tube should be placed immediately.

(B) The patient should be taken to the OR immediately for laparotomy since he is hemodynamically unstable with abdominal distention indicating an abdominal source of life-threatening hemorrhage.

(C) The patient should be intubated using in-line traction to protect his cervical spine before continuing the assessment.

(D) Because of the facial lacerations, there is a possibility of facial fractures making endotracheal intubation risky. An emergent cricothyroidotomy should be performed. /kri kō, thī, roi 'dätəm ē/

(E) A central line should be placed immediately to continue the resuscitation.

10. A 45-year-old male receives a cadaveric liver transplant for alcoholic cirrhosis. Postoperatively, the patient is taken to the surgical intensive care unit (SICU). There is concern for primary nonfunction of the allograft. Which of the following is a sign of this?

(A) coagulopathy with an INR of 2

(B) normalizing albumin level

(C) hyperglycemia requiring an insulin drip

(D) initial rise of transaminases

(E) high urine output

11. A 50-year-old man undergoes a sigmoid colectomy and colostomy for perforated diverticulitis of the midsigmoid colon. The surgeon reports a difficult dissection in the pelvis secondary to adhesions of the sigmoid colon to the abdominal wall. On postoperative day 1, the patient reports appropriate abdominal pain. His pulse is 100 and BP 120/60. He has made 400 mL of urine over the past 8 hours. The urine in the Foley bag is blood-tinged. He reports no problems with his urination preoperatively. What is the appropriate management?

(A) Remove the Foley catheter. The irritation of the catheter is probably causing the hematuria.

(B) Increase his IV fluids and add bicarbonate in case this is rhabdomyolysis.

(C) Start antibiotics for a urinary tract infection.

(D) Order an intravenous pyelogram to assess for ureteral injury.

(E) Send a prostate-specific antigen (PSA) to screen for a prostatic process.

12. A 75-year-old man undergoes a right colectomy for stage 3 colon cancer. He has a history of emphysema requiring chronic steroid use. He also has diabetes and coronary heart disease. On postoperative day 2, the surgeon is called because the patient acutely began to have a large amount of pinkish, serous drainage from the wound. There is no evidence of infection. Which of the following factors probably contributed to this complication?

(A) the surgeon used a running stitch to close the fascia instead of interrupted sutures

(B) coronary artery disease

(C) early mobilization of patient

(D) aggressive abdominal examination performed on postoperative day 1 by a medical student

(E) pulmonary disease

13. A 22-year-old male presents complaining of a 1-month history of progressive dysphagia. He reports occasional regurgitation of undigested food at night. His past medical history is noncontributory. The condition has worsened to the point that he is on a liquid diet. A contrast swallow study is shown in Figure 2-2. What is the best treatment for this patient?

FIG. 2-2 (Courtesy of H.J. Kim, MD.)

(A) proton pump inhibitors

(B) referral to a surgeon for a Nissen fundoplication

(C) calcium channel blockers

(D) serial esophageal sphincter dilations

(E) referral to a surgeon for esophagomyotomy

14. A 45-year-old woman undergoes an uncomplicated thyroidectomy for a goiter. Later that night, she becomes agitated and complains of difficulty breathing. The surgeon notices some neck swelling at the incision site, but the dressing is clean. What should the next step be?

(A) start oxygen by nasal cannula

(B) check STAT serum calcium level

(C) endotracheal intubation to protect her airway

(D) open the incision

(E) administer propranolol and morphine

15. A patient presents with a new neck mass. On examination, she has a palpable thyroid nodule and a palpable cervical lymph node on the same side. Needle biopsy of the thyroid nodule shows amyloid in the stroma. The treatment for this patient is which of the following?

(A) total thyroidectomy and modified neck dissection

(B) resection of the involved thyroid lobe, isthmusectomy, and removal of the palpable lymph node

(C) total thyroidectomy and radiation therapy

(D) resection of the involved lobe and part of the contralateral lobe, isthmusectomy, and removal of the palpable lymph node

(E) radioactive iodine administration

16. Which of the following statements is true about primary hyperparathyroidism?

(A) It is associated with chronic renal failure and is the result of hypocalcemia caused by hyperphosphatemia.

(B) Seen most commonly in patients with renal failure who undergo kidney transplantation.

(C) Commonly seen as a result of an adenoma in one of the parathyroid glands.

(D) Most patients present with renal stones, bone pain, or mental status changes.

(E) Is more common in men than women.

17. A 45-year-old man presents with suprapubic tenderness, fevers, and nausea. After a thorough evaluation, he is found to have acute cystitis and bladder stones. Which of the following bacteria is most likely responsible for this infection?

(A) *Staphylococcus aureus*

(B) *Pseudomonas*

(C) *Escherichia coli*

(D) *Proteus mirabilis*

(E) *Klebsiella* species

18. During laparoscopic abdominal procedures, the abdominal cavity is usually insufflated with carbon dioxide to a pressure of 15 mmHg. Increasing the intra-abdominal pressure to these levels produces which of the following physiologic responses?

(A) decreased afterload

(B) depressed cardiac output

(C) hypercarbia

(D) depressed diaphragm

(E) alkalosis

19. A 21-year-old male presents to the ED after sustaining a gunshot wound to the neck. After evaluation, it is determined that he has C6 quadriplegia. Which of the following activities will be limited by this injury?

(A) wrist extension

(B) elbow extension

(C) elbow flexion

(D) shoulder flexion

(E) raising his arms above his shoulders

20. Patients with septic arthritis of the hip joint usually present with which position?

(A) internal rotation and flexion

(B) internal rotation and extension

(C) internal rotation and abduction

(D) external rotation and flexion

(E) external rotation and abduction

21. Which of the following structures can be found *outside* of the spermatic cord during a hernia repair?

(A) direct hernia sac

(B) indirect hernia sac

(C) vas deferens

(D) testicular artery

(E) ovary

Questions 22 and 23

22. A 30-year-old male is brought to the ED after being hit in the head by a baseball. He is making incomprehensible sounds, but no words. He opens his eyes and withdraws to painful stimuli. His Glasgow Coma Scale score is:

(A) 10

(B) 9

(C) 8

(D) 7

(E) 6

23. The most appropriate next step in the treatment of this patient is:

(A) neurosurgery consultation

(B) intubation and mechanical ventilation

(C) CT scan of head to evaluate for intracranial blood

(D) administration of mannitol to prevent cerebral herniation

(E) blood and urine toxicology screens

24. A severely traumatized patient who has been receiving prolonged parenteral alimentation develops diarrhea, mental status changes, alopecia, and perioral and periorbital dermatitis. Administration of which of the following trace elements is most likely to reverse these complications?

    (A) iodine
    (B) zinc
    (C) selenium
    (D) silicon
    (E) tin

25. A man who underwent total thyroidectomy 24 hours ago now complains of a generalized "tingling" sensation and muscle cramps. Appropriate treatment would include which of the following?

    (A) intravenous infusion of calcium gluconate
    (B) administration of oxygen by mask
    (C) administration of an anticonvulsant
    (D) administration of a tranquilizer
    (E) neurologic consultation

26. Vital capacity is best described as the volume of air which is:

    (A) inhaled during normal respiration
    (B) expelled during passive expiration
    (C) remaining in the lungs after passive expiration
    (D) actively exchanging with pulmonary venous blood
    (E) able to be expelled following maximal inspiration

27. The most common site of aortic transection in deceleration injuries is which of the following?

    (A) the root of the aorta
    (B) at the level of the right innominate artery
    (C) at the level of the left innominate artery
    (D) near the origin of the left subclavian artery
    (E) in the middle portion of the descending thoracic aorta

28. Which of the following is the most common site for a gastrinoma?

    (A) gastric antrum
    (B) duodenum
    (C) pancreas
    (D) spleen
    (E) gallbladder

29. Avascular necrosis is most likely to occur in fracture dislocations involving which of the following?

    (A) the femoral head
    (B) the shaft of the femur
    (C) the shaft of the humerus
    (D) the scapula
    (E) the clavicle

30. A 38-year-old man, previously in good health, suddenly develops severe abdominal pain radiating from the left loin to the groin and associated with nausea, perspiration, and frequent urination. He is restless, tossing in bed, but has no abnormal findings. The most likely diagnosis is which of the following?

    (A) herpes zoster
    (B) left ureteral calculus
    (C) sigmoid diverticulitis
    (D) torsion of the left testicle
    (E) retroperitoneal hemorrhage

Questions 31 and 32

31. A 50-year-old man comes to the emergency room (ER) with a history of vomiting of 3 days' duration. His past history reveals that for approximately 20 years he has been experiencing epigastric pain that lasts for 2–3 weeks during spring and autumn. He remembers getting relief from pain by taking milk and antacids. Physical examination showed a fullness in the epigastric area with visible peristalsis, absence of tenderness, and normal active bowel sounds. What is the most likely diagnosis?

(A) gastric outlet obstruction

(B) small bowel obstruction

(C) volvulus of the colon

(D) incarcerated umbilical hernia

(E) cholecystitis

32. Which of the following metabolic abnormalities are typically found in the above patient?

(A) decreased antidiuretic hormone

(B) hypercalcemia

(C) hypokalemia

(D) hyperchloremia

(E) decreased aldosterone secretion

33. Gastrin secretion is enhanced by which of the following?

(A) antral distention

(B) antral acidification

(C) presence of fat in the antrum

(D) sympathetic nerve stimulation

(E) duodenal acidification

34. A patient is operated on with the presumptive diagnosis of acute appendicitis. However, at operation, the appendix and cecum are found to be normal. The terminal ileum though is red, edematous, and thickened with creeping of the mesenteric fat onto the ileum for a distance of approximately 30 cm. There is no dilation of the bowel proximal to the area of inflammation. The remainder of the small bowel is normal. What is the appropriate operative procedure?

(A) closure of the abdomen

(B) appendectomy

(C) ileostomy proximal to the area of involvement

(D) side-to-side ileotransverse colostomy

(E) right hemicolectomy

Question 35 and 36

35. A 25-year-old male presents to your office for evaluation of a testicular mass that he found in the shower. On examination, his left testicle is larger than his right with a firm palpable mass. A scrotal ultrasound confirms the presence of a solitary intraparenchymal testicular mass. Further management of his condition would include which of the following?

(A) close observation and repeat ultrasound in 3 months

(B) serum beta-human chorionic gonadotropin (HCG), alpha-fetoprotein (AFP), and lactate dehydrogenase (LDH)

(C) fine needle aspiration to determine if the mass is malignant

(D) transscrotal orchiectomy

(E) a 2-week course of antibiotics with follow-up clinical examination after completion

36. The most likely diagnosis in this patient is which of the following?

(A) benign fibroma

(B) epididymitis

(C) seminoma

(D) teratocarcinoma

(E) androblastoma

37. Which of the following is characteristic of Hirschsprung's disease?

(A) Constipation is the most frequent presenting feature.

(B) Severity of the symptoms corresponds with the extent of bowel involvement.

(C) Acetylcholinesterase activity is decreased in the aganglionic segment.

(D) The proximal colon is most commonly affected.

(E) It presents most commonly in young adults.

38. A 25-year-old male comes to the ER after a motor vehicle collision, complaining of vague left-sided abdominal pain. After initial evaluation, a CT of the abdomen is obtained as shown in Figure 2-3. Which of the following statements is true concerning the injury?

FIG. 2-3 (*Courtesy of H.J. Kim, MD.*)

(A) Hemodynamically unstable patients can be managed nonoperatively.

(B) Patients should be vaccinated against tetanus before hospital discharge.

(C) Splenic salvage is contraindicated in the presence of other major abdominal injuries.

(D) *Pseudomonas aeruginosa* is the most frequent organism responsible for postsplenectomy sepsis.

(E) Most patients require operative management.

39. A 50-year-old male presents with difficulty swallowing. Esophageal manometry demonstrates absence of peristaltic waves and a nonrelaxing lower esophageal sphincter (LES). Which of the following is the most likely diagnosis?

(A) Barrett's esophagus
(B) diffuse esophageal spasm
(C) achalasia
(D) Plummer-Vinson syndrome
(E) esophageal cancer

40. Which of the following statements is true regarding Barrett's esophagus?

(A) It is three times more common in women than men.

(B) Most cases are congenital in origin.

(C) The columnar-lined epithelial changes are always in direct continuity with the gastric epithelium.

(D) Surgical antireflux therapy does not necessarily result in regression of the Barrett's changes.

(E) Once the diagnosis of Barrett's esophagus is established, the patient does not need further biopsies on follow-up endoscopy.

Questions 41 and 42

A 49-year-old male presents with crushing substernal pain and rules out for a myocardial infarction. He is noted to have subcutaneous emphysema of the chest and neck and precordial crackles that correlate to his heartbeat but not his respirations.

41. Which of the following is the most likely diagnosis?

(A) spontaneous pneumothorax
(B) esophageal perforation
(C) pericarditis
(D) pneumopericardium
(E) pulmonary embolus

42. Which of the following approaches to management is most appropriate?

(A) This condition should always be managed operatively.

(B) The best diagnostic test is thoracic CT.

(C) Early endoscopy is contraindicated.

(D) Primary surgical repair is the first approach to treatment if the diagnosis is made within 24 hours.

(E) Anticoagulation should be started while the diagnostic workup proceeds.

43. A patient presents with a 24-hour history of periumbilical pain, now localized to the right lower quadrant. An abdominal CT scan is obtained in the ER, which is shown in Figure 2-4. Which of the following is considered a physical sign often associated with this diagnosis?

FIG. 2-4 (*Courtesy of H.J. Kim, MD.*)

(A) concave and empty right lower quadrant
(B) pain on flexion of the right hip
(C) flank bruising
(D) pain in right lower quadrant with palpation in left lower quadrant
(E) inspiratory arrest while palpating under the right costal margin

44. Following an uneventful appendectomy for acute appendicitis, the pathology report reveals the presence of a 1 cm carcinoid at the tip of the appendix. The patient has been otherwise asymptomatic. What is the most appropriate intervention?

(A) formal right hemicolectomy
(B) partial cecectomy—excision of the base of the cecum at the appendectomy site
(C) no further operative intervention required
(D) total abdominal colectomy with ileorectal anastomosis
(E) partial small bowel resection

45. A 64-year-old diabetic male undergoes a right hemicolectomy for an adenocarcinoma of the cecum. On the first postoperative night, he becomes tachycardic and is noted to have a temperature of 102.8°F. His surgical incision is tender

with erythema and murky discharge. Which of the following is the most important intervention?

(A) begin broad-spectrum antibiotics, Tylenol, and a cooling blanket
(B) open the wound and begin hyperbaric oxygen treatment
(C) apply sterile warm compress over the incision and replace dressing
(D) open the wound, send for Gram's stain of the fluid and emergent radical debridement
(E) postoperative fever evaluation including sputum, urine, and blood cultures

46. A 50-year-old diabetic man is treated as an outpatient with incision and drainage and oral clindamycin for an abscess and cellulitis of the skin on his back. About a week after completing his antibiotic he develops frequent, watery diarrhea. Which of the following is the most appropriate treatment of this complication?

(A) oral levaquin
(B) intravenous metronidazole
(C) oral vancomycin
(D) oral metronidazole
(E) intravenous vancomycin

47. A 62-year-old male on total parenteral nutrition (TPN) for 2 weeks following development of a postoperative enterocutaneous fistula has developed high, spiking temperatures up to 102.2°F over the last 8 hours. The only abnormal finding on physical examination is erythema and induration around his central line. The most appropriate management is which of the following?

(A) begin broad-spectrum antibiotics and observe for 24 hours
(B) obtain blood cultures through the central line, begin broad-spectrum antibiotics and await culture results
(C) remove catheter, send tip for culture and replace with a new central line over the guide wire
(D) remove catheter, send tip for culture and establish central line at another site
(E) remove catheter, send for culture and establish peripheral intravenous line

48. A 48-year-old male truck driver presents for evaluation of bright red rectal bleeding with bowel movements. He also has the feeling that something protrudes through his anus while he strains to move his bowels but that it withdraws into the bowel when he relaxes. He has no abdominal pain, weight loss, or other symptoms. A colonoscopy reveals no polyps or tumors but does note internal hemorrhoids. Which of the following is the best initial treatment for him?

    (A) high fiber diet, frequent sitz baths, and topical steroid ointment
    (B) rubber band ligation
    (C) sclerotherapy injection
    (C) infrared coagulation
    (E) surgical hemorrhoidectomy

49. Which of the following is true regarding anorectal abscess and fistula?

    (A) The most common cause is a subepithelial extension of a genital infection.
    (B) Conservative management should always be considered for fistula-in-ano as many heal spontaneously.
    (C) Most acute anorectal abscesses require a course of antibiotics.
    (D) The treatment protocol is not altered for patients with valvular heart disease.
    (E) Anal fistula is classified as intersphincteric, transsphincteric, suprasphincteric, or extrasphincteric.

50. The most common cause of surgery in a patient with Crohn's disease is which of the following?

    (A) carcinoma
    (B) fistula
    (C) bleeding
    (D) obstruction
    (E) abscess

51. A 26-year-old male presents with abdominal pain and bloody diarrhea. On examination, he has a low-grade fever and mildly tender abdomen. Lower endoscopy is performed which reveals edematous mucosa with contiguous involvement from the rectum to the left colon. Random biopsies are performed which reveals acute and chronic inflammation of the mucosa and submucosa with multiple crypt abscesses. There are no granulomas seen. What can you tell this patient about his condition?

    (A) He will likely require an operation.
    (B) There is no known cure.
    (C) The use of intravenous corticosteroids is contraindicated.
    (D) Perianal fistulas are characteristic.
    (E) There is a substantially increased long-term risk of developing colon cancer.

52. A 46-year-old female presents to your office with rectal bleeding, itching, and irritation. On examination, a 3-cm ulcerating lesion is seen in the anal canal. Biopsy of the lesion reveals squamous cell carcinoma (SCC). Which of the following is the most appropriate treatment?

    (A) chemotherapy and pelvic radiation protocol
    (B) low anterior resection
    (C) abdominal perineal resection
    (D) wide local excision of the lesion
    (E) wide local excision of the lesion and bilateral inguinal lymph node dissection

53. During initial exploration in a patient scheduled to undergo a right hemicolectomy for colon cancer, a deep 4-cm liver mass is seen in the right lobe of the liver. The left lobe appears to be normal. Intraoperative biopsy of the lesion is positive for metastatic colon cancer. The best management of this patient includes which of the following?

    (A) Immediately close the patient and refer for chemotherapy only.
    (B) Perform right hemicolectomy only.
    (C) Perform right hemicolectomy and right hepatic lobectomy.
    (D) Perform right hemicolectomy and wide excision of the liver lesion.
    (E) Perform liver resection only.

54. A mobile mass is found on rectal examination in a 77-year-old male with complaints of blood in his stool. On workup, he is found to have a

stage I (Dukes' A), well-differentiated adeno-carcinoma. The most appropriate intervention is which of the following?

(A) transanal excision
(B) abdominal perineal resection
(C) low anterior resection
(D) placement of endorectal wallstent
(E) neoadjuvant chemotherapy followed by transanal resection

55. A 27-year-old female whose father had a colon resection for adenocarcinoma undergoes her first colonoscopy. Over 100 small polyps are seen distributed mainly in her sigmoid and rectum. Multiple polyps are removed and histologic review reveals tubular adenomas with no evidence of atypia or dysplasia. The most appropriate next step in her management is which of the following?

(A) total proctocolectomy with ileoanal J pouch reconstruction
(B) surveillance colonoscopy in 5 years
(C) surveillance colonoscopy every 2 years until all polyps are removed
(D) flexible sigmoidoscopy with representative biopsy every 6 months for 2 years, then yearly for 3 years, then every 3–5 years
(E) abdominal perineal resection with sigmoid resection and end colostomy

56. Biopsy of a 4-cm sessile polyp of the cecum during a routine screening colonoscopy reveals it to be a villous adenoma with atypia. Attempt at piecemeal snare polypectomy through the colonoscope is unsuccessful. Which of the following is the most appropriate management?

(A) right hemicolectomy
(B) colonoscopy with electrocoagulation of the tumor
(C) colonoscopy with repeat biopsy in 6 months
(D) open surgery with colotomy and excision of polyp
(E) external beam radiation

Questions 57 through 59

57. A 56-year-old man comes to the hospital. For the past 5 days he has had colicky abdominal pain, vomiting, abdominal distention, and constipation. The most appropriate measure, after IV hydration and nasogastric decompression, in the initial management of this patient is which of the following?

(A) upper GI endoscopy
(B) supine and erect x-rays of the abdomen
(C) abdominal sonography
(D) antiemetic agents
(E) promotility drugs

58. He undergoes barium enema examination. The findings on barium enema, shown in Figure 2-5, are most compatible with which of the following diagnoses?

FIG. 2-5 (Courtesy of H.J. Kim, MD.)

(A) mechanical small bowel obstruction
(B) intussusception
(C) volvulus
(D) carcinoma of the colon
(E) diverticulitis

59. During definitive surgical treatment of the lesion shown on the barium enema, the left ureter is accidentally transected at the level of the pelvic brim. What is the most appropriate management of this complication?

    (A) ureteroneocystostomy
    (B) left to right ureteroureterostomy
    (C) anastomosis of the two cut ends over a "double J" stent
    (D) nephrectomy
    (E) ligation of the transected ends

60. A 60-year-old woman presents with an abnormal cluster of microcalcifications on a routine mammogram, and undergoes a needle-localized excisional biopsy. The pathology is shown in Figure 2-6. When counseling the patient regarding her surgical options, which of the following statements would be correct?

FIG. 2-6 (*Courtesy of H.J. Kim, MD.*)

    (A) Modified radical mastectomy differs from a Halsted mastectomy in that the pectoralis major is spared in the modified radical approach.
    (B) Modified radical mastectomy differs from Halsted mastectomy in that an axillary lymphadenectomy is not performed in the modified radical approach.
    (C) The anatomic limits of the modified radical mastectomy include the sternum medially and the anterior border of the serratus anterior muscle laterally.

    (D) Injury to the thoracodorsal nerve during mastectomy results in a "winged scapula."
    (E) Lymphedema occurs mainly as a complication of the Halsted radical mastectomy and should not be seen after modified radical mastectomy.

61. A 45-year-old man undergoes a distal esophagectomy for Barrett's esophagus. During his hospital course, a left chest tube is placed for an effusion. Milky white fluid is found to come out through the tube. Which of the following statements is most accurate about this condition?

    (A) Diagnosis can be confirmed by checking the lymphocyte count and triglyceride level in the fluid.
    (B) This condition requires immediate surgical intervention to repair.
    (C) The chest tube should be removed due to the possibility of an iatrogenic source of infection.
    (D) Usually found on the right if due to a traumatic source.
    (E) The use of TPN is contraindicated until the condition resolves.

62. A 60-year-old man with hypertension, hyperlipidemia, and peripheral vascular disease requires coronary artery bypass graft surgery. Which of the following vessels would be the most appropriate conduit for his coronary artery bypass graft?

    (A) left axillary artery
    (B) internal mammary arteries
    (C) ulnar artery
    (D) common femoral vein
    (E) femoral artery

63. The family of a patient recently diagnosed with esophageal cancer requests more information regarding the disease. You tell them which of the following?

    (A) The incidence of SCC of the esophagus is rising more rapidly than adenocarcinoma.
    (B) Premalignant conditions include caustic esophageal burns, Plummer-Vinson syndrome, and tylosis.

(C) It is more common in women than men.

(D) Smoking is not a risk factor for esophageal cancer.

(E) Barrett's esophagus increases the risk for esophageal SCC.

64. A 40-year-old woman presents with epigastric pain and is diagnosed with peptic-ulcer disease. A duodenal ulcer is seen on upper endoscopy. How would you counsel her regarding surgical management options?

(A) The ulcer is most likely secondary to a malignancy. Further workup is needed to rule out distant metastases before considering surgery.

(B) Surgery is the most effective first-line therapy.

(C) Recurrence rate of a duodenal ulcer 15 years after vagotomy and a drainage procedure is less than 5%.

(D) Patients operated on for intractability are more prone to developing postgastrectomy symptoms.

(E) Incidence of dumping syndrome is lower after highly selective vagotomy than after truncal vagotomy.

65. Which of these statements is true in regard to GI hormones?

(A) Vagal activation, antral distension, and antral protein are all stimuli for gastrin release.

(B) Secretin stimulates gastrin.

(C) Secretin is released from the antrum of the stomach.

(D) Cholecystokinin (CCK) release is stimulated by fat in the duodenum and results in release of insulin by the pancreas.

(E) CCK is released by the pancreas and relaxes the sphincter of Oddi.

66. A patient presents to the ED complaining of abdominal pain out of proportion to her examination. Initial vital signs are: BP 70/30, HR 120. The patient does report a prior history of abdominal pain after eating. Which of the following statements regarding this condition is most accurate?

(A) A CT scan which shows superior mesenteric artery (SMA) thrombosis or bowel wall thickening requires an immediate operation.

(B) The most common site of embolic event is the SMA.

(C) Nonocclusive mesenteric ischemia is treated with arterial bypass.

(D) Patients with cardiac arrhythmias are not at increased risk.

(E) After volume resuscitation, the initial diagnostic study for this patient is esophagogastroduodenoscopy (EGD).

67. A 59-year-old White male with a 40 pack-year history of smoking presents to your clinic complaining of three prior episodes of a "shade passing over his left eye" over the last 2 months. He reports that last week he experienced some weakness in his right arm, which resolved after 5 minutes. Appropriate management and counseling for this patient includes which of the following?

(A) Initial management of this patient should include bilateral cerebral vessel duplex ultrasonography.

(B) Explanation to him that he has had a stroke and will be referred to a neurologist for management.

(C) The most common cause of strokes in these patients is related to decreased blood flow.

(D) Presence of a carotid bruit confirms the diagnosis and may lead to operative intervention without the need for imaging studies.

(E) The presence of a 50% stenosis in the right carotid artery should lead to bilateral surgical repair.

68. A 65-year-old woman complains that she has become increasingly light-headed after playing golf. She also has had some cramping type pain in her left arm, which coincides with the episodes. She undergoes arteriogram and is found to have a stenotic lesion of her subclavian artery. Which of the following is true?

(A) The stenotic lesion is distal to the take off of the vertebral artery.
(B) It is unusual for these patients to have coronary artery disease as well.
(C) The patient's light-headedness is caused by an incomplete Circle of Willis.
(D) The operation of choice for this patient is a carotid-subclavian bypass.
(E) Radial pulses in this patient will be equal bilaterally.

69. A patient with a known family history of multiple endocrine neoplasia (MEN) I, now presents with intractable ulcer disease. Which of the following statements about his condition is most accurate?

(A) Diarrhea is a frequent complaint.
(B) Tumors are rarely multiple.
(C) Tumors are rarely malignant.
(D) An elevated fasting gastrin level is diagnostic for the Zollinger-Ellison syndrome.
(E) CT is useful in localizing the tumor in greater than 75% of patients.

Questions 70 and 71

70. A 60-year-old Asian male presents with early satiety and 40-lb weight loss over 3 months. Upper endoscopy shows an irregular mass in the antrum of the stomach. What can you tell him and his family about his situation?

(A) Weight loss indicates distant metastases, and surgical resection is not indicated.
(B) Antral tumors have a worse prognosis than tumors at other sites in the stomach.
(C) CT is the most effective imaging modality for determining TNM (tumor, nodes, and metastases) stage.

(D) 5-year survival for patients with gastric adenocarcinoma confined to the mucosa with no nodal metastasis approaches 90%.
(E) Chemotherapy is an effective treatment modality in stage IV gastric adenocarcinoma, with significant benefit in overall survival.

71. He follows up in the clinic a few days later, and you see that the results of the endoscopic biopsies are suggestive of a gastric lymphoma. Which of the following is true regarding this condition?

(A) The incidence of gastric lymphoma is increasing.
(B) Obstruction, perforation, and bleeding are common presenting symptoms.
(C) Upper endoscopy with biopsy is highly accurate for diagnosis.
(D) Gastric involvement of systemic lymphoma is best treated with gastric resection.
(E) Survival rates are dismal with overall prognosis similar to that seen in gastric adenocarcinoma.

72. You perform an upper endoscopy on a patient and find changes suggestive of Barrett's esophagus. How do you explain this to the patient and his family?

(A) Is a condition where the normal esophageal lining is replaced by columnar epithelium.
(B) Is a condition where the normal esophageal lining is replaced by dysplastic squamous cells.
(C) Two biopsies with histologic changes are needed to confirm the diagnosis.
(D) The main risk associated with Barrett's esophagus is bleeding.
(E) It is related to peptic ulcer disease.

73. On your surgery rotation you are assisting in a gastric surgical procedure. The attending surgeon asks you to describe the vascular supply to the stomach. You reply with which of the following?

(A) The right gastric artery arises from the celiac axis.

(B) The left gastric artery arises from the common hepatic artery.

(C) The right gastroepiploic arises from the right hepatic artery.

(D) The short gastric arteries arise from the splenic artery.

(E) The left gastroepiploic arises from the left gastric artery.

74. A patient with dyspepsia has a positive serologic test for *Helicobacter pylori* and is concerned that he could have an ulcer. Which of the following statements about *H. pylori* and ulcer disease would be most accurate?

(A) Gastric ulcers are usually caused by hypersecretion of acid, not bacteria.

(B) A positive IgG serology confirms an active infection with *H. pylori*.

(C) *H. pylori* is associated with both gastric and duodenal ulcers.

(D) Most patients with *H. pylori* have ulcers.

(E) The use of antibiotics alone is successful in eradicating *H. pylori*.

75. Which of the following patients is most likely to have symptoms of the carcinoid syndrome?

(A) patient with carcinoid tumor localized to the appendix

(B) patient with carcinoid tumor of the small intestine and a 3-cm nodule in the liver seen on CT scan

(C) patient with an apple core lesion seen on barium enema

(D) patient with adrenal mass and elevated levels of urinary vanillylmandelic acid (VMA)

(E) patient with a retroperitoneal carcinoid tumor

76. A patient undergoes a gastrectomy following a gunshot injury. How would you counsel him about postgastrectomy syndromes?

(A) Most patients tolerate gastrectomy without a change in their digestive habits.

(B) Dumping syndromes can be treated with high carbohydrate liquid diets.

(C) Cholestyramine is a treatment for postvagotomy diarrhea.

(D) Most patients with these syndromes require surgical intervention.

(E) Proton pump inhibitors are effective against alkaline reflux syndrome.

77. A 19-year-old female presents to the ED complaining of swelling in her left lower extremity. She reports that she had arthroscopy of the right knee about a week ago for a torn meniscus. The swelling started last night and is uncomfortable. Which of the following statements most accurately describes the situation?

(A) This condition is less likely to occur in women than men.

(B) The patient should be put on strict bed rest with leg elevation until her swelling resolves.

(C) Her surgically treated knee should be aspirated immediately to rule out a septic joint.

(D) Prophylaxis to prevent this complication includes subcutaneous heparin or daily coumadin.

(E) Directed lytic therapy is indicated for this patient if her lower extremity becomes bluish and has evidence of vascular compromise.

78. A 72-year-old woman undergoes a sigmoid colectomy for diverticulitis. Postoperatively, she develops a wound infection for which she is transferred to the ICU for 2 days because of hypotension. Which of the following would have had the most effect on reducing her risk of developing complications?

    (A) preoperative treatment of her concomitant urinary tract infection
    (B) nurses changing gloves in between their patient assessments so they don't have to wash their hands as often
    (C) using a preoperative antibiotic specific for *E. coli*, the most common intestinal flora
    (D) giving preoperative antibiotics immediately after the skin incision
    (E) treatment of the infected wound with an antibiotic only

79. A 40-year-old man presents with chronic diarrhea and peptic ulcer disease refractory to medical management with proton pump inhibitors. An octreotide scan is shown in Figure 2-7,

FIG. 2-7 (*Courtesy of H.J. Kim, MD.*)

which corresponds to an area near the head of the pancreas. Which of the following factors directly results in the release of the hormone produced by this tumor?

    (A) secretin
    (B) glucagon
    (C) antral pH <2.0
    (D) vagus nerve
    (E) somatostatin

80. An 18-year-old male is brought to the ED after sustaining a stab wound to the left chest that is medial and superior to the nipple. He was unresponsive at the scene and intubated by the emergency medical technician (EMT) team. His pulse is 140 and BP is 60/30 after receiving 1 L of lactated Ringers solution and 2 units of blood during his transport. On auscultation there are no breath sounds on the left. His trachea is midline. He has no evidence of neck vein distention. Which of the following statements is true?

    (A) Cardiac tamponade is unlikely since there is no evidence of neck vein distention.
    (B) A left chest tube should be placed immediately.
    (C) Given the probability of a cardiac injury, an emergent thoracotomy should be performed in the ED.
    (D) An aortic angiogram should be ordered immediately to assess for aortic injury.
    (E) No intervention should be performed until a chest x-ray is completed to provide more information.

81. A 23-year-old male is brought by ambulance to the ER after being found in a house fire. He was in a closed room with a large amount of smoke and has sustained burns to his face, torso, arms, and legs. His pulse is 120, BP 110/55, and SpO$_2$ 92% on 2 L of oxygen by nasal cannula. Which of the following statements is true?

    (A) The burns should be covered in cool, moist dressings.
    (B) An inhalation injury is unlikely since he is able to oxygenate on minimal supplementation.

(C) Fluids should be limited to prevent pulmonary edema after his smoke inhalation.

(D) This patient meets criteria for transfer to a dedicated burn center.

(E) Depth of the burn does not affect the management.

Questions 82 and 83

A 62-year-old man undergoes transplantation of a kidney from a cadaveric donor. The surgery is uncomplicated and his recovery proceeds well for the first week postoperatively. In the second postoperative week, he develops hypertension, peripheral edema, and decreased urinary output. He states that he has been taking his medications as ordered.

82. What is the most likely cause of this condition?

(A) hyperacute organ rejection
(B) acute organ rejection
(C) chronic organ rejection
(D) congestive heart failure
(E) failure of physician to restart him on his preoperative furosemide

83. What is the most appropriate management at this time?

(A) remove the donated kidney
(B) pulse steroid dose and increase immunosuppresion
(C) oral furosemide with follow-up in 1 week
(D) hospitalization for IV furosemide, angiotensin-converting enzyme (ACE) inhibitor, and close monitoring
(E) explain that the kidney transplant failed and that he needs to restart dialysis

Questions 84 and 85

A 23-year old male driver involved in a head-on motor vehicle collision is brought to the ER. On initial evaluation in the trauma unit, his blood pressure is 180/70 and his pulse is 56. After initial evaluation and resuscitation you obtain a CT scan of his head (see Figure 2-8).

FIG. 2-8 (Courtesy of H.J. Kim, MD.)

84. The patient in the above scenario is then transported to the ICU. The most appropriate initial evaluation and management would include which of the following?

(A) ensuring that his bed stays flat
(B) aggressive hydration with a hypotonic solution
(C) hyperventilation
(D) needle drainage of the hematoma
(E) MRI of the brain

85. The finding on the imaging study is most commonly associated with injury to which of the following?

(A) the bridging veins
(B) the middle meningeal artery
(C) the sagital sinus
(D) the temporal artery
(E) the epidural artery

86. A 49-year-old male underwent his last chemotherapy session for testicular cancer 3 weeks ago and now is complaining of shortness of breath. Which of the following drugs is most probably causing his problems?

    (A) doxorubicin
    (B) etoposide
    (C) cisplatin
    (D) bleomycin
    (E) vincristine

87. A 25-year-old African American female develops a large lesion on her ear lobe after having it pierced (see Figure 2-9). How would you advise this patient?

FIG. 2-9 *(Courtesy of H.J. Kim, MD.)* (Also see color insert.)

    (A) Surgical excision is curative.
    (B) This resulted from an infection that occurred when she had her ear pierced.
    (C) Recurrences of this problem are common.
    (D) She is likely to have reduced fertility.
    (E) Oral corticosteroids have been effective.

88. A 24-year-old male is involved in a house fire. His sputum is carbonaceous and he has suffered second- and third-degree burns to 65% of his total body surface area (TBSA). He is intubated in the ED without difficulty. A capnometer is placed at the end of the endotracheal tube and there is positive change in color. Examination of his chest reveals bilateral equal breath sounds. Suddenly he experiences ECG changes and goes into cardiac arrest. Which of the following drugs is most likely to be responsible for this event?

    (A) etomidate
    (B) rocuronium
    (C) succinylcholine
    (D) midazolam
    (E) ketamine

89. Which anatomic location is the most common site of extra-adrenal pheochromocytomas?

    (A) duodenum
    (B) inferior pole of the kidney
    (C) paraaortic area
    (D) parasplenic area
    (E) peripancreatic area

90. A 45-year-old man was kicked several times in the abdomen in a bar fight. He came to the ED and noted that he has not voided for 24 hours. Insertion of a Foley catheter revealed gross hematuria, which persisted after irrigation. A CT scan of the abdomen and pelvis is obtained that does not show any evidence of renal laceration. A CT cystogram is then obtained and is shown in Figure 2-10. Appropriate management of this injury includes which of the following?

FIG. 2-10 *(Courtesy of H.J. Kim, MD.)*

(A) urinary catheter drainage

(B) urinary catheter drainage with continuous bladder irrigation

(C) bilateral nephrostomy tubes

(D) exploratory laparotomy with oversewing of the bladder wall

(E) observation

Questions 91 and 92

A 54-year-old male presents to the ED with acute onset of severe abdominal pain. His history is significant for gnawing epigastric pain that radiates to the back for several months. Physical examination demonstrates mild hypertension and tachycardia as well as a rigid "board like" abdomen with generalized rebound tenderness and hypoactive bowel sounds. Rectal examination reveals dark hemoccult positive stools without gross blood.

91. Which of the following would be the next appropriate step in management?

(A) order upright chest and abdomen x-rays

(B) obtain a CT scan of the abdomen and pelvis

(C) plan for upper GI endoscopy

(D) take patient to the OR for immediate exploratory laparotomy

(E) schedule the patient to be seen in surgery clinic in 1 week

92. While you are in the process of working up the patient he becomes hypotensive and tachycardic. Bright red blood per rectum is now noted. The most likely explanation for his condition is which of the following?

(A) ruptured esophageal varices

(B) diverticulosis

(C) ruptured abdominal aortic aneurysm (AAA)

(D) ruptured splenic artery aneurysm

(E) erosion of the gastroduodenal artery

93. You are a second-year surgery resident and have just left work after a 30-hour shift. On your way home you witness a recent collision where there is an obviously injured pedestrian.

Several bystanders are providing care for the injured victim. You elect to keep driving. A witness at the scene recognizes you as a physician and reports you to the authorities for neglecting to stop to provide care. As a consequence of your actions, which of the following will most likely happen?

(A) You will lose your medical license.

(B) You will be found guilty of negligence in a court of law.

(C) You will have your medical license suspended.

(D) You will have no legal action taken against you.

(E) You will be subject to a malpractice suit.

Questions 94 and 95

94. A 35-year-old 80-kg male was transported to the regional burn center at your hospital after suffering second- and third-degree burns from the eruption of a brush fire fueled with gasoline. He was intubated by EMS to secure his airway for transport. On arrival, he is found to have burns across his face, anterior neck, chest, and anterior abdomen, as well as bilateral circumferential upper extremity burns. What do you estimate the total body surface area (TBSA) of his burns to be?

(A) 30%

(B) 35%

(C) 40%

(D) 50%

(E) 60%

95. Over the first 8 hours of his resuscitation, you estimate that he will require which of the following?

(A) 500 mL/h of isotonic fluid

(B) 600 mL/h of isotonic fluid

(C) 600 mL/h of hypertonic fluid

(D) 800 mL/h of isotonic fluid

(E) 800 mL/h of hypotonic fluid

Questions 96 and 97

You are called to the trauma bay to evaluate a 42-year-old male who suffered a blow to his knee at the construction site where he works. He is awake, alert, and his vital signs have been stable in transport. After completing your primary survey, you continue with your secondary survey and determine that his only injury is to his right leg. It is clear that he has suffered a posterior knee dislocation. As part of your examination, you determine that you cannot feel a pulse in his right foot.

96. Realizing that there is compromised blood supply to the patient's right foot, you immediately do which of the following?

   (A) Transport the patient to radiology for an arteriogram.
   (B) Relocate the knee into anatomical position and re-examine the pulse.
   (C) Take the patient directly to the OR to explore his popliteal artery.
   (D) Obtain an orthopedics consultation and order films to identify any fractures.
   (E) Determine the ankle brachial indices for his right and left foot.

97. Later that night after the patient had been treated and stabilized, you are called to the patient's room to evaluate severe pain in his right lower leg. Upon examining the patient, you determine that he has a bounding pulse in his right foot. However, the patient does state that he has a tingling sensation in his foot and he is in excruciating pain when you flex his foot. Which of the following should be the next step in his treatment?

   (A) Increase the dose of intravenous narcotics to help control the pain.
   (B) Prescribe an anti-inflammatory drug to enhance the effects of the narcotics.
   (C) Order a series of right foot x-rays looking for an occult fracture.
   (D) Obtain an emergent arteriogram looking for missed vascular injury.
   (E) Emergently take the patient to the OR.

98. You are called to the ER to assist with a series of trauma patients who arrived following a multiple vehicle accident. You are assigned to a 22-year-old male who was an unrestrained driver involved in a head-on collision. After you confirm the presence of an adequate airway and equal breath sounds bilaterally, you address his hypotension and tachycardia by giving 2 L of lactated Ringer's solution. His pulse remains elevated at 130 and his blood pressure is 92/55. His pelvic x-ray returns and demonstrates a widening of the pubic symphysis. In addition to continued fluid resuscitation, what is your next step in management?

   (A) reduce the pelvic volume with a sheet or pneumatic compression garment
   (B) exploratory laparotomy to isolate and control the hemorrhage
   (C) CT scan to evaluate for other source of hemorrhage
   (D) angiography to embolize pelvic vasculature
   (E) obtain additional pelvic x-rays for preoperative planning

99. You have been called to the ER to evaluate a 58-year-old female who presented to the hospital for evaluation of a painful left foot. She noticed the pain when she awoke in the morning. She has a history of painful calf muscles when she walks. On your examination, you notice that she has an irregular heart beat, and that she has no palpable pulses and no audible Doppler signals in her left foot. It is cool to the touch and she has some decreased sensation at her toes. Which of the following is the next best step in this patient's management?

   (A) an echocardiogram looking for atrial thrombus
   (B) initiation of a heparin infusion
   (C) duplex imaging of her arterial vessels in her left leg looking for acute occlusion
   (D) aortogram with left lower extremity runoff to determine the level of the vascular occlusion
   (E) initiate infusion of thrombolytics to dissolve the clot

100. You are asked to see a 74-year-old man who has been admitted for evaluation of abdominal pain. During his workup, he was found to have hemoccult positive stool and a CT scan that was concerning for a mass in his sigmoid colon. Which should be the next step in his treatment?

   (A) cardiology consultation for preoperative clearance

   (B) contrast enema to evaluate the lesion

   (C) colonoscopy to biopsy the mass and rule out synchronous lesions

   (D) sigmoidectomy to resect the mass and obtain mesenteric lymph nodes for staging

   (E) positron emission tomography (PET) scan to determine if the lesion is cancerous

101. You are seeing a 48-year-old female in follow-up in your clinic. She originally presented for evaluation of a suspicious nonpalpable lesion in her right breast that was seen on her annual mammogram. A stereotactic core biopsy was done. She now returns to your office to review the results of the pathology report that confirms the presence of lobular carcinoma in situ (LCIS). How do you counsel her at this time?

   (A) Tamoxifen can prevent this cancer from spreading but may increase your risk of developing cancer in the other breast.

   (B) You can consider nonoperative treatment with close observation, annual mammograms, and semiannual clinical examinations.

   (C) The recommended treatment is a right breast mastectomy.

   (D) Further staging workup at this time will include a chest x-ray and bone scan.

   (E) Because you are at such high risk for future cancers, bilateral mastectomies should be performed to prevent this from happening.

102. A 52-year-old female has been referred to you for consultation following a core biopsy of an area of calcifications seen on a screening mammogram. She has no family history of breast or ovarian cancer. She has not been taking hormone replacement therapy and has no reproductive risk factors. On physical examination, there is no palpable mass. The core biopsy results demonstrate atypical ductal hyperplasia. What should be the next step in her treatment?

   (A) close observation with semiannual mammograms and clinical examinations

   (B) treatment with tamoxifen for 5 years

   (C) needle localized excisional biopsy

   (D) unilateral mastectomy

   (E) bilateral mastectomy

103. You had previously seen a 24-year-old male in your office for evaluation of a suspicious looking mole. He had undergone a punch biopsy, which demonstrated a melanoma. He has no prior history of skin cancer, no family history of skin cancer, nor any history of blistering sunburns. Which of the following results in the pathology report are most predictive of outcome?

   (A) size of the melanoma

   (B) color of the melanoma

   (C) depth of the melanoma

   (D) presence of ulceration

   (E) site of the melanoma

104. You are asked to see a 64-year-old man with left lower quadrant abdominal pain that was admitted to the medicine service after a CT scan demonstrated diverticulitis of the sigmoid colon. There was no evidence for gross perforation and no abscess was identified. He had been admitted 6 months ago for the same problem and had an uneventful recovery. Which treatment do you recommend?

   (A) antibiotics only

   (B) antibiotics and sigmoidectomy prior to discharge

   (C) emergent sigmoidectomy

   (D) antibiotics and sigmoidectomy 1–2 weeks after discharge

   (E) antibiotics, interval colonoscopy, and subsequent sigmoidectomy

105. You are about to see a 52-year-old man in your office who presented with a 30-lb weight loss over the past 3 months and jaundice. He also has begun to develop early satiety and frequent vomiting. You had obtained a CT scan, which is shown in Figure 2-11. After reviewing the results of the scan, you discuss the diagnosis with him. He becomes angry and he demands that you operate immediately to remove the tumor. In response you do which of the following?

FIG. 2-11 (*Courtesy of H.J. Kim, MD.*)

(A) Schedule the patient for an urgent Whipple procedure.

(B) Explain that there is absolutely no role for surgery in his situation and that you have another patient to see.

(C) Tell the patient that he is terminal and he should focus on getting his affairs in order.

(D) Calmly review the diagnosis with the patient and help console him and his family before reviewing the options for management including potential clinical trials.

(E) Leave the room and have your nurse review local hospice services.

106. A 22-year-old male arrives in the trauma bay via ambulance. He was intubated in the field after suffering a gunshot wound to the head. On examination, he has both an entrance and exit wound suggesting a transcranial trajectory of the bullet. On physical examination, you note that there are no brain stem reflexes present and his pupils are fixed and dilated. Given his

age and health history, you believe he would be a good candidate for organ transplantation. When you discuss the patient's situation with the family, they do not mention organ transplantation. What should you then do?

(A) Explain to them the process of organ transplantation and its benefits to others.

(B) Withdraw mechanical ventilator support and allow the patient to expire.

(C) Add a narcotic drip to the patient's treatment in order to ease his pain prior to withdrawing mechanical ventilation.

(D) Contact the donor services agency to have a professional trained in addressing organ donation come to speak with the family.

(E) Contact the transplant team and prepare the patient for the OR because the organs are too vital to waste regardless of the family's wishes.

107. A 50-year-old male with a history of alcohol abuse presents with acute pancreatitis. Which of the following facts about the patient is included in Ranson's criteria?

(A) age of 65 years old
(B) elevated amylase
(C) thrombocytosis
(D) elevated lipase
(E) evidence of pancreatic necrosis on CT scan

108. A 55-year-old female presents to your office after a lung mass was found on a chest x-ray. She has undergone a series of imaging studies and has been referred to your office to determine if she is a candidate for surgery. With which of the following findings would she still be a candidate for potentially curative surgical resection?

(A) malignant pleural effusion
(B) contralateral mediastinal node involvement
(C) chest wall invasion
(D) liver metastases
(E) superior vena cava syndrome

109. A 70-year-old male presents with dysphagia, regurgitation of undigested food, and halitosis. You obtain a barium swallow study (see Figure 2-12). Which of the following is true regarding this condition?

FIG. 2-12 (*Courtesy of H.J. Kim, MD.*)

(A) Esophagoscopy is a critical portion of the preoperative workup.
(B) The diverticulum is situated posteriorly, just proximal to the cricopharyngeal muscle.
(C) The diverticulum will involve all layers of the esophageal wall.
(D) Treatment requires resection of the diverticulum.
(E) Vocal cord paralysis is most likely secondary to a traumatic endotracheal intubation at the time of surgery.

Questions 110 and 111

A 45-year-old woman, mother of four children, comes to the ER complaining of the sudden onset of epigastric and right upper quadrant pain, radiating to the back, associated with vomiting. On examination, tenderness is elicited in the right upper quadrant, bowel sounds are decreased, and laboratory data show leukocytosis as well as normal serum levels of amylase, lipase, and bilirubin.

110. What is the most likely diagnosis?

(A) acute cholecystitis
(B) perforated peptic ulcer disease
(C) myocardial infarction
(D) acute pancreatitis
(E) sigmoid diverticulitis

111. Which of the following is the most useful diagnostic test to confirm the diagnosis?

(A) two-way roentgenogram of the abdomen
(B) ultrasonography of the upper abdomen
(C) CT scan of the abdomen and pelvis with oral contrast
(D) HIDA (hydroxy iminodiacetic acid) scan
(E) magnetic resonance cholangiopancreatography (MRCP)

112. A 64-year-old male is referred to your office for evaluation of a pulsatile abdominal mass. His primary care physician orders a CT scan of the abdomen and pelvis (see Figure 2-13). Which of the following is true regarding the finding illustrated on the CT?

FIG. 2-13 (*Courtesy of H.J. Kim, MD.*)

(A) 75% of patients with this have a positive family history for this condition.
(B) Most patients with this will have aneurysms of peripheral vessels.
(C) When this is greater than 4 cm in diameter it should be repaired.
(D) Most are asymptomatic at presentation.
(E) Endovascular repair should be restricted to young healthy patients.

Questions 113 and 114

You have been asked to see a patient of one of your colleagues. He is a 67-year-old male with a long smoking history who has been having left foot pain at night. He tells you that dangling his feet over the bed relieves the pain. Previously, he had noted pain in his left calf with ambulation. Over the past several weeks, this pain has been worsening and the distance he could walk pain free had diminished.

113. After a through history and physical examination, which of the following would be your next step in diagnostic workup?

(A) three-view x-rays of his left foot and ankle
(B) left lower extremity arterial duplex
(C) lower extremity angiogram with runoff
(D) trial of pentoxifylline with 3-month follow-up
(E) CT angiogram to evaluate for aortoiliac occlusive disease

114. Which of the following is an indication for surgical revascularization?

(A) pain in both calves when walking that relieves with rest
(B) necrotic fifth toe
(C) presence of a localized focus of arterial stenosis seen on angiogram
(D) diabetic patient
(E) patient refusal to consider quitting smoking, as he has a greater risk of disease progression

115. A patient is evaluated for left-sided abdominal pain and undergoes a CT scan of the abdomen that shows renal calculi. The radiologist reports an incidental finding that is shown in Figure 2-14. She has never been symptomatic from this disease. All of her hepatobiliary serologies are within normal limits. Which of the following is an indication for elective surgical treatment?

FIG. 2-14 (*Courtesy of H.J. Kim, MD.*)

(A) patient is over 50 years old

(B) two small (<1 cm) stones and sludge present in gallbladder

(C) absence of calcifications in the gallbladder wall

(D) type II diabetes mellitus

(E) sickle cell disease

116. A 42-year-old male with a history of ulcerative colitis has been to the ER three times over the past 6 months complaining of right upper quadrant pain, fever, and jaundice. His total bilirubin has fluctuated from 0.5 to 4.2 over this time. Workup has included an endoscopic retrograde cholangiopancreatography (ERCP) with the findings as shown in Figure 2-15. Of which of the following should the patient be informed?

FIG. 2-15 (Courtesy of Douglas G. Adler, MD.)

(A) The symptoms will resolve if he undergoes a total colectomy.

(B) The only definitive treatment is liver transplantation.

(C) Hepatic ultrasound is the best modality to diagnose his condition.

(D) His disease is more commonly associated with irritable bowel syndrome.

(E) A bacterial pathogen is the responsible agent.

117. A 33-year-old female complains of a sore throat and general malaise over the past week after being treated for an upper respiratory infection. On examination, her thyroid gland is nodular and tender to palpation. Which of the following is the best treatment?

(A) penicillin G

(B) salicylates /səˈlisəˌlāt/

(C) fluconazole (Diflucan)

(D) subtotal thyroidectomy

(E) total thyroidectomy

118. Which of the following is the most appropriate treatment for a 32-year-old male with a toxic nodular goiter and compressive airway symptoms?

(A) radioactive iodine therapy

(B) propranolol

(C) propylthiouracil

(D) Lugol's solution

(E) total lobectomy

119. Several days following an uneventful laparoscopic cholecystectomy, the pathology report reveals gallbladder cancer that is invasive into the submucosa of the specimen. The most appropriate management is which of the following?

(A) observation and close follow-up

(B) chemotherapy with a 5-fluorouracil (5-FU)-based regimen

(C) laparotomy with 2–3 cm wedge resection of the gallbladder liver bed

(D) laparotomy with 2–3 cm wedge resection of the gallbladder liver bed and regional lymphadenectomy including the portal and hepatic nodal basins

(E) radiation to the gallbladder liver bed

120. A 19-year-old college student is found to have an elevated serum calcium on routine physical examination. She has a family history of hypercalcemia that has not resulted in any known symptoms. Further workup reveals a slightly elevated serum parathyroid hormone with depressed levels of serum phosphate. A 24-hour urine calcium excretion is obtained and is low. Which of the following is the correct diagnosis?

(A) familial hypocalciuric hypercalcemia (FHH)
(B) primary hyperparathyroidism
(C) secondary hyperparathyroidism
(D) tertiary hyperparathyroidism
(E) metastatic bone cancer

121. A 42-year-old male with extensive Crohn's disease undergoes a near complete resection of the ileum. A deficiency of which of the following vitamin is likely to result?

(A) niacin
(B) thiamine
(C) vitamin B_{12}
(D) vitamin C
(E) vitamin B_6

Questions 122 and 123

A 34-year-old male undergoes an uneventful excision of a parathyroid adenoma. The following postoperative day, he complains of numbness around his lips.

122. Which of the following is the most likely cause of this symptom?

(A) hypocalcemia secondary to hypomagnesemia
(B) hypocalcemia due to acute renal failure
(C) hypocalcemia due to hungry bone syndrome
(D) hypocalcemia due to inadvertent injury to the recurrent laryngeal nerve
(E) postoperative hematoma of the neck

123. Which of the following is the most appropriate intervention?

(A) oral calcium gluconate
(B) intravenous rehydration with normal saline
(C) intravenous magnesium sulfate infusion
(D) blood transfusion
(E) reassurance and close observation

124. A CT scan in a patient with a temperature of 102.1°F and a history of an abdominal aortic graft reveals fluid around the graft. Which of the following is the most appropriate treatment?

(A) IV antibiotics and repeat CT scan in 24–48 hours
(B) CT-guided catheter drainage of fluid collection
(C) exploration with graft excision, irrigation, and replacement with fresh graft
(D) exploration with graft excision and construction of axillobifemoral graft
(E) open exploration with debridement and drainage of fluid collection

Answers and Explanations

/ˌthȯrəˈkätəmē/

1. **(B)** Spontaneous pneumothorax is usually found in young males. A tall, thin habitus is common. Eighty-five percent of patients are found to have pulmonary blebs on the affected side. The correct management is placement of a chest tube, pain control, oxygen supplementation, and serial chest x-rays to monitor resolution. Thoracotomy is required if the pneumothorax does not resolve with a chest tube or if there is a persistent air leak. Bleb resection and pleurodesis is usually performed at the time of operation to prevent future bleb rupture and to promote adhesion of the lung to the chest wall. Thoracotomy is also offered to patients after a recurrence to prevent future episodes. Fifty percent of patients will have a recurrence on the ipsilateral side after a spontaneous pneumothorax. (*Brunicardi et al., 2005, pp. 583–584*)

2. **(B)** Intussusception is usually seen in children 8–12 months of age. They present with paroxysmal, crampy abdominal pain, and sometimes emesis. "Currant-jelly" stools are sometimes seen. They usually report a history of GI viral infection in the recent past. Enlarged Peyer's patches are usually the lead point of the intussusception. Polyps, tumors, and Meckel's diverticulum are less frequent causes. On examination, these children may have a mass in the epigastrium or right upper quadrant with an absence of intestine in the right lower quadrant. This is referred to as "Dance's sign." The diagnostic tool of choice is air contrast enema. This is also therapeutic in 60–90% of cases. If the intussusception cannot be reduced by the enema, laparotomy is required to prevent bowel ischemia. Compromised bowel is resected at that time. Only 5% of children have a recurrence after successful reduction. (*Brunicardi et al., 2005, pp. 1493–1494*)

3. **(D)** Pyloric stenosis usually presents in the first 4–8 weeks of life. Parents usually report non-bilious emesis after feeding, which progresses to a projectile nature. Untreated, this will become a complete obstruction. On examination, an "olive sign" or mass in the right upper quadrant is often found. Ultrasound is the best radiologic test. These infants may present with dehydration and metabolic abnormalities from the emesis. The most common abnormality is hypokalemic, hypochloremic metabolic alkalosis. While surgical correction is urgent, it is not emergent. These infants should be resuscitated with IV fluids and their metabolic derangements corrected before an operation. The surgical treatment is a pyloromyotomy, which involves splitting the hypertrophic muscles of the pylorus while keeping the mucosa intact. This can be performed either open or laparoscopically. Patients are usually allowed to feed within hours of their operation. (*Brunicardi et al., 2005, pp. 1486–1487*)

/pīˌlȯrō mīˈätəmē/

4. **(A)** Any infant or child that presents with bilious emesis should be evaluated immediately for malrotation with midgut volvulus. This is a surgical emergency since the volvulus can compromise the vascular supply to the intestine. Malrotation is a congenital disorder wherein the normal prenatal rotation of the midgut is incomplete and results in the cecum remaining in the epigastrium with a narrow superior mesenteric artery(SMA) pedicle. When this happens, bands form between the cecum and the abdominal wall ("Ladd's bands"). A volvulus may result around the shortened mesentery, cutting off the vascular supply to the midgut and causing obstruction. In volvulus, patients present with acute onset of bilious emesis and later with bloody stools or hemodynamic instability. The diagnosis of malrotation can be best made with an upper GI contrast study, which will show the duodenojejunal

junction displaced to the right of midline. Sometimes this can also reveal volvulus. Patients with volvulus must be taken emergently to the OR to reduce the volvulus. If intestinal ischemia is advanced, a significant portion of small bowel may have to be removed, resulting in "short gut syndrome."

In this patient presenting with bilious emesis, malrotation with volvulus must be considered and addressed early. The correct answer is to get an upper GI contrast study to evaluate for malrotation and obtain a surgical consultation. Observation (choice C) may result in intestinal ischemia or death. Pyloric stenosis (choice B) presents with nonbilious emesis. Choice D refers to intussusception, which often presents with bloody stools but bilious emesis is unlikely. Necrotizing enterocolitis (choice E) can also present with bloody stools, but usually occurs in premature infants as they approach full enteral feeds. (*Brunicardi et al., 2005, pp. 1489–1491*)

5. **(B)** Meckel's diverticuli are usually found incidentally, although they can present with painless lower GI bleeding or inflammation (often confused with acute appendicitis). They are usually found within 2 ft of the ileocecal valve. They represent a remnant of the vitelline (or omphalomesenteric) duct and are found on the antimesenteric side of the ileum. They often contain ectopic gastric mucosa. Acid secretion from this leads to ileal ulceration and bleeding. They can be diagnosed using nuclear medicine scans (technetium pertechnetate) and the treatment is surgical resection. (*Brunicardi et al., 2005, pp. 1495–1496*)

6. **(D)**

7. **(C)**

Explanations 6 and 7

In patients with liver failure, the source of an upper GI bleed is esophageal varices in 50%, gastritis in 30%, and duodenal ulcers in only about 10%. Esophageal variceal bleeding is a potentially fatal complication of portal hypertension. The initial management should include fluid resuscitation and replacement of blood and clotting factors as needed. The second step is to control the source of bleeding. Medical management may include vasopressin or octreotide. Once the patient is stabilized, endoscopic evaluation of the bleeding is crucial. It can be both diagnostic and therapeutic. Endoscopic techniques for controlling hemorrhage can include sclerotherapy, banding, or balloon tamponade. If these methods are ineffective, or the patient has numerous recurrences, portal shunts can be considered. TIPS have increased in popularity as a method for portal decompression. This can be performed in the acute setting. Surgical shunts are also an option, but are primarily reserved for stable patients with recurrent bleeding episodes and not performed in an acutely unstable patient. Mesocaval shunts connect the SMV to the IVC in a variety of manners. Splenorenal shunts are actually the most common type of shunt. Nonselective shunts that completely divert portal blood flow from the liver can actually increase hepatic encephalopathy. Most surgeons prefer selective shunts, which preserve a component of hepatic blood flow and thus function. Synthetic graft material can be safely used to create the shunts. Postoperative mortality is directly related to the patient's preprocedure medical condition and degree of hepatic failure (i.e., Child class). (*Brunicardi et al., 2005, pp. 1154–1156*)

8. **(B)** Sentinel lymph node biopsy offers an alternative to full axillary dissection as a diagnostic tool in breast cancer with clinically negative axillary lymph nodes. Patients are injected with technetium-labeled sulfur colloid and isosulfan blue dye. A gamma probe is used along with the visual cues of the blue dye to identify the "sentinel node." The theory is that if this node is negative for malignancy, the rest of the axilla will be negative as well. This spares these patients from an unnecessary axillary lymph node dissection and the morbidity that it entails. Patients with a positive sentinel lymph node require further therapy. Contraindications to the procedure include palpable axillary lymph nodes (because the diagnosis of axillary metastasis is apparent), multicentric disease, and

a history of reaction to the blue dye (anaphylaxis and urticaria have been reported). If the lesion is very close to the axilla, there may be too much background radiotracer activity to discern the sentinel node. Lesions under the nipple are quite amenable to this procedure. There are several studies showing that the accuracy and success of this technique is related to surgeon experience. Surgeons are required to perform 20–30 procedures with some supervision or confirmation of results before relying completely on sentinel node biopsy. *(Cameron, 2004, pp. 635–636)*

9. **(C)** The first step in any trauma assessment is the primary survey. This consists of:

   A—airway maintenance
   B—breathing and ventilation
   C—circulation
   D—disability/neurologic status
   E—exposure/environment

The first priority in any trauma patient is to establish an airway. In an unconscious patient with decreased saturations, endotracheal intubation is indicated. While facial lacerations may indicate fractures, these patients can often be successfully orally intubated. This should be attempted first, but if this technique is unsuccessful, a cricothyroidotomy should be performed to secure the airway. Once an airway has been established, you can address breathing/ventilation by auscultating breath sounds and evaluating for end-tidal CO_2 using a capnometer. It is at this point where a life-threatening tension pneumothorax can be identified and treated. The next step is to evaluate the circulation. This includes getting adequate intravenous access. The patient described has two large-bore IVs, which should be sufficient for the initial resuscitation. Central venous access is indicated only if adequate access cannot be established peripherally. It is here that evaluation for intra-abdominal hemorrhage can be conducted using ultrasound or diagnostic peritoneal lavage. *(Moore, 2004, pp. 161–168)*

10. **(A)** Early clinical decline in a transplant patient is concerning for primary organ failure. This can be related to donor issues, technical issues,

or donor organ ischemia. Signs of liver dysfunction include hypoglycemia (as the liver is unable to perform gluconeogenesis), coagulopathy with elevated prothrombin times, elevated ammonia levels, acid-base changes (unable to clear lactate via the Cori cycle), hyperkalemia, and oliguria. All liver transplant patients have an initial rise in transaminases which should decrease over the first 48 hours. *(Mulholland et al., 2006, pp. 603–604)*

11. **(D)** Ureteral injuries are a well-known complication of pelvic surgery. The risk is greatly increased in the setting of inflammation, which can make the ureters difficult to identify. Intravenous pyelogram is a sensitive test for injury. CT scan and retrograde pyelogram are also diagnostic options. Injuries identified early are usually amenable to primary surgical repair, making early diagnosis essential. Delayed recognition usually results in a staged repair requiring urinary diversion with percutaneous nephrostomy tubes. *(Brunicardi et al., 2005, pp. 1525–1527)*

12. **(E)** Dehiscence refers to a separation of the fascial layer. Evisceration is when peritoneal contents extrude through the fascial separation. Malnutrition, obesity, diabetes, uremia, malignancy, immunologic abnormalities, steroid use, infection, and coughing which increases intra-abdominal pressures are all factors that increase the risk of wound dehiscence. Technical factors are also very important in preventing the dehiscence, but there is no proof that interrupted sutures are better than a running stitch for fascial closure. *(Brunicardi et al., 2005, pp. 235–238)*

13. **(E)** This patient has achalasia. This disorder is defined by a nonrelaxing lower esophageal sphincter (LES) and decreased peristalsis of the esophageal body. The "bird's beak" deformity is a classic sign with a dilated esophagus which tapers to a small area at the LES. Esophagomyotomy is the treatment of choice for long-standing disease. Serial botox injections and dilations can be used early in the disease process, however their long-term results are inferior to myotomy. Proton pump inhibitors can be used for gastroesophageal

reflux disease (GERD). A Nissen fundoplication is also a treatment for GERD. Calcium channel blockers are sometimes used to treat other esophageal motility disorders. *(Brunicardi et al., 2005, pp. 877–878)*

14. **(D)** One of the most feared complications of neck surgery is postoperative hemorrhage causing airway compromise. Any patient with neck swelling and dyspnea must be assessed for this emergently. The treatment is to immediately open up the neck wound to release the hematoma and relieve the tracheal compression. *(Brunicardi et al., 2005, p. 1429)*

15. **(A)** The needle biopsy revealing amyloid makes the diagnosis of medullary thyroid cancer. Patients often present with a neck mass and palpable lymph nodes (15–20%). Because of the aggressive nature of the malignancy and the fact that it is often multicentric, total thyroidectomy is the treatment of choice. Modified radical neck dissection is indicated in patients with palpable lymphadenopathy and in patients with tumors larger than 2 cm (since 60% of these patients will have lymph node involvement). Because medullary carcinoma originates from the thyroid C-cells, they do not respond to thyroxine or radioactive iodine therapy. *(Mulholland et al., 2006, pp. 1303–1304)*

16. **(C)** Primary hyperparathyroidism is usually the result of a parathyroid adenoma. It can also be associated with multiglandular hyperplasia. Secondary hyperparathyroidism is associated with the hyperphosphatemia, and resultant hypocalcemia, in chronic renal disease. Tertiary hyperparathyroidism is seen after kidney transplant. Most patients (about 80%) with primary hyperparathyroidism are asymptomatic. Symptoms can include renal stones, bone abnormalities, peptic ulcer disease, and mental status changes. It is more common in females, and the incidence increases with age. *(Mulholland et al., 2006, pp. 1319–1325)*

17. **(D)** *E. coli* is the most common culprit for acute cystitis, although it is often caused by enterococci, *S. aureus, Klebsiella, Pseudomonas,* and *Streptococcus epidermis. P. mirabilis* can split urea,

which results in alkaline urine and precipitation of calcium. Patients with this organism often present with bladder calculi. *(Brunicardi et al., 2005, p. 1540)*

18. **(C)** Increasing abdominal pressures for laparoscopic procedures has several systemic effects. By increasing the carbon dioxide, patients become hypercarbic and acidotic. There is decreased venous return and increased afterload. The peritoneum is distended and the diaphragm elevated. In patients with normal cardiac function, cardiac output is not affected until the abdominal pressures reach about 20 mmHg. *(Brunicardi et al., 2005, pp. 381–382)*

19. **(B)** This patient should be able to perform any activity that requires innervation from C6 or above. The biceps and deltoid are innervated by C5, so he should be able to lift his arms above his head, have shoulder flexion, and elbow flexion. C6 innervates the extensor carpi radialis, so wrist extension should be preserved. The triceps rely on C7, so he would not be able to perform elbow extension. *(Mulholland et al., 2006, p. 2009)*

20. **(D)** The joint space is most relaxed when the hip is flexed and externally rotated. This tends to be the least painful position for patients with septic arthritis. *(Brunicardi et al., 2005, pp. 1677–1678)*

21. **(A)** A direct hernia comes through the medial inguinal canal floor and is found behind the spermatic cord. An indirect hernia passes though the internal inguinal ring, and thus can be found within the spermatic cord. The spermatic cord also contains the vas deferens, the testicular artery, lymphatics, and nerve fibers. *(Brunicardi et al., 2005, pp. 1358–1364)*

22. **(C)**

23. **(B)**

Explanations 22 and 23

The Glasgow Coma Scale is used to quantify a neurologic examination in patients with a head injury. It is based on three elements: eye opening, motor response, and verbal response. The total score ranges from 3 (worst) to 15 (best) with a score of 8 or lower indicating a coma. The scale is shown below. This patient has a score of 2(E) + 4(M) + 2(V) = 8.

This patient has evidence of a severe head injury. The initial step should be to protect his airway and prevent hypoxia, which could adversely affect his head injury. Thus, the initial step should be endotracheal intubation. Neurosurgical expertise, imaging to define the injury, and screens to rule out drugs or alcohol as contributions are all important, but should be performed after airway, breathing, and circulation are addressed. Mannitol is indicated in patients with evidence of herniation, such as those with pupillary dilatation. (*American College of Surgeons, 1997, pp. 181–206*)

GLASGOW COMA SCALE

	Score
Eye opening (E)	
Spontaneous	4
To speech	3
To pain	2
None	1
Motor response (M)	
Obeys commands	6
Localizes pain	5
Withdraws to pain	4
Abnormal flexion (decorticate)	3
Extension (decerebrate)	2
None (flaccid)	1
Verbal response (V)	
Oriented	5
Confused conversation	4
Inappropriate words	3
Incomprehensible sounds	2
None	1

24. **(B)** Symptoms of zinc deficiency include diarrhea, mental status changes, alopecia, and periorbital, perinasal, and perioral dermatitis. Persons who have cirrhosis, who are receiving steroids, who have excessive loss of GI secretions, or who are severely traumatized are at risk for zinc deficiency. Deficiency states resulting from inadequate ingestion of selenium, silicon, and tin have not been described. Deficiency of iodine produces hypothyroidism. (*Townsend et al., 2004, p. 156*)

25. **(A)** During total thyroidectomy, parathyroid glands may inadvertently be removed or their vascular supply interrupted. Hypoparathyroidism may then develop, the manifestations of which include tingling, muscle cramps, convulsions, and a positive Chvostek's sign (contraction of facial muscles after tapping the facial nerve). These symptoms are dramatically relieved by intravenous administration of calcium. Oral calcium and vitamin D are administered for long-term correction of hypocalcemia. (*Townsend et al., 2004, p. 987*)

26. **(E)** Vital capacity is an important measure of respiratory function. It is defined as the maximum volume of air a person can expel following a maximum inspiratory effort. When vital capacity is normal, significant restrictive pulmonary disease is not present. Acutely decreased vital capacity indicates decreased ventilatory reserve. (*Townsend et al., 2004, p. 1765*)

27. **(D)** In deceleration injuries, laceration involving the aorta most frequently occurs just distal to the left subclavian artery at the level of the ligamentum arteriosum. This is where the aorta is fixed and thus more susceptible to shear forces. The tear may be complete or partial. Diagnosis is difficult, but is suggested by a widened mediastinum on chest x-ray and confirmed with a CT scan of the chest or an aortogram. (*Townsend et al., 2004, pp. 2036–2037*)

28. **(C)** A gastrinoma, a gastrin-secreting tumor, produces Zollinger-Ellison syndrome, which is associated with markedly elevated gastric acid secretion and ulcer disease of the upper GI tract. The most common location for these tumors is the pancreas. However, they can be found in the gastric antrum, duodenum, spleen, and ovary. Removal of the gastrinoma can result in a cure. A thorough search must be made at the time of surgical exploration to locate the tumor, which in early stages will be small. The gastrinoma triangle, where 90% of gastrinomas are located, is defined as the area between the junction of the cystic and common bile ducts, the junction of the second and third portions of the duodenum, and the junction of the pancreatic neck and body. (*Townsend et al., 2004, pp. 1010–1015*)

29. **(A)** Avascular necrosis occurs following a fracture when the blood supply to a bone fragment is disrupted. The femoral head, humeral head, scaphoid, and talus are particularly vulnerable to this complication because of their precarious blood supply. A dense appearance of the bone on x-ray is a diagnostic clue. Radioisotope scanning can detect avascular necrosis at an earlier stage than is possible with roentgenography. *(Townsend et al., 2004, pp. 561–562)*

30. **(B)** Contraction of hollow organs against obstruction or excessive contraction causes colic. Typical ureteral colic is severe, sudden in onset, radiates from the loin to the groin, and is associated with an urge to urinate. Blood clots and calculi in the ureter can cause colic, the latter being more common. Urine examination demonstrates macroscopic or microscopic hematuria. *(Townsend et al., 2004, p. 2299)*

31. **(A)**

32. **(C)**

Explanations 31 and 32

In a patient who is known to have had symptoms of peptic ulcer disease for many years and presents with nausea and vomiting, one should consider gastric outlet obstruction. The obstruction can be the result of an exacerbation of the ulcer and subsequent edema or it can be secondary to scar tissue formation. These patients typically describe the sensation of epigastric fullness and demonstrate visible peristalsis going from left to right. A succussion splash may be audible. The history of periodicity and pain relief by taking antacids also favors a diagnosis of previous peptic ulcer disease. Patients with an umbilical hernia will have a mass in the region of the umbilicus. Patients with acute cholecystitis usually present with the sudden onset of pain, radiating to the back, with fever and chills. Volvulus of the sigmoid colon presents with constipation and abdominal distention but vomiting is a late feature. Small bowel obstruction would be associated with a history of colicky abdominal pain, nausea, and vomiting. Additionally, patients with small bowel

obstruction usually have hyperactive high-pitched bowel sounds on examination. *(Townsend et al., 2004, pp. 1283–1284, 1295)*

With persistent vomiting, the patient becomes dehydrated and hypovolemic. Loss of hydrogen ions, potassium, and chloride in the vomited gastric contents leads to alkalosis, hypokalemia, and hypochloremia. In response to the hypovolemia, adrenocortical and renal mechanisms are stimulated to conserve sodium at the expense of potassium and hydrogen ions. Excretion of potassium in the urine further aggravates the hypokalemia. The kidneys then compensate by exchanging hydrogen ions for potassium, which results in a paradoxical aciduria and self-perpetuating metabolic alkalosis. *(Townsend et al., 2004, p. 80)*

33. **(A)** Gastrin secretion is increased by vagal stimulation, antral distention, and by the presence of protein in the antrum. Antral acidification (pH = 1.5) decreases gastrin secretion by a feedback mechanism. The same is true with duodenal acidification. *(Townsend et al., 2004, p. 1270)*

34. **(B)** From the description, the diagnosis in this patient is acute regional enteritis. The incidental finding of regional enteritis in patients operated on for the presumed diagnosis of acute appendicitis is treated medically unless there is proximal obstruction. The risk of operating on patients with regional enteritis is the formation of a fistula and/or abscess, especially if the area to be resected is involved with the disease process. However, if the cecum and the appendix are not involved, it is advisable to perform an appendectomy. In this instance, it would be safe and eliminate acute appendicitis from the differential if his symptoms recurred. *(Townsend et al., 2004, p. 1394)*

35. **(B)**

36. **(C)**

Explanations 35 and 36

Testicular cancer is the most common malignancy in men between the ages of 15 and 35. It typically presents as unilateral scrotal swelling.

On examination, it is important to distinguish intraparenchymal masses (usually malignant) from extraparenchymal masses (usually benign). This is easily done with scrotal ultrasound. Upon the diagnosis of an intraparenchymal testicular mass, a staging CT scan of the chest, abdomen, and pelvis should be obtained. It is reasonable to evaluate the serum levels of beta-HCG and AFP as they may be elevated in 80–85% of patients with nonseminomatous germ cell tumors. LDH, on the other hand, can be elevated in patients with seminomas and can be of prognostic significance. Finally, if elevated, these serum markers can serve as a means to monitor the presence of residual disease and should be measured after resection of the tumor.

Additionally, the mass should be excised in order to establish a histologic diagnosis. A radical orchiectomy should be performed from an inguinal approach. Less invasive approaches such as biopsies or a scrotal approach to the tumor should be avoided as they can alter the lymphatic drainage and potentially adversely affect overall outcomes.

The majority of testicular tumors occurring in young adults are malignant tumors. The tumors may originate from germinal or nongerminal cells. Approximately 95% of testicular tumors are germinal tumors. These include seminomas (the most common), embryonal cell carcinomas, choriocarcinomas, and teratocarcinomas. On the other hand, Leydig cell tumors and androblastomas originate from nongerminal cells and may produce excess testosterone. Benign tumors such as fibroma can occur but are rare. *(Townsend et al., 2004, pp. 2311–2316)*

37. **(A)** Although constipation is the most common presenting feature of Hirschsprung's disease, some patients suffer from diarrhea. The severity of symptoms does not correlate well with the extent of bowel involvement. Enterocolitis, a major cause of death, requires vigorous treatment. This complication can occur even after removal of the aganglionic segment of the bowel. Increased acetylcholinesterase activity has been noted in the serum, affected aganglionic bowel, and erythrocytes of afflicted persons. Eighty

percent of affected infants are male. *(Townsend et al., 2004, pp. 2113–2114)*

38. **(C)** Because of the risk of postsplenectomy sepsis, attempts should be made for splenic salvage when possible. Most patients are managed nonoperatively. Nonoperative management is contraindicated in the presence of hypotension or persistent bleeding. If patients are treated operatively, attempts are still made at splenic salvage if possible instead of splenectomy. Attempts at splenic salvage are contraindicated in hemodynamically unstable patients or patients with multiple concomitant injuries, as it prolongs the operation and increases blood loss. The risk of postsplenectomy sepsis from encapsulated organisms persists throughout life, but the highest incidence is in the first 2 years following splenectomy. Patients should be vaccinated against *Pneumococcus, Meningococcus,* and *Haemophilus influenzae* prior to discharge from the hospital. *(Cameron, 2004, pp. 970–974)* /ɪnˈkapsəˌlāt/

39. **(C)** Esophageal achalasia is characterized by the findings of aperistalsis/atony and a failure of the LES to relax normally, resulting in esophageal dilatation proximally with a functional obstruction at the LES. Long-standing achalasia results in the characteristic barium swallow finding of a "bird's beak." Iatrogenic or tumor-related elevation of LES pressure can result in a "pseudoachalasia," but should have normal peristaltic patterns on manometry. Patients with Barrett's esophagus may have a "cobblestone" appearance on barium swallow, with normal peristalsis, and do not characteristically demonstrate esophageal dilatation; LES pressures may be normal or low. Finally, patients with Plummer-Vinson syndrome develop cervical dysphagia due to iron-deficiency anemia; patients often present with cervical esophageal webs and can be at higher risk for developing esophageal squamous cell carcinoma. *(Cameron, 2004, pp. 14–18)*

40. **(D)** Barrett's esophagus is a condition in which the normal stratified squamous esophageal mucosa is replaced by a columnar-lined epithelium. It is often the result of chronic GERD. If

left untreated, patients can develop dysplasia and esophageal adenocarcinoma. As such, they require lifelong endoscopic surveillance with repeated biopsies. Barrett's esophagus is more common in men than women, in Caucasians more than African-Americans, and the prevalence increases with age. Although effective medical and surgical antireflux therapies can cause regression of symptoms, the Barrett's esophagus segment rarely regresses and the potential for dysplasia or adenocarcinoma is not eliminated. *(Cameron, 2004, pp. 36–37)*

41. **(B)**

42. **(D)**

Explanations 41 and 42

"Hamman's crunch" is precordial crackles heard on auscultation that correlate with heart sounds in the setting of mediastinal emphysema and is suggestive of esophageal perforation. When present along with subcutaneous emphysema of the chest and neck, pneumomediastinum from an esophageal perforation is the most likely diagnosis. The most common cause of esophageal perforation is iatrogenic, but it may be spontaneous (Boerhaave's syndrome) or secondary to a malignancy or stricture. Diagnosis is often made after clinical suspicion by endoscopy or a swallow study with water-soluble contrast. If diagnosed early (within 24 hours), a primary repair is the first approach to treatment. Closure is dependent on the amount of infected or necrotic tissue, tension on the anastomosis, etiology of the perforation, and the ability to adequately drain the contaminated areas. Late perforations may be complicated in their management, requiring several procedures or diversion to provide for adequate healing. *(Cameron, 2004, pp. 10–14)*

43. **(D)** The diagnosis of acute appendicitis can often be made based on the history and physical findings. The sequence of symptoms classically begins with anorexia followed by periumbilical pain that localizes to the right lower quadrant after 6–12 hours. The onset on nausea and emesis occur after the development of abdominal pain. If the patient has an appetite

or if bouts of vomiting begin before the onset of abdominal pain, the diagnosis should be reconsidered. In this patient, the acute appendicitis has progressed to a rupture resulting in a localized right lower quadrant abscess (marked with arrow in Figure 2-16).

FIG. 2-16 *(Courtesy of H.J. Kim, MD.)*

The signs of acute appendicitis are also characteristic. On examination, tenderness is often maximal at McBurney's point, located approximately one-third the distance from the anterior superior iliac spine to the umbilicus. Other physical signs include Rovsing's sign (pain initiated in the right lower quadrant upon palpation in the left lower quadrant), Dunphy's sign (increased pain with coughing), the obturator sign (pain on internal rotation of the hip), and the psoas sign (pain during extension of the right hip). Dance's sign (concave and empty right lower quadrant) is associated with ileocecal intussusception. Grey-Turner's sign is bruising of the flanks and may occur in severe, acute pancreatitis due to subcutaneous tracking of inflammatory, peripancreatic exudate along the retroperitoneum. Murphy's sign is defined as inspiratory arrest secondary to pain when palpating under the right costal margin. It is associated with a diagnosis of acute cholecystitis. *(Brunicardi et al., 2005, pp. 1119–1125)*

44. **(C)** Carcinoids are the most common neoplasm of the appendix and arise from Kulchitsky cells, a type of enterochromafin cell. Aside from the appendix, the next most frequent site of involvement is the small bowel followed by

the rectum. Appendiceal and rectal carcinoids are almost never associated with carcinoid syndrome unless metastatic disease is present. Small bowel carcinoids are more commonly multifocal, metastatic, and associated with carcinoid syndrome.

The majority of appendiceal carcinoids are located at the tip and the extent of surgical resection depends on the size and resulting malignant potential. Lesions less than 1 cm rarely metastasize and therefore require only simple appendectomy as in this question. Lesions greater than 2 cm require a right hemicolectomy due to the high potential for metastasis. Partial small bowel resection is indicated for a carcinoid of the small intestine. Partial cecectomy and total abdominal colectomy are not appropriate options. *(Brunicardi et al., 2005, p. 1134)* /sē'sek təmē/

/kə'lek təmē/

45. **(D)** Postoperative wound infections usually occur between the fifth and eighth postoperative days. Evidence of a wound infection within the first 24 hours after surgery should alert the physician to the possibility of necrotizing fasciitis. Necrotizing fasciitis is a life-threatening infection most commonly caused by clostridial myositis and hemolytic streptococcus. In addition to spiking temperature, the patient may be septic with tachycardia, leukocytosis, and hemodynamic instability. On examination of the wound, crepitus (gas in the soft tissue) and a dishwater-appearing effluent may be apparent. /'nekrə,tīzing/

/,fashē 'ītəs/

Early diagnosis by opening the wound and sending a Gram's stain is critical. The Gram's stain will reveal a mixed flora of gram-negative rods and gram-positive cocci. Although broad-spectrum antibiotics are indicated, definitive treatment requires emergent aggressive debridement of the affected tissues. Hyperbaric oxygen treatment has no role in the acute management of necrotizing fasciitis.

Diabetic patients are especially prone to necrotizing fasciitis. Fournier's gangrene is a type of necrotizing fasciitis that affects the groin and perineum. The mortality rate can be as high as 75%. *(Brunicardi et al., 2005, pp. 353–354, 434–435)* /,perə'nēəm/

46. **(D)** Nearly all broad-spectrum antibiotics may result in superinfection of the colon with *Clostridium difficile.* This anaerobic enteric pathogen produces a toxin that causes necrosis of the colonic mucous membrane resulting in enterocolitis (pseudomembranous colitis). The infection can occur several weeks after the discontinuation of the inciting antibiotic. The presentation varies from mild diarrhea to systemic illness with abdominal pain, fever, and leukocytosis. Severe cases may progress to colonic dilatation and perforation.

Lower endoscopy reveals the characteristic yellow pseudomembranes, which represent ulceration and necrosis. The diagnosis is confirmed with either colonic wall biopsy for the organism, or more commonly with identification of the toxin in stool samples.

Orally administered metronidazole is the treatment of choice. Oral vancomycin is also effective, but it is reserved for refractory cases due to its side effect profile and expense. *(Townsend et al., 2004, pp. 277–278)*

47. **(D)** A high index of suspicion is warranted for catheter sepsis in any patient who has had a central line for several days and suddenly spikes a high fever. The catheter site may have erythema, induration, tenderness, and purulent discharge extruding from the skin. Often, however, the skin appears normal. A thorough search for other possible sources of fever including pulmonary, intra-abdominal, urinary, and wound infections is always prudent.

Catheter sepsis can be life threatening and early intervention is essential. Peripheral and central blood cultures should be obtained and the catheter must be removed promptly. It is contraindicated to replace the catheter over a guide wire because the skin tract is infected. It is not mandatory to treat with antibiotics unless the fever persists or signs of sepsis are present. *(Townsend et al., 2004, p. 267)*

48. **(A)** Internal hemorrhoids are highly vascularized submucosal cushions located in the anal canal. They are classified as first degree if no prolapse is present; second degree if prolapse occurs with spontaneous reduction; third degree if they require manual reduction; and fourth degree if they are irreducible. Treatment is based on the symptoms and degree of prolapse.

Nearly all patients with first- and second-degree hemorrhoids should initially be placed on a trial of conservative measures including a bowel management program with high fiber diet to avoid straining and constipation, frequent warm baths, and an anti-inflammatory topical cream. If symptoms continue, both rubber band ligation (a small rubber band is placed at the neck of the hemorrhoid resulting in eventual death and detachment of tissue) and infrared coagulation (controlled burn of the vessels at the neck of the hemorrhoid) are good alternatives to surgical therapy. For refractory first- and second-degree hemorrhoids, most third-degree and all fourth-degree hemorrhoids, surgical hemorrhoidectomy is the treatment of choice.

A thrombosed external hemorrhoid is a blood clot resulting in painful swelling of the tightly held anoderm. In most cases conservative management is indicated. Excision is reserved for patients with debilitating pain or signs of necrosis. (*Townsend et al., 2004, pp. 1490–1491*)

49. **(E)** The most common cause of anorectal fistula and abscess is infection of the anal glands, which empty into the anal canal at the level of the dentate line. Classification of anal fistula is based upon the relationship of the epithelialized tract to the anal sphincter muscle and can be intersphincteric (most common), transsphincteric, suprasphincteric, and extrasphincteric (least common). A symptomatic fistula is an indication for surgery because it rarely heals spontaneously.

Despite popular teaching, there is little use for antibiotics in the primary treatment of anal abscess. As a rule, surgical drainage is required and antibiotics are only indicated if cellulitis is present. However, those patients who are immunocompromised, have valvular heart disease, or poorly controlled diabetes should always be considered for antibiotics. (*Townsend et al., 2004, pp. 1495–1499*)

50. **(D)** Crohn's disease is a chronic inflammatory disease of the GI tract of unknown etiology. Both medical and surgical treatments are palliative in nature—there is no known "cure."

Approximately 70% of patients with Crohn's disease will require an operation during their lifetime. The most common indication for surgery is recurrent bowel obstruction, followed by perforation with abscess and fistula formation. (*Townsend et al., 2004, pp. 1348–1349*)

51. **(E)** Ulcerative colitis is a diffuse inflammatory disease of the colon and rectum with unknown etiology. Unlike Crohn's disease, surgical removal of the entire colon and rectum provides a complete cure. Nonetheless, many patients are treated successfully with medical therapy including corticosteroids and can avoid the potential complications of surgery and lifelong ileostomy.

Ulcerative colitis usually presents as bloody diarrhea, fever, and abdominal pain. The disease process begins in the rectum, advances proximally in a contiguous fashion, and affects the superficial layers of the colon wall. Crohn's disease is located anywhere from the mouth to anus, has skip lesions, and is transmural in nature. Histologically, superficial inflammation with crypt abscesses is most indicative of ulcerative colitis, whereas deeper involvement with granulomas and fissures are most characteristic of Crohn's disease. Both diseases may present with extraintestinal manifestations such as arthritis, skin lesions, and hepatic dysfunction, but perianal disease with fistula formation is characteristic of Crohn's disease.

Patients with ulcerative colitis have a 10–20% risk of developing colon cancer within 20 years after diagnosis. The incidence is also increased in those with Crohn's disease but to a lesser extent. Surveillance colonoscopy is essential in patients with long-standing disease. (*Townsend et al., 2004, pp. 1425–1441*)

52. **(A)** Anal carcinoma can arise from several epithelial cell types in the anal canal including squamous, basaloid, cloacogenic, and mucoepidermoid. For early, superficial lesions less than 2 cm, an attempt can be made to excise the lesion completely with negative margins. Otherwise, the standard of care is a multimodality chemoradiation protocol, which classically includes mitomycin C and 5-FU in combination with external beam radiation therapy to the tumor

and the pelvic and inguinal lymph nodes. The long-term survival rate after chemoradiation alone compares favorably with radical surgery. Abdominal perineal resection is reserved for persistent or recurrent disease. Low anterior resection refers to resection of the upper and middle rectum and plays no role in the treatment of anal cancer.

Inguinal lymph node dissection is not indicated. Any clinically suspicious node should be biopsied, and if positive, treated with radiation. Thus, even a small anal cancer with a positive lymph node should be treated with chemotherapy instead of surgery. (Townsend et al., 2004, pp. 1509–1510)

53. **(B)** Colon cancer is the most common metastatic lesion of the GI tract to the liver. Approximately 50% of patients with colorectal cancer will have liver involvement. Generally, synchronous liver metastasis should not be resected during the initial operation for the primary tumor. Only a solitary, small, peripherally located lesion in a hemodynamically stable patient would be an acceptable indication for a wedge resection. Otherwise, the planned colon resection should be completed. A second procedure can be planned after a thorough metastatic evaluation is completed using various diagnostic modalities such as intraoperative ultrasound, CT, MRI, and/or PET scan.

A delay of weeks to months between surgeries has not been shown to have a negative impact on long-term survival. The delay may help select patients who may benefit the most and exclude those who develop widespread metastatic disease during the interval.

Chemotherapy only is inappropriate because, even in the presence of metastatic disease, the primary colon carcinoma should be resected to prevent later complications such as bleeding, perforation, or obstruction.

The 5-year survival rate following resection of isolated hepatic metastasis from colorectal cancer now exceeds 50%. (Feig et al., 2006, pp. 341–342)

54. **(A)** Local treatment of rectal cancer is the treatment of choice in selected individuals with low-lying rectal cancers. The lesion must be mobile, nonulcerated, within 10 cm of the anal verge, less than 3 cm in diameter, less that one-fourth the circumference of the rectal wall, and stage T1 or T2 on endorectal ultrasound.

Transanal excision is the most straightforward technique of local treatment. It entails full thickness excision of the lesion into the perirectal fat with adequate margins. For early lesions into the submucosa only (T1), no adjuvant therapy is required unless poor prognostic features are present on final pathology (poorly differentiated or lymphatic/vascular invasion). If the lesion penetrates the muscular wall (T2), adjuvant radiation therapy with or without chemotherapy is indicated following surgical removal. Overall, the disease free survival rate is 80%.

Dukes originally proposed a staging classification for colon cancer. Dukes' A lesions are confined to the bowel wall, Dukes' B lesions extend beyond the wall involving the serosa or fat, and Dukes' C lesions have accompanying regional lymph node involvement. TNM staging is now probably the most widely used system for staging. (Feig et al., 2006, pp. 290–291)

Stage I	T1 – invades submucosa
	T2 – invades muscularis propria
Stage II	T3 – invades through muscularis propria into subserosa
	T4 – invades into contiguous organs
Stage III	Any T with presence of positive lymph nodes
Stage IV	Distant metastatic disease present

55. **(A)** The patient described has familial adenomatous polyposis (FAP). FAP is a rare autosomal dominant inherited form of colorectal cancer that results from a germline mutation in the APC gene. The disease is characterized by the presence of >100 polyps in the large intestine, as well as extraintestinal manifestations such as epidermoid cysts, desmoid tumors, and osteomas. All patients with FAP will develop colorectal cancer if left untreated. The average age of diagnosis is 29 and the average age of the development of cancer is 39.

Once diagnosed, the most definitive treatment requires complete removal of the entire colon and rectum in a timely fashion.

Surveillance colonoscopy is not protective against the development of cancer regardless of the frequency. The surgical procedure of choice is a proctocolectomy with permanent ileostomy or creation of an ileoanal anastomosis with ileal reservoir such as a J-pouch. Abdominal perineal resection with sigmoid colectomy leaves a significant portion of colon in situ with subsequent risk of developing colon cancer. *(Brunicardi et al., 2005, p. 1087)*

56. **(A)** Villous adenoma is a premalignant condition. The incidence of carcinoma in a polyp depends on the histology type and size of the polyp. Tubular adenomas are the most common type of polyps (60–80%), but are the least likely to harbor carcinoma (less than 5% if smaller than 1 cm in diameter). Villous adenomas are the least common type, but overall the most likely to contain malignant foci (50% if greater than 2 cm in diameter).

In this patient, a formal right hemicolectomy is indicated due to the high probability of finding cancer in the specimen. A lesser operation, such as open or laparoscopic polypectomy, would then require a second operative procedure if cancer is present. Colonoscopic fulguration of such a large lesion carries a high risk for perforation and would not allow histologic examination. Observation with repeat colonoscopy in 1 year is also inappropriate. *(Townsend et al., 2004, pp. 1448–1451)*

57. **(B)**

58. **(D)**

59. **(C)**

Explanations 57 through 59

This patient presents with classic symptoms of a bowel obstruction. The diagnosis is often made by a thorough history and physical examination. Following the initial evaluation, an acute abdominal x-ray series should be obtained, which includes supine and erect views of the abdomen. The diagnosis is confirmed with the presence of dilated loops of bowel with the presence of air-fluid levels. These plain films may also suggest the location of the obstruction (small vs. large intestine). Abdominal ultrasonography has limited role in the diagnosis or management of intestinal obstruction. Serum electrolyte determination helps in identifying the electrolyte disturbances that have taken place. Fluid loss needs to be corrected with rehydration, and nasogastric suction helps in decreasing abdominal distention. Upper GI endoscopy would increase distention, and is contraindicated. Antiemetics should not be given until a definitive diagnosis is made, and then only if indicated; promotility agents have little to no role in the management of a patient with bowel obstruction, and may even be contraindicated. *(Townsend et al., 2004, pp. 1336–1340)*

An annular constricting lesion with overhanging edges is typical of annular carcinoma of the colon. Mechanical small bowel obstruction results in multiple air-fluid levels in distended small bowel loops. Intussusception produces a "corkscrew" appearance on barium enema, and sigmoid volvulus produces a "bird's beak" appearance. In diverticulitis, extravasation of barium outside the lumen of the colon typically is seen. *(Mulholland et al., 2006, pp. 1111, 1132–1133, 1917)*

The ureters may be injured during pelvic operations. The principles of ureteral repair include early recognition, debridement of nonviable tissue, and tension-free anastomosis over an internal ureteral stent. The type of repair largely depends on the location of injury.

If the injury occurs above the pelvic brim, the best option is primary end-to-end repair over a double J stent. If there is a large defect precluding a tension-free anastomosis, a ureteroureterostomy (anastomosis to the opposite ureter) should be considered. However, this may result in injury to the uninvolved kidney and is reserved as a second-line option.

When the injury occurs below the pelvic brim, ureteroneocystostomy (ureteral reimplantation into the bladder) is the procedure of choice. Ligating the transected ends should be reserved for unstable patients. In this scenario, a nephrostomy tube is required as a temporizing measure until definitive repair *(Cameron, 2004, pp. 978–980)*

60. **(A)** The Halsted radical mastectomy involves removal of all breast tissue, lymphadenectomy, and removal of the pectoralis major. The modified radical mastectomy preserves the pectoralis major muscle thus decreasing the morbidity of the surgery with the same survival. The modified radical mastectomy does include a lymph node dissection. The anatomic limits of the modified radical mastectomy include the sternum medially, the subclavius muscle superiorly, the inframammary fold inferiorly, and the latissimus dorsi muscle laterally. The surgeon must identify the thoracodorsal nerve and the long thoracic nerve, which innervate the latissimus dorsi muscle and the serratus anterior muscle, respectively. Damage to the long thoracic nerve results in a "winged scapula." After a complete dissection of level I, II, and III lymph nodes, the use of radiation therapy needs to be critically evaluated because of the long-term morbidity of lymphedema. *(Brunicardi et al., 2005, pp. 488–491)*

61. **(A)** Damage to the thoracic duct can be seen as a complication following distal esophagectomy or any procedure that involves dissection into the cervical region. It is most commonly seen on the left if iatrogenic. Aspiration of an odorless, milky fluid from the chest cavity is diagnostic, although increased lymphocyte counts and triglyceride levels in the fluid help confirm the diagnosis. Normal chyle flow is around 2 L a day. Therefore, a chylous leak can result in nutritional depletion as well as decreased systemic lymphocytes to fight infection. The first therapy is placement of a chest tube to drain the chyle and to allow for approximation of the lung against the mediastinum. Stopping oral intake and starting total parental nutrition is usually tried for 7–10 days to see if there is spontaneous resolution of the leak. If conservative measures fail, ligation of the thoracic duct can be performed. *(Brunicardi et al., 2005, pp. 602–603)*

62. **(B)** Finding a conduit for use in coronary artery bypass grafting can sometimes be a challenge

since these patients often have diffuse atherosclerotic disease. The left internal mammary artery is most commonly used. Bilateral internal mammary arteries can be used, however this increases the chances of sternal healing problems. Saphenous vein grafts are used in patients with multivessel disease, although this may not be an option in patients with deep vein thrombosis (DVT), venous insufficiency, or arterial insufficiency to the legs (because they will not heal the harvest wound). Radial arteries, the right gastroepiploic artery, and inferior epigastric arteries have also been used. *(Mulholland et al., 2006, pp. 1488–1489)*

63. **(B)** Esophageal cancer is increasing in incidence in North America, largely due to the rise in incidence of esophageal adenocarcinoma. Premalignant lesions for esophageal cancer include: Barrett's changes, radiation esophagitis, caustic esophageal burns, Plummer-Vinson syndrome, leukoplakia, esophageal diverticula, ectopic gastric mucosa, and tylosis. It is more common in men, and smoking is clearly a risk factor along with alcohol. Barrett's esophagus requires frequent surveillance examinations with biopsies and increases the risk for adenocarcinomas of the esophagus at the gastroesophageal junction. *(Cameron, 2004, pp. 44–49)*

64. **(E)** The indications for surgery for duodenal ulcers include intractability, hemorrhage, obstruction, and perforation. Initial management includes dietary and behavior modification, H_2 blockade, proton pump inhibitors, and treatment for *H. pylori*. Duodenal ulcers are rarely secondary to a malignancy and are related to acid production, unlike gastric ulcers, which have a higher incidence of association with malignant processes. Surgical approaches include: vagotomy (truncal, selective, highly selective), vagotomy combined with antrectomy, or subtotal gastrectomy. There are varying rates of perioperative morbidity and effectiveness reported in the literature. Recurrence rates after vagotomy and pyloroplasty alone approach 30%, in long-term follow-up. The complication of dumping after a highly selective vagotomy is significantly lower than truncal vagotomy. A drainage procedure after

highly selective vagotomy is unnecessary, and vagal denervation of the proximal stomach reduces receptive relaxation. (*Cameron, 2004, pp. 71–76*)

65. **(A)** Gastrin is the humoral mediator of the gastric phase of secretion, and the release of gastrin is stimulated by antral distention, antral protein/amino acids, and by the vagus itself. Gastrin stimulates gastric acid secretion, promotes gut motility, and is a trophic factor for gut mucosa. Secretin is released by duodenal mucosal S cells in response to acid and promotes water and bicarbonate secretion from the pancreas. CCK is released in the gut by intestinal mucosal I cells and stimulates emptying of the gallbladder, increases bile flow, and relaxes the sphincter of Oddi. CCK has a structure very similar to gastrin. (*Townsend et al., 2004, pp. 1269–1276*)

66. **(B)** Severe abdominal pain is the hallmark presentation of acute mesenteric ischemia. The pain is often described as being out of proportion to examination. It is most often caused by an embolic event to the SMA. Patients with cardiac arrhythmias are at greater risk for having an embolic event. Nonocclusive mesenteric ischemia is thought to be due to reactive arterial vasoconstriction and is not a surgically correctible disease. CT scan findings of SMA thrombosis or gas in the bowel wall would necessitate emergency surgery. (*Mulholland et al., 2006, pp. 1614–1618*)

67. **(A)** This patient is experiencing multiple transient ischemic attacks (TIAs) associated with carotid artery disease. TIAs last only a few minutes, while RINDs (reversible ischemic neurologic deficit) typically resolve after 24 hours, and strokes result in long-term deficit. The symptoms are typically related to embolic events rather than reduced blood flow. The finding of carotid bruit on examination is more sensitive for coronary artery disease than it is for carotid disease. The initial workup for these patients should be bilateral carotid duplex ultrasound. Operative repair is indicated for asymptomatic patients with >60% stenosis as well as symptomatic patients. (*Mulholland et al., 2006, pp. 1591–1601*)

68. **(D)** This patient is presenting with subclavian steal syndrome, which is caused by subclavian stenosis proximal to the take off of the verterbral artery. Exertion of the extremity causes blood to be shunted away from the brain to the arm resulting in vertigo or even syncope. These patients usually have diminished radial pulses on the affected side and also have other evidence of atherosclerotic disease. A carotid-subclavian bypass is the operation of choice for these patients. (*Rutherford Vascular Surgery, 6th ed., p. 1288, 1301, 1988*)

69. **(A)** The Zollinger-Ellison syndrome was described in 1955, in two patients with the triad of gastroduodenal ulcerations, gastric hypersecretion, and nonbeta islet cell tumors of the pancreas. Gastrinomas arise from neuroendocrine cells and represent the third most common neuroendocrine tumors (after carcinoids and insulinomas). These tumors are associated with MEN I. These tumors occur predominantly in the pancreas, duodenum, antrum, and peripancreatic lymph nodes, but can also occur at distant sites like the ovary. Isolated tumors are found in 50%, and multiple tumors in 50%, but there is a higher incidence of multiple tumors in MEN I. Tumors are malignant in 50%, with metastases to the regional lymph nodes and the liver. Once the diagnosis has been established, tumor localization can be achieved with indium-labeled octreotide scan, CT with fine cuts through the pancreas, ultrasound, MRI, or selective angiography. None of these tests are highly sensitive, and often the tumors are not localized until the time of exploration and intraoperative-directed ultrasonography. (*Cameron, 2004, pp. 76–79*)

70. **(D)**

71. **(A)**

Explanations 70 and 71

Gastric adenocarcinoma is associated with dismal overall prognosis, with long-term survival seen only in patients with early stage disease. Surgical resection remains the mainstay of potentially curative therapy, with poor responses to chemotherapy in the majority of clinical trials. Patients often present with vague epigastric discomfort, occult GI bleeding/anemia, anorexia, weight loss, and even hematemesis/vomiting. Patients are staged with endoscopic ultrasound, which is the most effective imaging modality for determining T and N stage. CT may also be useful for determining nodal metastases, but is more accurate for determining distant metastases (liver). Antral tumors may have a better prognosis than more proximal gastric tumors, with a decreased incidence of nodal metastases. Five-year survival rates for stage I disease is excellent, approaching 80–90% in both the Western countries and in Asia. However, 5-year survival rates are dismal for stage III and stage IV disease, and most Western series report overall 5-year survival rates for gastric cancer of 10–21%. *(Feig et al., 2006, pp. 205–219)*

In contrast to gastric adenocarcinoma in the United States, the incidence of gastric lymphoma is rising. Gastric lymphoma accounts for two-thirds of GI lymphomas. Symptoms are similar to gastric adenocarcinoma, but obstruction, perforation, and massive bleeding are very uncommon symptoms. Because gastric lymphoma spreads by submucosal infiltration, mucosal biopsies at the time of upper endoscopy can often be nondiagnostic. Repeated biopsies to obtain submucosal tissue are needed to establish a diagnosis. Treatment protocols vary among institutions, but most often center on chemotherapy; surgical resection of isolated or localized gastric lymphoma can be curative, but is rarely seen. Fortunately, survival rates for gastric lymphoma are much better than those seen in gastric adenocarcinoma, with cure rates of 70% seen in patients with stage IE and IIE disease treated with chemotherapy alone. *(Feig et al., 2006, pp. 232–233)*

72. **(A)** Barrett's esophagus is related to GERD. It is found proximal to the LES and is thought to be a result of constant acidic exposure. It is a condition where the normal esophageal squamous cell epithelium is replaced by columnar epithelium, similar to intestinal metaplasia. A single biopsy is all that is needed to confirm the diagnosis. In fact, many biopsies should be taken

during endoscopy if the diagnosis is suspected in an effort to find dysplasia. The risk of malignant degeneration is the most important risk associated with Barrett's esophagus. *(Brunicardi et al., 2005, pp. 860–861)*

73. **(D)** The main blood supply to the stomach comes from the right gastric artery (from the hepatic artery), the left gastric artery (from the celiac axis), the right gastroepiploic artery (from the gastroduodenal artery), the left gastroepiploic (from the splenic artery), and the short gastric arteries from the splenic artery. *(Brunicardi et al., 2005, pp. 935–937)*

74. **(C)** Duodenal ulcers are usually associated with hypersecretion of acid, whereas gastric ulcers may be related to breakdown of the mucosal protective mechanisms or to malignancy. Type I gastric ulcers are the most common. They are usually associated with altered mucosal defense and not hypersecretion of acid. Type II gastric ulcers are caused by a duodenal ulcer and the resulting pyloric obstruction. Type III gastric ulcers are found proximal to the pylorus and are associated with hypersecretion and duodenal ulcers. *H. pylori* is found in 95% of duodenal and 80% of gastric ulcer patients. However, only 10% of people who carry the bacteria actually manifest ulcer disease. Serologic testing does not determine the presence of an active infection. Active infections can be determined by endoscopic biopsy sampling or the use of urease breath testing. All currently recommended regimens to eradicate *H. pylori* utilize both antibiotics and acid suppression. *(Brunicardi et al., 2005, pp. 953–959)*

75. **(E)** Carcinoid syndrome is seen in less than 10% of patients with metastatic carcinoid disease. It is seen in patients with elevated serotonin levels, which is metabolized by the liver. Thus, only patients with massive hepatic metastasis or with tumors that bypass the hepatic filter—such as a retroperitoneal tumor—show symptoms. 5-Hydroxyindoleacetic acid (5-HIAA) levels can be tested in the urine to give the diagnosis (urinary vanillylmandelic acid [VMA] is indicative of a pheochromocytoma). An apple core lesion on the colon is most

likely to be a large adenocarcinoma, which would not be associated with carcinoid symptoms. Common symptoms of carcinoid syndrome include flushing, diarrhea, right heart failure, and asthma. Weight loss and liver failure are uncommon symptoms. *(Mulholland et al., 2006, pp. 814–817)*

76. **(C)** Most patients have a change in their digestive habits after gastrectomy. These symptoms are actually related to the vagotomy done with the operation. The majority of patients learn to manage their symptoms with only a small amount requiring surgical intervention. Dumping syndrome is associated with abdominal pain, nausea, vomiting, dizziness, and palpitations related to the quick hyperosmolar emptying into the small intestine. These symptoms can be managed by eating small, low carbohydrate meals throughout the day. Postvagotomy diarrhea is related to the rapid transit of unconjugated bile salts and is effectively treated with cholestyramine. Proton pump inhibitors are not a useful therapy for alkaline reflux. *(Brunicardi et al., 2005, pp. 985–990)*

77. **(E)** This patient has developed a DVT of her left leg. This is a complication following surgery that can be prevented in part by the use of subcutaneous heparin and sequential compression devices. Coumadin is not used as a prophylaxis, but rather as a treatment modality. Risk factors for developing DVTs include female gender, obesity, orthopedic surgery, use of oral contraceptives, smoking, and long periods of being sedentary. Her knee should be aspirated if she has a red, hot, or swollen joint; as these symptoms are not mentioned and the DVT is in the leg opposite to the surgically treated joint, aspiration is not necessary at this time. *(Mulholland et al., 2006, pp. 1781–1786)*

78. **(A)** Wound infection is a complication of surgery that can lead to a great deal of morbidity and longer hospital stay. Prevention of wound infection includes perioperative antibiotics, which should be at their peak tissue concentration at the time of skin incision. This means they should be given at least 30 minutes prior to incision. Patients who have other infections, such as urinary tract infections, are at increased risk for wound infection. Bowel surgery exposes the wound to the normal intestinal flora, the most common being *Bacteroides*. Washing hands is an essential part of preventing spread of infectious pathogens between patients. Using gloves is not a substitute for good hand hygiene. Once a wound is infected, it must be opened and drained. Antibiotic therapy alone is not adequate. *(Mulholland et al., 2006, pp. 165–170)*

79. **(D)** This patient has a gastrinoma, seen in Zollinger-Ellison syndrome, and should also be evaluated for possible MEN I. Gastrin is a GI hormone that is released from the antral G cells of the stomach to regulate acid secretion by the gastric parietal cells. It is released when the stomach gets the signal that is needed to initiate the digestion process, and also acts to stimulate chief cells to secrete pepsinogen and to increase gastric mucosal blood flow. Known stimulants for the release of gastrin include: vagal stimulation, calcium, alcohols in the stomach, proteins/amino acids in the stomach, antral distention, and gastric pH greater than 3. Antral pH less than 2 inhibits gastrin release, as does somatostatin. Secretin has no effect or decreases gastrin levels in healthy patients, but it increases gastrin release in patients with Zollinger-Ellison syndrome. Glucagon has little or no effect on gastrin release. *(Mulholland et al., 2006, pp. 885–887)*

80. **(B)** One of every four trauma deaths in North America is due to thoracic trauma. Many deaths from thoracic trauma can be prevented with prompt diagnosis and treatment of injuries. The first step in the evaluation of any trauma patient is the primary survey, or ABCDE (airway, breathing, circulation, disability, exposure). First you would evaluate the airway. In this case, an endotracheal tube was placed at the scene. It would be important to evaluate this airway's adequacy of placement using a capnometer to assess end-tidal CO_2 and auscultation of the breath sounds. Next you would assess breathing. Auscultation in this patient reveals an absence of breath sounds on the left. This must be resolved before moving

on to circulation. This could be the result of placing the endotracheal tube in too far into the right mainstem, which is easily checked by withdrawing the endotracheal tube 2 cm. The other possibilities are life-threatening emergencies, including a tension pneumothorax or a hemothorax. Given the fact that the patient is unstable and there is a history of penetrating chest trauma, a chest tube should be placed immediately without the delay of a chest x-ray. A tube thoracostomy in this patient will be diagnostic and also therapeutic. A hypovolemic patient with cardiac tamponade may not have neck vein distension. ED thoracotomies should only be performed in a pulseless patient. All other patients requiring thoracotomy should go to the OR. This patient is unstable and as such should not be taken to angiogram. (*American College of Surgeons, 1997, pp. 125–141*)

81. **(D)** Like other trauma patients, the initial management of burn patients is crucial in improving survival and function. Inhalation injury should be suspected in anyone with a history of confinement in smoke, facial burns, singed eyebrows or nasal hairs, carbonaceous sputum, or carboxyhemoglobin levels greater than 10%. These patients sometimes look stable initially but soon develop airway edema. These patients should be placed on high-flow oxygen and observed closely. There should be a very low threshold for endotracheal intubation to protect the airway. Burn patients require large volume fluid resuscitation that should begin immediately. If patients develop pulmonary edema, they should be intubated. Fluid resuscitation should not be withheld to prevent intubation. Heat loss is also a major concern in burn patients who have lost their thermoprotective skin covering. They should be wrapped in warm, moist dressings. Depth of burn affects management in resuscitation efforts, as well as need for debridement or escharotomy, and should be evaluated in every patient. The American Burn Association recommends transfer to a burn center for patients with:

- Partial thickness and full thickness burns of >10% of total body surface area (TBSA in patients with age <10 years old or >50 years old

- Partial or full thickness burns of >20% in patients of any other age
- Partial or full thickness burns involving face, hands, feet, genitalia, or perineum
- Full thickness burns of >5% TBSA in any age group
- Significant electrical or chemical burns
- Inhalation injury (*American College of Surgeons, 1997, pp. 273–288*)

82. **(B)**

83. **(B)**

Explanations 82 and 83

In transplant immunology, a wide variety of immune effector mechanisms are responsible for rejection. Acute rejection typically occurs in the first few days to weeks after organ transplantation. The primary mediator of this immune response is the T cell. Treatment of acute rejection usually involves pulse dose steroids and increased immunosuppression. Other forms of rejection include hyperacute rejection and chronic rejection. Hyperacute rejection is the result of preformed antibodies and occurs within hours of transplantation and leads to graft loss. Chronic rejection occurs on the scale of months to years after transplantation and is characterized by fibrosis and loss of normal histologic architecture. (*Mulholland et al., 2006, pp. 547–548*)

84. **(C)**

85. **(B)**

Explanations 84 and 85

The management of elevated intracranial pressure following traumatic injury has been extensively studied. Several interventions have been shown to be of benefit in the acute setting. The pressure can be relieved through mechanical means such as elevating the head of the bed to 30 degrees or by direct drainage of cerebrospinal fluid via a ventricular catheter. Administration of a hyperosmotic solution such as mannitol can decrease intracranial pressure by reducing brain water, increasing plasma volume and reducing blood viscosity. Additionally, if the ICP is refractory to these interventions, it is reasonable to consider a barbiturate coma or potentially a decompressive craniectomy. Hyperventilation is used only in the acute setting to keep $PaCO_2$ around 35 mmHg, which functions to decrease intracranial pressure by decreasing intracranial blood volume through vasoconstriction. MRI would not be indicated initially, as it would not change your management.

Severe head injuries are a frequent problem encountered in the field of trauma. CT scans are the primary diagnostic modality used to evaluate patients with suspected head injuries. Elevated intracranial pressure is a frequent result of severe brain injury either from brain swelling or mass effect from expanding hematomas. Subdural hemorrhages (Figure 2-17) typically have a crescent shape and extend across suture lines covering the entire surface of one hemisphere. These are usually the result of the disruption of bridging veins. Epidural hematomas (Figure 2-18) on the other hand have a biconvex lens appearance on CT scan. They typically develop after an injury to the middle meningeal artery. Brain injury is generally greater in patients with subdural hematomas than in those with epidural hematomas. *(Townsend et al., 2004, pp. 2152–2157)*

FIG. 2-18 *Epidural*

FIG. 2-17 *Subdural*

86. **(D)** Bleomycin is known to cause pulmonary fibrosis. Doxorubicin toxicity is predominantly manifested by leucopenia and cardiotoxicity. Etoposide is a podophyllotoxin derivative that inhibits topoisomerase which normally unwinds DNA and is associated with myelosuppression. Cisplatin is a platinum alkylating agent that can be nephrotoxic and ototoxic. Vincristine is a microtubule inhibitor that can result in peripheral neuropathy. *(Brunicardi et al., 2005, p. 280)*

87. **(C)** Keloids occur at the site of injury, predominately in people with dark skin who have a genetic predisposition. The keloid is a form of benign tumor that consists of an overabundance of collagen that extends beyond the margins of the incision. Treatment options have only moderate success and include excision of the keloid with intralesional steroid injections. Recurrences of keloids, both at the original site and with subsequent injury/incision elsewhere in the body, are common. They are not associated with decreased fertility or other systemic processes. *(Mulholland et al., 2006, pp. 94–95)*

88. **(C)** Succinylcholine is a depolarizing neuromuscular blocking agent that can cause

arrhythmias including bradycardia and junctional rhythms because of vasotonic effects. Additionally, succinylcholine is associated with a transient hyperkalemia that can be profound in patients with burns or those who have experienced significant crush injury and result in cardiac arrest. *(Brunicardi et al., 2005, p. 1858)*

89. **(C)** Pheochromocytomas arise from neuroectoderamal cells and are most often found within the adrenal medulla. Ten percent of all pheochromocytomas are located outside of the adrenal gland along the embryologic path of the adrenal gland. The most common site of an extra-adrenal pheochromocytoma is in the paraaortic area. *(Mulholland et al., 2006, p. 1346)*

90. **(D)** Bladder ruptures are highly associated with pelvic fractures. They typically present with hematuria and are typically evaluated with CT cystogram in the setting of trauma. The management of the injury is defined by the location of the rupture. If the rupture remains contained in the extraperitoneal space the treatment is Foley catheter drainage, which allows the bladder to heal spontaneously. However, if the patient has an open pelvic fracture or has other intra-abdominal injuries requiring operative exploration, the bladder injury should also be repaired. If imaging of the urinary tract demonstrates rupture of the bladder contents into the peritoneal cavity, operative exploration with a two-layer closure of the defect is the standard of care. A suprapubic catheter is then placed to help protect the repair. *(Townsend et al., 2004, pp. 2295–2296)*

91. **(A)**

92. **(E)**

Explanations 91 and 92

The patient's history of gnawing epigastric pain is consistent with ulcer disease. His presentation is that of a perforated duodenal ulcer. The most appropriate first step is to obtain upright plain films of the chest and abdomen to look for free intraperitoneal air. Although the patient is in mild distress, he is not toxic and it is reasonable to confirm your suspicion with

radiologic studies. If the plain films did not demonstrate free air and the patient remained hemodynamically stable, a CT scan of the abdomen and pelvis may be indicated to try to make the diagnosis. However, if the patient did show signs of increasing toxicity and evidence for sepsis, such as hypotension or mental status changes, it would be reasonable to proceed with an exploratory laparotomy to make the diagnosis. Upper endoscopy is not indicated in the acute management of a perforated duodenal ulcer and this patient is currently in significant distress and discharging to home with delayed follow-up is unwise.

The patient most likely has a posterior perforation of a duodenal ulcer that has eroded into the gastroduodenal artery causing bleeding per rectum, tachycardia, and hypotension. Diverticulosis is a common cause of bright red blood per rectum in elderly patients but is often painless and not consistent with the presentation of this patient. A ruptured AAA generally presents with hypotension and profound shock. A distended abdomen and pulsatile mass can be found on physical examination. Ruptured esophageal varices present with upper GI bleeding and hematemasis and are most often associated with patients who have chronic liver disease. *(Cameron, 2004, pp. 71–76)*

93. **(D)** As a practicing physician, you are not required to stop at an accident and care for the injured, as you have not established a doctor-patient relationship. As such, there are no legal requirements for physicians to assist in the care of accident victims outside of their employment (i.e., hospital, ER, clinic). It is also important to realize that under the Good Samaritan law, individuals who provide aid to the injured or ill are protected from prosecution for unintentional injury or wrongful death. It is also important to be familiar with local laws. For example, in some states, this law only applies to people who are trained in basic first aid. (The state of Vermont requires any bystander to render aid until proper authorities arrive). In the situation presented above, you most probably would not be faulted for not assisting in

the care of the injured person and there would be no grounds for legal action.

94. (C)

95. (D)

Explanations 94 and 95

Burn injuries can be very serious and very intimidating for the patient and physician alike. In an ER setting, the most efficient way to estimate the extent of the burn injury is to use the "rule of nines." In determining the percentage of the TBSA that is involved, it is important only to consider second- and third-degree burns in this calculation. In this system, the head and neck are 9%; each arm represents 9%; the anterior trunk, posterior trunk, and each lower extremity carry a value of 18%; the genitalia are estimated to be 1%. For the patient in this question, the burns cover his anterior face and neck (4.5%), anterior trunk (18%), and bilateral upper extremities (18%) for a TBSA of approximately 40%. Having identified the extent of the thermal damage, it is critical to initiate resuscitation immediately. The thermal injury itself causes the release of many inflammatory mediators that result in a profound capillary leak. As a result of this profound increase in capillary permeability, the patient's intravascular volume and thus overall perfusion can drop rapidly and dramatically. In order to compensate, burn patients will require aggressive fluid resuscitation. Furthermore, as in any trauma situation, the fluid used in the initial resuscitation should be isotonic such as Ringer's lactate. The Parkland formula (4 mL/kg/%TBSA) is a common equation used to estimate the fluid needs in the first 24 hours for thermal injuries. Typically, one-half of this total volume is given in the first 8 hours. In this particular case, an 80-kg man with 40% TBSA burns would require 12.8 L of fluid in the first 24 hours. So for the first 8 hours, you would plan to run isotonic fluid at 800 mL/h. (*Moore, 2004, pp. 1083–1085*)

96. (B)

97. (E)

Explanations 96 and 97

It is important to consider vascular injuries in the setting of extremity trauma. This is particularly true in the setting of fractures, dislocations, or penetrating trauma in the vicinity of major vascular structures. When evaluating patients for traumatic vascular injuries, the first step is evaluation of peripheral pulses. This should be done after the initial resuscitation in order to rule out hypovolemia as the source for diminished peripheral perfusion. In the presence of fractures or dislocations, if diminished or absent pulses are identified, it is critical to reduce the fracture or the dislocation and then re-evaluate the perfusion. By placing the bony structures in the anatomical position, you rule out a kink in the vessel as the source of the arterial obstruction. After reduction or relocation, if the pulse is still absent or diminished compared to an uninjured extremity, then further investigation of the vasculature is indicated.

In the case described, posterior knee dislocations have a very high incidence of concomitant popliteal artery injury. If vascular compromise is identified after relocation of the knee, operative exploration is indicated for emergent repair of the popliteal artery with a venous interposition graft. It would not be indicated in this setting to delay operative repair for an arteriogram. Arteriograms are indicated in the evaluation of extremity trauma if there are diminished distal pulses after restoring anatomical alignment and the ankle-brachial indices are <0.9.

If a vascular injury is identified, one must always consider the possibility of compartment syndrome following reperfusion of the extremity. The most sensitive physical finding is pain on passive flexion of the muscles. The most common sight for compartment syndrome is the calf. There are four compartments within the lower leg and, in the presence of prolonged ischemia, crush injuries or combined arterial and vascular injuries, you must have a high suspicion for compartment syndrome. In the postoperative setting following repair of a traumatic vascular injury, increased pain in the calf is concerning. Furthermore, evidence for compartment syndrome such as tense swelling, pain on passive flexion, or altered sensation without evidence of acute vascular occlusion requires emergent four compartment fasciotomies to prevent further tissue loss. *(Mulholland et al., 2006, pp. 462–465)*

98. **(A)** The x-ray described demonstrates an open book pelvic fracture. This type of injury can often be associated with significant hemorrhage. It is most commonly seen in frontal impacts involving anterior-posterior compression. The majority of the bleeding occurs from the tearing of pelvic veins in the posterior of the pelvis. The initial treatment for open book pelvic fractures is to reduce the pelvic volume to decrease the amount of hemorrhage. In the trauma bay, this can easily be accomplished by wrapping a sheet around the superior iliac crests and twisting the sheet tight using a dowel or by applying the pneumatic compression garment. These are useful techniques in the short term, but definitive treatment will be necessary. This involves formal repair of the pelvis with external fixation or open reduction and internal fixation. If hemorrhage persists despite reduction of the pelvic fracture, pelvic angiography would be the next step in the treatment algorithm to attempt to identify the source of the hemorrhage and embolize the vessel. Given the difficulty of identifying a bleeding vessel in an expanding pelvic hematoma, exploratory laparotomy is not recommended. Finally, an unstable patient should never be transported for imaging studies. *(Moore, 2004, pp. 787–790)*

99. **(B)** Acute arterial occlusion is a surgical emergency. However, the most important intervention is immediate heparinization. The infusion of heparin will help prevent extension of the clot. Furthermore, it will help to keep collateral vessels open. If the patient is stable enough to undergo operative intervention, a catheter embolectomy would be the procedure of choice. Physical examination findings including vascular examination and level of temperature change and altered sensation can help identify the level of the occlusion prior to operative intervention. Duplex ultrasound is not necessary to isolate the occlusion. Arteriograms are more useful in the OR following the embolectomy. Finally, if small vessel occlusion occurs, catheter-directed thrombolytics can

help restore distal perfusion. Once perfusion to the threatened limb has been restored, the workup to identify the thromboembolic source should be obtained. Typical sources for emboli include atrial thrombus, valvular disease, aortic aneurysms, or iliac artery atherosclerotic disease. *(Mulholland et al., 2006, pp. 1649–1655)*

100. **(C)** In the workup of a lesion identified within the colon, the gold standard for diagnosis is colonoscopy. Colonoscopy allows for biopsy of the tissue to establish a diagnosis of cancer prior to removing the mass. Furthermore, it also enables examination of the rest of the colon to rule out synchronous lesions. Barium enemas continue to have a role in diagnosis, but are more useful identifying the level of the lesion particularly in the setting of obstruction. You would not proceed straight to surgical resection unless the patient presented with an obstruction. Finally, PET scans have no role in the diagnosis of colon cancer. *(Townsend et al., 2004, pp. 1457–1459)*

101. **(B)** LCIS is a benign diagnosis and alone does not have a risk of progression to an invasive cancer. However, a diagnosis of LCIS does increase the risk for development of future breast cancer at a rate of about 1% per year. It is important to remember that the risk is increased for both breasts. It has been shown that chemoprevention with tamoxifen can decrease the incidence of breast cancer by 49%. It is also sufficient to follow this population closely with annual mammograms and semiannual clinical examinations. Prophylactic bilateral mastectomies are an option and result in a 90% decrease in the risk of subsequent breast cancer. Since a diagnosis of LCIS increases the risk of cancer in both breasts, a mastectomy of the affected side is insufficient treatment. *(Cameron, 2004, pp. 649–650)*

102. **(C)** The management of a breast lesion has become more complex as our knowledge regarding breast cancer development and treatment has continued to grow. The gold standard for evaluation of a suspicious lesion on mammogram is a core needle biopsy. This can be performed on palpable lesions directly, but can also be used on nonpalpable lesions using ultrasound or stereotactic guidance. A diagnosis of

atypical ductal hyperplasia cannot be established on core biopsy alone. Studies have demonstrated that nearly 20% of patients with this diagnosis on core biopsy go on to have evidence of ductal carcinoma in situ or invasive ductal carcinoma after excisional biopsy. As such, if a core biopsy demonstrates evidence for atypical ductal hyperplasia, the standard of care is to proceed with an excisional biopsy to establish the diagnosis. Once this diagnosis has been confirmed, management decisions can be made including close observation with frequent screening mammograms, chemoprevention with tamoxifen, or prophylactic bilateral mastectomy. A unilateral mastectomy is not an option as a diagnosis of atypical ductal hyperplasia increases the risk of breast cancer in both breasts. (*Townsend et al., 2004, pp. 880–886*)

103. **(C)** When assessing the prognosis for a patient diagnosed with melanoma, there are many factors that are involved. Tumor thickness, the presence of ulceration, the location of the lesion, the age of the patient, and the gender can all contribute. The most predictive factor is the tumor thickness. There are two measurement systems that have been developed to classify melanoma. The Clark level refers to the depth of invasion of the melanoma in terms of the anatomical layers of the skin. A second system, known as the Breslow depth, simply measures the overall tumor thickness in millimeters. Since the Breslow depth is more reproducible among pathologists, it has proven to be more accurate in the prediction of outcomes. (*Townsend et al., 2004, pp. 784–786*)

104. **(E)** Diverticulitis is categorized based on its complications. Uncomplicated diverticulitis is defined as inflammation of colonic diverticuli that does not involve free intraperitoneal perforation, abscess formation, fistula formation, or colonic obstruction. This entity can be managed as an outpatient but may require inpatient admission if the pain is severe. The treatment of choice is broad-spectrum antibiotics. The majority of patients will respond well to this intervention. However, as the incidence of recurrence increases the rate of complications also rises. Therefore, it is recommended

that surgical resection be performed after the second episode of diverticulitis. Prior to the operative intervention, it is important to rule out the presence of cancer. A colonoscopy should be performed after resolution of the inflammation and prior to surgical resection. It is much more sensitive than a barium enema. The operation is typically delayed until 4–6 weeks following discharge from the hospital. This provides adequate time for resolution of the inflammation and enables an adequate workup, which includes a colonoscopy. (*Townsend et al., 2004, pp. 1418–1420*)

105. **(D)** Informing a patient of a new diagnosis of cancer can be a very challenging and emotional experience for both the patient and the physician. It is important to maintain composure and not to rush. Certainly in the setting of a terminal cancer, the news can be devastating. The discussion that will follow this kind of information will often be lost as the patient copes with the news. In these situations, it is important to give the patient time to grieve. It is also important to be prepared to spend adequate time with the patient and family in order to review any questions. Finally, it is not unreasonable, if the patient is in agreement, to give them time to process this information and to discuss the diagnosis with their family before presenting them with management options. It is poor practice to avoid these confrontations, and a new diagnosis of cancer should be presented to the patient by a physician in a face-to-face manner if possible. It is also important to have information for the patient to take home in the form of handouts, pamphlets, or Internet resources, in order to help them continue to come to terms with the diagnosis and the current management options that are available.

106. **(D)** Organ donation can often be a very sensitive topic. As the transplant waiting lists continue to grow, the process of approaching the family of potential organ donors has been of great interest. In this setting, it is important to provide adequate information in a nonthreatening manner. Even today with donor cards, living wills, and so on, there can still be conflict between the patient and family, or even

amongst family members, with regard organ transplantation. An individual who has been trained to discuss organ transplantation with grieving families best addresses this sensitive topic. Furthermore, regardless of the decision after appropriate discussions are held, it is vital to respect the family's choice.

107. **(A)** Ranson's criteria represent a series of chemical clinical measurements that can be used to estimate the prognosis of an acute episode of pancreatitis. These markers are not meant for diagnosis of pancreatitis, but rather can be used to help gauge the severity of the disease and subsequently triage patients to the appropriate level of care. The criteria are measures of events that occur at admission and over the first 48 hours of hospitalization (see table below). Patients who meet three to four of the criteria have an estimated mortality of 15% and approximately 50% will require admission to the ICU. Essentially, all patients with five or more criteria will need to be cared for in the ICU, while patients with seven to eight positive criteria have a >90% mortality. It is important to note that amylase, lipase, and platelet counts are not considered in these criteria. *(Brunicardi et al., 2005, pp. 1236–1239)*

Admission	Initial 48 h
Age >55 years	Hematocrit fall >10
WBC >16,000	BUN elevation >5mg/100 mL
Glucose >200 mg/100 mL	Calcium <8 mg/100 mL
LDH >350 IU/L	PaO$_2$ <60 mmHg
AST (SGOT) >250 U/100 mL	Base deficit >4 meq/L
	Fluid sequestration >6 L

108. **(C)** Tumor resectability in lung cancer is generally determined by (1) whether or not the resection is technically feasible and (2) whether or not the resection will result in improved survival. In general, invasion of the tumor into structures that are vital to life would classify the tumor as unresectable. For example, the presence of superior vena cava syndrome in the setting of lung cancer is generally the result of tumor growing into the superior vena cava, which cannot be surgically removed. Those

patients should be treated with chemotherapy and radiation. For lung cancer, the presence of distant metastatic disease is a contraindication to surgical resection. Distant metastasis is defined by the presence of tumor in distant organs, such as brain, bone, or liver, as well as distant nodal involvement. In the treatment of lung cancer, this can be confusing when evaluating patients with lymph node metastases because the presence of positive *ipsilateral* medastinal nodes is not a contraindication to surgery, while positive *contralateral* mediastinal nodes indicates disseminated disease. With regards effusions, the presence of a pleural effusion in and of itself does not dictate the method of treatment, but identification of malignant cells within the effusion indicates noncurability and those patients should be treated medically. On the other hand, patients who present with local invasion of the tumor into the chest wall can potentially be cured of the disease with en bloc resection. Finally, involvement of more than one lobe has no bearing on prognosis as long as the patient's preoperative ventilation parameters will allow for safe resection. *(Townsend et al., 2004, pp. 1773–1788)*

109. **(B)** Pharyngoesophageal (Zenker's) diverticulum is the most common diverticulum of the esophagus, and is an example of a pulsion diverticulum. It is a false diverticulum and consists of the mucosa and submucosa protruding through the esophageal musculature. A true diverticulum would involve all three layers. It is situated posteriorly just proximal to the cricopharyngeal muscle, at a weak point in the esophagus. Symptoms include dysphagia, spontaneous regurgitation of undigested food/pills, noisy swallowing, and halitosis. The most serious complication of a Zenker's diverticulum is aspiration leading to pneumonia or a lung abscess. The diagnostic test of choice is a barium swallow. Both AP and lateral views are essential to estimate the size of the diverticulum and determine the side of deviation. Treatment mandates a cricopharyngeal myotomy in order to relieve the increased pressure at the upper esophageal sphincter that is responsible for the development of the diverticulum. Surgical management of the diverticulum

/ˈæpə.ˈsē/

itself could involve a resection or a diverticu-lopexy, which allows the pouch to spontaneously drain. Esophagoscopy with biopsy to rule out cancer is only indicated preoperatively if there is evidence of ulcers or mass defects on the barium swallow. EGD should be considered postopera-tively because of a high association of GERD with Zenker's diverticula. Complications of sur-gery include infection, recurrence, vocal cord paralysis secondary to injury to the recurrent laryngeal nerve, and esophagocutaneous fistulas. *(Townsend et al., 2004, pp. 1105–1107)*

110. (A)

111. (B)

Explanations 110 and 111

Cholelithiasis is much more common in women than men. In addition to gender, the develop-ment of gallstones can also be affected by age, weight, family history, and pregnancy. Gallstones often remain asymptomatic, but they can cause symptoms when they cause obstruction of the cystic duct. The result of this obstruction is biliary colic, which is experienced as epigastric pain radiating to the back and can be associated with nausea and vomiting. The presence of tenderness to palpation in the right upper quadrant, fever, and leukocytosis would suggest acute cholecys-titis, a complication of gallstones.

In a patient suspected of having complica-tions of gallstones, the best test for evaluation is ultrasonography. Ultrasonography is highly sensitive in detecting gallstones and also pro-vides details about the thickness of the gall-bladder wall, the presence of pericholecystic fluid, and also the presence or absence of tenderness over the gallbladder during the examination (sonographic Murphy's sign). A two-way roentgenogram of the abdomen is much less sensitive, detecting only 20% of gall-stones. A CT scan of the abdomen with IV and PO contrast can be sensitive in detecting the inflammatory changes associated with acute cholecystitis, but it is much more expensive and time consuming when compared to ultrasound. A HIDA scan, although sensitive and specific in the right setting, is generally reserved for

more complicated cases where the diagnosis is unclear. Failure to visualize the gallbladder with HIDA scan in 1 hour indicates either par-tial or complete cystic duct obstruction and confirms the diagnosis of acute cholecystitis. However, this should not be the first-line test in evaluating a patient for acute cholecystitis. Finally, an MRCP can be very useful in evalu-ating the biliary tree and the presence of chole-docholithiasis in a patient with cholecystitis and an elevated bilirubin, but does not have a role in the diagnosis of acute cholecystitis. *(Townsend et al., 2004, pp. 1608–1611)*

112. (D) AAA is most common in the infrarenal aorta (shown by the arrow in Figure 2-19). Fifteen to twenty-five percent of patients with an AAA have a first-degree relative with clini-cally apparent AAA. Fifteen percent of patients with an AAA will have an aneurysm of a peripheral vessel. Risk factors include age, gender, smoking, family history, and collagen vascular diseases such as Marfan syndrome. The risk of rupture of an AAA >5 cm is approx-imately 5–10% per year. At this point, the risk of rupture begins to outweigh the risk of open operative repair. Therefore, most patients with an aneurysm that has exceeded 5 cm in antero-posterior diameter should undergo repair. The role for endovascular repair of AAA continues to evolve. Recently, the benefits of this proce-dure in terms of decreased operative morbidity, mortality, length of stay, and recovery time

FIG. 2-19 *(Courtesy of H.J. Kim, MD.)*

have been established while the long-term durability of this less invasive repair is still being evaluated. Endovascular repair has become a valuable tool in the treatment of AAA, but as the long-term outcomes are still uncertain, it is not yet the procedure of choice for young patients with this disease. *(Rutherford Vascular Surgery, 6th ed., pp. 1408–1425)*

113. (B)

114. (B)

Explanations 113 and 114

The symptoms described by the patient are classic for rest pain. Patients often experience pain at night while lying in bed, and the pain improves with dependent positioning of the affected extremity. Initial evaluation of this patient should be an arterial duplex study of the vessels of the affected leg. This noninvasive test can provide great detail on the extent of the disease and the location of hemodynamically significant obstruction. Furthermore, it will help determine if inflow obstruction is present in the aorta or iliac vessels. It is crucial in these patients to determine if the arterial obstruction involves the aortoiliac vessels or is confined to the lower extremity vasculature. After determining the location of the atherosclerotic lesion, you can proceed with a traditional angiogram, CT angiogram, or even an MRI/MRA to evaluate the vessels in order to plan your intervention.

The management of peripheral arterial occlusive disease is determined in part by the severity of the symptoms. Patients with limb-threatening ischemia, indicated by rest pain, tissue necrosis, and nonhealing wounds, should be considered for revascularization. On the other hand, patients with intermittent claudication, usually described as an "ache" in the calf, should first be managed conservatively. This includes institution of lifestyle modifications such as smoking cessation, walking programs, and medical therapy with pentoxifylline or cilostazol. However, patients with severe intermittent claudication that is lifestyle limiting should be considered for surgical revascularization.

In the era of endovascular surgery, the treatment of intermittent claudication has begun to evolve. Many patients with this disease are being treated with angioplasty, stents, or even atherectomy. The long-term effects of these interventions are still unknown and therefore the gold standard therapy remains surgical revascularization. *(Mulholland et al., 2006, pp. 1649–1653)*

115. (E) The incidental finding is a gallstone within the gallbladder without evidence for inflammation. For most patients with asymptomatic cholelithiasis, a cholecystectomy is not routinely performed. Only 20–30% of these patients will develop symptoms within 20 years. Moreover, only 1–2% per year will develop serious symptoms or complications from their gallstones. However, certain patients are at greater risk for developing complications and should be considered for elective cholecystectomy. This population includes patients with stones greater than 2.5 cm in size since they are at greater risk for obstruction. Children with cholelithiasis have a high frequency of becoming symptomatic and also should be considered for early intervention. In patients with sickle cell disease, acute cholecystitis can induce a sickle crisis, which can complicate surgery and as such should undergo elective cholecystectomy. Finally, the finding of calcifications in the gallbladder wall, also known as a "porcelain gallbladder" is associated with increased risk of gallbladder carcinoma and an elective cholecystectomy should be considered. Diabetes mellitus is associated with increased surgical risks with both emergent and elective cholecystectomy, and therefore diabetics should not be recommended for surgery for asymptomatic gallstones. *(Mulholland et al., 2006, pp. 981–982)*

116. (B) Sclerosing cholangitis is a chronic progressive disease of the liver in which an inflammatory process results in intrahepatic and/or extrahepatic biliary strictures. The disease is progressive and may eventually result in biliary cirrhosis and portal hypertension. Sclerosing cholangitis is strongly associated with ulcerative colitis and, to a lesser extent, with Crohn's disease. The precise cause is unknown; however, it has been suggested that it may result from a local response to viral infection.

The diagnosis should be considered in a patient with inflammatory bowel disease who presents with abnormal liver function tests and a clinical picture of jaundice, intermittent right upper quadrant pain, nausea, vomiting, and fever. The diagnosis is traditionally established by ERCP demonstrating characteristic biliary strictures alternating with areas of dilatation that has been referred to as a "string of beads." The appropriate management of sclerosing cholangitis is supportive, with no known medical cure. Definitive treatment of the underlying ulcerative colitis with total colectomy does not prevent progression of the disease. In patients with diffuse and advanced parenchymal disease, hepatic transplantation is the only known cure. *(Cameron, 2004, pp. 428–432)*

117. **(B)** Subacute thyroiditis (giant cell, granulomatous, or de Quervain's thyroiditis) is an acute inflammatory disease of the thyroid gland. The cause is thought to be viral and it is often preceded by an upper respiratory tract infection. Patients may also experience a viral prodrome marked by muscle aches, fever, and general malaise. The thyroiditis is characterized by constant and often severe pain over the gland that is aggravated with swallowing. It often presents as a sore throat. Physical examination reveals a firm, nodular, and tender thyroid gland with overlying erythema and warmth. Patients may have symptoms of hyperthyroidism due to the release of thyroid hormone from the gland, secondary to the inflammation.

The disorder is usually self-limited and treatment focuses on conservative measures for pain control. Salicylates and nonsteroidal anti-inflammatory agents are successfully used in mild to moderate cases. For severe pain and swelling, oral glucocorticoids such as prednisone may be required. If symptoms of hyperthyroidism are present, beta-adrenergic blockage may also be needed. Antithyroidal medications are ineffective because the hyperthyroidism is not caused by increased thyroid hormone synthesis. *(Cameron, 2004, p. 599)*

118. **(E)** Toxic nodular goiter, also known as Plummer's disease, is a consequence of one or more thyroid nodules secreting inappropriately high levels of thyroid hormone independently of thyroid-stimulating hormone (TSH) control. Hyperthyroidism in patients with toxic nodular goiter is milder than in those with Graves' disease, and the condition is not accompanied by extrathyroidal manifestations such as ophthalmopathy, pretibial myxedema, vitiligo, or thyroid acropathy.

Patients with toxic multinodular goiter are older at presentation than those with Graves' disease. The thyroid gland characteristically has one or more nodules on palpation. Local symptoms of compression, such as dysphagia and dyspnea, may occur. The diagnosis is suggested by a thorough history and physical examination and confirmed by documenting suppressed serum TSH level and raised serum thyroid hormone level.

Therapy with antithyroid medications or beta-blockers may help alleviate symptoms but is not definitive, especially if the patient possesses local symptoms of compression. Radioiodine therapy is not as effective as in Graves' disease because of lower uptake. I^{131} ablation may be used in patients who are unsuitable for surgery but, because of the high failure rate, local resection is considered the treatment of choice. For solitary nodules, nodulectomy or thyroid lobectomy is the treatment of choice. *(Brunicardi et al., 2005, p. 1409)*

119. **(A)** Carcinoma of the gallbladder accounts for 2–4% of GI malignancies. Fewer than 1% of patients undergoing biliary tract operations have carcinoma either as an anticipated diagnosis or as an incidental finding. The calcified "porcelain" gallbladder is associated with a 20% incidence of gallbladder carcinoma.

Signs and symptoms of carcinoma of the gallbladder are generally indistinguishable from those associated with cholecystitis and cholelithiasis. They include abdominal discomfort, right upper quadrant pain, nausea, and vomiting. Most long-term survivors are patients who underwent cholecystectomy for cholelithiasis and in whom the malignancy was an incidental finding on the pathology report. The management of these patients is based on the depth of tumor penetration into the wall of the gallbladder. No further surgical intervention is required if the tumor invades superficially into the mucosa and submucosa. These patients are placed on surveillance programs. However, if the lesion penetrates deeper into the muscularis or perimuscular connective tissue of the gallbladder wall, a radical second procedure is undertaken which includes radical lymphadenectomy and partial hepatic resection.

If a malignancy is identified at the time of initial surgery, removal of the regional lymph nodes, partial liver resection and, in some cases, pancreaticoduodenectomy are indicated. *(Brunicardi et al., 2005, pp. 1214–1215)*

120. **(A)** FHH, or familial benign hypercalcemia, is a rare condition characterized by asymptomatic or mildly symptomatic hypercalcemia. It is inherited as an autosomal dominant trait and the parathyroid glands are usually normal in size. The basis for the development of FHH appears to be mutations in the calcium-sensing receptor gene which regulates the parathyroid gland set point and modulates the extracellular calcium concentration. The condition may be mistaken for primary hyperparathyroidism because, in both conditions, the serum calcium and parathyroid hormone levels are elevated with a concomitant low serum phosphate. The distinction is made by obtaining a 24-hour urine calcium excretion level. In patients with FHH, the urine calcium level is low, whereas in primary hyperparathyroidism the level is high. The distinction is important, as patients with primary hyperparathyroidism benefit from surgery and those with FHH do not. *(Cameron, 2004, p. 602)*

121. **(C)** The distal small bowel (ileum) is the site of absorption of fat-soluble vitamins (vitamins A, D, E, and K) as well as vitamin B_{12}. Vitamin B_{12} binds with intrinsic factor, a glycoprotein secreted from parietal cells of the gastric fundus and body. Specific receptors in the terminal ileum take up the B_{12} intrinsic factor complex. Vitamin B_{12} deficiency leads to megaloblastic anemia. The patient will require monthly vitamin B_{12} injections. *(Brunicardi et al., 2005, p. 1024)*

122. **(C)**

123. **(A)**

Explanations 122 and 123

Hungry bone syndrome refers to hypocalcemia following surgical correction of hyperparathyroidism in patients with severe, prolonged disease, as serum calcium is rapidly taken from the circulation and deposited into the bone. Symptoms usually occur within 24–48 hours following parathyroidectomy, when calcium levels reach a nadir. Early symptoms include numbness and tingling in the perioral area, fingers, or toes. Advanced symptoms include nervousness, anxiety, and increased neuromuscular transmission evidenced by positive Chvostek's and Trousseau's signs, carpal pedal spasm, and hyperactive tendon reflexes. In severe cases, one may develop a prolonged QT interval on ECG.

Patients who manifest any signs or symptoms of hypocalcemia always require intervention. In severely symptomatic patients, treatment should begin with intravenous calcium gluconate. Mildly symptomatic patients may be given oral calcium in the form of calcium lactate, calcium carbonate, or calcium gluconate. If hypocalcemia remains despite calcium supplementation, additional therapy with vitamin D may be needed. Supplemental calcium and vitamin D therapy should be continued until serum calcium levels return to normal. *(Brunicardi et al., 2005, p. 1448)*

124. **(D)** The triad of fever, abdominal fluid collection, and history of abdominal graft surgery indicates the development of a graft infection. The most common organism isolated is *S. aureus*. It is a rare, but morbid, complication, with mortality rates as high as 36%. The infection may rapidly result in sepsis, hemorrhagic shock, and septic embolization.

The standard treatment is early detection and surgical removal of the infected graft, with primary closure of the aorta and creation of an extra-anatomical reconstruction—most commonly an axillofemoral bypass. Such a bypass carries its own morbidities, including risk of limb loss, aortic stump blowout, and pelvic ischemia. *(Bliziotis et al., 1999, pp. 136–140)*

BIBLIOGRAPHY

American College of Surgeons. *Advanced Trauma Life Support Program for Doctors*, 6th ed. Chicago, IL: American College of Surgeons, 1997.

Bliziotis IA, Kapaskelis AM, Kasiakou SK, et al. Limitations in the management of aortic graft infections. *Am J Surg* 1999;178(2):136–140.

Brunicardi FC, Anderson DK, Billiar TR, et al., eds. *Schwartz's Principles of Surgery,* 8th ed. New York, NY: McGraw-Hill, 2005.

Cameron JL, ed. *Current Surgical Therapy*, 8th ed. St. Louis, MO: C.V. Mosby, 2004.

Feig BW, Berger DH, Fuhrman GM, eds. *The M.D. Anderson Surgical Oncology Handbook,* 4th ed. Philadelphia, PA: Lippincott Williams & Wilkins, 2006.

Moore EE, Feliciano DV, Mattox KL, et al., eds. *Trauma,* 5th ed. New York, NY: McGraw-Hill, 2004.

Mulholland MW, Oldham KT, Lillemoe KD, et al., eds. *Greenfield's Surgery: Scientific Principles and Practice,* 4th ed. Philadelphia, PA: Lippincott Williams & Wilkins, 2006.

Rutherford R. *Vascular Surgery.* 6th ed. Philadelphia, PA: W.B. Saunders, 2005.

Townsend CM, Beauchamp RD, Evers BM, et al., eds. *Sabiston Textbook of Surgery: The Biological Basis of Modern Surgical Practice,* 17th ed. Philadelphia, PA: W.B. Saunders, 2004.

CHAPTER 3

Pediatrics
Questions

Questions 1 and 2

1. A newborn male is brought to you in the neonatal intensive care unit (NICU). On physical examination, you notice that the infant has deficient abdominal musculature and undescended testes. Your suspicion is high for a certain condition. You presumptively diagnose the child with which of the following?

   (A) VATER association
   (B) Cushing's triad
   (C) Potter's syndrome
   (D) Jones criteria
   (E) Eagle-Barrett syndrome

2. Upon further imaging, what associated finding would be expected?

   (A) posterior urethral valves on a voiding cystourethrogram (VCUG)
   (B) hydrocephalus on head ultrasound
   (C) cardiomegaly on chest x-ray (CXR)
   (D) bilateral adrenal enlargement on abdominal ultrasound
   (E) tracheoesophageal fistula on an upper gastrointestinal (UGI) series

3. What is the most sensitive indicator of pneumonia in a child?

   (A) tachycardia
   (B) tachypnea
   (C) hypotonia
   (D) vomiting
   (E) coughing

4. A 12-month-old male child is brought to your office for a well-child examination and immunizations. You have been following the child since delivery and are aware that he has acquired immune deficiency syndrome (AIDS) and a markedly reduced T-cell count. Which of the following vaccinations should he not receive?

   (A) diphtheria, tetanus, and acellular pertussis (DTaP)
   (B) diphtheria tetanus (dT)
   (C) hepatitis B
   (D) injectable polio vaccine (IPV)
   (E) varicella

Questions 5 and 6

While working in the emergency room you see a 14-month-old boy brought in with apparent leg pain. His parents tell you that he has recently been learning to walk and that this injury is the result of a fall. You obtain the following x-ray (see Figure 3-1).

FIG. 3-1 *(Reproduced, with permission, from Schwartz DT, Reisdorff EJ. Emergency Radiology. New York, NY, p. 181.)*

5. What is your interpretation of the x-ray?

    (A) dislocation of the ankle
    (B) a "chip" fracture of the proximal tibia
    (C) a spiral fracture of the distal tibia
    (D) a buckle fracture involving the distal tibia and fibula
    (E) a transverse fracture of the distal tibia

6. What is the mechanism that likely resulted in this injury?

    (A) twisting on a planted leg while learning to walk
    (B) forced rotation of the leg by another person (child abuse)
    (C) fall from a piece of furniture or stairs
    (D) inversion of the ankle
    (E) motor vehicle accident while not restrained in a car seat

Questions 7 and 8

A 16-year-old sexually active woman is being seen in the emergency department. She is complaining of vaginal discharge. She has a temperature of 99.5°F, but is otherwise well. On pelvic examination, you see a mucopurulent cervical discharge with scant blood. Samples of the discharge are sent to the laboratory for culture. There are no cervical ulcers noted. She does not have any medical allergies.

7. Which of the following is the most common sexually transmitted infection in adolescents?

    (A) herpes simplex virus (HSV)
    (B) chlamydia
    (C) gonorrhea
    (D) human immunodeficiency virus (HIV)
    (E) syphilis

8. For this patient, what is the most appropriate regimen for initial therapy?

    (A) azithromycin (Zithromax) 1 g orally once and ceftriaxone (Rocephin) 125 mg intramuscular (IM) once
    (B) amoxicillin/clavulanic acid (Augmentin) 500 mg orally twice a day for 7 days and ceftriaxone 125 mg IM once
    (C) metronidazole (Flagyl) 500 mg orally twice a day for 7 days and amoxicillin/clavulanic acid 500 mg orally twice a day for 7 days
    (D) ceftriaxone 125 mg IM once
    (E) azithromycin 1 g orally once and metronidazole 500 mg orally for 7 days

Questions 9 and 10

An 8-month-old boy is brought to the clinic by his mother because he has been lethargic, fussy, and not feeding well over the past several days. The mother has been working two jobs so the baby has been cared for by her boyfriend for the past month. She is very worried because he has not been smiling and vocalizing as much as he normally does and he has not been able to lift his head.

9. What is the most common cause of injury in the first year of life?

   (A) falls down stairs
   (B) child abuse
   (C) motor vehicle collisions
   (D) dog bites
   (E) other children

10. Which of the following findings on physical examination is suggestive of child abuse?

   (A) superficial abrasions on the shins of a 5 year old
   (B) retinal hemorrhages visualized on funduscopy in a 4 month old
   (C) a laceration on the forehead of a 6 year old
   (D) a partial dislocation of the elbow in a 3 year old
   (E) a linear skull fracture in a 9-year-old boy

Questions 11 through 15

You are called to see a newborn in the nursery because the nurse is concerned that the baby may have Down syndrome.

11. Which of the following signs is associated with Down syndrome?

   (A) café au lait spots
   (B) high arched palate
   (C) ambiguous genitalia
   (D) hypotonia
   (E) club feet

12. After confirming that the child does indeed have Down syndrome, the parents ask you what problems their baby may have in the future. With which of the following is the infant most likely to have problems?

   (A) renal failure
   (B) hypothyroidism
   (C) osteoporosis
   (D) hemophilia
   (E) lens dislocation

13. The infant begins to have progressively large amounts of bilious emesis. The infant feeds well and has only a small amount of abdominal distention. What is the most likely diagnosis?

   (A) pyloric stenosis
   (B) Hirschsprung disease
   (C) biliary atresia
   (D) duodenal atresia
   (E) milk protein allergy

14. If you were to perform an abdominal x-ray, what is the most likely finding that would be seen?

   (A) "double-bubble" sign
   (B) scimitar sign
   (C) normal gas patterns
   (D) free fluid in the abdomen
   (E) pneumatosis intestinalis

15. What is the most common central nervous system (CNS) complication of Down syndrome?

   (A) seizures
   (B) hydrocephalus
   (C) microcalcifications
   (D) berry aneurysms
   (E) mental retardation

Questions 16 and 17

A father and son come to your office because of persistent diarrhea. They relate the presence of watery diarrhea for over 2 weeks. They noted that the diarrhea began after returning from a Boy Scout camping trip in the Rocky Mountains. The diarrhea has waxed and waned for 2 weeks. It is nonbloody and foul smelling. They have had increased flatulence and mild abdominal cramping.

16. What is the most likely etiology of their diarrhea?

    (A) enterotoxigenic *Escherichia coli*
    (B) *Giardia lamblia*
    (C) *Rickettsia rickettsii* (Rocky Mountain spotted fever [RMSF])
    (D) rotavirus
    (E) Norwalk virus

17. What would be the most appropriate treatment?

    (A) oral ciprofloxacin
    (B) oral metronidazole
    (C) bismuth subsalicylate (Pepto-Bismol)
    (D) an antidiarrheal agent only; no antimicrobials necessary
    (E) oral rehydration only

Questions 18 through 20

A 5-year-old male is admitted to the hospital following a 3-week history of spiking fevers and fatigue. Your examination reveals pale mucous membranes and skin. You also find splenomegaly.

18. You are concerned about a possible malignancy. What is the most common malignancy of childhood?

    (A) medulloblastoma
    (B) Wilms' tumor
    (C) leukemia
    (D) neuroblastoma
    (E) rhabdomyosarcoma

19. This child has an extensive evaluation by the Hematology-Oncology consultants. Their evaluation excludes the presence of a malignancy. The extensive evaluation did reveal that the child has a WBC count of 22,000 with 41% monocytes and 12% "atypical" lymphocytes. His hematocrit is 28% and erythrocyte sedimentation rate (ESR) is 5. This child likely has which of the following diseases?

    (A) Lyme disease
    (B) acute Epstein-Barr virus (EBV) infection
    (C) systemic lupus erythematosus (SLE)
    (D) juvenile rheumatoid arthritis (JRA)
    (E) acute hematogenous tuberculosis (TB)

20. The best course of care for this young man would be which of the following?

    (A) initiate high-dose aspirin therapy (100 mg/kg/day)
    (B) initiate "renal sparing" course of oral prednisone
    (C) a repeat bone marrow evaluation with AFB (acid fast bacilli) staining and mycobacterial cultures
    (D) obtain serum for Lyme enzyme immunoassay(EIA) testing and begin an empiric course of doxycycline
    (E) obtain EBV serologies (IgM and IgG) and treat symptomatically with comfort measures

21. While in the emergency department you see a 3-week-old infant. The mother says that the child felt warm earlier in the day and has not been eating very well. The infant has a temperature of 100.9°F and has mildly decreased tone. What is the most appropriate initial management?

    (A) Give acetaminophen and reassess in a few hours.
    (B) Draw a blood culture, recommend increased fluid intake, and follow-up for re-examination in 24 hours in the primary pediatrician's office.
    (C) Admit to the hospital and perform a full "sepsis workup."
    (D) Draw a blood culture, give a shot of ceftriaxone (Rocephin) to cover for any infections and follow-up in 24–48 hours.
    (E) Get a urine culture and begin trimethoprim/sulfamethoxazole (Septra).

Questions 22 and 23

You see a 2-month-old infant in the emergency department for vomiting. The mother says that the baby has been spitting up more over the past few days and has become more irritable. She denies any fever, diarrhea, or change in formula. The mother tells you that there is a family history of "heartburn" and that her other children have all spit up. The infant has some emesis in the emergency department that seems to be formula mixed with some bile. The infant is intermittently irritable and sleepy.

22. What is the most concerning diagnosis that this could be?

    (A) biliary atresia
    (B) malrotation
    (C) pyloric stenosis
    (D) imperforate anus
    (E) diaphragmatic hernia

23. Which of the following would be the most appropriate initial test?

    (A) abdominal computed tomography (CT)
    (B) barium enema
    (C) abdominal ultrasound
    (D) UGI series with small bowel follow through
    (E) radionuclide scan

Questions 24 and 25

An 8-year-old male presents to your office complaining of a 1-week history of painful knee and elbow joints. On examination, you find a painful, hot, and swollen knee. He also has multiple erythematous macules with pale centers on his trunk and extremities. The laboratory work you order reveals elevated antistreptococcal antibodies.

24. What is the most likely diagnosis?

    (A) JRA
    (B) septic arthritis
    (C) acute rheumatic fever (ARF)
    (D) child abuse
    (E) SLE

25. Which of the following information is required to make this diagnosis?

    (A) The child must currently have a fever.
    (B) The child must have arthritis.
    (C) The presence of a group A streptococcal (GAS) infection must be documented.
    (D) The child may have chorea alone.
    (E) Aspiration of fluid from the swollen knee is required to confirm the diagnosis.

Questions 26 and 27

On a Monday morning you see a 12-year-old otherwise healthy boy in the emergency department. The parents brought the boy in because they noticed that he started to have an abnormal gait in the past few days. He seems to be shuffling his feet. The boy complains that his legs feel heavy and are tingling. He relates that his arms feel fine. His past history is significant for attention deficit/hyperactivity disorder (ADHD) for which he is taking methylphenidate. He denies trauma or taking any other medicines or drugs. On examination, he is afebrile with normal vital signs. His entire physical examination is normal with the exception of the examination of his lower extremities. He has 3/5 strength throughout both of his lower extremities with a normal muscle mass. His all joints have a full range of motion, without any pain or swelling. His reflexes are absent and he describes some paresthesias of his feet and ankles.

26. What is the most likely diagnosis?

    (A) methylphenidate toxicity
    (B) acute inflammatory demyelinating polyneuropathy (Guillain-Barré syndrome)
    (C) acute poliomyelitis
    (D) malingering (school avoidance)
    (E) polymyositis

27. Which of the following is the most appropriate initial management plan?

    (A) hospitalization and close observation for progression of his weakness
    (B) high-dose corticosteroids
    (C) gastric lavage and activated charcoal
    (D) outpatient family counseling
    (E) plasmaphoresis

28. You are called to see a 12-hour-old male infant who was born to a 19-year-old G_1 woman with no prenatal care. She presented to the emergency room completely dilated and crowning. The baby was born minutes later. On examination, the baby is febrile and tachypneic. A CXR confirms the presence of pneumonia. What is the most likely infectious agent?

   (A) group B *Streptococcus* (GBS)
   (B) HSV
   (C) *E. coli*
   (D) respiratory syncytial virus (RSV)
   (E) *Streptococcus pneumoniae*

Questions 29 and 30

A 4-year-old is brought to your office by his mother for evaluation. She is concerned because the child has been spiking fevers and pulling on his left ear. Your examination reveals a bulging and erythematous tympanic membrane (TM).

29. Which of the following is most likely to be the cause of his illness?

   (A) *Haemophilus influenzae*, type B (HIB)
   (B) *Moraxella catarrhalis*
   (C) *Mycoplasma pneumoniae*
   (D) GAS
   (E) *S. pneumoniae*

30. You determine that the child should receive antibiotics. The initial antibiotic of choice should be?

   (A) amoxicillin
   (B) azithromycin (Zithromax)
   (C) erythromycin
   (D) trimethoprim/sulfamethoxazole (Septra)
   (E) tetracycline

31. Which of the following has a carrier state that is not considered contagious?

   (A) *E. coli*
   (B) HSV
   (C) *Chlamydia trachomatis*

   (D) GAS
   (E) RSV

Questions 32 and 33

You are working in the emergency department and are called to perform a lumbar puncture on a 3-month-old infant who presented with fever and lethargy. The spinal fluid that you obtain is turbid. The laboratory reports that there are 200 WBCs and 5 RBCs per high-power field (HPF). Ninety-five percent of the WBCs in the spinal fluid are neutrophils.

32. Which of the following is the most probable cause of this illness?

   (A) GBS
   (B) HSV
   (C) GAS
   (D) *S. pneumoniae*
   (E) *E. coli*

33. If the laboratory result showed that 98% of the WBCs in the spinal fluid were lymphocytes, what would be the most likely etiology of the infection?

   (A) *Mycobacterium tuberculosis*
   (B) HSV
   (C) *C. trachomatis*
   (D) RSV
   (E) nonpolio enteroviruses

34. You are working in a community clinic on a Native American reservation. A mother brings in her 8-year-old son for an ophthalmic evaluation. On examination, you find bilateral corneal ulceration and decreased visual acuity. What is the most common infectious cause of blindness in the world?

   (A) HSV
   (B) *C. trachomatis*
   (C) GAS
   (D) *S. pneumoniae*
   (E) *E. coli*

Questions 35 through 37

A 4-year-old girl is brought in to the office by her mother. She developed chicken pox about 6 days ago. She appeared to be recovering well but mother became concerned because she was persistently scratching at several of the lesions and they were not healing. On examination, the child is afebrile and generally well appearing. On examination of her skin you see the following image (see Figure 3-2).

FIG. 3-2 *(Reproduced, with permission, from Wolff K, Johnson RA, Suurmond R. Color Atlas and Synopsis of Clinical Dermatology, 5th ed. New York, NY: McGraw-Hill, 2005, p. 589.)* (Also see color insert.)

35. What is the most likely current diagnosis?

   (A) tinea corporis
   (B) impetigo
   (C) warts
   (D) contact dermatitis
   (E) reactivated chicken pox

36. What is the most likely responsible agent?

   (A) *Trichophyton rubrum*
   (B) poison ivy
   (C) human papilloma virus
   (D) GAS
   (E) varicella-zoster virus

37. What would be the most appropriate treatment?

   (A) topical triamcinolone 0.1% cream
   (B) topical nystatin cream
   (C) oral acyclovir
   (D) oral cephalexin
   (E) no treatment is necessary as this is a self-limited condition

Questions 38 through 40

38. A well-appearing 6-year-old presents to your office with a chief complaint of bruising. The parents report that the child had a cold 2 weeks ago but completely recovered. The child is sitting on the examining table, in no distress, discussing her favorite cartoons. On examination, you find mucosal bleeding and bruises on the child's arms and chest. You order a complete blood count (CBC) that has the following results: WBC 12,000, hemoglobin 11 g/dL, and a platelet count of 45,000. What is the most likely cause of this child's bleeding and bruising?

   (A) immune thrombocytopenic purpura (ITP)
   (B) Henoch-Schönlein purpura (HSP)
   (C) Evans syndrome
   (D) meningococcemia
   (E) hemolytic uremic syndrome (HUS)

39. After discussing various options with a regional pediatric hematologist and the patient's parents, your most appropriate initial management would be which of the following?

   (A) a platelet transfusion at the regional children's hospital
   (B) an IM dose of methylprednisolone as an outpatient
   (C) reassurance to the parents with close outpatient follow-up
   (D) intravenous immunoglobulin (IVIG) at the regional children's hospital
   (E) bone marrow biopsy at the regional children's hospital

40. Following your initial evaluation and treatment, you see the child for follow-up in 1 week. She continues to appear well but still has obvious purpura and her platelet count is now 17,000. All other cell lines are normal. Of the options listed below, what is your most appropriate management at this time?

    (A) admission to the regional children's hospital for a platelet transfusion
    (B) admission to the children's hospital for a splenectomy
    (C) reassurance to the parents and close outpatient follow-up
    (D) admission to the children's hospital for IVIG and steroids
    (E) whole-blood transfusion with several hours of observation to ensure that there is no transfusion reaction

41. A 4-year-old child is brought to your office because of a sudden onset of irritability, weakness, and pallor. The mother tells you that both of her children have been experiencing episodes of vomiting and diarrhea. Your physical examination reveals a blood pressure of 115/80, dry mucus membranes, petechiae, and diffuse abdominal pain. The following laboratory work is obtained:

    Urinalysis: microscopic hematuria and proteinuria
    Blood urea nitrogen (BUN)/creatinine (Cr): 20/1.0 mg/dL
    Hemoglobin: 7 g/dL
    Peripheral blood smear: fragmented RBCs
    Prothrombin time (PT), partial thromboplastin time (PTT): normal
    Coombs' test: negative

    What is the most likely diagnosis?

    (A) ITP
    (B) HSP
    (C) Evans syndrome
    (D) meningococcemia
    (E) HUS

Questions 42 and 43

42. A mildly mentally retarded 9-year-old girl is brought to your office for acne. On examination, she does not actually have acne but has small flesh colored papules along her nasolabial fold. Her past history is significant for having had a first (afebrile) seizure last year. The mother reminds you that she has a faint birthmark on her hip that is pale and becomes more prominent in the summer, when the child's skin tans. Examination of this area reveals a 5-cm oval patch that is hypopigmented. Which condition would she most likely have?

    (A) Sturge-Weber syndrome
    (B) neurofibromatosis, type 1 (von Recklinghausen disease)
    (C) tuberous sclerosis
    (D) CHARGE association
    (E) Beckwith-Wiedemann syndrome

43. In evaluating her first seizure, a head CT was performed. Which finding would be most consistent with her diagnosis?

    (A) frontal cortical atrophy with dysplastic vessels
    (B) periventricular "tubers"
    (C) diffuse white matter calcifications
    (D) hydrocephalus from aqueductal stenosis
    (E) poor gray-white differentiation

44. Which of the following conditions usually causes hypoglycemia at birth?

    (A) Sturge-Weber syndrome
    (B) neurofibromatosis, type 1 (von Recklinghausen disease)
    (C) tuberous sclerosis
    (D) CHARGE association
    (E) Beckwith-Wiedemann syndrome

45. A 10-month-old infant has a dysplastic right external ear, some preauricular tags, and a small notch (coloboma) in the iris and lower lid. Which condition does he likely have?

    (A) VATER association
    (B) neurofibromatosis, type 1 (von Recklinghausen disease)

(C) retinoic embryopathy

(D) CHARGE association

(E) DiGeorge syndrome

46. While working in the emergency department in the winter, you examine a 3-week-old female infant. The baby is accompanied by her mother and father. They report that the baby has been congested for the past 24 hours. The parents have been taking the infant's temperature rectally and report that it has been normal. The infant was a born at 35 weeks' gestation and was delivered by caesarian due to preeclampsia. On examination, you see a well-appearing infant with a respiratory rate (RR) of 46 and a heart rate (HR) of 112. The TMs are normal and the lung fields are clear to auscultation. The mother relates that she has had a "cold" for the past few days. The father reports that he smokes, but only outside. As part of your evaluation you perform a nasopharyngeal swab for RSV antigen, which comes back positive. The best course of action for this infant is which of the following?

(A) full sepsis workup with empiric intravenous antibiotic

(B) IM RSV-IVIG administration

(C) admit to the hospital for IV ribavirin for 5 days

(D) admit to the hospital for observation

(E) begin prophylactic oral amoxicillin

Questions 47 and 48

A term infant <u>male</u> is born after an uncomplicated vaginal delivery. The mother's prenatal labs were negative with the exception of being GBS positive at 36 weeks' gestation. The mother received two doses of ampicillin prior to delivery and did not have a fever. The infant had APGAR scores of 9 at 1 minute and 9 at 5 minutes. The infant was brought to the newborn nursery and appears well.

47. The most appropriate management of the infant would be which of the following?

(A) Draw a CBC and blood culture, but do not start empiric antibiotics.

(B) Give the baby a prophylactic dose of ampicillin.

(C) Routine care.

(D) Cultures of blood, urine, and spinal fluid and wait for culture results before starting antibiotics.

(E) Cultures of blood, urine, and spinal fluid and begin empiric antibiotics before getting culture results.

48. The father tells you that he has hemophilia. His wife neither has hemophilia nor is a carrier. What does this mean for the baby?

(A) The baby has a 50% chance of having hemophilia.

(B) The baby neither has hemophilia nor is a carrier of the hemophilia gene.

(C) The baby is a carrier of the hemophilia gene but does not have the disease.

(D) The baby has a 25% chance of being a carrier for hemophilia.

(E) The baby has a 50% chance of being a carrier for hemophilia.

49. A mother brings her 4-year-old son to your office, relating that he fell earlier that morning while at the playground. She says that the boy tripped over another child and landed on his outstretched hands. On examination, the boy has some mild swelling around his left wrist, and he says that it hurts when you palpate it. What is the most appropriate next step?

(A) Call the department of Children's Protective Services to investigate the accident.

(B) Attempt a nursemaid's elbow reduction.

(C) Perform anterior-posterior (AP) and lateral x-rays of the left wrist and elbow.

(D) Wrap the wrist in an Ace wrap, and put the arm in a sling.

(E) Order a magnetic resonance imaging (MRI) of the wrist looking for a growth plate injury.

Questions 50 and 51

A mother brings her baby girl for a 9-month well-child visit. You have been following her since birth. Her growth chart is shown in Figure 3-3. Her vital signs and examination are otherwise normal.

50. The growth pattern is most consistent with which of the following?

    (A) congenital growth hormone (GH) deficiency
    (B) constitutional short stature
    (C) constitutional growth delay
    (D) familial short stature
    (E) nutritional failure to thrive (FTT)

Birth to 36 months: Girl
Length-for-age and Weight-for-age percentiles

NAME _____

RECORD # _____

Published May 30, 2000 (modified 4/20/01).
SOURCE: Developed by the National Center for Health Statistics in collaboration with
the National Center for Chronic Disease Prevention and Health Promotion (2000).
http://www.cdc.gov/growthcharts

FIG. 3-3 *(Reproduced from National Center for Health Statistics in collaboration with the National Center for Chronic Disease Prevention and Health Promotion 2000).*

51. What would be the best next step for management of this infant?

(A) a detailed dietary history with calculation of calories per kg per day
(B) serum levels of GH
(C) serum levels of somatomedin-C (insulin like growth factor-1 [ILGF-1])
(D) detailed family history with specific attention to the mother's and father's height
(E) UGI series to evaluate for malabsorption

Questions 52 through 55

You see a 3½-year-old child in the emergency department who has had fever for the past week. The parents relate that their son has some swollen glands, fever, and now seems to be getting a rash on his arms. On examination, you find an uncomfortable appearing young boy whose vital signs are normal with the exception of a temperature of 104°F. You note that he has a red posterior oropharynx with dry, cracked lips. His TMs are normal. He has mild conjunctival injection bilaterally without any discharge. His chest is clear, and his heart sounds are normal. He does not have any hepatosplenomegaly. His has a lacy, confluent macular rash on his chest and upper arms, with mild peeling of the tips of his fingers.

52. What is the most likely diagnosis?

(A) group A beta-hemolytic streptococcal pharyngitis
(B) hand-foot-mouth disease (Coxsackie viral infection)
(C) Kawasaki disease
(D) ITP
(E) erythema infectiosum (parvovirus B-19 infection)

53. Which laboratory result would be most consistent with the diagnosis?

(A) an elevated platelet count
(B) a positive rapid strep test
(C) a low platelet count
(D) elevated viral IgM titers
(E) a low ESR

54. What is the most appropriate treatment at this point?

(A) no medicine is needed, only supportive care
(B) an IM dose of long-acting penicillin (LA Bicillin)
(C) oral acyclovir
(D) IVIG
(E) topical lidocaine gel 1%

55. What is the most worrisome complication of this disease?

(A) encephalitis
(B) coronary artery aneurysm
(C) cardiac valve dysfunction
(D) intracerebral hemorrhage
(E) hemorrhagic stroke

Questions 56 and 57

You see a 3-week-old infant in your office for an acute visit. She was born via spontaneous vaginal delivery following a term, uncomplicated prenatal course. The parents are concerned because they have seen some streaks of blood in her diaper over the past few days. The infant's stools have been soft and not difficult to pass. The parents relate that she is eating 2 oz every 2 hours of a cow's milk based formula.

56. What is the carbohydrate source in most infant formula?

(A) casein
(B) lactose
(C) human milk fortifier
(D) coconut oil
(E) soy oil

57. What is the most likely cause of the blood in her stool?

(A) Meckel diverticulum
(B) group B streptococcal colitis
(C) cow's milk protein intolerance
(D) pseudomembranous colitis
(E) lactose intolerance

Questions 58 through 60

In January, you see an 18-month-old boy in the middle of the night in the pediatric emergency department. The father relates that 1 hour ago his son started coughing. The father describes the cough as barking ("seal" like). The child has mild stridor at rest, but otherwise is not in respiratory distress. His RR is 45 breaths per minute. He has a temperature of 103.4°F.

58. What is the most likely diagnosis?

   (A) epiglottitis
   (B) croup
   (C) pneumonia
   (D) sinusitis
   (E) bronchiolitis

59. What is the most common etiology of this illness in children?

   (A) HIB
   (B) RSV
   (C) influenza, type B
   (D) parainfluenza, types 1 and 2
   (E) *S. pneumoniae*

60. What is the most common x-ray finding in this illness?

   (A) swollen adenoids
   (B) the "thumb" sign
   (C) a lobar pulmonary infiltrate
   (D) a deviated tracheal air column
   (E) the "steeple" sign

Questions 61 and 62

61. Parents bring their 12-year-old son to your clinic for evaluation. The child states that he gets teased a lot in school because of his short stature. His weight and height are below the 10th percentile for his age. His parents are of average height. Following your physical examination, you determine that he has tanner stage 1 development and his bone age is that of a 9-year-old male. His examination is otherwise normal. What is the most likely diagnosis?

   (A) familial short stature
   (B) constitutional growth delay
   (C) deficiency in GH
   (D) chronic renal failure
   (E) vitamin D deficiency

62. Which of the following is a true statement regarding the assessment of a child with short stature?

   (A) An advanced bone age indicates that the child's final height will be greater than his peers.
   (B) A slower growth velocity means the child will have more time to "catch up."
   (C) A spot GH level is a good test in screening for GH deficiency.
   (D) Somatomedin-C (ILGF-1) will be low in a child with GH deficiency.
   (E) The most common cause of short stature in children is chronic renal disease.

Questions 63 and 64

A mother brings her 15-year-old son in for a preparticipation sports physical examination. She feels that her son has not yet undergone pubertal changes and that makes her concerned.

63. Which of the following is a true statement regarding puberty delay?

   (A) The onset of puberty in males is earlier than that in females.
   (B) A puberty delay is not considered pathologic unless accompanied by short stature.
   (C) Hypothyroidism can be a cause of pubertal delay.
   (D) Males do not have a true adrenarche as females do.
   (E) The most common cause for pubertal delay is pan-hypopituitarism.

64. Which of the following physical examination findings is usually the first sign of the onset of puberty in males?

   (A) increased testicular volume
   (B) increased skeletal muscle mass

(C) deepening of the voice

(D) increased facial hair

(E) physiologic gynecomastia

Questions 65 and 66

A mother brings her 2¹/₂-year-old daughter to your office for evaluation of frequent urination. The mother relates that the daughter seems to be urinating more frequently, up to 8–10 times in a day, over the past week. The girl complains of pain when she urinates, but the urine does not have any different odor to it. The mother says that the girl otherwise seems fine and still loves to take her bubble bath at night. The girl does not have a fever, weight loss, diarrhea, or vomiting.

65. What is the most appropriate next step in evaluating this girl?

(A) fingerstick blood sample for random serum glucose

(B) plain abdominal x-ray

(C) clean urine sample for urinalysis and urine culture

(D) vaginal examination for discharge and cultures

(E) synchronized serum and urine osmolality

66. What is the most likely diagnosis?

(A) pyelonephritis

(B) chemical urethritis

(C) retained vaginal foreign body

(D) type 1 diabetes mellitus

(E) diabetes insipidus

67. A mother relates seeing worms in her 3-year-old's stool. She describes them as 1-cm long white threads that seemed to be moving. What is the most likely infectious etiology for this finding?

(A) *Ascaris lumbricoides*

(B) *Diphyllobothrium latum*

(C) *Taenia solium*

(D) *Toxocara canis*

(E) *Enterobius vermicularis*

68. Deficiency of which of the following is the most common nutritional cause of anemia?

(A) calcium

(B) vitamin B₁₂ deficiency

(C) iodine

(D) iron

(E) vitamin C

69. A 9-month-old male infant is brought to your office for evaluation of new skin lesions. The mother tells you that she recently had to return to work, and the child is now in day care. He has since developed new erythematous facial plaques (see Figure 3-4). She also reports that the child has been irritable with chronic diarrhea. On examination, the child has dry scaly plaques symmetrically distributed in the perianal and perioral areas. Which deficiency does this child likely have?

FIG. 3-4 *(Reproduced, with permission, from Wolff K, Johnson RA, Suurmond R. Color Atlas and Synopsis of Clinical Dermatology, 5th ed. New York, NY: McGraw-Hill, 2005:456.)*

(A) calcium

(B) zinc

(C) iodine

(D) iron

(E) vitamin C

70. Which of the following is regulated by the parathyroid gland?

    (A) calcium
    (B) zinc
    (C) iodine
    (D) iron
    (E) vitamin B$_{12}$

Questions 71 and 72

A 6-month-old male infant presents to your clinic because the mother is concerned that he is not eating well and he has been constipated. The mother tells you that her prenatal course and delivery were uneventful. On physical examination, the infant has a puffy face, large tongue, and persistent nasal drainage.

71. Which of the following conditions is most likely to present with these findings?

    (A) rickets
    (B) scurvy
    (C) hypothyroidism
    (D) microcytic anemia
    (E) adrenocortical insufficiency

72. The above condition can be caused by a deficiency of which of the following?

    (A) iron
    (B) vitamin C
    (C) vitamin D
    (D) iodine
    (E) cortisol

Questions 73 through 75

A 4-year-old child is seen in the emergency department after having a seizure at home. This is the first time that this has happened. The mother says that the child was sitting on the couch watching television when she suddenly became limp, started drooling, and having generalized tonic-clonic movements of her arms and legs. The mother relates that the child felt like she was "burning up" and that the tonic-clonic activity stopped after a few minutes. The mother says that the child is otherwise healthy, does not take any medicines, and has never been

hospitalized. The child's immunizations are up-to-date, and she has no known drug allergies. On examination, the vital signs are temperature of 104°F, BP 97/49, HR 112, and RR 26. The child is sitting on the examination table playing with stickers and drawing. She has a mild amount of clear nasal congestion but her examination is otherwise normal. When asked, the child replies that she feels fine.

73. What is the most likely diagnosis?

    (A) bacterial meningitis
    (B) first seizure in an epilepsy syndrome
    (C) viral encephalitis
    (D) typical febrile seizure
    (E) hypocalcemic tetany

74. Which test(s) should be performed while the child is in the emergency department to evaluate the cause of these seizures?

    (A) electroencephalogram (EEG)
    (B) no testing is needed
    (C) noncontrast head CT
    (D) lumbar puncture
    (E) blood and urine cultures

75. Which of the following medications would be most appropriate to be given to the child while in the emergency department?

    (A) acetaminophen (Tylenol) for fever as needed
    (B) phenytoin (Dilantin)
    (C) phenobarbital
    (D) diazepam (Valium)
    (E) ceftriaxone (Rocephin)

76. A 2-week-old infant is brought to the office for a check-up. The father relates that they have no concerns except that the baby seems to have tearing from his left eye. They also point out some swelling at the edge of his left eye. The infant is eating, sleeping, stooling, and voiding well. On examination, you find a $1/2 \times 1/2$ cm firm nodule inferior to the medial canthus of the left eye. What does this most likely represent?

(A) dermoid cyst

(B) nasolacrimal duct obstruction

(C) mucocele

(D) accessory lacrimal gland

(E) frontal encephalocele

Questions 77 through 79

A 14-year-old boy is brought to the emergency department for evaluation of fever and headache. The mother relates that her son has had a worsening headache for 5–6 days. She says that she took him to a walk-in clinic, and he was put on amoxicillin for a sinus infection. His headaches have been getting worse and that he is now having fevers as high as 103.6°F. The mother says that he normally is very active and that he currently has a summer job at a local park clearing out underbrush. Since he has become ill, he has had such a decrease in energy that he cannot go to work. He has had a decrease in his appetite and has been sleeping more. He denies any sore throat, abdominal pain, chest pain, dysuria, vomiting, or diarrhea. On examination, he is an uncomfortable young man whose vital signs are: temp. 101.9°F, RR 26, HR 124, and BP 79/56. His head, ear, eye, nose, and throat examination reveals normal TMs, a mildly erythematous hypopharynx, and some shotty cervical lymphadenopathy. His lungs are clear. His cardiac examination is normal. His liver edge is palpable just below the right costal margin and is mildly tender. His spleen is not palpable. His skin examination is normal with the exception of scattered petechiae around his ankles and wrists. A CBC reveals WBC 13,000 with 65% segs and 22% lymphs, hematocrit of 35, and platelet count of 95,000. His electrolytes reveal a Na 125, K 5.1, Cl 102, and bicarbonate 21. His BUN and Cr are normal.

77. What is his most likely diagnosis?

(A) enteroviral encephalitis

(B) measles

(C) Still disease

(D) RMSF

(E) Kawasaki syndrome

78. The best treatment course would include which of the following?

(A) continue amoxicillin only

(B) begin oral doxycycline

(C) add acyclovir to the amoxicillin

(D) begin oral corticosteroids

(E) stop all antimicrobials

79. What additional testing would be warranted at this point?

(A) serum rickettsial titers

(B) ESR

(C) C-reactive protein (CRP)

(D) enteroviral polymerase chain reaction (PCR) on cerebrospinal fluid (CSF)

(E) head CT without contrast

Questions 80 through 82

A 4$^1/_2$-year-old girl is brought to your office during summertime hours for ear pain. She has been swimming at camp for the past few days and now has copious cloudy discharge from her left external auditory canal with pain on movement of the pinna.

80. What is the most likely diagnosis?

(A) otitis media with perforation of the TM

(B) mastoiditis

(C) otitis externa (OE)

(D) foreign body in the ear canal

(E) tempero-mandibular joint dysfunction

81. What organism is the most common cause of this infection?

(A) methicillin-resistant *Staphylococcus aureus* (MRSA)

(B) *S. pneumoniae*

(C) *Pseudomonas* species

(D) nontypable *H. influenzae*

(E) GAS

82. What is the best course of treatment for this patient?

   (A) amoxicillin PO

   (B) erythromoycin PO

   (C) erythromycin topical

   (D) cefuroxime PO

   (E) neomycin/polymyxin B/hydrocortisone topical

Questions 83 through 85

Parents bring you a 9-month-old boy they recently have adopted from western Russia. They have sparse medical records of the child's past. They do know that the boy was the result of a sexual assault on the mother and was given up at birth. The child has been in a "baby home" for 5 months. The records which accompanied the boy indicate that there had been some testing done. These tests include HIV, hepatitis B and C serologies, and a rapid plasma reagin (RPR), all of which are negative at 8 months of age. There is what appears to be a Russian immunization record as well. It seems to indicate that the child has had three diphtheria, tetanus, pertussis (DTP), three oral polio, and three hepatitis B vaccinations. There is also an indication that BCG (Bacille Calmette-Guérin) was given.

83. The parents are interested in having the boy tested for infections. What is the most appropriate evaluation at this time?

   (A) No need to repeat the serologies because they have been done within the past month.

   (B) Collect stool for ova and parasites only.

   (C) Repeat all serologies (HIV, hepatitis B, hepatitis C, RPR) now.

   (D) Perform a full sepsis workup (blood culture, urine culture, CSF culture).

   (E) Screen for infections using CBC.

84. The parents are concerned about fetal alcohol syndrome (FAS). Which physical feature is most consistent with FAS?

   (A) smooth philtrum

   (B) single palmar crease

   (C) hypertelorism

   (D) synophrys (confluent eye brows)

   (E) low set ears

85. You place a purified protein derivative (PPD) and the parents come back in 48 hours to have it read. The response is 15 mm of induration. The boy does not have any respiratory symptoms at this time. What is the most appropriate response to this information?

   (A) Collect three morning sputum and send for acid-fast stain and TB culture.

   (B) Give a repeat BCG vaccine.

   (C) Do nothing as the PPD is considered negative given the prior BCG vaccination.

   (D) Perform a CXR and begin isoniazid (INH) for 9 months if the x-ray is negative.

   (E) Perform a CXR and begin "triples" (INH, rifampin, pyrazinamide) even if the x-ray is negative.

Questions 86 and 87

A 9-year-old boy comes to the clinic for evaluation of a rash. The boy says that he began developing some blisters on his cheek the night prior. He says that over the past few days he has spent time outside with his friends "down by the creek." The rash appears to be a linear crop of vesicles beginning in front of his left ear and extending to the corner of his mouth. There is no erythema, and he describes them as quite pruritic. He has not had any fever, vomiting, or changes in his hearing.

86. What does this rash most likely represent?

   (A) HSV infection of the facial nerve (Ramsey-Hunt syndrome)

   (B) bullous impetigo

   (C) allergic contact dermatitis (Rhus dermatitis)

   (D) erythema chronica migrans

   (E) cutaneous larval migrans

87. Along with good skin hygiene, which of the following is the best treatment plan for this child?

    (A) topical diphenhydramine for comfort
    (B) oral diphenhydramine for pruritus
    (C) topical and oral antibiotics which would cover *Staphylococcus* and *Streptococcus*
    (D) topical high-potency fluorinated steroid
    (E) oral acyclovir

Questions 88 through 90

A 16-year-old woman comes to see you for a yearly physical examination. Her only concern is that her periods are very irregular, and she desires oral contraceptives to regulate them. She relates that menarche was at 12 years, of age and that her periods have always been irregular. On examination, she is a markedly obese woman with a body mass index of 35 and with normal linear growth. She has some coarse facial hair down both of her checks as well as cystic acne along her hairline. On the nape of her neck she is noted to have acanthosis nigricans. She has tanner 4 breast development as well as tanner 4 pubic hair. Her urinalysis in the office is normal.

88. What is the most likely cause of her irregular periods?

    (A) hypothyroidism
    (B) polycystic ovarian syndrome (PCOS)
    (C) late-onset congenital adrenal hyperplasia (CAH)
    (D) Cushing syndrome
    (E) testosterone insensitivity

89. Which of the following would confirm your diagnosis?

    (A) ultrasound of the pelvis showing multiple ovarian follicles ("string of pearls" sign)
    (B) a low serum thyroid-stimulating hormone (TSH) level
    (C) an elevated serum prolactin level

    (D) elevated high-density lipoprotein (HDL) with low triglycerides
    (E) normal glucose tolerance test

90. What would be the best intervention to achieve the best long-term outcome in this woman?

    (A) Begin low-dose subcutaneous insulin to prevent diabetes mellitus.
    (B) Begin daily corticosteroid therapy to suppress testosterone secretion.
    (C) Begin a regimen of lifestyle changes, including dietary and exercise alterations.
    (D) Begin levothyroxine (Synthroid) for control of weight gain.
    (E) Oophorectomy to decrease hormone levels.

91. What is the major mode of transmission of HIV infection in young children today?

    (A) biting
    (B) blood transfusion
    (C) vertical transmission
    (D) horizontal transmission
    (E) sexual abuse

92. A 17-year-old is brought by emergency medical services to the emergency room in a postictal state after a witnessed grand mal seizure. No family member is available and the patient is unable to answer questions. A friend who is with him says that he takes some medicine for seizures, but he doesn't know the name. On examination, you note that he has prominent gingival hyperplasia. Of the medications listed below, which one is he most likely to be taking?

    (A) phenobarbital
    (B) valproic acid
    (C) carbamazipine
    (D) phenytoin
    (E) levitiracetam (Keppra)

Questions 93 and 94

A 4-year-old boy returns for his second visit to the emergency room. Three days ago he was brought in with a 4-day history of fever up to 102°F. At that time, his physical examination was significant for injection of the oropharynx and an enlarged left anterior cervical lymph node. His left TM was non-bulging and nonerythematous. He was sent home on amoxicillin with a diagnosis of streptococcal pharyngitis. He returns today with a persistent fever, edema of both hands, bilateral conjunctivitis, and a polymorphous truncal rash.

93. What is the most likely diagnosis?

(A) rickettsial infection
(B) drug hypersensitivity reaction
(C) measles
(D) Kawasaki disease
(E) Scarlet fever

94. What is the treatment for this condition?
(A) a tapering dose of prednisone
(B) high-dose aspirin and IVIG
(C) IVIG alone
(D) admission to the hospital for IV antibiotics and fluids
(E) a 2-week course of antibiotics and a shot of prednisone

95. Parents bring their 6-year-old son to the emergency room following an acute onset of vomiting and combative behavior. The parents state that the child has recently had chickenpox. They have been giving him medication to reduce his fever, which has been as high as 102°F. Which medication is the likely cause of his current condition?

(A) acetaminophen
(B) aspirin
(C) amoxicillin
(D) ibuprofen
(E) diphenhydramine

96. Use of which medication can result in enamel staining of primary teeth?

(A) erythromycin
(B) ciprofloxacin (Cipro)
(C) cephalexin
(D) trimethoprim/sulfamethoxazole (Septra)
(E) tetracycline

97. A 10-year-old male has a history of seizures which are controlled with dilantin. The child also has asthma and often uses an albuterol inhaler. Which of the following asthma medications can lower the seizure threshold in children?

(A) theophylline
(B) salmeterol
(C) beclomethasone
(D) montelukast
(E) nedocromil

98. A 10-year-old boy presents to your clinic with right knee pain for 2 weeks. He is physically active at school and plays soccer and basketball. He describes pain in his knees when he runs or jumps. He denies any recent trauma. His physical examination is normal except for mild edema and tenderness over the right tibial tubercle. What is the most likely diagnosis?

(A) slipped capital femoral epiphysis
(B) Osgood-Schlatter disease
(C) patellar tendonitis
(D) iliotibial band friction syndrome
(E) septic joint

99. A concerned mother brings in her 18-month-old infant girl. The baby's developmental milestones have been normal. The mother states that there is a "funny glint" in her baby's eyes. She also states that sometimes the infant's eyes look crossed. Which of these supports the diagnosis of a serious life-threatening disease?

(A) Baby reaches for small objects.
(B) Baby fusses when each eye is covered.
(C) Bright red reflex in one eye, a white reflex in the other.
(D) Baby rubs both eyes.
(E) Baby holds objects close to inspect them.

100. A 4-year-old boy is brought to the emergency room by his mother after the child spontaneously admitted to swallowing part of a toy. The child is unable to describe what he ate further, although he appears to be in no distress. His vital signs are normal and his respiratory and abdominal examinations are unremarkable. The child is hungry and is demanding to eat something. A CXR reveals what appears to be a watch battery ("button battery") in the patient's esophagus. What is the best course of action in this situation?

(A) admit the child to the hospital and allow him to eat

(B) admit the child to the hospital but keep him in a fasting state

(C) induce vomiting

(D) emergency endoscopy

(E) discharge the patient with instructions to look in his stools for the battery to confirm passage

101. An 18-month-old boy is taken to his family doctor for evaluation of easy bruising and decrease range of motion of the right knee. On examination, he had multiple large ecchymoses, mostly in the lower extremities, and a right knee hemarthrosis. He has not had surgery or family history of a bleeding disorder. Initial blood tests reveal a prolonged activated partial thromboplastin time (aPTT) with a normal PT and platelet count. What further tests should be ordered to make a diagnosis in this boy?

(A) factor VII

(B) factors II, VII, IX, and X

(C) bleeding time

(D) factors XI, IX, VIII

(E) factor I and II

102. Which of the following are currently recommended for all children for every well-child visit?

(A) serum lead levels

(B) hematocrit

(C) PPD

(D) full physical examination

(E) urinalysis

Answers and Explanations

1. **(E)**

2. **(A)**

Explanations 1 and 2 |ˈkrip'tȯrˌkȯˌdiz̄m/

The constellation of cryptorchidism, posterior urethral valves, and abnormal abdominal musculature is called Eagle-Barrett syndrome. Another name is prune belly syndrome. The greatest morbidity comes from the poor amniotic fluid production, due to bladder outlet obstruction, with a resulting pulmonary hypoplasia. Cushing's triad are hypertension, bradycardia, and widened pulse pressure. This is seen as terminal findings associated with increased intracranial pressure. VATER association has multiple anomalies, none of which are the three mentioned. VATER is a mnemonic which stands for **V**ertebral anomalies, **A**nal atresia (imperforate), **T**racheo-**E**sophageal fistula, and **R**enal anomalies (the R also indicated **R**adial anomalies). It is sometimes referred to as VACTERL association in which the C indicates **C**ardiac anomalies with the L indicating **L**imb anomalies. Potter's syndrome is bilateral renal agenesis. This condition is fatal, due to marked pulmonary hypoplasia. The Jones criteria are used in the diagnosis of ARF. *(Rudolph et al., 2003, pp. 1737–1738)*

3. **(B)** Tachypnea is the most sensitive clinical parameter for diagnosing a lower respiratory tract infection. The child may have tachycardia from a fever or anxiety but, typically, not simply from pneumonia. Coughing is common in children with pneumonia but it is not specific for lower respiratory tract infections, as it can also be seen in upper and lower respiratory tract infections. *(Rudolph et al., 2003, p. 1980)*

4. **(E)** All of the vaccines mentioned, except varicella, are killed or synthetic vaccines. Varivax is an attenuated varicella strain (OKA) from Japan. Live virus vaccines are contraindicated in the case of AIDS with a markedly reduced T-cell count. The IPV is the inactivated version of the live polio vaccine, oral polio vaccine (OPV). *(American Academy of Pediatrics, 2003, pp. 11–14)*

5. **(C)**

6. **(A)**

Explanations 5 and 6

The x-ray provided shows a nondisplaced spiral fracture of the distal tibia. This is also known as a toddler's fracture. This fracture can occur when the toddler begins to walk and twists on a planted leg. This torque can result in a spiral fracture of the planted tibia. There usually is no dislocation of the ankle joint and minimal displacement of the fracture. A chip fracture of the metaphysis is a common fracture seen in abused infants and is commonly termed as a "bucket-handle" or "corner" fracture. A buckle fracture is a common accidental fracture seen in falls from a height. *(Rudolph et al., 2003, p. 2451)*

7. **(B)**

8. **(A)**

Explanations 7 and 8

This young woman has cervicitis, but without evidence of pelvic inflammatory disease (PID). Chlamydia is the most common bacterial cause of sexually transmitted diseases in the United States and the most likely etiology of this patient's infection. Gonorrhea would be the next most likely cause and, frequently, there will be coinfection with the two pathogens. The simplest outpatient treatment for these two would be a single 1-g oral dose of azithromycin and a

125-mg IM dose of ceftriaxone. This regimen will ensure complete compliance, which is crucial. Treatment of her sexual partners would also be recommended. Another cause of cervicitis is trichomoniasis, for which metronidazole, either for 1 week of 500 mg bid or a single 2-g oral dose, would be recommended therapy. Of the suggested answers, option A is the only one which would cover the two most common infectious agents. *(Centers for Disease Control and Prevention, 2002, pp. 32–34)*

9. **(B)**

10. **(B)**

Explanations 9 and 10

There are nearly 900,000 victims of child abuse in the United States each year. An inflicted injury is the most common cause of injury in the first year of life. As a child becomes more mobile, falls and motor vehicle accidents become increasingly more common. Other children are a very rare cause of serious injury in childhood. *(Department of Health and Human Services, 2002)*

Brain injury that results from violent shaking of the infant is known as Shaken baby syndrome. These infants can present with seizures, a bulging fontanelle, or irritability presenting a clinical picture similar to that of a septic infant. Intracranial injury is evident on CT or MRI and with a funduscopic examination revealing retinal hemorrhages. Accidental bruises are usually found over bony areas such as shins, knees, elbows, and forehead. Linear fractures of the skull can result from low-energy blunt trauma over a wide surface area of the skull. Nursemaid's elbow is a common condition in young children and generally affects children under 5. It occurs when a child is pulled up too hard by the hand or wrist resulting a in a partial dislocation of the elbow. *(Rudolph et al., 2003, pp. 464–466)*

11. **(D)**

12. **(B)**

13. **(D)**

14. **(A)**

15. **(E)**

Explanations 11 through 15

The most common finding in a newborn with Down syndrome is hypotonia. Other common findings include single palmar crease, flat facial profile, macroglossia, and wide space between the first and second toes. Hypotonia in the newborn period should prompt close evaluation and follow-up. Café au lait spots are associated with neurofibromatosis. High arched palates are associated with fragile X syndrome. Ambiguous genitalia are commonly seen in CAH. *(Jones, 1997, pp. 8–13)*

Children with Down syndrome are at an increased risk for hypothyroidism. It may be hard to detect without routine laboratory screening as they will commonly have mental retardation and developmental delay as part of their syndrome. Hypothyroidism may not be present in the immediate newborn period and requires, at a minimum, annual testing throughout the child's life. The other findings listed are not specifically associated with Down syndrome. Lens dislocation is commonly found with Marfan syndrome or homocysteinuria. *(Jones, 1997, pp. 8–13)*

Children with Down syndrome have an increased prevalence of duodenal atresia. Pyloric stenosis is uncommon to see in the newborn period. It tends to present with nonbilious vomiting usually after 2–4 weeks of age. Hirschsprung disease (aganglionosis coli) presents with constipation and failure to pass stool. Infants with Hirschsprung disease commonly will not pass stool in the first days of life. Biliary atresia is a progressive cause of jaundice in an infant. It is the most common cause of a cholestatic jaundice in the newborn period. Emesis is not typically associated with biliary atresia. Milk protein allergy is a common cause of bloody stools in the first few months of life, but does not have bilious emesis associated with it. *(Jones, 1997, pp. 8–13)*

The double-bubble sign is typically seen in duodenal atresia. It represents gas in the stomach and the first part of the duodenum. This finding can also be seen in children with malrotation with a midgut volvulus. A midgut volvulus may also have bilious emesis as well, but malrotation is not specifically associated with Down syndrome. Pneumatosis intestinalis is the radiographic appearance of dissected air in the intestinal wall. It is seen in necrotizing enterocolitis (NEC). Scimitar sign is seen on CXR and is indicative of anomalous pulmonary veins. (*Rudolph et al., 2003, p. 203*)

The mean IQ of children with Down syndrome is 50 (the average is 20–85). Children with Down syndrome are not at greater risk of CNS malformations. There is not an increased presence of calcifications or of aneurysms. Five percent of children with Down syndrome can have a seizure disorder, making it a less common finding than mental retardation. Hydrocephalus is not increased in children with Down syndrome. (*Jones, 1997, pp. 8–13*)

16. (B)

17. (B)

Explanations 16 and 17

G. lamblia is a common protozoan which can be acquired by ingesting unfiltered water. It is seen frequently in people who drink fresh stream water. It is a cause of chronic, non-bloody diarrhea. There is typically a large amount of gas and cramping associated with *Giardia* infections. RMSF does not typically cause a gastroenteritis. Children with RMSF will commonly have fevers, headaches, and a petechial rash. Rotavirus and Norwalk viruses typically cause acute, self-limited gastroenteritis. The diarrhea is nonbloody, nonmucousy, and typically lasts a few days. (*American Academy of Pediatrics, 2003, pp. 283–285*)

The most appropriate treatment for giardiasis is oral metronidazole. Oral rehydration is an important mainstay in the treatment of diarrhea of any cause but is not a specific treatment for giardiasis. Ciprofloxacin is commonly used for traveler's diarrhea caused by *E. coli.*

18. (C)

19. (B)

20. (E)

Explanations 18 through 20

The most common malignancy in childhood is leukemia/lymphoma. The most common solid tumors of childhood are CNS tumors, followed by neuroblastoma and Wilms tumors. (*Rudolph et al., 2003, p. 1583*)

The mildly elevated WBC with lymphocyte predominance with the presence of "atypical" lymphocytes would indicate that his child most likely has acute EBV infection (infectious mononucleosis). This acute EBV infection is usually subclinical in younger children, but can be manifested by acute hemolytic anemia and splenomegaly. Testing for the diagnosis of EBV includes EBV DNA PCR and heterophile antibody response testing (monospot test). Diagnosis usually is made based upon serology testing for anti-EBV IgG and IgM levels. There is no specific therapy indicated for the acute EBV infections. (*American Academy of Pediatrics, 2003, pp. 286–288*)

Acute Lyme disease is very uncommon in children. The early stages of acute Lyme disease is characterized by a distinctive rash (erythema migrans). This is then followed by a multiple annular rash of disseminated Lyme disease. Often seen in this stage is cranial nerve palsies, specifically a facial nerve (CN VII) palsy. Late Lyme disease is characterized by recurrent arthritis and arthralgia. Serologic testing is only recommended if there is a very high clinical index of suspicion, unlike this child. (*American Academy of Pediatrics, 2003, pp. 428–433*)

Acute systemic-onset JRA (Still disease) can present in a child of this age in a nonspecific manner (i.e., fever of unknown origin). Children with Still disease will typically have dramatic elevations in acute-phase reactants (i.e., ESR). This child's ESR being 5 would go against JRA. (*Rudolph et al., 2003, pp. 480–481*)

SLE would be unexpected in a child of this age, specifically a male. There are no features of this vignette which would indicate the need for confirmatory testing in this child. Likewise, the low ESR would not be consistent with acute SLE. *(Rudolph et al., 2003, pp. 486–489)*

TB presents in children mostly as acute lower respiratory tract infection or subacute lymphadenitis (scrofula). In infants, an aggressive meningitis is a global cause of significant morbidity and mortality. Acute hematogenous TB is not a condition seen in otherwise healthy children. *(American Academy of Pediatrics, 2003, pp. 678–698)*

21. **(C)** A fever in the first 4–6 weeks of life needs to be treated very aggressively. There are no reliable clinical or laboratory findings currently available that can discriminate between a nominal viral illness and a serious bacterial infection. In the newborn period, fever may be the only indicator of bacteremia or meningitis. Any rectal temperature greater than 100.5°F should trigger a full sepsis workup. This should include cultures of the blood, urine, and spinal fluid. In this age range, empiric antimicrobials should be initiated that should cover for GBS, *E. coli*, and *Listeria monocytogenes*. A commonly used regimen is ampicillin and gentamicin. Many would also include empiric acyclovir in this age range. In infants, the routine use of antipyretics should be discouraged. A blood culture alone is not an adequate screening tool for meningitis. While a urinary tract infection (UTI) is a common cause of infection in infants, a more complete evaluation would be warranted. *(Fleisher and Ludwig, 2000, pp. 725–736)*

22. **(B)**

23. **(D)**

Explanations 22 and 23

Bilious emesis in an infant is malrotation until proven otherwise. Malrotation can lead to a midgut volvulus. The volvulus can result in bowel ischemia and necrosis. This makes bilious emesis in a newborn a concerning finding. Pyloric stenosis would cause nonbilious emesis. Imperforate anus would present with the failure of stool passage. Diaphragmatic hernia will present with poor feeding, drooling, and respiratory embarrassment.

The best radiographic test in the diagnosis of malrotation is an UGI contrast study with small bowel follow through. This will identify the duodenum and its location relative to the ligament of Treitz. The characteristic finding in a midgut volvulus is the "corkscrew" sign, which is seen as contrast media traverses the kinked intestine. An abdominal CT may show malrotation but is less specific for it. Barium enema and radionuclide scans have no role in the diagnosis of malrotation. *(Rudolph et al., 2003, p. 203)*

24. **(C)**

25. **(D)**

Explanations 24 and 25

ARF is clinically diagnosed by using the Jones criteria. The Jones criteria are separated into major and minor findings. The major criteria are arthritis (not simply arthralgia), carditis, Sydenham chorea, erythema marginatum, and subcutaneous nodules. The minor criteria include the presence of a fever, arthralgias, documentation of a GAS infection (either currently or in the past), or laboratory evidence of inflammation (increased ESR). Two major criteria, or one major and two minors, are required for the diagnosis of ARF. The only exception to this rule is that the presence of Sydenham chorea alone will make the diagnosis. While the documentation of a prior, or current, GAS infection is compelling, it is not a requirement for the diagnosis of ARF. Children with rheumatic fever are not considered contagious. *(Rudolph et al., 2003, pp. 1901–1904)*

26. **(B)**

27. **(A)**

Explanations 26 and 27

Acute inflammatory demyelinating polyneuropathy, commonly called Guillain-Barré syndrome, is an ascending paralysis with a hallmark of absent reflexes. There may also be some nominal sensory deficits as well, but they are not as striking as the paresis. Methylphenidate toxicity usually results in seizures and tachycardia. In children with malingering, reflexes are usually present, as they are not under cognitive control. Reflexes are also present in children with polymyositis. Children with polymyositis will usually have fever and muscle pain with weakness, as well. With the use of the polio vaccines (OPV or IPV), poliomyelitis is no longer present in wild type in the United States.

Guillain-Barré is usually a self-limited disease. The most common complication is respiratory failure. The paresis usually advances for 48–72 hours and then will slowly recede. The use of corticosteroids is not recommended. Plasmaphoresis is used in the following situations: progressive paresis, nonambulatory patients, or bulbar or respiratory involvement. As this child's disease has plateaued at the time of evaluation, plasmaphoresis would be of little benefit. *(Fenichel, 1997, pp. 176–202; Rudolph et al., 2003, pp. 2281–2283)*

28. **(A)** GBS is the most common cause of infection in the newborn infant, followed by *E. coli* and *L. monocytogenes*. GBS is the most common cause of pneumonia, septicemia, UTI, and meningitis. The risk of early-onset (within the first 7 days of life) GBS infection can be reduced with the antenatal administration of appropriate antimicrobials. The use of perinatal antimicrobials has no effect on the occurrence of late-onset (after 7 days of life) GBS disease. *(American Academy of Pediatrics, 2003, pp. 584–591)*

29. **(E)**

30. **(A)**

Explanations 29 and 30

The most common cause of otitis media in children is pneumococcus (*S. pneumoniae*). This is also the most common cause of sinusitis and pneumonia. Otitis media is usually seen in conjunction with an upper respiratory tract infection. *(American Academy of Pediatrics, 2003, pp. 490–500)*

Pressure from extensive use of antimicrobials has resulted in a dramatic increase in penicillin resistance in pneumococcus. Amoxicillin remains the recommended initial antibiotic of choice for the treatment of otitis media in children. In an effort to reduce the incidence of antibiotic resistance, and because of the high spontaneous cure rate of otitis media, many authorities are advocating withholding antimicrobial treatment unless symptoms persist for several days in spite of symptomatic treatment.

31. **(D)** GAS pharyngitis ("strep throat") is a common cause of tonsillitis requiring antibiotics. GAS continues to be very susceptible to penicillin, which still remains the treatment of choice. Occasionally, children will have a persistently positive throat culture for GAS and are considered carriers. This carrier state is not a risk for rheumatic disease and is felt not to be contagious to others. The presence of *E. coli* in the intestinal tract is considered colonization and not carrier state. An example of an enteric bacteria which does have a carrier state would be *Salmonella typhi* (typhoid fever). *(American Academy of Pediatrics, 2003, pp. 573–584)*

32. **(D)**

33. **(E)**

Explanations 32 and 33

In children over 1 month of age, the most common causes of bacterial meningitis are *S. pneumoniae* and *Neisseria meningitidis*. HIB was also a frequent cause of this disease prior to the widespread use of the HIB vaccine. GBS, *E. coli*, and HSV would be more common causes of CNS infections in neonates. *(McMillin et al., 1999, Chap. 142)*

Nonpolio enteroviruses are the most common causes of aseptic meningitis in childhood. There are approximately 65 nonpolio enteroviruses, including the Coxsackieviruses, echoviruses, and enteroviruses. Children are the main susceptible population and transmission is from child to child, via fecal-oral or oral-oral (respiratory) contact. Meningitis may result from viremic spread of the virus. Treatment of this is supportive. *(McMillin et al., 1999, Chap. 199)*

34. **(B)** The most common infectious cause of blindness in the world is trachoma. Trachoma

is the chronic effect of a *C. trachomatis* infection acquired in the perinatal period. The most common cause of blindness in the world is non-infectious (glaucoma and diabetic retinopathy). (*American Academy of Pediatrics, 2003, pp. 238–243*)

35. (B)

36. (D)

37. (D)

Explanations 35 through 37

The image provided shows a classic case of impetigo. This is a common skin infection of childhood. It frequently occurs following a case of chickenpox and is due to the child picking or scratching at the varicella lesions, resulting in a secondary bacterial infection. GAS infection is the most common cause of impetigo associated with varicella infections. It is markedly more prevalent than the next most common infectious agent, *S. aureus*. Tinea corporis, often due to *T. rubrum*, is also known as ringworm. It classically is a circular lesion with a red, raised border, and central clearing. Contact dermatitis, from exposure to an irritant such as poison ivy, often causes plaques of erythema and edema with superimposed vesicles. This is also frequently secondarily infected with GAS from scratching. Warts, caused by the human papilloma virus, do not typically appear as the lesions in the image.

Of the options listed, oral cephalexin would be the most appropriate initial therapy. Most GAS isolates are sensitive to first-generation cephalosporins, such as cephalexin. Topical steroids are useful for inflammatory or allergic conditions, topical nystatin for a fungal infection (such as tinea corporis) and oral acyclovir can be used early in the course of a varicella infection. (*Fitzpatrick et al., 2001, p. 18, 696; American Academy of Pediatrics, 2003, pp. 573–584, 598–610*)

38. (A)

39. (C)

40. (D)

Explanations 38 through 40

The hallmark of immune (also known as idiopathic) thrombocytopenia purpura (ITP) is the otherwise healthy appearing child with isolated thrombocytopenia. ITP is the most common cause of isolated thrombocytopenia in childhood. It occurs with equal frequency in both boys and girls. The presence of thrombocytopenia in a patient with otherwise normal cell lines, and a normal physical examination is enough to make the diagnosis, so further evaluation, such as a bone marrow biopsy, is unnecessary. Which children to treat and which treatment to use are areas of controversy in the management of ITP. Most acute ITP will resolve spontaneously, so many will recommend observation for children who appear well, are asymptomatic, and have platelet counts above 30,000. Platelet transfusions should be reserved only in the instance of ongoing or imminent bleeding.

When a decision is made to treat, usually when the platelet count falls below 20,000, there are several options available. Treatment involves using IVIG, steroids, anti-D immunoglobulins, or combinations thereof. Combinations of medications may work synergistically. Prednisone is often used initially, as it can be given orally and is inexpensive. Typically, it will be tapered over 2 weeks to 3 months. By using combination therapy when needed, splenectomy can be avoided in the vast majority of cases. When it is necessary, it should be delayed, if at all possible, for at least a year after diagnosis. (*Hoffman et al., 2000, pp. 2102–2104*)

41. (E) HUS is, as the name implies, the combination of a microangiopathic hemolytic anemia and acute renal failure. It is commonly associated with *E. coli* O157/H7 gastroenteritis. HUS is one of the most common causes of acquired renal failure in children. (*Rudolph et al., 2003, pp. 1696–1698*)

42. (C)

43. (B)

Explanations 42 and 43

Children with tuberous sclerosis (tuberous sclerosis complex, TSC) can develop nasolabial fold angiofibromas (commonly referred to adenoma sebaceum). These can be mistaken for acne in an adolescent and is seen in over 80% of adolescents with TSC. Other cutaneous findings include peri- and subungual fibromas, ash leaf spots (hypomelanocytic macules), and shagreen patches. Skin findings are seen in 75% of cases of tuberous sclerosis. Tuberous sclerosis can also have CNS cortical defects and "tubers," which may be foci of seizure activity. The "tubers" have a classic periventricular distribution. Mental retardation is very common in varying degrees. (*Jones, 1997, pp. 506–507*)

Sturge-Weber syndrome (also known as leptomeningeal angiomatosis) is a port wine stain, typically with V1 or V2 distribution, with an underlying leptomeningeal blood vessel dysplasia. These dysplastic vessels will typically result in an underlying cortical atrophy. This cortical atrophy can be a nidus for seizures and can be seen on a CT scan of the head. (*Jones, 1997, pp. 495–497*)

Neurofibromatosis, type 1 is polymorphous neurocutaneous syndrome. The most common findings are café au lait spots, which may be present at birth and worsen during puberty. (*Jones, 1997, pp. 495–497*)

Beckwith-Wiedemann syndrome and CHARGE association are discussed further in explanations 44 and 45.

44. (E) Of the listed syndromes, only Beckwith-Wiedemann syndrome has neonatal hypoglycemia as part of its clinical spectrum. The constellation of macroglossia, hypoglycemia, and visceral organomegaly (hepatosplenomegaly) is a common finding in children with Beckwith-Wiedemann syndrome. The presence of an omphalocele in a newborn would also be concerning for Beckwith-Wiedemann syndrome. (*Jones, 1997, pp. 164–165*)

45. (D) The term CHARGE is a mnemonic standing for **C**oloboma, **H**eart malformations, **A**tresia choanae, **R**etarded (growth and mental), **G**enital anomalies, and **E**ar anomalies.

The colobomas are usually seen in the iris, but can be seen in the eyelids and the nasolabial folds as well. The heart anomalies of CHARGE association are usually ventricular septal defects and tetralogy of Fallot. (*Jones, 1997, pp. 668–669*)

46. (D) The majority of otherwise healthy infants who get RSV infections will tolerate the course without complications. Some rare complications can occur in infants with risk factors, which include prematurity; cardiac or pulmonary disease or immune system dysfunction. Premature infants are at particular risk for apnea. It is prudent to observe premature infants for apnea in the first few days of their RSV infection. A full sepsis workup would not be warranted in an otherwise well-appearing, afebrile, infant. RSV-IVIG is not indicated for acute management of RSV infections. Likewise, it is unwarranted to begin antimicrobial therapy without a clear indication. (*American Academy of Pediatrics, 2003, pp. 560–566*)

47. (C)

48. (B)

Explanations 47 and 48

The most common bacterial infection in the newborn period is GBS. GBS is commonly cultured in the adult vaginal tract, and its vertical transmission can be interrupted with maternal antimicrobial treatment prior to delivery of the infant. Mothers are commonly treated in labor with penicillin, ampicillin, clindamycin, or azithromycin in an attempt to interrupt transmission to the infant while passing through the birth canal. If antimicrobial prophylaxis is initiated greater than 4 hours prior to delivery, the rate of early-onset GBS disease is dramatically decreased. The current recommendation for term infants of GBS-positive women who have received antibiotics in labor (at least two doses or ≥4 hours prior to delivery) is observation without testing or antibiotics. (*American Academy of Pediatrics, 2003, pp. 584–591*)

Classic hemophilia is an X-linked recessive bleeding diathesis. Hemophilia is inherited on the maternal lineage from carrier (or affected) mothers. This infant, being a male, would receive his X chromosome from his mother. He is, therefore, not at risk for having hemophilia. Further, being an X-linked trait, there cannot be a male "carrier" state. *(Rudolph et al., 2003, pp. 1570–1573)*

49. **(C)** Falling on outstretched arms is one of the most common injuries among school-aged children. This can result in a buckle, or torus, fracture of the distal radius and/or ulna. This is a common accidental mechanism and should not, by itself, raise suspicions for an inflicted injury. AP and lateral x-rays of the wrist and elbow would be diagnostic of this type of injury. Nursemaid's elbows occur from a pulling or twisting mechanism to the upper extremity and are not the result of falls. An MRI of this injury would be overkill. *(Fleisher and Ludwig, 2000, p. 1455)*

50. **(E)**

51. **(A)**

Explanations 50 and 51

This infant's growth pattern is most consistent with nutritional FTT. This is often termed "nonorganic" FTT. This term is used for conditions in which the child, usually an infant, begins to fall off of the standardized growth curves. The growth curve in this vignette shows that this infant's weight has trailed off while her length has remained stable. Causes of poor growth that are hormonal in nature will tend to have blunted growth velocity (decreased linear growth) that results in infants and children with short stature and normal weight. Short stature refers to deceased linear growth (i.e., length or height). The infant in this vignette does not have short stature, as her linear growth is normal. A child with GH deficiency would be expected to have a decreased linear growth velocity (height) with a weight that remains relatively stable.

The next best step in the evaluation of this infant would hinge on understanding the total calories that this infant is consuming. A measure of the appropriate caloric intake is related

in terms of calories per kilogram per day. This will give a metric to measure whether infants are getting appropriate nutritional intake. Obtaining a serum GH level is an unreliable way to look at an infant's growth due to its pulsatile nature. While a serum somatomedin-C (ILGF-1) may be a more accurate measure of GH activity, in this child a level will likely not reveal much useful information. In children with malnutrition or caloric deprivation, a somatomedin-C level may be depressed due to decreased body mass. If there were a family history of short stature, that would be manifested with poor linear growth, which is not the case in this vignette. While a malabsorption may be a cause of FTT, an UGI series would not be the modality to evaluate for it. *(Zenel, 1997, pp. 371–378)*

52. **(C)**

53. **(A)**

54. **(D)**

55. **(B)**

Explanations 52 through 55

Kawasaki disease (mucocutaneous lymph node syndrome) is a disease of unclear etiology. The salient diagnostic features include fever for greater than 5 days, cervical lymph node greater than 1 cm, nonpurulent conjunctivitis, oral changes (cracking lips or "strawberry tongue"), polymorphous rash to the trunk, and changes to the hands and feet (peeling of the fingers or toes or edema of the hands or feet). This may be confused with group A beta-hemolytic streptococcal pharyngitis, which usually is not associated with conjunctivitis. Coxsackie viral infection is commonly seen as the "hand-foot-mouth" disease, with shallow ulcers on the palms, soles, and in the mouth. There is nominal fever associated, and conjunctivitis is uncommon. Parvovirus B-19 (erythema infectiosum, "fifth disease") is commonly called "slapped cheek" disease because of the exanthem of bright red cheeks. Adenopathy and conjunctivitis are not features of this infection.

Acute phase reactions are often elevated late in the course of Kawasaki disease. The most common blood test result would be a dramatically elevated platelet count. It is usually greater than 750,000 and can be greater than 1,000,000. An ESR is also likely to be elevated, not low. A positive rapid strep test would lead one more toward acute GAS disease.

The treatment of choice for Kawasaki disease is IVIG and aspirin. IVIG infusion is usually over 12 hours and will commonly result in rapid defervescence and clinical improvement. Treatment of Kawasaki disease is important as it will prevent long-term sequelae. A common side effect of IVIG is aseptic meningitis.

Nearly a quarter of untreated children will develop coronary artery dilatation. This is most common cause of acquired heart disease in children younger than 5 years of age. The coronary artery dilatation can result in aneurysm formation and myocardial infarction. *(Rudolph et al., 2003, pp. 844–845)*

56. (B)

57. (C)

Explanations 56 and 57

Most infant formulas are cow's milk based. The most common form of carbohydrate in these infant formulas is lactose. Soy formulas use corn syrup and/or sucrose as their source of carbohydrate. Casein is a form of protein. Human milk fortifier is a supplement added to breast milk for the premature infant and is a combination of protein and carbohydrate. *(Rudolph et al., 2003, pp. 1329–1333)*

GBS colitis is an uncommon disease in infants. Cow's milk protein intolerance is a common cause of blood-streaked stool in an infant on cow's milk based formulas. Lactose intolerance is very uncommon in an infant and usually causes chronic, nonbloody diarrhea. Pseudomembranous colitis would be a consideration in a child with diarrhea who recently had been on antibiotics. *(Fleisher and Ludwig, 2000, p. 1445)*

58. (B)

59. (D)

60. (E)

Explanations 58 through 60

This case is a common presentation for viral croup, with the symptoms of a seal-barking cough, stridor, tachypnea, and fever in the winter. Pneumonia must also be considered with tachypnea, cough, and fever, but it is less likely to cause stridor and may not have the seal-bark type of cough. Sinusitis may cause cough and fever, but would be more likely to have a purulent nasal discharge and less likely to have the typical croupy cough. Bronchiolitis due to RSV is a common cause of wintertime cough and fever. It is less likely to have stridor and more likely to have wheezing. Children with epiglottitis are typically found in the "tripod position" and may be drooling. It is, fortunately, becoming rare with the widespread use of the *H. influenzae* vaccine.

Parainfluenza types 1 and 2 account for 60–70% of all viral croup. HIB was a common cause of epiglottitis, but is now rare because of widespread vaccinations. Influenza B and RSV can cause croup, but not as commonly as parainfluenza types 1 and 2. *S. pneumoniae* would be the most common bacterial cause of pneumonia or sinusitis. *(American Academy of Pediatrics, 2003, pp. 454–455)*

The steeple sign is subglottic narrowing of the trachea seen on an AP view of the trachea or a CXR. The trachea is seen to narrow, almost to a point, like the steeple of a church. Swollen adenoids are difficult to identify in lateral neck x-rays. The presence of swollen adenoids is unrelated to the airway narrowing seen in croup. The thumb sign is a swollen epiglottis seen with epiglottitis. A lobar pulmonary infiltrate may be seen with a typical bacterial pneumonia. *(Fleisher and Ludwig, 2000, p. 745)*

61. (B)

62. (D)

Explanations 61 and 62

Short stature in an adolescent is a common reason for visiting the pediatrician or endocrinologist. Most short stature in adolescence is constitutional growth delay. These children will have normal growth velocity and delayed bone age. Growth is normal for the first 4–12 months, then decelerates to below the fifth percentile. These children will catch up to their peers in a slightly delayed fashion. Frequently, other family members have a history of short stature in childhood, delayed puberty, and eventual normal stature as adults. In contrast, children with familial short stature have a normal bone age and regular onset of puberty. These children will maintain their short stature as adults. Somatomedin-C (ILGF-1) is commonly used as a surrogate measure for the end-organ effect of the pulsatile GH release. In children with GH deficiency, the end-organ effect will be a low somatomedin-C level. An advanced bone age (advanced bone maturation) usually results in shorter final height. Chronic renal failure is a cause of growth delay, but not a common one. *(Behrman, 2004, p. 1851; Rudolph et al., 2003, pp. 2014–2017)*

63. **(C)**

64. **(A)**

Explanations 63 and 64

Pubarche in females is usually earlier than in males. Delayed puberty alone may be a pathologic condition; its presence in conjunction with short stature makes a pathologic state more likely. Males do, indeed, have adrenarche. Panhypopituitarism is a cause of puberty delay, but not a common one. Undiagnosed hypothyroidism can be a cause of pubertal delay, and thyroid function testing should be a part of the routine evaluation of this problem.

The onset of puberty in males is usually signaled by an increase in testicular volume. This is commonly seen in conjunction with lengthening of the phallus and thinning of the scrotal skin. As a result of puberty, the other findings (deepening of the voice, increased muscle mass, and increased facial hair) may be seen, but the first of the listed findings to appear is increased testicular volume. In females, puberty is usually signaled by the enlargement of breast buds. *(Rudolph et al., 2003, pp. 2093–2105)*

65. **(C)**

66. **(B)**

Explanations 65 and 66

Polyuria in a prepubertal female may indicate the presence of a UTI. A UTI must be excluded as the first step. Polyuria may also indicate vulvovaginitis. Vulvovaginitis in a prepubertal female is usually irritation and hygiene related. The presence of dysuria with the polyuria would make the utility of checking a fingerstick glucose, as a screening test for diabetes, low yield.

The nightly use of bubble baths makes chemical urethritis the most likely cause of this girl's polyuria and dysuria. Diabetes mellitus would present typically with polyuria, polydipsia, weight loss, and decrease in energy. There would also be no dysuria unless there were a concomitant UTI. Diabetes insipidus is a very rare disease in childhood and would be unlikely in an otherwise healthy girl. The presence of a retained foreign body (typically toilet paper) is usually seen in conjunction with a vaginal odor and discharge as well. *(Rudolph et al., 2003, pp. 607–611)*

67. **(E)** Pinworms (*E. vermicularis*) are common nematodes (roundworms) found in children. It usually is a benign, incidental finding, but can present with perianal pruritus or small, white, threadlike worms on visual examination. Ascariasis is the most common roundworm infection in humans, but these worms are larger. *T. canis* (dog roundworm) is another nematode and is the cause of visceral larval migrans. *D. latum* (fish tape worm) and *Taenia solium* (pork tape worm) are cestodes, which are long, flat worms. *(American Academy of Pediatrics, 2003, pp. 486–487)*

68. **(D)** Iron deficiency is a common finding. Most proprietary infant formulas have iron supplementation. Infants who are strictly

breast fed may require oral iron supplementation. A total body iron deficiency can result in a microcytic, hypochromic anemia. Testing of total serum iron, ferritin, and total iron binding capacity can help clarify the body iron stores. *(Rudolph et al., 2003, pp. 1525–1528)*

69. **(B)** The absence, or malabsorption, of zinc from the diet will result in zinc deficiency. The clinical entity is called acrodermatitis enteropathica. Symptoms may manifest during the transition from breast milk to cow's milk. The typical dermatologic manifestations of this are symmetrically distributed perianal and perioral (in a horseshoe pattern) dermatitis. The skin lesions are eczematous, dry, scaly, or psoriasiform. Children with vitamin C deficiency present with petechial hemorrhages of the skin and mucus membranes. Hypocalcemia does not include specific dermatologic changes. Tetany is a classic manifestation of hypocalcemia. Skin pallor is the most important sign of iron deficiency. Children with inadequate iodine in their diet may develop hypothyroidism. *(Behrman, 2004, p. 2249; Rudolph et al., 2003, p. 1326)*

70. **(A)** Parathormone (PTH), with vitamin D, is a major regulator of the serum levels of calcium. PTH is made in the chief cells of the four parathyroid glands and exerts effects mainly on the bone and kidneys to maintain adequate serum levels of calcium. *(Rudolph et al., 2003, pp. 2142–2149)*

71. **(C)**

72. **(D)**

Explanations 71 and 72

Hypothyroidism results from inadequate thyroid hormone production or a defect in thyroid hormone receptor activity. Hypothyroidism can be congenital or acquired. Most infants with congenital hypothyroidism are asymptomatic at birth. Feeding difficulties, choking spells, and somnolence often present during the first month of life. Respiratory distress can also occur in part due to the large tongue and nasal obstruction. On physical examination,

you may find a large abdomen, umbilical hernias, subnormal temperature, cold skin, murmurs, or bradycardia. Iodine is absorbed in the GI tract as iodide. Iodide is concentrated in the thyroid gland and four atoms are incorporated into each molecule of thyroxine. Profound dietary deficiency of iodine will result in hypothyroidism and is the most common cause of goiter in the world.

Rickets results from a deficiency of vitamin D. This condition predominately affects the long bones and skull. Vitamin C deficiency results in scurvy, a condition with impaired collagen formation. The clinical manifestations may include changes in the gums, loosening of teeth, brittle bones, and swollen joints. Pallor is the most important sign of iron-deficiency anemia. Children may also have the desire to ingest unusual substances such as ice or dirt. Finally, hyponatremia and hypoglycemia are the prominent presenting signs of adrenal insufficiency in infants. *(Behrman, 2004, pp. 184–186, 1872–1875; Rudolph et al., 2003, p. 2059)*

73. **(D)**

74. **(B)**

75. **(A)**

Explanations 73 through 75

Febrile seizures are the most common cause of seizures in childhood. These are classically seen early in an illness and when there is a rapid rise in the child's temperature. These seizures usually last less than 2–3 minutes (typical febrile seizures last no longer than 15 minutes) and have a very mild, short, postictal phase. Children who have seizures that are the result of bacterial meningitis will not subsequently be normal.

For typical febrile seizures, in an otherwise healthy and well-appearing child, no evaluation (outside of treating any underlying cause of the fever) is warranted. Blood and urine cultures would not be necessary in evaluation of the seizures, but they may be warranted in evaluation of the fever. An EEG and head CT will nearly universally be normal and are unwarranted.

A single typical febrile seizure routinely does not require any anticonvulsant therapy. If the child has had multiple febrile seizures, or the seizures are not typical, anticonvulsant therapy may be entertained. Prophylactic anticonvulsant therapy is usually initiated after the third febrile seizure. Occasionally, children may have convulsions associated with fevers which do not fall into the typical features. Some criteria which would make a febrile seizure atypical would be prolonged duration (greater than 15 minutes) and a prolonged postictal state (greater than 30–60 minutes). (Fenichel, 1997, pp. 18–19)

76. **(B)** Relative immaturity of the lacrimal drainage system can result in the accumulation of debris in the nasolacrimal duct. This will manifest as a swelling inferior to the middle canthus. Dermoid cysts in children are commonly found as a subcutaneous nodule on the lateral portion of the eyebrow. Mucoceles are usually found as fleshy papules on the inner portion of the lower lip. Frontal encephaloceles are midline in location. (Rudolph et al., 2003, pp. 2366–2367)

77. **(D)**

78. **(B)**

79. **(A)**

Explanations 77 through 79

The clinical scenario describes a classic presentation of RMSF (infection with R. rickettsii). Typical symptoms include a summertime fever, headache, petechial rash, thrombocytopenia, and hyponatremia. This may be mistaken for a systemic enteroviral infection, or enteroviral encephalitis, but the presence of thrombocytopenia and hyponatremia would exclude this diagnosis. Still disease (systemic-onset JRA) would have an elevation of acute-phase reactants, including the WBC and platelet count. Fourteen years old is an unlikely age for Kawasaki disease, and the acute phase reactants would likewise also be elevated.

RMSF is a very serious infectious illness. Appropriate antimicrobial therapy, usually doxycycline, needs to be started as soon as the diagnosis is seriously considered, as this can prevent some of the more severe sequelae. The use of systemic corticosteroids has no place in the management of RMSF. Confirmation of RMSF is serologic. Rising IgG titers or the presence of IgM titers to R. rickettsii is a confirmation of RMSF. (American Academy of Pediatrics, 2003, pp. 532–534)

80. **(C)**

81. **(C)**

82. **(E)**

Explanations 80 through 82

The constellation of ear pain, pain with movement of the pinna, and cloudy discharge from the ear canal in a child who has been swimming frequently is most probably OE, also known as "swimmer's ear." Perforated TMs can occur, often as the result of an untreated otitis media, a foreign body inserted deep in the ear or from barotrauma. This can cause ear pain and may have a cloudy drainage if the perforation is the result of otitis media. Neither otitis media nor perforated TMs typically cause pain on movement of the pinna. Mastoiditis is a rare infection that usually results from extension of an untreated otitis media into the mastoid air cells. The common findings on examination would be an acute otitis media and tenderness over the mastoid area behind the ear. Temporomandibular joint dysfunction can cause ear pain, but the common finding is tenderness anterior to the ear, not pain with movement of the ear or drainage from the ear canal. It would also be uncommon in a child this age.

The most common cause of acute OE is *Pseudomonas aeruginosa*. Treatment for acute OE will involve topical antimicrobials which cover *P. aeruginosa*, often in combination with a topical steroid. A commonly used treatment consists of eardrops containing neomycin, polymyxin B, and hydrocortisone (Cortisporin Otic), four drops into the affected ear four times a day for 7–10 days. Alternative therapy consists of oflaxacin drops twice a day into the affected ear for 7–10 days. For chronic OE, yeast becomes a more important pathogen, and therapy should be directed as such. *(Fleisher and Ludwig, 2000, p. 1571; Rudolph et al., 2003, pp. 1255–1256)*

83. (C)

84. (A)

85. (D)

Explanations 83 through 85

Repeating all serologies is important. The prior negative testing should be included in the medical record, but should not dissuade one from confirming the result. The collection of stool for ova and parasites (O + P) is an important evaluation but should not be the only testing performed. A CBC is not an adequate screen for infections. *(American Academy of Pediatrics, 2003, pp. 173–180)*

The diagnosis of FAS includes findings of characteristic facies, growth retardation, and CNS impairment. The characteristic facies of FAS includes flat philtrum, thin upper vermilion border, short palpebral fissures, micrognathia, microphthalmos, and microcephaly. *(Jones, 1997, pp. 555–558)*

BCG is a common vaccine administered in countries outside of the United States. The presence of a positive reaction to a PPD in a child who has had a prior BCG is still concerning. The presence of a 15-mm reaction is considered positive and warrants a CXR and initiation of anti-TB treatment. The negative CXR would indicate TB exposure, and INH alone is recommended. Sputum collection is usually unwarranted in asymptomatic children. *(American Academy of Pediatrics, 2003, pp. 642–660)*

86. (C)

87. (B)

Explanations 86 and 87

This represents an allergic contact dermatitis. The allergen is the oil on the leaf of certain plants (poison ivy). The reaction is a delayed-type hypersensitivity reaction (type 4) and may take up to 72–96 hours after exposure to fully manifest.

Limited allergic contact dermatitis will usually warrant limited therapy. Oral antihistamines, taken on an as-needed basis, can provide effective symptomatic relief. Topical antihistamines are usually not effective and, if added to oral antihistamines, can result in toxic effects. Steroids should be used sparingly on the face, and high-potency steroid should not be used at all on the face. Secondary infection is unlikely if good skin hygiene is used. *(Fleisher and Ludwig, 2000, pp. 1134–1136)*

88. (B)

89. (A)

90. (C)

Explanations 88 through 90

This clinical vignette describes an adolescent female with PCOS. PCOS is commonly seen in obese adolescent females with anovulatory menstrual cycles, hirsutism, and generalized virilization (acne). Commonly, PCOS patients will have glucose insensitivity and manifest features of type II diabetes mellitus.

The diagnosis of PCOS may be difficult to ascertain. A pelvic ultrasound demonstrating "polycystic ovaries" (the string of pearls sign) may be quite helpful. Girls with PCOS will typically have elevated triglycerides, low HDL cholesterol, and a suppressed prolactin. As indicated above, PCOS girls also often have glucose insensitivity and an abnormal glucose tolerance test.

The most effective therapy in PCOS involves lifestyle alterations (weight loss and exercise) and hormonal regulation of ovulation. The hypoglycemic agent metformin is now being used to assist in the management of PCOS. Occasionally, subcutaneous insulin may be effective in controlling hyperglycemia, but this will not prevent diabetes mellitus. *(Rudolph et al., 2003, pp. 249–252)*

91. (C) Vertically transmitted, or perinatally acquired, HIV is the most common mode of transmission in pediatric patients. Maternal health, maternal viral load, third trimester antiretroviral therapy, and mode of delivery all affect the rate of perinatal acquisition. (*American Academy of Pediatrics, 2003, pp. 360–382*)

92. **(D)** Gingival hyperplasia is a common side effect of chronic phenytoin administration. This will resolve with cessation of the medication. None of the other anticonvulsants listed will result in this problem. (*Rudolph et al., 2003, p. 1292*)

93. **(D)**

94. **(B)**

Explanations 93 and 94

Kawasaki disease is the second most common systemic vasculitis in children. The diagnosis requires the presence of fever for at least 5 days and four of the five criteria: bilateral conjunctivitis (generally nonpurulent); oropharyngeal mucosal changes including pharyngeal injection, strawberry tongue, or injection or fissuring of the lips; nonfluctuant cervical lymphadenopathy, usually unilateral; polymorphous rash that is primarily truncal; and changes of the peripheral extremities, including edema or erythema of hands and feet, or desquamation of the finger/toes, usually beginning periungally.

The treatment of Kawasaki disease consists of high-dose aspirin and IVIG as a single dose infused over 12 hours. The role of corticosteroid as treatment is controversial. This therapy was abandoned after an initial report citing increased rates of coronary artery aneurysms. A few recent studies reveal successful treatment with methylprednisolone in children who failed therapy of IVIG, but it is not first line. (*Rudolph et al., 2003, pp. 844–845*)

95. **(B)** Historically, Reye's syndrome was a cause of hepatitis and encephalitis. It was seen in children with influenza or varicella who were given aspirin. Widespread knowledge of this issue, resulting in an almost complete cessation of the use of aspirin in children, has made Reye's syndrome a very rare occurrence. (*Rudolph et al., 2003, p. 1490*)

96. **(E)** Gray or brown teeth staining can be seen with the use of tetracycline in children who still have their primary teeth. Tetracyclines are usually safe as a single course in normal doses in younger children. The use of tetracyclines in children is typically safe after 8 years of age. Teeth staining can also be seen in the children of women who took tetracycline while pregnant. (*Rudolph et al., 2003, p. 878*)

97. **(A)** Theophylline, a methylxanthine, has an excitatory effect on the CNS. This serious side effect, in conjunction with its very narrow therapeutic window, has made theophylline use very uncommon. The use of any of the other medications listed would be recommended before consideration of the use of theophylline. (*Fleisher and Ludwig, 2000, pp. 924–925*)

98. **(B)** Osgood-Schlatter disease is a repetitive stress injury to the inferior end of the patellar tendon at its insertion into the tibial tubercle. These patients are usually young, athletic males between the ages 10 and 15 years. The diagnosis is made when a young male presents with knee pain that increases with exercise without a history of trauma. Treatment consists of rest, activity restriction, and anti-inflammatory agents. Slipped capital femoral epiphysis occurs most commonly in African American obese adolescent males. It refers to a slipping of the epiphysis off the metaphysis. The "slipping" is caused by weakening of the perichondral ring of the growth plate, which allows the epiphysis and metaphysis to gradually or acutely displace from each other. This results in pain in the groin, thigh, or knee as well as a limp. Treatment is primarily operative internal fixation. Patellar tendonitis is caused by injury to the patellar tendon. Most of these patients have tenderness in the inferior portion of the patella and complain of chronic anterior knee pain. Iliotibial band friction syndrome causes lateral knee pain in runners. (*Rudolph et al., 2003, p. 2432, 2438*)

99. **(C)** Leukocoria, a white pupillary reflex, can be caused by several conditions. The most serious, and potentially life threatening, is retinoblastoma. Retinoblastoma is a malignant

neoplasm of the retina that may appear as a white mass extending into the vitreous, a mass lesion underlying a retinal detachment or as a diffusely spreading lesion. Retinoblastomas may be unilateral, bilateral, or multifocal. The diagnosis is usually made between 1 and 2 years of age. Other causes of leukocoria may include retinopathy of prematurity, congenital cataracts, toxocarisis (a nematode infection), or Coats disease (a retinal vascular abnormality). The treatment of retinoblastoma may involve surgery, chemotherapy, or other modalities such as cryotherapy and photocoagulation. *(Kunimoto et al., 2004, Sect. 8.1)*

100. **(D)** The child has ingested a button battery which has lodged in the esophagus. This constitutes a medical emergency and immediate emergency endoscopy is warranted. Button batteries can cause severe esophageal injury and tissue necrosis via electrical current discharge as well as burns from alkali chemicals contained within the battery itself. Severe burns and perforation can occur within hours. Admission for observation is inadequate, and vomiting should not be induced as this could promote aspiration of the battery or gastric contents. Emergency surgery should be reserved for patients in whom endoscopy fails. The patient cannot be discharged with a button battery in the esophagus. *(Hay et al.,2003, p. 349)*

101. **(D)** The PTT represents the time for clot formation after adding calcium, phospholipids, and kaolin to citrated blood. It is prolonged by heparin, direct thrombin inhibitors, a deficiency or inhibitor for factors in the intrinsic and common pathway (i.e., factors II, V, VIII, IX, X, XI, XII) as well as lupus anticoagulant, vitamin K deficiency, or severe liver disease.

The PT represents the time for clot formation after the addition of thromboplastin (tissue factor) and calcium to citrated blood. It is prolonged with deficiencies of the extrinsic and common pathway factors II, V, VII, X, or fibrinogen; liver disease; vitamin K deficiency and Warfarin use. *(Kottke-Marchant, 1994, pp. 809–853; Sallah and Kato, 1998, pp. 209–210)*

102. **(D)** While all of the screenings listed may be appropriate for children with varying symptoms, only a full physical examination is recommended by the American Academy of Pediatrics for ALL well-child visits. *(Pediatrics 2000;105(3):645–646)*

BIBLIOGRAPHY

American Academy of Pediatrics. *The Red Book, 2003 Report of the Committee on Infectious Diseases*, 26th ed. Elk Grove Village, IL: American Academy of Pediatrics, 2003.

American Academy of Pediatrics: Committee on Practice and Ambulatory Medicine. Recommendations for Preventive Pediatric Health Care. *Pediatrics.* Mar 2000; 105:645-646.

Behrman RE, Kliegman RM, Jensen HD. *Nelson Textbook of Pediatrics*, 17th ed. Philadelphia, PA: W.B. Saunders, 2004.

Centers for Disease Control and Prevention. Sexually transmitted diseases treatment guidelines 2002. *MMWR* 2002;51(RR-6):32–34.

Department of Health and Human Services. *Child Maltreatment.* Washington, DC: Administration on Children, Youth, and Families, 2002.

Fenichel GM. *Clinical Pediatric Neurology*, 3rd ed. Philadelphia, PA: W.B. Saunders, 1997.

Fitzpatrick TB, Johnson RA, Wolff K, et al. *Color Atlas and Synopsis of Clinical Dermatology*, 4th ed. New York, NY: McGraw-Hill, 2001

Fleisher GR, Ludwig S, eds. *Textbook of Pediatric Emergency Medicine*, 4th ed. Baltimore, MD: Lippincott Williams & Wilkins, 2000.

Hay WW, Hayward AR, Levin MJ, Sondheimer JM. *Current Pediatric Diagnosis and Treatment,* 16th ed. New York, NY: McGraw-Hill, 2003.

Hoffman R, Benz EJ, Shattil SJ, et al. *Hematology: Basic Principles and Practice*, 3rd ed. Philadelphia, PA: Churchill Livingstone, 2000.

Jones KL, ed. *Smith's Recognizable Pattern of Human Malformations*, 5th ed. Philadelphia, PA: W.B. Saunders, 1997.

Kottke-Marchant K. Laboratory diagnosis of hemorrhagic and thrombotic disorders. *Hematol Oncol Clin North Am* 1994;8:809–853.

Kunimoto DY, Rapuano CJ, Friedberg MA, et al. *The Wills Eye Manual: Office and Emergency Room Diagnosis and Treatment of Eye Disease*, 4th ed. Philadelphia, PA: Lippincott Williams & Wilkins, 2004.

McMillin JA, Feigin RD, Warshaw JB, et al. *Oski's Pediatrics: Principles and Practice*, 3rd ed. Philadelphia, PA: Lippincott Williams & Wilkins, 1999.

Rudolph CD, Rudolph AM, Hostetter MK, et al., eds. *Rudolph's Pediatrics*, 21st ed. New York, NY: McGraw-Hill, 2003.

Sallah S, Kato G. Evaluation of bleeding disorders. A detailed history and laboratory tests provide clues. *Postgrad Med* 1998;103:209–210.

Zenel JA. Failure to thrive: a general pediatrician's perspective. *Pediatr Rev* 1997;18:371–378.

CHAPTER 4

Obstetrics and Gynecology
Questions

1. A 23-year-old female presents to the emergency department (ED) with "abdominal cramping," nausea, and vaginal bleeding. A human chorionic gonadotropin (hCG) level returns 5150 mIU/mL. A vaginal probe ultrasound is performed and notes no evidence of an intrauterine pregnancy, normal appearing ovaries, a mild amount of fluid in the cul-de-sac, and no evidence of ectopic gestation. The ED physician can exclude which diagnosis from the differential?

   (A) spontaneous abortion
   (B) ectopic pregnancy
   (C) singleton intrauterine pregnancy
   (D) ruptured ovarian cyst (corpus luteum)
   (E) molar pregnancy

2. Following tubal ligation what percentage of pregnancies are ectopic?

   (A) 1%
   (B) 5%
   (C) 30%
   (D) 50%
   (E) 75%

3. A 31-year-old female presents to her physician complaining of rapid onset of hirsutism, deepening of the voice, irregular menses, clitoral enlargement, and acne. Which of the following is the most likely cause of this clinical presentation?

   (A) polycystic ovary syndrome (PCOS)
   (B) Cushing syndrome
   (C) type II diabetes mellitus
   (D) androgen secreting tumor
   (E) congenital adrenal hyperplasia

4. A 23-year-old female presents to her obstetrician/gynecologist (OB/GYN) complaining of inability to conceive. She has regular menstrual cycles, and her husband's semen analysis is normal. She undergoes a hysterosalpingogram that shows evidence of bilateral distal tubal obstruction. Which of the following is the most likely cause of acquired tubal damage?

   (A) appendicitis
   (B) pelvic inflammatory disease (PID)
   (C) salpingitis isthmica nodosa (SIN)
   (D) Asherman's syndrome
   (E) ruptured ovarian cyst

5. A 17-year-old female presents with delayed puberty. Her mother reports her daughter has never menstruated. On examination, the patient is 59 in. (4 ft 11 in.) tall and is shown in Figure 4-1. Which of the following tests is most likely to confirm the diagnosis?

FIG. 4-1 (*Courtesy of Kathy Hullfish, MD.*)

(A) karyotype
(B) follicle-stimulating hormone (FSH)
(C) luteinizing hormone (LH)
(D) cranial magnetic resonance imaging (MRI)
(E) growth hormone (GH)

6. In order to prevent unintended pregnancy following an episode of unprotected intercourse, by when is it recommended that "emergency" oral contraception should be initiated?

(A) 12 hours
(B) 24 hours
(C) 48 hours
(D) 72 hours
(E) 1 week

7. A 61-year-old female is diagnosed with osteoporosis by a screening dual-energy x-ray absorptiometry (DEXA) scan. Which of these is a risk factor for postmenopausal osteoporosis?

(A) black race
(B) lack of exercise
(C) obesity
(D) multiparity
(E) late menopause

8. A 5-year-old girl presents for evaluation of breast development, history of multiple bone fractures, and vaginal bleeding. Physical examination is notable for "café au lait" spots on her skin, tanner stage 2 breasts, and she appears tall for her age. What is the most likely cause of precocious puberty in this child?

(A) acromegaly
(B) McCune-Albright syndrome
(C) ovarian cyst
(D) ingestion of her mother's oral contraceptives
(E) hyperparathyroidism

9. A 39-year-old obese female presents with irregular menstrual periods, mild acne and hirsutism, and acanthosis nigricans on the nuchal fold, axilla, and intertriginous areas (inner upper thighs). You suspect PCOS. Which of the following laboratory tests would be most important to perform to rule out a likely confounding diagnosis?

(A) 2-hour oral glucose tolerance test
(B) testosterone
(C) prolactin
(D) dehydroepiandrosterone sulfate (DHEAS)
(E) LH and FSH

10. A 17-year-old female presents with primary amenorrhea. On physical examination, she has normal secondary sexual characteristics, scant pubic and axillary hair, and a blind ending vaginal pouch. A pelvic MRI indicates inguinal gonads and no uterus. Her karyotype is 46,XY. Which of the following is the most likely etiology of primary amenorrhea in this patient?

(A) Müllerian agenesis (Mayer-Rokitansky-Küster-Hauser syndrome)

(B) Klinefelter syndrome

(C) androgen insensitivity

(D) Turner mosaic

(E) Kallmann syndrome

11. A 15-year-old female presents to the emergency room (ER) with acute onset right lower quadrant pain and nausea. She recently became sexually active and is "in the middle" of her menstrual cycle. Physical examination is notable for generalized guarding, rebound, and 8/10 pain in both lower quadrants. A pelvic examination shows no vaginal discharge, a normal appearing cervix, and general pelvic tenderness, but the examination is limited by the patient's guarding. Her complete blood count is notable for a borderline elevated white blood cell (WBC) count, and a urinary β-hCG is negative. Pelvic ultrasound shows a 2-cm simple appearing cyst on the right ovary and a mild amount of fluid in the cul-de-sac. A computed tomographic (CT) scan cannot definitively visualize the appendix, confirms the presence of a 2-cm cystic structure in the right ovary, and otherwise notes normal anatomy. Which of the following is the most appropriate next step?

(A) diagnostic laparoscopy

(B) pelvic MRI

(C) intravenous antibiotics

(D) admission for serial physical examinations and pain control

(E) discharge home on oral antibiotics

12. An amenorrheic 17-year-old female is diagnosed with Kallmann syndrome. Blood testing of this patient would indicate which of the following results?

(A) FSH, LH, normal estradiol

(B) high FSH, high LH, low estradiol

(C) normal FSH, normal LH, normal estradiol

(D) low FSH, low LH, normal estradiol

(E) low FSH, low LH, low estradiol

13. A woman complains of amenorrhea for several months following a dilation and curettage. Which of the following is the most likely reason?

(A) occult perforation of uterus during the procedure

(B) intrauterine scarring

(C) infection of the endometrium (endometritis)

(D) iron-deficiency anemia from blood loss during the procedure

(E) premature menopause

14. Implantation of the embryo into the endometrium occurs how many days after ovulation?

(A) 1

(B) 2

(C) 4

(D) 6

(E) 10

Questions 15 and 16

A 24-year-old G₁ presents to you for initiation of obstetric care. She informs you that she is on a medication that was prescribed for acne. The drug is listed as category X in your pharmacy book.

15. The pregnancy risk factor category X for a drug indicates which of the following?

(A) Controlled human studies demonstrate no risk to a fetus.

(B) This drug should never be used by a pregnant female under any circumstances.

(C) Evidence of human teratogenic risk exists but in some cases the known risks may be outweighed in some serious situations, such as life-threatening disease.

(D) Animal reproduction studies have not demonstrated fetal risk but there are no controlled human studies to assess the risk.

(E) Animal reproduction studies have demonstrated risk to a fetus and no controlled human studies are available.

16. The patient reports that she is going to continue the medication because she would be too embarrassed to go to work if her acne were to return. You counsel the patient about the possible risks of this approach but she desires to proceed. You counsel the patient that her best option may be to terminate the pregnancy and continue the medication. Allowing her to make this decision is an example of which of the following?

    (A) beneficence
    (B) autonomy
    (C) breach of confidentiality
    (D) malfeasance
    (E) justice

17. A 26-year-old female with recurrent pregnancy loss undergoes a laparoscopy and hysteroscopy. She is found to have a Müllerian anomaly with a heart-shaped uterus that has two uterine horns but one common cervix. What is the name of the uterine anomaly?

    (A) didelphic
    (B) septate
    (C) unicornuate
    (D) bicornuate
    (E) Müllerian agenesis (Mayer-Rokitansky-Küster-Hauser syndrome)

18. A patient with a persistent headache following a postpartum hemorrhage is diagnosed with Sheehan's syndrome. If the patient were subsequently amenorrheic and infertile, what treatment would you recommend to assist this patient to conceive?

    (A) gonadotropin releasing hormone (GnRH) pump
    (B) clomiphene citrate
    (C) dopamine agonist
    (D) in vitro fertilization
    (E) gonadotropins (FSH and LH)

19. A 44-year-old female has a history of endometriosis resulting in chronic pelvic pain. She presents to you 6 months after her total abdominal hysterectomy and bilateral salpingo-oophorectomy. She reports continued pelvic pain. Which of the following would be your

most appropriate recommendation for medical management?

    (A) GnRH
    (B) oral estrogens
    (C) oral progestins
    (D) tamoxifen
    (E) GnRH antagonist

20. The predicted length of the follicular phase of a patient with a consistent 34-day menstrual cycle is which of the following?

    (A) 14 days
    (B) depends on the length of the luteal phase
    (C) 16 days
    (D) 18 days
    (E) 20 days

21. Which of the following can induce menstrual bleeding in a 21-year-old anovulatory, amenorrheic woman with PCOS?

    (A) administration of progestins
    (B) administration of estrogens
    (C) withdrawal of progestin therapy
    (D) withdrawal of estrogen therapy
    (E) danazol

22. A 63-year-old woman with a grade 2 endometrioid adenocarcinoma of the uterus diagnosed by endometrial biopsy is taken to the operating room for surgical treatment with a total abdominal hysterectomy, bilateral salpingo-oophorectomy, and pelvic and paraaortic lymphadenectomy. No complications are noted intraoperatively. On postoperative day 1, the patient complains of numbness in her medial thigh. Your neurologic examination suggests absence of cutaneous sensation to the medial thigh and an inability to adduct her hip. Which of the following is the most likely etiology for this clinical presentation?

    (A) femoral nerve injury
    (B) genitofemoral nerve injury
    (C) pudendal nerve injury
    (D) obturator nerve injury
    (E) peroneal nerve injury

23. A 41-year-old woman, recently diagnosed with a 2-cm, stage IB1 cervical cancer, undergoes a radical hysterectomy, bilateral salpingo-oophorectomy, and retroperitoneal pelvic lymph node dissection. Her surgery and post-operative course are uncomplicated. Four weeks postoperatively, she presents to the ER complaining of left leg swelling and left lower quadrant abdominal pain. On physical examination, she is afebrile, has a normal WBC count, and you palpate a 5 × 4 cm mass in the left lower quadrant. You order a pelvic ultrasound that shows a 5 × 5 cm simple cyst in the left lower quadrant. Which of the following is the most likely diagnosis?

(A) deep venous thrombosis (DVT)
(B) pelvic abscess
(C) lymphocyst
(D) ovarian cyst
(E) diverticular abscess

Questions 24 and 25

A 38-year-old woman presents to the ER with heavy vaginal bleeding. A pelvic examination using a speculum to visualize the cervix reveals a large, friable, fungating cervical mass. On bimanual examination, the mass extends to the right pelvic sidewall. A biopsy from a recent gynecologic visit reveals invasive squamous cell carcinoma of the cervix. An abdominal/pelvic CT scan shows enlarged pelvic lymph nodes and right hydronephrosis. Her hematocrit (HCT) in the ER is 24%, but she is hemodynamically stable with a BP of 124/70 and a pulse of 73. The cervical mass is actively bleeding.

24. Which of the following is the most appropriate immediate management of the vaginal bleeding in the ER?

(A) vaginal packing soaked with Monsel solution
(B) vitamin K
(C) transfusion of fresh frozen plasma (FFP)
(D) uterine massage
(E) supportive care with transfusion of packed red blood cells

25. Your initial treatment of the vaginal bleeding in the ER only partially controls the bleeding, and she is requiring frequent retreatment. The best definitive treatment to control the bleeding at this time is which of the following?

(A) emergency bilateral hypogastric artery ligation
(B) uterine artery embolization
(C) emergency high-dose radiation therapy
(D) emergency radical hysterectomy
(E) loop excision electrocautery procedure (LEEP)

Questions 26 and 27

26. A 42-year-old woman who previously underwent a vaginal hysterectomy for persistent cervical dysplasia presents to your office for vaginal cytology. Her vaginal cytology is shown in Figure 4-2. Which of the following is the most appropriate next step in management?

FIG. 4-2 (*Courtesy of Kathy Hullfish, MD.*) (Also see color insert.)

(A) repeat vaginal cytology in 6 months
(B) observation
(C) random vaginal biopsies
(D) intravaginal estrogen cream followed by repeat cytology
(E) colposcopic examination of the vaginal canal

27. On speculum examination, you visualize a 1×1 cm lesion at the left vaginal fornix. The lesion is acetowhite, slightly raised, with coarse punctation and bizarre branching vessels. You take a biopsy of the lesion and the pathology returns consistent with vaginal intraepithelial neoplasia (VAIN) 3, suspicious for invasion. Which of the following is your next step in management?

(A) carbon dioxide (CO_2) laser
(B) wide local excision of the lesion
(C) intravaginal 5-flourouracil (5-FU)
(D) intravaginal estrogen cream
(E) total vaginectomy

28. A 61-year-old postmenopausal woman, who has been on continuous combined hormone replacement therapy for 5 years, presents to your office complaining of vaginal bleeding. Which of the following is the most appropriate next step in her management?

(A) pap smear
(B) endocervical curettage (ECC)
(C) pelvic ultrasound
(D) endometrial biopsy
(E) dilation and curettage

29. You are consulted by a 55-year-old asymptomatic postmenopausal woman who has been on tamoxifen for 2 years following a diagnosis of breast cancer. She has no other risk factors for endometrial cancer but she was searching the Internet and found information about the risks of tamoxifen therapy. She inquires about endometrial cancer screening. You tell her that for asymptomatic woman on tamoxifen, the screening recommendations for endometrial cancer are which of the following?

(A) yearly pelvic ultrasounds
(B) yearly endometrial biopsies
(C) yearly gynecologic examinations
(D) yearly pelvic CT scans
(E) yearly hysteroscopy

30. In your internal medicine clinic you are caring for a 42-year-old woman with hereditary nonpolyposis colon cancer (HNPCC), Lynch syndrome II, which is a hereditary, autosomal dominant, cancer syndrome that results from a mutation in a mismatch deoxyribonucleic acid (DNA) repair gene. These patients have a lifetime risk of colon cancer nearly 60–80%, but are also at risk for several other malignancies. For which gynecologic malignancy is this woman most at risk?

(A) ovarian cancer
(B) breast cancer
(C) cervical cancer
(D) vulvar cancer
(E) endometrial cancer

31. A 37-year-old woman (gravida 3, para 3) presents with a 4-month history of postcoital spotting. On pelvic examination, you visualize a 2-cm friable lesion on the anterior lip of the cervix. The next most appropriate step is which of the following?

(A) colposcopy
(B) pap smear
(C) office biopsy of the cervical lesion
(D) cervical cone biopsy
(E) metronidazole vaginal cream followed by re-examination

Questions 32 through 34

32. A 22-year-old nulliparous woman who desires future fertility is found to have a pap smear consistent with high-grade squamous intraepithelial lesion (HGSIL). Initial management should be which of the following?

(A) routine pap smear in 1 year
(B) random cervical biopsies
(C) colposcopy
(D) endometrial biopsy
(E) human papilloma virus (HPV) testing

33. The test you performed above was inadequate. What would be your next step in management?

    (A) transvaginal ultrasound (TVUS)
    (B) endometrial dilation and curettage
    (C) ECC
    (D) cold knife cervical conization
    (E) repeat pap smear in 3 months

34. The final pathology report indicates a single focus of squamous carcinoma invasive into the cervical stroma to a depth of 2.0 mm. An ECC is negative. There is no lymphvascular space invasion, and the cone margins are negative. The most appropriate therapy for this patient is which of the following?

    (A) radiation therapy
    (B) simple hysterectomy with pelvic lymphadenectomy
    (C) radical hysterectomy with pelvic lymphadenectomy
    (D) radical trachelectomy
    (E) observation with close follow-up

35. A 39-year-old woman with a long-standing history of normal pap smears undergoes a total abdominal hysterectomy for a large uterine fibroid and menorrhagia. Six months after her hysterectomy she had a negative vaginal pap smear from the vaginal apex. She presents to your clinic today for a routine physical examination. Based on the American College of Obstetricians and Gynecologists recommendations, when should this patient have pap smears?

    (A) yearly
    (B) every 3 years
    (C) every 5 years
    (D) never again
    (E) only if she develops risk factors

36. A 56-year-old thin, White woman, who has recently undergone a total abdominal hysterectomy, bilateral salpingo-oophorectomy, and pelvic lymphadenectomy for a stage IB,

grade 1, endometrioid tumor of the uterus, presents to your office complaining of hot flashes and vaginal dryness. She wants advice about the use of estrogen replacement in women treated for endometrial cancer. Which of the following is the best treatment for this woman?

    (A) psychotherapy
    (B) estrogen replacement therapy
    (C) increased soy intake
    (D) combination hormone replacement therapy
    (E) referral to an endometrial cancer support group

Questions 37 and 38

A 43-year-old Black female (gravida 3, para 3) with a previous tubal ligation, presents to your office complaining of increasing menorrhagia, dysmenorrhea, and fatigue over the past 6 months. On examination, her vital signs are normal, and on abdominal examination you palpate a firm, mobile mass just below the umbilicus. On pelvic examination, there is a moderate amount of old blood coming from the cervical os. A urine pregnancy test is negative, her last pap smear was normal and her spun HCT today is 28%.

37. Which diagnostic test would be most cost-effective in confirming a diagnosis?

    (A) pelvic MRI
    (B) abdominal plain films
    (C) pelvic ultrasound
    (D) hysterosalpingogram
    (E) office laparoscopy

38. Which pharmacologic agent would potentially result in an improvement in her HCT and help to decrease uterine size?

    (A) oral contraceptive pills (OCPs)
    (B) medroxyprogesterone
    (C) nonsteroidal anti-inflammatory agents
    (D) narcotics
    (E) GnRH agonists

Questions 39 and 40

A 76-year-old White female (gravida 8, para 8) presents to her family practitioner complaining of vaginal pressure, dyspareunia, urinary incontinence, and difficulty emptying her bladder for the past 4 weeks. Seven years ago she had a prolapsed "bladder tacking" procedure. Her postvoid residual urine in the office measures 250 mL. The most notable finding on pelvic examination is seen in Figure 4-3.

FIG. 4-3 (*Courtesy of Kathy Hullfish, MD.*) (Also see color insert.)

39. What is the most likely etiology of her urinary retention?

(A) detrusor overactivity
(B) bladder outlet obstruction
(C) urinary tract infection (UTI)
(D) menopause
(E) spinal cord tumor

40. Which of the following would be the most appropriate action to take at this time?

(A) referral for immediate surgery
(B) abdominal and pelvic CT scan
(C) urinalysis (UA) with culture and sensitivity
(D) prescription for oxybutynin (Ditropan)
(E) urodynamic studies

Questions 41 and 42

A 14-year-old nulligravid female is brought to the ER by her parents with a 12-hour history of severe, intermittent left lower quadrant pain. She has had nausea and vomiting for the past 2 hours. On history, the patient experienced menarche at age 12 and denies past or current contact with a sexual partner. Her last normal menstrual period was 3 weeks ago. On examination, she is afebrile, pulse 100, BP 110/70, respiratory rate (RR) 20. She is visibly uncomfortable. She has no costovertebral tenderness, has diminished bowel sounds, her abdomen is nondistended, and exhibits rebound and guarding in both lower quadrants. She is unable to tolerate a pelvic examination due to pain. Laboratory values are as follows: WBC 13, HCT 39, β-hCG (–), UA (–). A pelvic ultrasound shows a normal nonpregnant uterus, normal right adnexa, and an 8-cm left adnexal mass with a 3-cm solid component.

41. Which of the following would be the next appropriate step in managing this patient?

(A) abdominal and pelvic CT scan
(B) social work referral for possible sexual abuse
(C) obtain liver enzymes, amylase, and lipase
(D) consultation for immediate surgical intervention
(E) discharge to home with pain medications

42. The most likely etiology of this patient's pain is which of the following?

(A) ectopic pregnancy
(B) acute appendicitis
(C) ovarian torsion
(D) pancreatitis
(E) somatization disorder

Questions 43 and 44

A 22-year-old White female (gravida 2, para 1, abortus 1) comes to your office with a 3-week history of lower abdominal pain and increased vaginal discharge. She has a prior history of an ectopic pregnancy at age 16. Her last menstrual period (LMP) was 7 days ago, and she has had unprotected vaginal intercourse with a new sexual partner several times over the past few weeks. Her temperature is 38.0°C; her vital signs are stable. She has bilateral lower quadrant tenderness but no peritoneal signs. On speculum examination, she has foul smelling green discharge emanating from her cervix. She has cervical motion tenderness on bimanual examination and is tender in both adnexae. Her wet mount shows copious white cells. Her urine β-hCG is (–).

43. Which of the following would be the most appropriate treatment regimen for this patient?

   (A) metronidazole PO for 5 days
   (B) gentamicin IV × one dose
   (C) ceftriaxone intramuscular (IM) plus doxycycline PO for 14 days
   (D) Diflucan PO × one dose
   (E) ampicillin PO qid × 14 days

44. Most cases of PID are associated with which of the following?

   (A) gonorrhea alone
   (B) chlamydia alone
   (C) *Candida albicans*
   (D) herpes simplex virus
   (E) polymicrobial aerobic and anaerobic bacteria from the lower genital tract

45. A 43-year-old morbidly obese woman presents to your office with a 3-week history of increasing vulvar burning. She has had no new sexual partners or practices. She has not noticed any change in her vaginal discharge. She has attempted to medicate herself with over-the-counter antifungals, herbal creams, and old antibiotics, none of which have provided relief. On examination, her entire labia majora and minora are markedly erythematous and tender to the touch. Her vaginal mucosa appears to have normal rugae. Her vaginal pH is normal and whiff test is negative. The wet mount shows a few WBCs and normal squamous cells. What is the most likely diagnosis?

   (A) chemical dermatitis
   (B) bacterial vaginosis

   (C) PID disease
   (D) atrophic vaginitis
   (E) lichens sclerosis et atrophicus

46. A concerned mother brings her 5-year-old daughter to the ER because she noticed redness around her daughter's genital region while bathing her last night. The child has not complained of any discomfort, itching, bleeding, or inappropriate contact with other adults. On external inspection of her labia, you see the fusion of the labia minora and generalized erythema. The most appropriate treatment would be which of the following?

   (A) surgical excision
   (B) vaginoscopy and biopsies
   (C) ice packs and sitz baths
   (D) lidocaine ointment
   (E) topical estrogen cream

Questions 47 through 49

A 70-year-old White woman has been faithful about taking 1200 mg of calcium, 400 IU of vitamin D supplements, and performing weight-bearing exercise on a daily basis. Her hip T score from her current DEXA scan has changed from –2.0 SDs to –2.55 SDs compared with last year's test.

47. At this time, which of the following do you recommend?

   (A) an oral bisphosphonate
   (B) weekly GnRH injections
   (C) discontinuation of her vitamin D
   (D) glucocorticoid therapy
   (E) IM testosterone

48. Which of the following statements is correct?

   (A) With osteoporosis, serum calcium is low.
   (B) With hyperparathyroidism, serum calcium is normal.
   (C) With Paget disease, serum calcium is low.
   (D) With renal failure, serum calcium is low.
   (E) With osteomalacia, serum calcium is high.

49. Which of the following is associated with a reduced risk of osteoporotic fractures?

    (A) family history of hip fractures
    (B) estrogen deficiency
    (C) body mass index of greater than 23
    (D) tobacco use
    (E) vision problems

50. A 25-year-old nulligravid female, whose LMP was 4 weeks ago, is seen by her OB/GYN for a left breast mass. The patient discovered it 2 weeks ago while in the shower. Her maternal aunt died of breast cancer at age 60, and the patient is very worried about this new finding. On examination, a mobile, nonerythematous, 3-cm nonsolid feeling mass is palpated in the left upper outer quadrant of her left breast. There is no nipple discharge, and the axillary lymph nodes are nonpalpable. Her right breast examination is normal. The patient wants you to schedule a mammogram that same day. Your response is which of the following?

    (A) A surgical biopsy should be performed instead.
    (B) A needle core biopsy can be done at the same time of her mammogram.
    (C) Ultrasound would be a better imaging modality for her situation.
    (D) In-office cyst aspiration is reassuring if the fluid is bloody.
    (E) Antibiotics can treat her mastitis.

51. A 63-year-old Black female presents to your office complaining of leaking urine. She gets up at night five times to urinate and occasionally loses urine en route to the toilet. During the daytime, she urinates every 45 minutes "to help prevent the leakage." She denies loss of urine with coughing or sneezing. She has not had dysuria or any other pelvic floor complaints. She has a family history of diabetes. She drinks several caffeinated beverages throughout the day. On examination, her postvoid residual urine is normal, and a urine dipstick shows 3+ glucose but is otherwise negative. Her abdominal and pelvic examinations are normal. Which of the following do you recommend?

    (A) surgery for her incontinence
    (B) antibiotics for a UTI
    (C) diuretic therapy
    (D) timed voids, decrease in caffeine intake, and screening for diabetes
    (E) referral to a urologist for cystoscopy

52. A 31-year-old (gravida 1, para 1) female had a forceps-assisted vaginal delivery 3 months ago. Her infant weighed 4250 g. During the delivery she sustained a fourth degree perineal injury that was repaired. She now complains of fecal incontinence and foul vaginal discharge when her stools are loose, which happens several days a week. The most likely etiology for her fecal incontinence and foul vaginal discharge would be which of the following?

    (A) Crohn's disease
    (B) a perianal abscess
    (C) a vaginal hematoma
    (D) a retained vaginal foreign body
    (E) a rectovaginal fistula

Questions 53 through 55

You are asked to perform a high school physical examination for a 16-year-old female patient. She is on the track team. By history, she is healthy except for the fact that she has been amenorrheic for 4 months. She denies current or past sexual activity. On examination, she is 5 ft 9 in. tall and weighs 115 lbs. Her heart rate is 50 bpm. She has dry skin with lanugo. She has several sores in her mouth and obvious dental caries. She has several scratches on the backs of her hands. She is tanner stage III on breast examination. Her pelvic examination is remarkable for findings of urogenital atrophy. Her urine β-hCG is negative.

53. Which of the following would be the most likely diagnosis for this patient?

    (A) domestic abuse
    (B) eating disorder
    (C) hyperthyroidism
    (D) herpes simplex virus serotype I
    (E) congenital adrenal hyperplasia

54. At this point in time, appropriate management of this patient would include which of the following?

    (A) laboratory assessment of electrolytes and an electrocardiogram
    (B) intensive care unit (ICU) admission
    (C) antipsychotic medication
    (D) reassurance
    (E) IM Depo-Provera injection

55. This patient is at risk for developing which of the following?

    (A) schizophrenia
    (B) renal failure
    (C) morbid obesity
    (D) osteoporosis
    (E) cholecystitis

Questions 56 and 57

A 22-year-old female (G_3P_{0020}) presents to your office for an initial obstetric visit in her third pregnancy. She reports a sure LMP date approximately 6 weeks ago, with a history of regular cycles. Her two previous pregnancies ended in spontaneous abortions. She denies any significant medical or surgical history. She denies use of alcohol, tobacco, or illicit drugs, though she does report a history of IV drug use as a teenager. She is a full-time student. She reports that twins run in her family, but she does not have any family history of diabetes, hypertension, or congenital anomalies. On review of her prenatal labs that have already been drawn, you find that her human immunodeficiency virus (HIV) antibody test (enzyme-linked immunosorbent assay [ELISA]) is positive. Her test results are otherwise normal.

56. Which of the following indicates how you counsel the patient?

    (A) This result is a false positive due to pregnancy, and she does not need any further testing.
    (B) She is infected with HIV and will need to begin treatment right away.

    (C) She will require an additional, confirmatory test to determine whether or not she has HIV.
    (D) She may have HIV, but she should wait until after she delivers her baby to have further testing.
    (E) Because it has been years since she participated in high-risk behaviors, she is unlikely to have HIV.

57. Which of the following is recommended to reduce the risk of perinatal transmission of HIV from mother to infant?

    (A) A scheduled cesarean delivery can reduce the risk of transmission if the maternal viral load is greater than 1000 copies/mL.
    (B) All pregnant women with HIV should receive highly active antiretroviral therapy regardless of severity of HIV infection.
    (C) No treatment is required; the risk of perinatal transmission of HIV is quite low.
    (D) All patients with HIV should be required to have a cesarean delivery.
    (E) Treatment of opportunistic infections such as *Pneumocystis carinii* pneumonia in the mother is most important in reducing the perinatal transmission of HIV.

58. A 34-year-old Black (G$_1$) female presents to your clinic for an obstetric visit at 16 weeks estimated gestational age (EGA). She has a sure LMP and her estimated date of delivery (EDD) is in December. She is generally healthy and has not had any surgeries. She denies history of sexually transmitted diseases or abnormal pap smears. She has no significant family history. She does not smoke or use alcohol or illicit drugs. She works as an administrative assistant.

Her prenatal labs are as follows: blood type O+, antibody screen negative; hepatitis B surface antigen negative; HIV antibody negative; Rubella nonimmune; rapid plasma regain (RPR) nonreactive; pap smear within normal limits; urine culture negative.

Based on her laboratory results and history, you recommend that she receive which of the following injections during her pregnancy?

(A) measles, mumps, and rubella (MMR) vaccine
(B) influenza vaccine
(C) hepatitis B vaccine series
(D) RhoGAM injection
(E) poliomyelitis vaccine

Questions 59 and 60

A 19-year-old (G$_2$P$_{1001}$) female at 35^4/$_7$ weeks EGA presents for a routine prenatal visit. Her pregnancy has been uncomplicated. She reports good fetal movement and denies vaginal bleeding, loss of fluid, or contractions. She is excited about the arrival of her baby and is planning to breast-feed. Her past medical history is significant for chlamydia that was treated approximately 1 year ago. She is otherwise healthy. Her blood pressure today is 110/60. Fundal height is appropriate. UA is negative.

59. The patient would like to discuss options for postpartum birth control. Which of the following would be an appropriate and effective option for postpartum birth control for this patient?

(A) combined OCP
(B) intrauterine device (IUD)
(C) progesterone-only pill

(D) no birth control is necessary as the patient will be breast-feeding
(E) rhythm method

60. The patient wants to know what complications she might experience from breast-feeding. You tell her that the most common complication of breast-feeding is mastitis. If she were to develop mastitis, which of the following treatments would be recommended?

(A) dicloxacillin by mouth plus discontinuation of breast-feeding
(B) discontinuation of breast-feeding only
(C) Flagyl by mouth plus discontinuation of breast-feeding
(D) dicloxacillin by mouth with continued breast-feeding
(E) no treatment is required for mastitis

Questions 61 through 63

A 30-year-old (G$_2$P$_{0101}$) female presents to the clinic for a new obstetric visit. She has an unknown LMP. She reports that she discovered she was pregnant when she took a urine pregnancy test at home a month ago. She vaguely recalls having a period about 2 months ago, but is not sure exactly when that occurred. She reports that she is generally healthy. She had a previous delivery at 36 weeks EGA, though she reports her doctor was not really sure about her due date in that pregnancy. She reports that she had a normal spontaneous vaginal delivery in her previous pregnancy, and the child is healthy. Her postpartum course was complicated by depression, which has since resolved and not recurred. She denies history of sexually transmitted diseases or abnormal pap smears. She has no surgical history. She does not smoke, drink alcohol, or use illicit drugs. She does not have any family history of hypertension, diabetes, twins, or congenital anomalies. She does report that her mother has a history of depression.

61. Which of the following tests will provide the most useful information to determine this patient's EDD?

(A) pelvic examination
(B) serum FSH and LH

(C) serum quantitative β-hCG level

(D) measurement of fundal height

(E) pelvic ultrasound

62. Given the patient's history of postpartum depression as well as her family history of depression, her risk of postpartum depression after this pregnancy is approximately what percentage?

(A) 50% or greater

(B) 5%

(C) 10%

(D) 20%

(E) less than 1%

63. Postpartum psychosis is a serious disorder that can occur in the early postpartum period. Patients with which of the following medical conditions are at increased risk of postpartum psychosis?

(A) multiparity

(B) anxiety disorder

(C) thyroid disease

(D) bipolar disorder

(E) advanced maternal age

Questions 64 and 65

A 24-year-old White (G_1P_{1001}) female presents to your office 6 weeks after a normal spontaneous vaginal delivery at term. She reports that she has been unable to breast-feed her baby despite help from her pediatrician and a lactation consultant. On further questioning, you elicit that she has also experienced nausea, weakness, and weight loss. In addition, she reports dizziness when getting out of bed in the morning. On your examination, she has a waxy texture to her skin and periorbital edema. You also note decreased axillary and pubic hair, which she reports is a change for her.

64. She most likely has which of the following diagnoses?

(A) postpartum depression

(B) normal postpartum changes

(C) Sheehan syndrome

(D) PCOS

(E) medication reaction

65. This condition is most commonly associated with which of the following?

(A) obesity and increased facial hair

(B) postpartum hemorrhage

(C) acute thrombosis

(D) no specific association is known, this condition is idiopathic

(E) serotonin imbalance

Questions 66 through 68

A 28-year-old White G_1 woman presents to your office for an initial obstetric visit. Her LMP is certain and allows you to estimate a 9-week gestational age today. She denies bleeding, cramping, or other symptoms of concern. She is excited about being pregnant. She has already started taking her prenatal vitamins with folic acid. She reports no significant past medical history. In fact, she states that she has not been to a doctor in many years because she has not had any problems. She has had no surgeries. She does not smoke. She drank alcohol socially prior to pregnancy but has not consumed any alcohol since she became pregnant. She has family history of hypertension, but no other significant history is elicited.

On physical examination, her blood pressure is 110/60. She is healthy appearing, and there are no significant findings on examination. Your pelvic examination confirms uterine size consistent with stated dates. As part of a routine laboratory evaluation, you decide to check a thyroid-stimulating hormone (TSH). The TSH is 0.4 μIU/mL (normal range 0.5–5.5) and a free T4 of 1.8 ng/dL (normal range 0.7–2.0).

66. You counsel the patient that she most likely has which of the following?

(A) hypothyroidism

(B) hyperthyroidism

(C) normal thyroid function, with laboratory values altered by hormone interactions associated with pregnancy

(D) a drug reaction altering thyroid function

(E) a thyroid nodule

The patient returns to the clinic for routine prenatal visits. At approximately 28 weeks' gestational age, you decide to recheck her thyroid levels. At this visit, her TSH is 0.1 µIU/mL, her total T4 is 15 ng/dL (normal range 4.5–12.5), and her free T4 is 2.4 ng/dL.

67. What is the most likely cause of this patient's hyperthyroidism?

    (A) toxic adenoma
    (B) multinodular goiter
    (C) hyperemesis gravidarum
    (D) lymphocytic thyroiditis
    (E) Grave's disease

68. What is the most appropriate management of this condition?

    (A) thyroid ablation with radioactive iodine
    (B) prescription for propylthiouracil (PTU)
    (C) prescription for propranolol
    (D) subtotal thyroidectomy
    (E) no intervention is necessary as the problem will go away after the pregnancy

Questions 69 through 71

A 25-year-old nulligravid woman presents as a new patient to your gynecology practice. She has recently moved to the area. She is a healthy woman with no medical problems and is currently using oral contraceptives without problems. She informs you that she and her husband are planning to start a family within the next year. On review, you find her family history is unremarkable, but she informs you that her husband's sister has cystic fibrosis.

69. What is the approximate prevalence of cystic fibrosis carrier state in White individuals?

    (A) 1 in 10
    (B) 1 in 25
    (C) 1 in 50
    (D) 1 in 100
    (E) 1 in 200

70. Given that the husband's sister has cystic fibrosis, what is the likelihood that he is a carrier?

    (A) 100% chance of being a carrier
    (B) 67% (2 in 3) chance of being a carrier
    (C) 50% (1 in 2) chance of being a carrier
    (D) 25% (1 in 4) chance of being a carrier
    (E) his chance of being a carrier is no greater than the general population

71. If she and her husband were both known to carry a cystic fibrosis gene mutation, what would be their likelihood of having a child with cystic fibrosis?

    (A) 100%
    (B) 75%
    (C) 50%
    (D) 33%
    (E) 25%

Questions 72 and 73

A 35-year-old woman with two prior term pregnancies presents for her first prenatal visit at 12 weeks' gestation. She recalls having had hypertension near the end of her first pregnancy. She believes her blood pressure has been normal since, but admits that she rarely seeks preventive health care visits, and that her last examination by a physician was more than 2 years ago. Today, you find her blood pressure to be 160/100.

72. Which of the following antihypertensive agents would be contraindicated for management of her hypertension during pregnancy?

    (A) labetalol
    (B) alpha-methyldopa
    (C) enalapril
    (D) nifedipine
    (E) hydralazine

73. Her blood pressure comes under good control after initiating medication and remains well controlled until the 36th week, when her blood pressure is noted to have risen again to 170/110. She is also noted to have 3+ proteinuria on urine dipstick testing. For which of the following complications is she at risk?

    (A) eclampsia
    (B) fetal macrosomia
    (C) abnormal progress of labor
    (D) postpartum hemorrhage
    (E) breech presentation

74. Which of the following agents is considered the first-line therapy for prevention of eclamptic seizures?

    (A) diazepam
    (B) phenytoin
    (C) magnesium sulfate
    (D) phenobarbital
    (E) carbamazepine

75. A woman with type 1 diabetes is at increased risk for having a fetus with which of the following congenital anomalies?

    (A) gastroschisis
    (B) duodenal atresia
    (C) cleft lip and palate
    (D) congenital heart defects
    (E) diaphragmatic hernia

76. Which of the following statements about diabetes in pregnancy is true?

    (A) The risk of spontaneous abortion is not increased when compared to women without diabetes.
    (B) The risk of congenital anomalies rises in relation to the maternal hemoglobin A1C.
    (C) The rate of stillbirth is unchanged when compared with nondiabetic women.
    (D) The risk of cesarean birth is unchanged when compared to nondiabetic women.
    (E) Glycemic control is not related to fetal macrosomia.

77. A pregnant woman presents to the ER at 20 weeks' gestation with an acute exacerbation of her chronic bronchial asthma. She complains of a cold of 1 week's duration and admits that she lost her inhaler 2 weeks ago. Her examination reveals a temperature of 38°C, RR of 40, pulse of 110, and fetal heart rate of 150. Her lung examination is notable for diffuse expiratory wheezes and a prolonged I:E ratio. She is utilizing accessory muscles for breathing, which appears labored. Which of the following statements regarding asthma in pregnancy is true?

    (A) Asthma exacerbations are more common in pregnant women than in nonpregnant women of similar age.
    (B) Influenza vaccination is contraindicated in pregnancy.
    (C) Peak expiratory flow rate monitoring is unreliable for monitoring disease state during pregnancy.
    (D) In pregnant women, the arterial partial pressure of carbon dioxide ($PaCO_2$) is decreased on arterial blood gases compared to nonpregnant individuals.
    (E) Due to potential risks of fetal radiation exposure, chest radiography should not be performed to evaluate for underlying pneumonia in women with asthma exacerbation.

78. Which of the following maternal cardiac conditions is associated with the highest mortality rate during pregnancy?

    (A) mitral stenosis, New York Heart Association class 1–2
    (B) corrected tetralogy of Fallot
    (C) porcine prosthetic heart valve
    (D) mechanical prosthetic heart valve
    (E) pulmonary hypertension

79. Which of the following statements regarding seizures in pregnancy is true?

   (A) Women with a seizure disorder are at increased risk for eclampsia.
   (B) Carbamazepine would be a better anti-convulsant during pregnancy, as it is associated with lower risk of congenital anomalies.
   (C) Women who take valproate during pregnancy are at increased risk for both open neural defects and congenital heart disease.
   (D) Women who require multidrug therapy to control their seizures are at no greater risk for congenital anomalies than women on monotherapy.
   (E) It has been clearly demonstrated that women taking anticonvulsants benefit from higher doses of folic acid for prevention of neural tube defects.

80. The background of major congenital anomalies in a general obstetric population is closest to which of the following numbers?

   (A) 0.1% (1 in 1000)
   (B) 0.5% (5 in 1000)
   (C) 1% (10 in 1000)
   (D) 3% (30 in 1000)
   (E) 7% (70 in 1000)

81. A patient presents to your office for an annual gynecologic examination. She is an obese, post-menopausal, White female who reports a 4-month history of vulvar pruritis. Otherwise, she is without complaint. On examination, she is noted to have a whitened plaque-like area involving the posterior fourchette. The area is nontender, raised, and approximately $2.0 \times 2.0 \times 0.5$ cm. What is the next step in the management of this patient?

   (A) Prescribe a topical antimonilial cream.
   (B) Obtain a viral culture for herpes simplex type II.
   (C) Perform a vaginal wet mount.
   (D) Obtain a punch biopsy from the center of the lesion.
   (E) Prescribe a topical steroid cream.

82. A 27-year-old nulligravid single White female presents to your office for an annual examination. In taking her history, you learn that her mother died of ovarian cancer at the age of 63. There is no other family history of breast or ovarian cancer. The patient asks you to tell her what she can do to reduce her own ovarian cancer risk. What is the most effective strategy appropriate for this patient to reduce her risk?

   (A) bilateral laparoscopic salpingo-oophorectomy
   (B) daily aspirin use
   (C) oral contraceptive therapy
   (D) bilateral tubal ligation
   (E) avoidance of breast-feeding following pregnancy

83. A 37-year-old multiparous White female, s/p bilateral tubal ligation, reports a family history remarkable for a mother diagnosed with bilateral breast cancer at the age of 43, from which she ultimately died, and a sister diagnosed with epithelial ovarian cancer at the age of 47, for which she is currently undergoing chemotherapy. Secondary to this worrisome family history, the patient elected to undergo genetic testing and was found to be a BRCA1 carrier. In view of her carrier status, you inform her of which of the following?

   (A) She has a 30–50% lifetime risk for the development of ovarian cancer.
   (B) She has a 10% lifetime risk for the development of breast cancer.
   (C) If she develops ovarian cancer, it will likely be 10–15 years later than the normal onset of ovarian cancer seen in the general population.
   (D) She is at increased risk for the development of hereditary nonpolyposis colorectal cancer (Lynch family syndrome type II).
   (E) She has a lower risk for the development of Fallopian tube cancer than the general patient population.

84. A 62-year-old female with newly diagnosed International Federation of Gynecology and Obstetrics (FIGO) stage IIIC epithelial ovarian cancer is without evidence of visible remaining disease following a total abdominal hysterectomy, bilateral salpingo-oophorectomy, complete omentectomy, bilateral pelvic and paraaortic lymph node sampling, and rectosigmoid resection with reanastomosis. She is seen now for further treatment planning. The appropriate adjuvant therapy indicated in this setting is which of the following?

(A) external radiation

(B) the patient has no visible remaining disease and thus requires no further therapy

(C) implanted radiation seeds

(D) chemotherapy

(E) oral progestin

85. A 64-year-old White female presents to your office with complaints of vulvar pruritis and pain. You examine her and find an ulcerated lesion in the medial aspect of the left labia majora, 3.0 × 1.5 cm, that is thickened and indurated. You biopsy this lesion and the findings confirm a squamous cell carcinoma of the vulva. The groin nodes are palpably normal bilaterally. The next step in the patient's management would be which of the following?

(A) wide local excision of the lesion

(B) chemotherapy

(C) radiation therapy

(D) radical vulvectomy with ipsilateral inguinofemoral lymphadenectomy

(E) laser ablation

86. A 37-year-old female presented to your office with an ultrasound report suggestive of bilateral ovarian masses. You take her to the operating room for an exploratory laparotomy and note the left ovary to be replaced by an 8 × 9 cm neoplastic process. The right ovary appears to have a small 2 × 2 cm cystic process, similar in appearance to the left ovary, involving only a small portion of the right ovary. After obtaining pelvic and upper abdominal washings, you remove the left ovary and then perform a cystectomy on the right ovary, removing all visible disease without

rupture. The frozen section on both resected specimens reveals a serous tumor of low malignant potential (LMP). The best procedure for the patient at this point is which of the following?

(A) termination of the procedure; await final pathology report on the resected specimens

(B) total abdominal hysterectomy and right salpingo-oophorectomy

(C) omentectomy and peritoneal biopsies

(D) omentectomy, peritoneal biopsies, selected pelvic and peritoneal lymph node sampling

(E) terminate procedure and prescribe postoperative chemotherapy

87. A 65-year-old female presents with ascites, multiple peritoneal implants, and a large abdominopelvic mass. At laparotomy, she is found to have omental disease, splenic metastases, retroperitoneal lymphadenopathy, and bilateral pelvic masses with rectosigmoid involvement posteriorly and bladder involvement anteriorly. The appropriate surgical management for this patient would be which of the following?

(A) bilateral salpingo-oophorectomy, followed by postoperative chemotherapy

(B) total abdominal hysterectomy and bilateral salpingo-oophorectomy, followed by postoperative chemotherapy

(C) complete omentectomy, retroperitoneal lymphadenectomy, total abdominal hysterectomy, and bilateral salpingo-oophorectomy, followed by postoperative chemotherapy

(D) peritoneal stripping, splenectomy, complete omentectomy, retroperitoneal lymphadenectomy, total abdominal hysterectomy, and bilateral salpingo-oophorectomy, followed by postoperative chemotherapy

(E) rectosigmoid resection with reanastomosis, peritoneal stripping, splenectomy, complete omentectomy, retroperitoneal lymphadenectomy, total abdominal hysterectomy, and bilateral salpingo-oophorectomy, followed by postoperative chemotherapy

88. A thin, 37-year-old patient undergoes a total abdominal hysterectomy and bilateral salpingo-oophorectomy for chronic menometrorrhagia. The procedure lasts 2 hours. A Balfour retractor is utilized intraoperatively to assist with exposure. On the morning of postoperative day 2, the patient stands to get out of bed and collapses on the floor, her right lower extremity is unable to support her weight. You are called to examine her. Your neurologic examination suggests an absence of deep tendon reflex in the right lower extremity, absence of cutaneous sensation to the anterior and medial thigh, and an inability to flex at the hip and extend at the knee. Which of the following is the most likely etiology for this presentation postoperatively?

(A) DVT
(B) intraoperative compression injury of the femoral nerve
(C) intraoperative stroke
(D) intraoperative transection of the sciatic nerve
(E) undiagnosed diabetes

Questions 89 through 91

You are called by the labor and delivery nurse to evaluate the fetal monitoring strip of a patient. She is a 24-year-old G_1 female at 40 weeks' gestation who went into spontaneous labor earlier today. She is currently on IV oxytocin (Pitocin). You review the fetal monitoring strip shown in Figure 4-4.

89. What fetal heart rate condition does this monitor strip reveal?

(A) late decelerations
(B) early decelerations
(C) variable decelerations
(D) hyperstimulation
(E) fetal tachycardia

90. What physiologic process causes this to occur?

(A) uteroplacental insufficiency
(B) umbilical cord compression
(C) compression of the fetal head
(D) maternal fever
(E) fetal acidosis caused by too frequent uterine contractions

FIG. 4-4

4483AA0   25830   4483AA0

FIG. 4-4 (Continued)

91. What is the most appropriate management at this point?

(A) reduction in the dose of oxytocin

(B) place the woman on oxygen 10 L via facemask

(C) reposition the patient from her back to her left side

(D) acetaminophen to reduce maternal temperature

(E) reassurance and continuation of current care

92. Preconception counseling is an important component of health care encounters with reproductive age women. As a general recommendation, women of childbearing age should be advised to consume what dose of folic acid for prevention of neural tube defects?

(A) 0.1 mg

(B) 0.4 mg

(C) 1 mg

(D) 4 mg

(E) folic acid has only been shown to prevent the recurrence of neural tube defects in women who have previously had an affected child

Questions 93 and 94

93. A healthy 38-year-old G_4P_{3003} presents for amniocentesis. The karyotype returns as shown in the Figure 4-5. What is the diagnosis?

    (A) Down syndrome
    (B) Patau syndrome
    (C) Edwards syndrome
    (D) Turner syndrome
    (E) Klinefelter syndrome

94. You counsel the patient that which of the following was likely her biggest risk factor for the development of this karyotype?

    (A) cigarette smoking
    (B) lack of folic acid supplementation
    (C) maternal age at conception
    (D) family history
    (E) alcohol consumption

Questions 95 through 97

95. A 16-year-old nulligravid high school student is on your afternoon office schedule for a "talk visit." She was seen last year by one of your colleagues for an initial GYN evaluation. She is healthy and has no medical problems. Today she tells you that she and her new boyfriend had intercourse the night before, and the condom they were using broke. Your initial course of action should include which of the following?

    (A) placing an IUD
    (B) requesting that her parents be told of the situation
    (C) an examination and offer of sexually transmitted infections testing
    (D) performing a new obstetric workup
    (E) empirically treating her with ceftriaxone and doxycycline

96. The patient requests a prescription for "Plan B" emergency contraception. You tell her which of the following?

    (A) The medication is not effective after 24 hours.
    (B) Your office does not dispense prescriptions as such to minors.
    (C) She should first seek permission from her parents.

1   2   3   4   5

6   7   8   9   10   11   12

13   14   15   16   17   18

19   20   21   22   X   Y

FIG. 4-5 *(Courtesy of Dr. Nancy R. Schneider.)*

(D) The first dose must be taken within 72 hours of intercourse.

(E) The medication will cause an abortion.

97. She tells you that earlier in the day she had called her family doctor, who wouldn't call in a prescription because it was "against his personal beliefs." Your response should be which of the following?

(A) Prescribing health care providers must always prescribe it upon patient demand.

(B) It is within his right to decline giving treatments he deems outside his belief system, but he is ethically obliged to help her find a provider who does dispense Plan B.

(C) Plan B is available over the counter for all patients.

(D) You will report him to the state medical board.

(E) In situations regarding pregnancy, the physician is entitled to follow his personal ethical beliefs and has no obligation to assist a patient in seeking care that is outside of these beliefs.

Questions 98 and 99

You are asked to see an inpatient for a gynecologic consultation. The patient is an 85-year-old female who was admitted s/p her third stroke. She has a history of dementia, coronary artery disease, insulin-dependent diabetes, and hypertension. She resides in a local nursing home and normally requires extensive nursing assistance as she is unable to care for herself. While in the hospital, the nursing staff observed a small amount of new vaginal bleeding. Her past OB/GYN history is unknown and no family members are immediately available for clarification. On physical examination, she is lying comfortably in bed, awake but not oriented to person, place, or time. She is unable to speak coherently, and becomes combative when you attempt to examine her abdomen. She quiets down when you step out of the room.

98. Which of the following would be the most appropriate next step?

(A) Request that the nursing staff place her in restraints.

(B) Administer intravenous sedation.

(C) Take her to the operating room to perform an examination under anesthesia.

(D) Attempt to contact her family to assist in further decision making.

(E) Contact her primary attending physician and tell her that no further workup should be done in a patient in this condition.

99. You then receive a telephone call from someone who says she is the patient's granddaughter, inquiring as to the patient's status and your recommendations. What should be your response?

(A) "Your grandmother is very sick. We will be taking her to the operating room this afternoon. Would you please give us permission to do that over the telephone?"

(B) "In order to respect patient confidentiality and privacy, I am unable to discuss patient-related issues without explicit permission from her or her designated decision maker."

(C) "In her current condition, I believe that she has too many other medical problems to workup her vaginal bleeding. I will not be seeing her again unless something changes."

(D) "Please call back later after we have completed her examination."

(E) "I cannot give you information over the phone but could give you any information that you want if you come to the hospital and can prove to us that you are related to the patient."

Answers and Explanations

1. **(C)** Differentiating between an ectopic pregnancy, an early intrauterine pregnancy, or a miscarriage is a common dilemma for the ED physician. Transabdominal ultrasound (TAUS) requires a β-hCG level of 6500 mIU/mL before an intrauterine gestation can be confidently visualized. Transvaginal ultrasound (TVUS) is the most accurate means of confirming intrauterine pregnancy and gestational age during the early first trimester. TVUS can help detect signs of intrauterine pregnancy approximately 1 week earlier than TAUS because it has a lower discriminatory zone (β-hCG level between 1000 and 1500 mIU/mL). A TAUS that does not detect an intrauterine gestational sac with a β-hCG level higher than 6500 mIU/mL or a TVUS examination that does not detect an intrauterine gestational sac when the β-hCG level is higher than 1500 mIU/mL suggests an ectopic pregnancy. The literature provides a wide range of sensitivities and specificities for transvaginal ultrasonography in the detection of ectopic pregnancy. Sensitivities range from 69 to 99%, and specificities range from 84 to 99.6%. *(Anne-Marie and Beth, 2005, pp. 1707–1714; Beckmann et al., 2002, pp. 192–194)*

2. **(C)** Following tubal ligation pregnancy occurs about 1% of the time. This depends on the method used and the expertise of the surgeon. In general, 30% of pregnancies following tubal ligation are ectopic. A patient who presents with a positive pregnancy test following tubal ligation should be considered an "ectopic until proven otherwise." *(Beckmann et al., 2002, p. 353)*

3. **(D)** Androgen excess syndromes are common and usually characterized by one or more of the following problems: hirsutism, acne, weight gain, or irregular menses. PCOS is the most common disorder of androgen excess. Other syndromes that often result in signs and symptoms of androgen excess in adults include Cushing syndrome and late-onset congenital adrenal hyperplasia. The classic presentation of a patient with an androgen-secreting tumor of the ovary or adrenal gland involves the rapid onset of symptoms. Late-onset congenital adrenal hyperplasia and an androgen-secreting tumor are the only disorders of androgen excess usually resulting in clitoromegaly. *(Beckmann et al., 2002, pp. 475–480)*

4. **(B)** PID is the most common cause of Fallopian tube damage. It is a polymicrobial infection that originates from upward spread of infecting organisms through the cervix and into the uterus, Fallopian tubes, or peritoneal cavity. The two most common pathogens are *Neisseria gonorrhea* and *Chlamydia trachomatis*; however, microorganisms that comprise the vaginal flora (e.g., anaerobes, *Gardnerella vaginalis*, *Haemophilus influenzae*, enteric gram-negative rods, and *Streptococcus agalactiae*) also have been associated with PID. Symptoms of PID include lower abdominal pain, dyspareunia, fever, back pain, and vomiting, as well as symptoms of lower genital tract infection such as abnormal vaginal discharge or bleeding, itching, and odor. In some women, symptoms are mild or even absent. Risk factors for PID include the presence of a sexually transmitted infection, a previous episode of PID, sexual intercourse at an early age, high number of sexual partners, and alcohol use. Empiric treatment of PID should be initiated in sexually active young women and other women at risk for STDs if they are experiencing pelvic or lower abdominal pain, if no cause for the illness other than PID can be identified, and if one or more of the following minimum criteria are present on pelvic examination: cervical motion tenderness OR uterine tenderness OR adnexal tenderness. Other common causes of acquired tubal damage include endometriosis, previous pelvic surgery, and a ruptured appendix. *(Beckmann et al., 2002, pp. 500–501)*

5. **(A)** Numerous causes lead to delayed puberty. Common features of Turner syndrome include short stature, sexual infantilism, "shield" chest, "webbed" neck, high arched palate, increased carrying angle of the arms (cubitus valgus), short fourth metacarpal, and streak gonads. The diagnosis of Turner syndrome requires the presence of typical phenotypic features and the complete or partial absence of a second X chromosome. Diagnosis should be considered in individuals with primary or secondary amenorrhea and in adult women with unexplained infertility, particularly when such individuals also are short in stature. Although the FSH would be elevated in Turner syndrome, it would not differentiate among the many causes of ovarian failure. In childhood, GH therapy is standard to prevent short stature as an adult. Estrogen replacement therapy usually is required, but starting too early can compromise adult height. Estrogen usually is started from age 12 to 15 years. *(Beckmann et al., 2002, p. 458)*

6. **(D)** The U.S. Food and Drug Administration (FDA) has approved the use of oral contraceptives as an effective method of postcoital contraception, often termed emergency contraception. The most common regimens involve two to four oral contraceptive tablets, depending on the dosage of the brand used, repeated 12 hours later. Progestin-only regimens are also highly effective. Initiating treatment greater than 72 hours after the event of unprotected intercourse is associated with a lower success rate. *(Beckmann et al., 2002, pp. 343–344)*

7. **(B)** Risk factors for postmenopausal osteoporosis include cigarette smoking, thinness, early menopause (natural or surgical), nulliparity, northern European heritage, some medications (e.g., glucocorticoids), high alcohol or caffeine intake, low dietary calcium consumption, and a family history of osteoporosis. Dietary calcium and vitamin D supplementation and exercise (preferably weight bearing) are the classic lifestyle changes recommended to prevent or treat osteoporosis. *(Beckmann et al., 2002, pp. 487–488)*

8. **(B)** The McCune-Albright syndrome is due to a G-protein mutation in the alpha-subunit that causes constitutive stimulatory activity of the tissues. Affected tissues are autonomously active. McCune-Albright syndrome classically consists of a triad of café au lait skin spots, cystic bone lesions (polyostotic fibrous dysplasia), and autonomous endocrine hyperfunction resulting in sexual precocity. A dominant ovarian cyst develops independent of stimulation by gonadotropins and it secretes estradiol, resulting in sexual precocity and skeletal maturity. Therefore, the finding of elevated estradiol levels and suppressed or undetectable gonadotropins is diagnostic. Affected individuals also may have hyperthyroidism, hypercortisolism, pituitary gigantism, or acromegaly. *(Speroff et al., 1999, p. 395; Stenchever et al., 2001, p. 269)*

9. **(A)** PCOS is the most common endocrine disorder of reproductive age women. Common symptoms include oligo- or amenorrhea, acne, hirsutism, infertility, and weight gain. Common tests used to support the diagnosis of PCOS include LH to FSH ratio, testosterone, DHEAS, and pelvic ultrasound.

    Acanthosis nigricans is a raised, velvety, tan skin lesion commonly seen on the back of the neck, in the axilla, and the intertriginous areas. Acanthosis nigricans is associated with hyperinsulinemia and is a sign that the patient is at significant risk for prediabetes and frank diabetes. Up to 30% of patients with suspected PCOS have prediabetes, and 8% are frank type II diabetics.

    PCOS is a diagnosis of exclusion and requires ruling out other possible confounding diagnoses. Given the obesity and acanthosis nigricans in this patient, a 75-g, 2-hour oral glucose tolerance test would be recommended. Other common confounding diagnoses in patients with PCOS include late-onset congenital adrenal hyperplasia (screened with a serum 17-hydroxyprogesterone), Cushing syndrome (screened with a 24 hour urinary free cortisol, or overnight dexamethasone suppression test), and thyroid disease. *(Beckmann et al., 2002, pp. 475–477)*

10. **(C)** Androgen insensitivity is an inherited disease resulting from the lack of functional androgen receptors. Gonadal function is that of

normal testicles; however, there is no end-organ effect due to the lack of any functional receptors. Because the gonads produce Müllerian inhibiting substance (MIS), the Müllerian structures regress. Primary amenorrhea is therefore a common cause for presentation to a physician. Normal female secondary sexual characteristics and external genitalia result due to the absence of any effect of endogenous androgens and the production of small, but adequate, amounts of estrogen, mostly from peripheral conversion of androstenedione. *(Stenchever et al., 2001, pp. 1106–1107)*

11. **(A)** Acute pelvic pain is a difficult diagnostic dilemma. An acute abdomen can result from appendicitis, ovarian torsion, ruptured ovarian cyst, ectopic pregnancy, PID, diverticular abscess, and other causes. Misdiagnosis of PID is common and the most likely diagnosis confused with PID is appendicitis. In the setting where the etiology of the acute abdomen is not certain, a laparoscopy is indicated both for diagnostic and, in many cases, therapeutic purposes. A pelvic MRI or serial examinations would further delay the diagnosis. In the case of ovarian torsion or appendicitis, rapid diagnosis and treatment is critical to optimize outcomes. *(Beckmann et al., 2002, pp. 373–374)*

12. **(E)** Kallmann syndrome is a genetic problem due to failure of migration of olfactory and GnRH secreting neurons to make their appropriate connections in the brain. Classically, this leads to anosmia (inability to smell), delayed puberty, and amenorrhea. The GnRH is not secreted, and pituitary FSH and LH release does not occur. In the absence of stimulation the ovaries do not produce significant estrogen. This is an example of hypogonadotropic hypogonadism, also termed hypothalamic amenorrhea. *(Stenchever et al., 2001, p. 1106)*

13. **(B)** Asherman syndrome describes intrauterine synechiae (scarring) of the uterine cavity following a surgery of infection of the uterine endometrium. Asherman syndrome is seen following uterine surgery (such as a uterine curettage or myomectomy), septic abortion, or other endometrial cavity infection. The damaged endometrium scars together lead to impairment of the endometrial function. This may result in amenorrhea, dysmenorrhea, infertility, or miscarriage. If the scarring causes obstruction of outflow of menstrual tissue, then hematometra and dysmenorrhea can occur. Severe scarring leads to complete obliteration of the uterine cavity. *(Stenchever et al., 2001, pp. 1109–1110)*

14. **(D)** Following ovulation, fertilization of the egg by the sperm occurs in the Fallopian tube. The embryo then divides and grows as it migrates down the Fallopian tube and into the uterine cavity. As early as 6 days postovulation the embryo implants in the uterine endometrium. Trophoblast invasion then occurs allowing the embryo to burrow into the endometrium. A uteroplacental circulation is established by 11–12 days after ovulation allowing β-hCG to be detectable in maternal serum or urine. *(Stenchever et al., 2001, pp. 7–9)*

15. **(B)**

16. **(B)**

Explanations 15 and 16

The pregnancy risk factor category assists the physician and patient to understand the safety of the use of a medication during pregnancy. The summary of the categories is as follows: category A—controlled human studies demonstrate no risk to a fetus. Category B—animal-reproduction studies have not demonstrated fetal risk but there are no controlled human studies to assess the risk. Category C—animal-reproduction studies have demonstrated risk to a fetus and no controlled human studies are available. Category D—evidence of human teratogenic risk exists but in some cases the known risks may be outweighed in serious situations, such as life-threatening disease. Class X—this drug should never be used by a pregnant female under any circumstances. *(Beckmann et al., 2002, p. 96)*

The principle of autonomy states that the patient has the right and capability to control the course of her medical care and to participate in the decision-making process. *(Marx et al., 2006, Chap. 205)*

17. **(D)** Müllerian anomalies result from either the lack of proper fusion or resorption of the paramesonephric (Müllerian) ducts during organogenesis. Vertical abnormalities occur when the invaginating urogenital sinus—extending in a cranial direction from the introitus—and the Müllerian structures—extending caudally—fail to canalize appropriately. Longitudinal defects occur when the two paramesonephric ducts either do not fuse appropriately or following fusion the intervening tissue is not reabsorbed completely. A didelphic uterus represents lack of fusion, and the patient has a duplicated cervix and each cervix is connected to a separate uterine horn. A unicornuate uterus results from aplasia of one of the paramesonephric ducts so that only one cervix connecting to a single uterine horn is found. A bicornuate uterus results from failure of the paramesonephric ducts to fuse cranially resulting in a single cervix but two separate uterine horns. A septate uterus occurs when fusion is completed but reabsorption of the intervening tissue is incomplete. *(Stenchever et al., 2001, pp. 260–264)*

18. **(E)** Sheehan syndrome describes damage to the pituitary gland classically resulting from hypotension following a postpartum hemorrhage. The clinical picture is variable due to the fact that the damage may involve one or more of the various cellular subtypes in the pituitary gland that secrete either adrenocorticotropic hormone (ACTH), GH, prolactin, TSH, or LH/FSH. An amenorrheic patient with a history of Sheehan's syndrome would not be expected to have functional pituitary gonadotropes so a GnRH pump or clomiphene citrate would not be useful because they both rely on a functional pituitary gland. Replacement of gonadotropins (LH and FSH) would be the best treatment option. *(Stenchever et al., 2001, p. 1116)*

19. **(C)** There are a number of effective medical therapies for pain due to endometriosis. These include GnRH agonists, danazol, progestins, and oral contraceptives. Surgical menopause requires the use of GnRH agonists or antagonists in order to suppress of ovarian function. Unopposed estrogen would be contraindicated in this patient because of its stimulatory effect on any remaining endometriosis. Tamoxifen has not demonstrated efficacy in the treatment of endometriosis. Progestins are effective at improving endometriosis symptoms due to their atrophic effect. *(Stenchever et al., 2001, pp. 542–552)*

20. **(E)** The luteal phase of the menstrual cycle, defined as beginning with the LH surge and ending with onset menses, is normally fixed at 14 ± 2 days. Therefore, the length of the follicular phase can fairly accurately be determined by subtracting 14 days from the total length of the cycle. In this case, the length of the follicular phase is: $34 - 14 = 20$ days. *(Beckmann et al., 2002, pp. 444–454)*

21. **(C)** A patient who is anovulatory due to PCOS would be expected to have normal estrogen production. However, without corpus luteum formation following ovulation there is no significant progesterone production. Therefore, the discontinuation of a period of progestin therapy would initiate menstrual flow. *(Beckmann et al., 2002, p. 467)*

22. **(D)** In gynecology, the obturator nerve (L2-L4) is most commonly injured during retroperitoneal surgery for gynecologic malignancies. In this case, a pelvic lymph node dissection for endometrial cancer involves a retroperitoneal dissection into the obturator fossa to remove the obturator lymph nodes. The nodal tissue of the obturator fossa obscures the location of the obturator nerve and predisposes it to injury. Postoperatively, patients with an injury to the obturator nerve will present with sensory loss to the upper medial thigh and motor weakness in the hip adductors.

  If an obturator nerve injury is recognized intraoperatively, immediate repair is the recommended treatment. However, with postoperative recognition, as in this case, treatment includes physiotherapy with neuromuscular electrical stimulation and electromyographic biofeedback, and exercise. Obturator nerve injury is a highly treatable condition, and complete recovery of motor strength is generally the result after physical therapy.

  The femoral nerve is the most commonly injured nerve at the time of gynecologic surgical procedures, and it is usually injured at the time of laparotomy from inappropriate placement of lateral retractor blades. Patients with injury to the femoral nerve will present with diminished or absent deep tendon reflexes, inability to straight leg raise, flex at the hips, or extend the knee. There may also be a loss of cutaneous sensation over the anterior thigh and the medial aspect of the thigh and calf.

The genitofemoral nerve (L1, L2) runs along the ventral surface of the psoas muscle, lateral to the external iliac artery. If removed or damaged, patients present with numbness of the ipsilateral mons pubis, labia majora, and skin overlying the femoral triangle. This nerve conducts sensory information only, thus there is no loss in motor function.

The pudendal nerve (S2-S4) also conducts sensory information only. Injury to the pudendal nerve results in a loss of sensation to the perineum.

The common peroneal nerve branches off the posterior tibial branch of the sciatic nerve just above the popliteal fossa and runs superficially across the lateral head of the fibula and down the lateral calf. This nerve can be compressed when patients are inappropriately placed in the lithotomy position with stirrups. Compression of the peroneal nerve results in a foot drop and lateral lower extremity numbness or paresthesia. *(Irvin et al., 2004, pp. 374–382)*

23. **(C)** The incidence of lymphocyst formation following radical hysterectomy and pelvic lymphadenectomy ranges as high as 30%, but is less than 5% if only symptomatic cysts are counted. Risks for lymphocyst formation include lymphadenectomy, radiation therapy, lymph node metastases, and closure of the pelvic peritoneum. From a surgical standpoint, closure of the pelvic peritoneum traps the lymph fluid in the retroperitoneal space and prevents absorption by the peritoneal membrane. Most lymphocysts are small, asymptomatic, and clinically insignificant. Large lymphocysts can produce serious consequences including venous obstruction with DVT, ureteral obstruction, leg edema, and pain. Bilateral lymphocysts can cause obstructive renal failure. The diagnosis is made most easily and accurately by pelvic ultrasound. Large or symptomatic pelvic lymphocysts can almost always be managed by percutaneous drainage with a pigtail catheter placed under CT or ultrasound guidance.

A pelvic DVT following gynecologic surgery should be in the differential for this patient. Typically, DVT following pelvic surgery is asymptomatic, but the appearance of leg edema, pain, or tenderness in the calf, popliteal space, or inguinal triangle is highly suspicious. Erythema and fever are uncommon. A pelvic DVT is uncommon compared to a more distal DVT in the lower extremity venous system. Women with a pelvic DVT will not have the classic symptoms associated with a calf DVT. The diagnostic test to evaluate for a DVT would be a lower extremity venous duplex ultrasound.

In the absence of fever, an elevated WBC or diagnostic evidence of a bacterial infection in the cystic structure seen on pelvic ultrasound, the diagnosis of pelvic abscess cannot be confirmed. Typically, a pelvic abscess arises within the first 7–14 days postoperatively. The cardinal clinical signs are fever, leukocytosis with a left shift, abdominal/pelvic pain, malaise, ileus, and perhaps a poorly defined mass. CT scan or ultrasound confirms the diagnosis.

An ovarian cyst is unlikely in this patient since she has had her ovaries surgically removed, and because the occurrence of the cyst occurred so rapidly following surgery. Occasionally, patients can have an ovarian remnant syndrome in which a remnant of the ovary was incidentally left at the time of surgery. Women who have this syndrome can then develop symptomatic benign or malignant ovarian mass in this remnant of ovarian tissue.

In the absence of fever, leukocytosis, or gastrointestinal (GI) symptoms, the diagnosis of diverticular abscess cannot be confirmed. Treatment for a diverticular abscess includes intravenous antibiotics directed against gram-negative anaerobic bacteria, followed by surgical drainage or resection. *(Morrow and Curtin, 1996; Braunwald et al., 2001, pp. 831–2)*

24. **(A)**

25. **(C)**

Explanations 24 and 25

A woman with advanced cervical cancer may present emergently with heavy vaginal bleeding. Often, the bleeding can be controlled for 24 hours by packing the vagina with a packing soaked in Monsel solution. The patient is kept on bedrest, and the packing is changed every 24 hours. If packing the vagina does not control the bleeding, then emergent radiation therapy is warranted if the patient has not had previous radiation treatment. Hemorrhage is usually controlled within 24–48 hours of initiating external beam therapy.

If radiation therapy fails, then the next best treatment is arterial embolization of either the uterine or hypogastric arteries. However, embolization may result in tumor hypoxia and decrease the sensitivity of the tumor to radiation. Arteriography with embolization may allow visualization of the bleeding vessel with direct embolization of the source. Arterial embolization has several risks including infarction of distal tissue, infection, and femoral artery thrombosis. If embolization is not available or not successful, bilateral hypogastric artery ligation is an option.

In this patient, surgical therapy with radical hysterectomy is not an appropriate treatment because this patient's disease has spread beyond the cervix. This procedure would result in transection of the tumor and lead to further bleeding complications. This patient has at least a stage IIIB tumor, and the best treatment for her is chemoradiation. (*American College of Obstetricians and Gynecologists, 2001*)

26. (E)

27. (B)

Explanations 26 and 27

VAIN is frequently found in women who have a history of cervical dysplasia. Although the etiology of VAIN has not been thoroughly elucidated, like cervical intraepithelial neoplasia (CIN), it is thought that HPV is the carcinogenic agent. Thus, when vaginal cytology is abnormal, the evaluation is very similar to that of an abnormal pap smear. It is important to assess the histologic severity and the extent of the lesion. To do this, the next step in management is a thorough colposcopic evaluation of the entire vaginal canal, especially because many patients will have multifocal disease. During colposcopy the application of acetic acid (4%) is useful. The speculum should be fully inserted to visualize the upper vagina and then slowly removed while rotating the speculum, being careful to view the entire vaginal mucosal surface. Most vaginal lesions are not grossly visible. However, a raised white epithelium may occasionally be seen. If a lesion is visible, then directed biopsy of the lesion is indicated to confirm the diagnosis.

The image provided shows HGSIL. In the presence of high-grade vaginal cytology, repeat cytology in 6 months, and observation are not viable management options given the concern for carcinoma in situ or for invasive carcinoma of the vagina. Random vaginal biopsies are also not likely to be helpful since they will most likely miss the involved area and lead to a false negative result. Intravaginal estrogen cream is reserved for postmenopausal women with vaginal atrophy and low-grade VAIN without evidence of invasion. Estrogen is not a treatment for VAIN 3, or high-grade VAIN.

Other acceptable treatments for VAIN include wide local excision or partial vaginectomy, laser ablation, 5-FU, and total vaginectomy. Before deciding on a therapy, several factors should be considered including the patient's age and hormonal status, the grade of the lesion, the presence or suspicion of invasion, and the location, extent, and multifocality of the lesion. In this case, the patient is 42 years old and premenopausal, with a high-grade lesion suspicious for invasion that is relatively small and localized. Therefore, wide local excision is the best treatment option. Laser and 5-FU, which are obliterative procedures, should be avoided in the presence of invasion or a suspicion for invasion. If invasion can be ruled out, then these options are reasonable. Finally, a total vaginectomy should be reserved for very large lesions, multifocal lesions that involve the entire vaginal mucosa, suspicion for invasion, or failure of other treatment modalities. In this young, premenopausal, sexually active woman with a localized lesion, a total vaginectomy is an overaggressive treatment for her disease. *(Wharton et al., 1996, pp. 325–345; Wright and Chapman, 1992, pp. 180–190)*

28. **(D)** Vaginal bleeding in a postmenopausal woman may be caused by numerous etiologies including an endometrial polyp, endometrial hyperplasia, atrophic endometrium, a submucosal fibroid, or endometrial cancer to name a few. In this group of women, endometrial cancer must be ruled out. Although this woman may need a pap smear as part of her routine gynecologic screening, a pap smear is inadequate to rule out the diagnosis of endometrial cancer. ECC is a sampling of the endocervical canal, not of the endometrium. Thus, again, an ECC is not adequate to rule out endometrial cancer. The ECC is more commonly used in the workup for cervical dysplasia to assess extension into the cervical canal. A thickened endometrial stripe on pelvic ultrasound can aid in making the diagnosis of an endometrial abnormality, but the ultrasound itself is not diagnostic for endometrial cancer. A thickened endometrium on ultrasound may be the result of a submucosal fibroid, hyperplasia, a polyp, or endometrial cancer. A dilation and curettage is an outpatient surgical procedure that involves dilation of the cervix and a thorough sampling of the endometrium with a curette. This procedure will obtain adequate endometrial tissue to make a diagnosis of tissue. In general, this procedure is reserved for patients in which endometrial biopsy is unsuccessful or for patients who have continued symptoms with a negative endometrial biopsy. Endometrial biopsy is a simple office procedure for sampling the endometrium, and it is 95% accurate. Thus, it is the preferred method of sampling the endometrium to rule out endometrial cancer. *(Good, 1997, pp. 345–349)*

29. **(C)** The current American College of Obstetricians and Gynecologists guidelines for screening women on tamoxifen for endometrial cancer state that no screening except for routine yearly gynecologic examinations should be performed in asymptomatic women. In symptomatic women with vaginal bleeding on tamoxifen therapy, endometrial biopsy is recommended. Tamoxifen directly affects the endometrium, and a pelvic ultrasound will reveal a thickened endometrium in 75% of asymptomatic women. The most common changes to the endometrium include benign cystic glandular dilation, stromal edema, endometrial hyperplasia, and polyps. Approximately 20–30% of women will develop benign endometrial and endocervical polyps. Women on tamoxifen have a two- to threefold increased risk for endometrial cancer. Given the high rate of benign changes in the endometrium from tamoxifen, the usefulness of TVUS and endometrial biopsy is drastically diminished. In the setting of tamoxifen, ultrasound has only a 9% positive predictive value. However, the negative predictive value is 99%, meaning that if the ultrasound is normal, you may be 99% certain that there is no disease present. CT scans in general are less effective than ultrasound at evaluating the endometrial cavity, and they are not recommended for screening. Hysteroscopy will allow direct visualization with directed biopsy of the abnormal endometrium. However, again, the majority of lesions in women on tamoxifen will be benign, and a large number of hysteroscopies would be performed with the detection of very few cancers. Thus, this is not cost-effective and is a low yield diagnostic procedure in this group of women. Also, there is some debate as to whether hysteroscopy in the presence of endometrial cancer increases the risk for positive cytology and leads to a seeding of the peritoneal cavity with endometrial cancer cells by effusing cancer cells from the endometrium out through the Fallopian tubes into the abdominal cavity. *(Barakat, 1998, pp. 195–207)*

30. **(E)** Women with HNPCC, Lynch syndrome II have a 20–40% lifetime risk of endometrial cancer. These women tend to get endometrial cancer at a much earlier age (median 46 years) compared to the general population (median 63 years). These women are also at risk for carcinomas of the ovary, breast, stomach, small bowel, pancreas, biliary tract, and transitional cell tumors of the urinary tract. Because of the inordinately high risk for endometrial and ovarian

cancer in these patients, prophylactic hysterectomy and bilateral salpingo-oophorectomies are offered to women with this syndrome after the completion of childbearing. *(Vasen et al.,1996, pp. 1020–1027)*

31. **(C)** An office biopsy of the cervical lesion should be taken immediately when a gross lesion is seen on physical examination. For smaller, less distinct lesions, colposcopy may be helpful in determining the best area to biopsy, but it is not always necessary for larger, distinct, gross lesions. A pap smear can be performed, but it cannot be relied on to detect invasive cervical cancer. Cervical cone biopsy is not indicated at this time, particularly because the diagnosis can be made by less invasive means with an office biopsy. Also, if a cone biopsy is performed and the cancer is invasive or more extensive than originally thought, a cone biopsy may affect the oncologist's ability to perform a radical hysterectomy or alter the effectiveness of vaginal brachytherapy. Finally, the use of metronidazole vaginal cream is not indicated in this patient since there is no evidence of a vaginal infection. *(Hillard, 1996, pp. 331–397)*

32. **(C)**

33. **(D)**

34. **(E)**

Explanations 32 through 34

Current American Society for Colposcopy and Cervical Pathology (ASCCP) guidelines for treating a pap smear consistent with HGSIL is to perform colposcopy with directed biopsies if a lesion is seen. Routine pap smear in 1 year is an unacceptable option for this patient given her increased risk for developing cervical cancer. Random biopsies have a high false negative rate if there is no visible lesion to biopsy, thus, are not helpful. The pap smear is a screening test of the cervix, not the endometrium. There is no reason to suspect that this patient has endometrial pathology, therefore, an endometrial biopsy is not warranted. HPV testing is not recommended for high-grade pap smears. All high-grade pap smears require further investigation with colposcopy regardless of HPV status.

If colposcopy is unsatisfactory, meaning no lesion is identified, the full transformation zone is not visualized or the full extent of the lesion is not identified, then a diagnostic excisional procedure is warranted. A loop excisional electrocautery procedure (LEEP) would be appropriate. However, note that if your suspicion for cancer is high, the cauterized edges from a LEEP procedure can complicate the pathologic assessment of positive margins. A cold knife cervical conization can be performed in the operating room as an outpatient surgery and provides the best surgical specimen for pathologic evaluation. In this case, a TVUS, endometrial dilation, and curettage, and ECC are all inappropriate options since they do not accurately evaluate the cervix, which is the primary site of concern. *(JAMA 2002; 287, pp. 220–2129)*

This patient has, by definition, microinvasive cervical cancer. Approximately 10–15% of patients in the United States with stage I cervical cancer will have a microinvasive cancer. Microinvasive cancer is defined as stage IA with invasion limited to a depth of 5 mm with lateral extent not to exceed 7 mm. Stage IA is further subdivided into stage IA1 with stromal invasion less than 3 mm and IA2 with invasion 3–5 mm in depth. Young patients with microinvasive squamous cell carcinoma of the cervix who desire future fertility can be treated with conization alone, provided that certain strict criteria are met. The cone specimen should be properly excised and then evaluated by an experienced pathologist. The tumor must meet the criteria for stage IA1 disease with invasion less than 3 mm and a lateral extent less than 7 mm. The cone margins must be negative, and there should be no lymphvascular space invasion.

Patients with stage IA1 disease who do not desire future childbearing should be treated with a simple hysterectomy. Thus, the other options including radiation, simple or radical hysterectomy with pelvic lymphadenectomy, or radical trachelectomy would be overtreatment for this patient, and they would not preserve her fertility. *(Winter, 1998, pp. 433–436)*

35. **(E)** This patient, who had a hysterectomy for a benign condition, no longer needs pap smear screening as long as she is monogamous and does not develop risk factors for cervical dysplasia. The incidence for vaginal dysplasia after hysterectomy for benign disease is approximately 0.13%. Invasive carcinoma of the vagina is rare, and screening for this cancer is not cost-effective. However, women who had a hysterectomy for cervical dysplasia or cancer are at increased risk for vaginal dysplasia and should continue to have vaginal pap smears. It is also reasonable to reinitiate pap smear screening in women who had a hysterectomy for benign disease if they have new sexual partners or new risk factors. A pap test is also indicated if patients present with vaginal spotting or bleeding. *(McIntosh, 1998, pp. 14–18)*

36. **(B)** The use of estrogen replacement in women previously treated for endometrial cancer represents a recent change in practice. For many women, the improvement in quality of life and the reduction in osteoporosis outweigh the possible risks of stimulating tumor growth. Most patients are diagnosed early with endometrial cancer and successfully treated with surgery. As a result, the risk-benefit ratio of estrogen replacement in these women has been re-examined. In a recent survey of the Society of Gynecologic Oncologists, 83% of the respondents approved estrogen replacement in stage I, grade 1 endometrial cancer. Data on the use of estrogen replacement therapy in women with endometrial cancer are limited primarily to retrospective studies. Three retrospective studies have concluded that estrogen replacement therapy is not detrimental to patients after treatment for endometrial cancer. There exists no data on which to base specific recommendations about estrogen replacement in these patients. The decision must involve a candid discussion about risks and benefits to the patients and be individualized to each patient, taking into consideration the stage, grade, and histology of the tumor and their current

hypoestrogenic symptoms and risk factors for osteoporosis. The delivery method of estrogen is also not clear. Some patients may want to use more natural products like soy, although the relief of symptoms with soy varies considerably. Others may complain more of vaginal dryness, and a vaginal estrogen cream may be more appropriate. The benefit of adding progesterone and giving patients combined hormone replacement therapy is also unclear. *(ACOG Committee on Gynecologic Practice Number 126—August 1993. Int J Gynaecol Obstet. 1993 Oct;43(1):89.)*

37. **(C)**

38. **(E)**

Explanations 37 and 38

Pelvic ultrasound is the least invasive and most cost-effective test to diagnose uterine fibroids. MRI is useful but not always readily available and much more expensive. Plain radiographs would not be helpful, and office laparoscopy is impractical and potentially dangerous given the presumed size of her uterus. A hysterosalpingogram would only note filling defects within the uterine cavity and miss intramural or subserosal fibroids. *(Buttram and Reiter, 1981, pp. 433–445)*

GnRH agonists have been used widely for preoperative treatment of uterine fibroids. They work by inducing amenorrhea, which improves hematologic parameters and decreases uterine volume. Although nonsteroidal anti-inflammatory drugs (NSAIDs) may help decrease bleeding for some patients with fibroids, they have not been reliably shown to decrease fibroid size. The other agents (OCPs, progesterone, and narcotics) do not have these effects and generally are not effective in treating dysfunctional uterine bleeding caused by anatomic lesions such as fibroids. *(Stovall et al., 1995, pp. 65–71)*

39. **(B)**

40. **(C)**

Explanations 39 and 40

When pelvic organs prolapse occurs beyond the level of the hymen, anatomic obstruction of urine occurs in approximately 30% of patients. Over time, urinary stasis from obstruction can lead to UTIs. Detrusor hypocontractility, not overactivity, can be another long-term sequela of chronic urinary retention, enhanced by a stretch injury to the postsynaptic parasympathetics in the bladder wall. Menopause alone is not a risk factor for retention, and a spinal cord tumor is not likely in this patient without specific neurologic complaints or findings on physical examination.

Due to urinary stasis, she is at risk for a UTI. Left untreated, she could develop obstructive uropathy and/or pyelonephritis. Surgery is an option, but not without the prior consideration of nonsurgical options such as a pessary or intermittent clean, self-catheterization (if the problem were to persist). In the event of chronic retention, radiographic imaging would help to assess for upper tract obstruction (i.e., hydronephrosis). Oxybutynin is not appropriate, as it could compound urinary retention. Urodynamic studies could be helpful in the future to ascertain the exact cause of her retention (obstruction from the prolapse vs. chronic detrusor insufficiency vs. neurogenic bladder), but is not the first action to consider. *(Coates et al., 1997, pp. 217–221; Weinberger, 2003, pp. 64–65)*

41. **(D)**

42. **(C)**

Explanations 41 and 42

This patient is demonstrating acute peritoneal signs that require surgical intervention. Adding additional testing, either with radiology or more laboratory assessment would not alter the management at this point in time. Although some patients with chronic pelvic pain have a history of sexual or physical abuse, an assessment in the acute emergent setting does not take initial priority.

Although ovarian torsion can be enigmatic in its presentation, this patient demonstrates classic signs of intermittent pelvic pain and an ovarian cyst with a solid component. The 8-cm increase in ovarian size is likely due to vascular congestion from occlusion of the blood supply. Early intervention is more likely to result in salvaging viable tissue before the onset of irreversible tissue necrosis. The absence of fever and other GI symptoms, along with a left lower quadrant mass on ultrasound goes against the possibility of appendicitis or pancreatitis. Her pregnancy test is negative which generally excludes an ectopic pregnancy. *(Corfman et al., 2001, pp. 676–677)*

43. **(C)**

44. **(E)**

Explanations 43 and 44

PID is actually a spectrum of inflammatory disorders of the upper female genital tract. It includes endometritis, salpingitis, tubo-ovarian abscess, and pelvic peritonitis. While the sexually transmitted bacteria *N. gonorrhea* and *C. trachomatis* are often implicated, vaginal flora, including anaerobes, *G. vaginalis*, *H. influenzae*, gram-negative rods, and others, are also associated with PID. The clinical diagnosis of acute PID can be difficult and imprecise. There is a wide range of variation in signs and symptoms, and many women have very mild or subtle symptoms only. Because of the difficulty with diagnosis and the potential for damage to reproductive health with even mild PID, one must keep a low threshold for the diagnosis. Empiric treatment for PID should be considered in sexually active young women, or other women at risk for STDs, if there is uterine, adnexal, or cervical motion tenderness, and no other cause of illness can be identified. Additional criteria that support a diagnosis of PID include temperature >101°F, mucopurulent cervical or vaginal discharge, presence of WBCs on wet prep of vaginal secretions, elevated ESR, elevated C-reactive protein, and documentation of infection with gonorrhea or chlamydia.

The treatment of PID should provide broad-spectrum coverage of gonorrhea, chlamydia, anaerobes, gram-negatives, and streptococci. Treatment should be initiated as soon as a presumptive diagnosis is made. Hospitalization should be considered when surgical emergencies (such as appendicitis) cannot be excluded, the patient is pregnant, the patient cannot tolerate or does not respond to outpatient treatment, the patient has severe illness (nausea, vomiting, and high fever), or the patient has a tubo-ovarian abscess. Sexual partners of women with PID should be evaluated and appropriately treated as well. *(Centers for Disease Control: www.cdc.gov/mmwr/preview/mmwrhtml/rr5106a1.htm)*

45. **(A)** History is critical in the evaluation and management of vulvar diseases. Given the fact that this patient has had exposures to numerous topical medications, it is likely that she has contact dermatitis of the vulva. Given the lack of hyphae on her wet mount and no apparent abnormal vaginal discharge, a candidal infection is less likely. She is obese and not in the average age range for menopause, thus atrophic findings are unlikely. The wet mount lacks clue cells that establish the diagnosis of bacterial vaginosis. *(Stenchever et al., 2001, pp. 487–488)*

46. **(E)** Labial agglutination is a clinical diagnosis, with a greater prevalence occurring in pediatric or elderly patients. Forced manipulations of the genital region are to be avoided, as the condition readily responds to topical estrogen therapy. *(Bacon, 2002 pp. 327–331)*

47. **(A)**

48. **(D)**

49. **(C)**

Explanations 47 through 49

This patient meets criteria for the diagnosis of osteoporosis, with a T score falling below –2.5 standard SD. A T score indicates the number of standard deviations below or above the average peak bone mass in young, healthy adults of the same gender. Bisphosphonate therapy has been shown to reduce vertebral and hip fracture risk in up to 50% of women with documented osteoporosis. GnRH therapy and

discontinuation of her vitamin D therapy would worsen, not improve, this patient's bone density. Although testosterone may arrest further bone loss, the side effects of the medication are too great compared to any potential benefit. *(Schnitzer et al., 2000, pp. 1–12)*

For women who have osteoporosis the serum calcium level is generally normal. In premenopausal osteoporosis, or more severe cases of bone loss/fractures, the presence of metabolic bone disease should be considered. In hyperparathyroidism the serum calcium is elevated. With renal failure, as with osteomalacia, serum calcium is low. The serum calcium level is normal, and the alkaline phosphatase level is elevated in patients with Paget disease. *(Barbieri, 1998)*

The use of tobacco, a family history of mother or maternal grandmother with hip fractures, postmenopausal state without estrogen replacement, vision problems, and a body mass index of less than 23 are all increased risks for fractures. A body mass index of greater than 23 does not represent an increased risk for fracture. *(Ullom-Minnich, 1999, pp. 194–202)*

50. **(C)** By history and physical examination, this patient most likely has a breast cyst. Given her age, mammography is not helpful due to the density of her breast tissue. Ultrasound is more helpful in detecting fluid-filled breast masses. In-office aspiration would be both diagnostic and therapeutic if the fluid was not bloody. *(Agency for Healthcare Research and Quality, 2001; Lister et al., 1998, pp. 490–492)*

51. **(D)** Clinically, this patient is exhibiting signs and symptoms of overactive bladder syndrome, or urge incontinence. Her risk factors include her age, race, caffeine use, and potential abnormal glucose tolerance. Attention should first be directed toward treating any modifiable risk factors. She does not demonstrate findings or a history of stress urinary incontinence for which surgery might be appropriate. Diuretic therapy could worsen, rather than improve, her symptoms, and she does not have findings consistent with a UTI. *(Montella, 2002, pp. 293–306)*

52. (E) Maternal obstetric injury remains a major cause of rectovaginal fistula in women. For this patient, it is imperative to determine the presence or absence of a concomitant injury to the anal sphincter complex along with the possibility of a fistula. Crohn's disease can be a cause of abdominal pain, diarrhea, anal abscess formation, and fecal incontinence. It would be very unlikely, and highly coincidental, for it to present in this manner. Perianal abscesses can lead to anal fistula formation and subsequent fecal incontinence, but most commonly present with exquisite pain. Fistulas and fecal incontinence would be later complications. Neither a vaginal hematoma nor a retained vaginal foreign body would result in fecal incontinence. *(Strohbehn et al., 2001, pp. 429–438)*

53. (B)

54. (A)

55. (D)

Explanations 53 through 55

Menstrual disorders, primarily oligo- and amenorrhea, are particularly common among women with eating disorders and are thought to be the result of hypothalamic hypoestrogenism. This patient demonstrates estrogen deficiency (decreased breast size, urogenital atrophy). Her dental caries, oral sores, and hand sores might be a result of self-induced vomiting. Hyperthyroidism would be considered in the differential diagnosis of a young woman with weight loss and menstrual irregularities. In contrast to persons with a medical condition that causes weight loss, those with an eating disorder express a disordered body image and, often, a desire to be underweight.

This patient requires additional investigation to assess for the possibility of inpatient admission. Patients with a prolonged, severe eating disorder are at risk for developing dehydration, electrolyte imbalance (especially hypokalemia), cardiac dysrhythmias, and hypothermia. Hospitalization would be considered for those who are severely dehydrated, who have marked electrolyte abnormalities,

who are <75% of their ideal body weight, or who have a comorbid condition that would require hospitalization, such as a severe psychiatric disorder.

Although weight-bearing exercise favors bone formation, when excessive exercise and/or an eating disorder results in amenorrhea, estrogen levels fall. Subsequently, bone mineral density decreases. Persons with eating disorders are at increased risk for comorbid psychiatric conditions including depression, anxiety, obsessive-compulsive disorder, and personality disorders. *(Becker et al., 1999, pp. 1092–1098)*

56. (C)

57. (A)

Explanations 56 and 57

Screening for HIV should be offered to all pregnant women as part of routine prenatal care. Screening for HIV infection is done using an enzyme immunoassay (EIA). If the screening test is positive, it may be repeated. Once the screening test is determined to be positive, a Western blot assay or immunofluorescent antibody assay (IFA) is done as a confirmatory test. If the confirmatory test is positive, the patient is then considered to be infected with HIV. Pregnant patients should be treated for HIV by the same standards as any other adult with HIV, though some consideration is given to selection of antiretroviral medications that are safest in pregnancy. Appropriate HIV-related care should not be deferred because of pregnancy. For patients with significant HIV disease, the combination of elective scheduled cesarean and antiretroviral therapy has been shown to be more effective than antiretrovirals alone at reducing perinatal transmission of HIV. In the absence of any therapy, the risk of vertical transmission is estimated at 25%. With zidovudine therapy, the risk is decreased to approximately 5–8%. When zidovudine is given in combination with elective cesarean for appropriate patients, the risk is decreased to approximately 2%. In a recent meta-analysis, perinatal transmission occurred in only 1% of treated women with RNA viral loads less than 1000 copies/mL. Given the low risk of transmission in this group, it is unclear whether cesarean delivery would provide additional benefit. After reviewing this data, the American College of Obstetricians and Gynecologists Committee on Obstetric Practice has issued a Committee Opinion concerning route of delivery, recommending consideration of scheduled cesarean delivery for HIV-1-infected pregnant women with HIV-1 RNA levels >1000 copies/mL near the time of delivery. *(ACOG, 2000. pp. 233–5; Centers for Disease Control: www.cdc.gov; Gabbe et al., 2002, Chap. 40)*

58. **(B)** Influenza vaccination is recommended to all women who will be in the second or third trimester of pregnancy during the flu season. Poliomyelitis vaccination is not recommended for women in the United States unless they have some increased risk due to travel or exposure. MMR vaccination is contraindicated in pregnancy secondary to a theoretic risk of teratogenicity from the rubella vaccine. MMR should be given to this patient postpartum. RhoGAM is recommended routinely during pregnancy in Rh negative women who are unsensitized to Rh factor. In this case the patient is Rh positive. *(ACOG Compendium.Number 282, 2003; Centers for Disease Control: www.cdc.gov)*

59. **(C)**

60. **(D)**

Explanations 59 and 60

The patient would be best served by a progesterone-only pill as it will be less likely to interfere with breast milk production. The rhythm method cannot be reliably used in the early postpartum period as normal menstrual cycles may not have resumed. An IUD would be contraindicated in this patient because of her recent history of chlamydia infection. Patients may not ovulate during breast-feeding but should not rely on breast-feeding alone as a form of contraception, as pregnancy

can occur while breast-feeding. *(Koetsawang, 1987, pp. 115–127)*

Mastitis is a common complication of breast-feeding. It is characterized by fever, myalgias, and redness with pain in the affected breast. Antibiotic options include penicillin V, ampicillin, or dicloxacillin. Studies show that patients may continue to breast-feed while undergoing treatment for mastitis. *(Gabbe et al., 2002, Chap. 21; Thomsen et al., 1984, pp. 492–495)*

61. **(E)**

62. **(A)**

63. **(D)**

Explanations 61 through 63

The pelvic ultrasound is the most reliable measurement of fetal gestational age in the absence of accurate dating by LMP. A first trimester sonogram is thought to be reliable ±7 days. Given the patient's history, she is likely at least 2 months pregnant. hCG level at this gestation can be variable and is not a useful method of pregnancy dating. A pelvic examination is useful to help confirm likely dating, but is not a reliable means of determining EDD. FSH and LH levels have no role in determining pregnancy dating. *(Gabbe et al., 2002, Chap. 10; Savitz et al., 2002, pp. 1660–1666)*

The risk of postpartum major depression is estimated at 8–20% in all postpartum patients. In those with a previous history of postpartum depression, the risk is thought to be 50–100%. In patients who have had previous depression not associated with pregnancy, the risk of postpartum depression is 20–30%. Maternity blues is a milder psychological reaction that can occur in the early postpartum period and is thought to occur in 70+ % of all postpartum patients. Patients with a history of bipolar disease have a higher risk of recurrence in the postpartum period, and these patients often present with postpartum psychosis symptoms. *(Gabbe et al., 2002, Chap. 21; Gold, 2002, pp. 27–41; Nonacs and Cohen, 2003, pp. 547–562)*

64. (C)

65. (B)

Explanations 64 and 65

Sheehan syndrome is also known as postpartum pituitary necrosis. It is associated with severe blood loss during the early postpartum period. The patient with this syndrome may present acutely with hypotension and shock due to adrenal insufficiency, though often it presents as in this case, with the more gradual onset of symptoms. The most common initial presentation is the inability to lactate. Other symptoms may occur over months to years with the classic patient presenting with failure of lactation, rapid breast involution, amenorrhea, failure to regrow pubic and axillary hair, skin depigmentation, anorexia and nausea, lethargy, weakness, and weight loss. Signs and symptoms may present years after the event. Additionally, on physical examination, patients may have waxy skin, periorbital edema, and decreased skin pigmentation. Sheehan syndrome usually involves the anterior pituitary but can sometimes cause ischemia of the posterior pituitary. With posterior pituitary involvement, vasopressin secretion is diminished resulting in diabetes insipidus. Most cases involve the selective loss of hormone secretion of the anterior pituitary hormones, and the loss is usually incomplete. The clinical manifestation depends on the degree of deficiency and the hormones that are affected. GH deficiency is seen in the majority of patients with Sheehan syndrome followed by ACTH deficiency, hypogonadism, and hypothyroidism. *(Gabbe et al., 2002, Chap. 33; Nader, 2004, pp. 257–285)*

66. (C)

67. (E)

68. (B)

Explanations 66 through 68

In question 66, this patient likely does not have thyroid disease. She is asymptomatic, has a normal physical examination, and her free T4 is normal. hCG shares a chemical subunit with TSH. The circulating hCG can cause suppression of the thyroid. This is a transient change and does not represent true thyroid disease.

Graves' disease is the most common cause of hyperthyroidism in pregnancy. It is the cause of 90–95% of such cases. Patients may complain of rapid heartbeat, weight loss, and GI symptoms such as nausea and vomiting. On examination, you may palpate diffuse thyromegaly and may note exophthalmos. The other listed causes of thyrotoxicosis are much less common in pregnancy, accounting for the remaining 5–10% of cases.

Treatment of this problem is necessary because thyrotoxic women are at increased risk of perinatal mortality, preterm delivery, and maternal heart failure. Treatment is typically with PTU or methimazole. Propranolol can be used initially to reduce symptoms but does not address the underlying problem. Surgery should be reserved for women who do not respond to medical therapy. Radioactive iodine is contraindicated during pregnancy as it can ablate fetal thyroid tissue, leading to the possibility of congenital hypothyroidism. *(Neale & Burro, 2004, 31(2), pp. 893–905; American College of Obstetrics and Gynecology: ACOG Practice Bulletin. Clinical management guidelines for obstetrician-gynecologists. Number 37, August 2002. (Replaces Practice Bulletin Number 32, November 2001). Thyroid disease in pregnancy. Obstet Gynecol 2002 Aug; 100(2): 387–96)*

69. (B)

70. (B)

71. (E)

Explanations 69 through 71

Cystic fibrosis is the most common hereditary condition in Whites with a carrier frequency of 1 in 25. The American College of Obstetricians and Gynecologists, the American College of Medical Genetics, and the National Institutes of Health have recommended that cystic fibrosis carrier screening be offered to all White couples either pregnant or considering a pregnancy, and that the availability of screening be discussed with members of other ethnic groups who have a lower frequency of cystic fibrosis carrier state.

Cystic fibrosis is inherited in an autosomal recessive fashion, so for a couple in which both mother and father are carriers the risk of having an affected child is 25% or 1 in 4. In the case presented, in which the husband's sister has cystic fibrosis, his likelihood of being a carrier is 2 in 3 (since he has an affected sibling, both of his parents are obligate carriers, and since he is not affected, he is either a noncarrier [1 in 3] or a carrier [2 in 3]). This pattern is true for all autosomal recessive disorders. *(American College of Medical Genetics/American College of Obstetricians and Gynecologists/National Institutes of Health Standing Committee, 2001)*

72. (C)

73. (A)

Explanations 72 and 73

The angiotensin-converting enzyme inhibitors (and angiotensin receptor blockers) are contraindicated in pregnancy due to their potential to cause decreased fetal renal perfusion, ultimately resulting in fetal oliguria, oligohydramnios, renal tubular dysplasia, and neonatal anuric renal failure, as well as defects in ossification of the fetal skull. These adverse effects occur during the second and third trimesters of pregnancy. If a woman conceives while taking an angiotensin-converting enzyme inhibitor, she should be changed to another agent during the first trimester. *(Piper et al., 1992, pp. 429–432)*

Preeclampsia causes 50–70% of cases of hypertension in pregnancy. Mild preeclampsia is characterized by an increase in systolic BP of 30 mmHg, an increase in diastolic BP of 15 mmHg, or an absolute reading of 140/90 mmHg in a pregnant patient with minimal proteinuria and pathologic edema. A systolic BP greater than 160/110 mmHg with significant proteinuria (>5000 mg/24 h) and evidence of end-organ damage indicate severe preeclampsia. End-organ damage results from increased vascular reactivity, third spacing of fluids (including peripheral and

cerebral edema), and platelet activation. Complications include oliguria, the syndrome of hemolysis, elevated liver function tests, and low platelets (HELLP) and eclamptic seizures. Seizure prophylaxis is effective in both primary prevention of eclampsia and in prevention of recurrent seizures. Fetal macrosomia occurs more commonly in pregnancies complicated by diabetes. Abnormal labor progress and postpartum hemorrhage as well as breech presentation are not more common in pregnancies complicated by preeclampsia. *(Gabbe et al., 2002)*

74. (C) Magnesium sulfate has been demonstrated in randomized-controlled trials to be superior to any other anticonvulsant agent in prevention of initial eclamptic seizures and prevention of recurrence of eclampsia. Phenytoin would be considered the best alternative in patients who had an absolute contraindication to magnesium sulfate therapy (such as women with myasthenia gravis). *(Witlin and Sibai, 1998, pp. 883–889)*

75. (D) In general, women with diabetes mellitus are at increased risk for congenital abnormalities as well as spontaneous abortion, with the risk rising in direct relationship to the maternal hemoglobin A1C. The risk is particularly increased when the periconception hemoglobin A1C value exceeds 10%. In addition to congenital heart defects, which are increased approximately fivefold over the general population (2.5% vs. 0.5%), open neural defects are thought to be 10 times more common (1% vs. 0.1%). *(Gabbe et al., 2002; Reese and Hobbins, 1986, pp. 325–335)*

76. (B) Women with preexisting diabetes, both type 1 and type 2, are at increased risk both for spontaneous abortion and congenital anomalies, and the risk for these rises in direct relation to the maternal hemoglobin A1C concentration. In general, women with diabetes are at increased risk for late pregnancy complications, including stillbirth and cesarean delivery. The likelihood of fetal macrosomia (birth weight greater than 4000 g) increases with worsening degrees of maternal glycemic control; the macrosomic fetus is at increased risk for birth trauma, including shoulder dystocia and resultant Erb palsy. *(Albert et al., 1996, pp. 1424–1428)*

77. **(D)** Physiologic changes in respiration during pregnancy include reduced total lung capacity and functional residual capacity, increased inspiratory capacity and no change in the vital capacity. Increased progesterone causes a chronic hyperventilation, as reflected by a 30–40% increase in tidal volume and minute ventilation. This rise in minute ventilation results in a decrease in both alveolar and arterial carbon dioxide, with normal arterial partial pressure of carbon dioxide in pregnancy ranging between 27 and 32 mmHg. Overall, the risk of asthma exacerbation is not thought to be higher in pregnancy. The peak expiratory flow rate correlates well with the forced expiratory volume in 1 second, which is an excellent way of monitoring disease state in both pregnant and nonpregnant individuals. The Centers for Disease Control recommends vaccination against influenza during the appropriate season for all pregnant women who will be in the second and third trimester during the time of vaccine administration. This is a killed virus vaccine and has not been demonstrated to be associated with risk to the developing fetus. Similarly, the pelvic radiation dose of a single chest radiograph is approximately 50 mrad, which is well below the threshold of concern for fetal risk of 5 rad. (*Gabbe et al., 2002; Lucius et al., 1970, pp. 311–317*)

78. **(E)** Many women with underlying cardiac disease have increased risk for serious complications during the pregnancy, including maternal mortality. Clark et al. have classified maternal cardiac conditions into mortality groups. Group 1 conditions (including mild mitral stenosis, corrected tetralogy of Fallot, and porcine prosthetic valves) have a maternal mortality rate of less than 1%. Group 2 conditions, which include mechanical prosthetic heart valves, more severe degrees of mitral stenosis, uncorrected congenital heart disease, and mild Marfan syndrome, have a mortality rate of 5–15%. Group 3 conditions include those that have a mortality risk of 50% or higher and include pulmonary hypertension, complicated coarctation of the aorta, and Marfan syndrome with an abnormal aortic root. (*Foley MR, "Cardiac Disease" in Dildy GA, Belfort MA, et al. Critical Care Obstetrics, 4th ed. 2004, Malden, MA: Blackwell Publishing. 252–27*)

79. **(C)** All anticonvulsant drugs are associated with at least some risk of congenital abnormalities. Most anticonvulsants are classified as FDA category D, indicating that there is some demonstrated fetal risk but that the maternal benefits of taking the medication may outweigh the risks to the fetus. Carbamazepine, which for a time was thought to have a lower risk for fetal anomalies than other agents such as phenytoin, is now known to have a risk as high or higher. It particularly contributes to an increased risk when it is part of multidrug therapy for women with epilepsy. While the risk of neural tube defects is known to be elevated in women with epilepsy, and particularly those taking anticonvulsant drugs, no data exist to show that higher doses of folic acid will prevent neural tube defects in this group of women. The risk of open neural tube defects in women taking valproate is thought to be 1% (or 10 times the risk in the general population), and the risk of congenital heart disease is also increased. (*Lindhout and Schmidt, 1986, pp. 1392–1393; Nulman et al., 1997, pp. 18–24*)

80. **(D)** A major congenital anomaly is defined as one that is not compatible with survival or one that requires major corrective surgery to restore normal function. The risk of such anomalies in a general obstetric population is usually reported to be between 2 and 3%. If minor congenital anomalies are included, 7–10% of pregnancies will be affected. (*Wilson and Fraser, 1979*)

81. **(D)** The most common presenting symptom of vulvar cancer is vulvar pruritis. Women diagnosed with vulvar cancer typically experience a 6- to 12-month delay prior to diagnosis secondary to the hesitancy of physicians to biopsy the area in the office in order to establish a histologic diagnosis. Generally, women are prescribed antimonilial creams to address presumed intertriginous yeast infections, or topical steroid creams to relieve the inflammation and associated pruritis. Ultimately, in the absence of improvement, a biopsy will finally be performed and the diagnosis established.

Delay in diagnosis is the leading cause of preventable death in patients diagnosed with vulvar cancer, with the 5-year survival rate dropping off precipitously with advancing stage at diagnosis (*stage I 90%, stage II 80%, stage III 50%, stage IV 15%*). Physicians should have a very low threshold to biopsy cutaneous abnormalities noted on the external genitalia in any patient presenting for a problem visit, or for routine gynecologic care. (*Tyring, 2003, pp. S17–S23*)

82. **(C)** A meta-analysis of 20 studies published from 1970 to 1991 demonstrated a significant reduction in the risk of ovarian epithelial carcinoma with the use of oral contraceptives. The risk of ovarian cancer decreased with increasing duration of oral contraceptive use: a 10–12% decrease in lifetime risk was noted with 1 year of use, a 50% decrease in lifetime risk noted with 5 years of use, and an 80% decrease in lifetime risk associated with 10 years of use. Oral contraceptive therapy has consistently demonstrated in epidemiologic studies the ability to decrease a woman's lifetime risk for the development of ovarian cancer. It is the most effective means of primary prevention in women at high risk for the development of ovarian cancer, short of physically removing the ovaries themselves.

    Both hysterectomy and bilateral tubal ligation have been associated with a 30% decrease in the lifetime risk for the development of ovarian cancer. However, in women yet to complete their childbearing neither is a realistic option. Breast-feeding and increasing parity have been shown to decrease a woman's lifetime risk for the development of ovarian cancer. There are some data to suggest that anti-inflammatory medications (aspirin, NSAID) may decrease the risk of ovarian cancer, but this has yet to be substantiated in epidemiologic studies. (*Gross and Schlesselman, 1994, pp. 419–425*)

83. **(A)** Though 85% of cancers develop spontaneously, approximately 10–12% will arise in patients with an inherited chromosomal defect that places them at increased risk for the development of certain types of cancers. Patients with an inherited defect in a tumor suppressor gene encoded on chromosome 2, for example, have an increased risk for the development of breast, ovarian, endometrial, and ovarian cancers and suffer from a syndrome known as hereditary nonpolyposis colorectal cancer, or Lynch family syndrome type II. Patients with an inherited defect in a tumor suppressor gene encoded on chromosome 17 (BRCA1), on the other hand, have an increased lifetime risk for the development of predominantly breast and ovarian cancer.

    Patients with a BRCA1 chromosomal defect have a 30–50% lifetime risk for the development of ovarian cancer (compared to a 1.4% lifetime risk in the general patient population), a 60–80% lifetime risk for the development of breast cancer (compared to a 10% lifetime risk in the general patient), and an increased lifetime risk for the development of both Fallopian tube cancer as well as peritoneal carcinoma. These cancers generally arise in affected women 10–15 years earlier than when seen in nonaffected women.

    The risk for ovarian and breast cancer in carrier women is sufficiently high to warrant bilateral salpingo-oophorectomy once childbearing is complete, or by the age of 35, whichever comes first, as well as prophylactic bilateral mastectomy. An alternative to prophylactic surgery is a more vigilant screening program, with lifetime annual mammography beginning at the age of 25 and ovarian screening with annual or biannual ultrasound, CA-125 determination, and pelvic examination beginning at the age of 35. The efficacy of these screening programs is unproven. (*Roesser, 2003, pp. 591–594*)

84. **(D)** All patients diagnosed with ovarian cancer require postoperative chemotherapy, with the exception of FIGO stage IA and IB disease. There is some debate as to whether patients with stage IC disease require postoperative chemotherapy. Two large studies (ICON I, GOG 157) would suggest an improvement in overall survival among this group of patients when given postoperative chemotherapy following surgical debulking.

    For those patients requiring postoperative chemotherapy, the combination of carboplatin and paclitaxel represents the current standard. For several years, the combination of cisplatin and cyclophosphamide had been considered the treatment of choice. However, in 1993 a large prospective randomized trial compared cisplatin and cyclophosphamide to cisplatin and paclitaxel in patients with advanced stage disease and found the combination of cisplatin and paclitaxel to be associated with a 50% improvement in median survival. Though this came to be accepted as the new chemotherapeutic standard for the management of ovarian cancer, the nephrotoxicity and neurotoxicity associated with the cisplatin prompted a second large prospective randomized trial, GOG 158. This study compared the efficacy of cisplatin and paclitaxel to carboplatin and paclitaxel in patients with advanced stage disease following optimal surgical debulking. The study found the two arms to be equivalent and actually suggested that the carboplatin/paclitaxel arm may even be superior to the cisplatin/paclitaxel arm in terms of overall survival. This has since become the standard chemotherapeutic management for advanced stage ovarian cancer.

Melphalan, an alkylating agent, was previously used in the treatment of patients with advanced stage ovarian cancer (response rate 35–60%) but has since been replaced by more effective chemotherapeutic agents. Tamoxifen is not used in the primary treatment of ovarian cancer, but rather as a third- or fourth-line agent (response rate 11–18%). (*Ozols, 2000, pp. 3–7*)

85. **(D)** The management of vulvar cancer is primarily a surgical one. In the setting of small volume disease, wide local excision with 2–3 cm margins is generally sufficient. For patients to be candidates for such conservative management, the lesion must be <2 cm in width, <1 mm in depth, with no lymphatic or vascular space invasion and nonpalpable groin nodes.

The majority of patients presenting with vulvar cancer, however, will require a radical vulvectomy and inguinofemoral lymphadenectomy to resect the primary lesion, as well as to evaluate for evidence of metastatic spread. If the lesion is midline, with a midline lesion defined as one less than 2 cm lateral to an imaginary vertical line drawn through the clitoris, urethra, and anal verge, the potential for metastatic spread to either groin is sufficiently

high that both groins should undergo lymphadenectomy. If the lesion is lateralized, however, only the ipsilateral groin needs be dissected. If metastatic tumor is found in two or more groin nodes, postoperative radiation therapy to the involved groin(s) and ipsilateral pelvic nodes has been shown to improve survival. (*Marsden and Hacker, 2001, pp. 799–813*)

86. **(D)** Borderline tumors of the ovary, or tumors of low malignant potential (LMP), represent approximately 15% of all epithelial ovarian tumors. The average age at diagnosis is 40 years of age, 15–20 years earlier than is the average age at diagnosis for the invasive ovarian counterpart.

Roughly 50% of all borderline tumors are serous. Because most borderline serous tumors occur in women of reproductive age and are classified as stage I at the time of diagnosis, treatment is usually conservative. Most patients can be managed with cystectomy or oophorectomy alone; in fact, cystectomy is the treatment of choice in the presence of bilateral borderline ovarian cystic tumors, or when only one ovary remains and fertility is desired. If the patient is perimenopausal, postmenopausal, or has no desire for fertility, hysterectomy with bilateral salpingo-oophorectomy is recommended.

When the diagnosis of borderline tumor is made on the basis of an intraoperative frozen section evaluation, a complete staging procedure is still recommended in the event the final pathology report reveals an invasive cancer. The staging information will be critical in that setting in order to determine the stage of disease present and the need for chemotherapy postoperatively. Surgical staging should include pelvic and abdominal cytology, random peritoneal biopsies (right hemidiaphragm, paracolic gutters, ovarian fossa bilaterally, cul-de-sac, and bladder flap), partial omentectomy, and lymph node sampling.

Unlike invasive ovarian neoplasms, chemotherapy has not been shown to be helpful in the management of ovarian tumors of LMP. LMP tumors have such a low cellular turnover rate that any DNA damage that results following exposure to chemotherapy is easily repaired prior to S-phase associated DNA replication. *(Candiani et al., 1999, pp. 206–210)*

87. **(E)** Despite decades of effort aimed at improving methods of early detection and diagnosis, the majority of cases of cancer of the ovary are not diagnosed until the disease has spread beyond the ovary. The surgical management of epithelial ovarian cancer consists of attempts at maximal surgical cytoreduction at the time of surgical exploration. The surgical goal is to remove all disease, such that at the completion of the debulking procedure no visible remaining disease is present. In order to accomplish this goal, extensive surgical procedures are often required in those patients presenting with advanced stage disease.

Griffiths et al. reviewed the theoretical basis for cytoreductive surgery. Complete removal of bulky ovarian tumor masses improves patient survival when compared to inadequate or incomplete surgical cytoreduction, in three specific ways:

1. Maximal surgical debulking enables the resection of hypoxic tumor sanctuaries in which viable tumor cells have the ability to escape exposure to adequate concentrations of chemotherapy postoperatively.
2. Maximal surgical debulking enables the resection of large tumor masses containing chemoresistant tumor clones that do not respond well to any form of postoperative chemotherapy.
3. Maximal surgical debulking enables the resection of large tumor masses, thereby reducing the tumor burden to such an extent that all remaining cells in the G0 resting state will now return to the actively dividing cell cycle, where they are more amenable to chemotherapeutic damage and ultimate cell kill.

Numerous investigators (Griffiths, Munnell, Delclos and Quinlan, Hoskins, Eisenkop) have consistently confirmed the biggest single prognosticator predicting how well a patient will respond, and how long they will live, following treatment for ovarian cancer is the volume of disease remaining following their initial surgical debulking. Patients left with residual deposits

of disease >2 cm in diameter are considered suboptimally debulked and do no better than patients who have no surgical debulking procedure performed. Optimal surgical cytoreduction, on the other hand, is defined as no residual deposit of disease remaining greater than 1 cm in maximal dimension. The smaller the residual disease remaining (no deposit >.5 cm, no deposit >.25 cm, and so on), the longer the overall survival of the patient, with those left with no visible remaining disease having the longest overall survival of all as a rule. Given the immense amount of retrospective data supporting the importance of optimal surgical debulking in the patient's overall outcome and survival, all attempts must be made at the time of initial surgical cytoreduction to obtain an optimal debulking, preferably one with no visible remaining disease at completion. *(Mutch, 2002, pp. 3–8)*

88. **(B)** The femoral nerve is the most commonly injured nerve at the time of gynecologic surgical procedures. The nerve can be injured at the time of laparotomy through the inappropriate placement of lateral retractor blades with fixed or self-retaining retractors. The retractor blades, when placed too deeply within the lateral pelvis, have the potential to directly compress the psoas muscle and thereby, the femoral nerve within the psoas muscle. The more prolonged the nerve compression, the more pronounced and long lasting the injury postoperatively. The femoral nerve can also be injured at the time of vaginal surgery as a result of inappropriate lithotomy positioning, with extreme hip flexion and maximal knee extension most commonly associated with injury.

The femoral nerve is a component of the lumbosacral nerve plexus and provides both motor as well as sensory function. Injury to the femoral nerve will present with diminished or absent deep tendon reflexes, inability to straight leg raise, hip flex, or knee extend. There may also be a loss of cutaneous sensation over the anterior thigh as well as the medial aspect of the thigh and calf.

Neurologic injuries following gynecologic surgical procedures are rare, complicating approximately 1–3% of all gynecologic surgical procedures. Once these injuries occur, postoperative physical therapy is generally required, often with braces, until neurologic function returns. Careful attention to retractor blade placement at the time of laparotomy and to appropriate lithotomy positioning at the time of vaginal surgical procedures can minimize the potential for neurologic injury at the time of surgery.

DVT will generally present with asymmetric lower extremity swelling postoperatively, but without associated motor or sensory neurologic deficits. An undetected cerebrovascular accident intraoperatively will generally present with more widespread central deficits than the focal lower extremity deficit seen in this example. Injury to the sciatic nerve will present with a different constellation of neurologic deficits, including inability to extend at the hip, flex at the knee, ankle dorsiflex, and evert. Undiagnosed diabetes can present with a variety of neurologic sequelae including peripheral neuropathy, nephropathy, and retinopathy. Rarely will undiagnosed diabetic neuropathy present with such a focal deficit as seen in this case scenario. (*Irvin et al., 2004, pp. 374–382*)

89. (B)

90. (C)

91. (E)

Explanations 89 through 91

The fetal monitoring strip in these questions shows the presence of early decelerations. Early decelerations are characterized by a gradual decrease in the fetal heart rate and gradual return to the baseline in association with a contraction. The onset and recovery of the heart rate are coincident with the onset and recovery of the contraction. These are thought to be due to vagal stimulation due to fetal head compression. They are not associated with fetal hypoxia or acidosis and no intervention, other than continued careful labor monitoring, is indicated.

Variable decelerations are caused by umbilical cord compression. They are characterized by the abrupt decrease in heart rate. The onset of the deceleration frequently varies in successive contractions, and they generally last less than 2 minutes. Late decelerations are gradual decreases in heart rate that begin at or after the peak of the contraction and return to baseline after the contraction has ended. It is often the first fetal heart rate abnormality seen in uteroplacental-induced hypoxia. Any process that causes maternal hypotension, excessive uterine activity, or placental dysfunction can induce late decelerations. Fetal tachycardia is defined as a baseline fetal heart rate of >160 bpm and is considered severe if the rate is >180 bpm. The most common cause of this is maternal fever, but it can also be due to fetal compromise, arrhythmias, or certain medications. Hyperstimulation is a nonreassuring heart rate pattern caused by the presence of frequent uterine contractions. This occurs most commonly in labors that are being augmented with oxytocin. The initial management includes reduction in the dose, or discontinuation, of the oxytocin. (*Cunningham et al., 2001, pp. 336–344*)

92. (B) In randomized-controlled trials, the daily administration of 0.4 mg of folic acid in the periconception period was shown to prevent the first occurrence of open neural tube defects by approximately 70% as compared to placebo. For women who have previously had a fetus with an open neural defect, the recommended dose for prevention of recurrence is 4 mg and has been shown to have approximately 70% effectiveness in preventing recurrence. (*American College of Obstetricians and Gynecologists Practice Bulletin 44; Czeizel and Dudas, 1992, pp. 1832–1835*)

93. (A)

94. (C)

Explanations 93 and 94

Down syndrome is a trisomy of chromosome 21. It is the most common nonlethal trisomy. Patau syndrome is trisomy 13 and Edwards syndrome is trisomy 18. Turner syndrome is 45 X, a monosomy. Klinefelter syndrome is the presence of an extra X chromosome in a male resulting in 47 X-X-Y.

Down syndrome is the most commonly recognized genetic cause of mental retardation.

The risk of trisomy 21 is directly related to maternal age as a result of maternal nondisjunction. The risk of having a child with Down syndrome increases in a gradual, linear fashion until about age 30 and increases exponentially thereafter. Women who will be 35 years or older at the time of delivery should be offered chorionic villus sampling or second-trimester amniocentesis. Women younger than 35 years should be offered maternal serum screening at 16–18 weeks of gestation. The maternal serum markers used to screen for trisomy 21 are alpha-fetoprotein, unconjugated estriol, and hCG. The use of ultrasound to estimate gestational age improves the sensitivity and specificity of maternal serum screening. (*Cunningham et al., 2001, pp. 288–291*)

95. (C)

96. (D)

97. (B)

Explanations 95 through 97

Discussing the potential implications of her sexual activity is warranted, both in terms of potential pregnancy and risk of acquiring sexually transmitted infections. Making assumptions about her decision making (choices B and D) would breach the ethical principles of autonomy and confidentiality. (*American College of Obstetricians and Gynecologists, pp. 1–17*)

In August 2006, the FDA approved emergency oral contraception (Plan B) to be available over the counter for women ages 18 and older. Younger women must have a prescription from a health care provider. Plan B contains 0.75 mg of levonorgestrel in two doses taken 12 hours apart. It is to be used within 72 hours of unprotected intercourse. The mechanisms of action include delay in ovulation, insufficient corpus luteum function, and interference with sperm transport. It is not an abortifacient. (*American College of Obstetricians and Gynecologists, 2001*)

A physician is not obligated to provide treatments which conflict with his or her own personal belief system. Nonetheless, using ethical principles of autonomy, beneficence, nonmaleficence, veracity, and justice, physicians should discuss patients' requests for treatments in an attempt to reach common ground. If that is not possible, the physician should provide an alternative resource to address a patient's request. (*American College of Obstetricians and Gynecologists, pp. 1–17*)

98. (D)

99. (B)

Explanations 98 and 99

At this point in time, the patient would appear to be incapacitated, and unable to provide informed consent for herself. Given her baseline medical conditions, one would hope that the patient has a durable power of attorney for health care, with a designated surrogate decision maker. All attempts should be made to contact that person prior to initiating any procedures or surgery. It is unclear at this point in time as to whether or not this patient's dementia is being impacted by delirium. Restraints and/or additional sedation would not be appropriate unless the patient is posing a harm to herself or others. (*American College of Obstetricians and Gynecologists, p. 15*)

In 1996, Congress enacted the Health Insurance Portability and Accountability Act (HIPAA). It provides standards for health information transactions and security of patient data. Under the HIPAA regulations, Health care providers must obtain the individual's written consent prior to disclosure of health information except in the management of emergencies or if the consent can be inferred from a patient with impaired communication. In this situation, where the patient is not capable of giving this consent, efforts should be made to identify a surrogate decision maker. As that person has not yet been identified, it would be appropriate to ask the caller if she could assist in identifying a previously designated decision maker. However, it would not be appropriate to disclose protected information to her at this time. *Office for Civil Rights - HIPAA Medical Privacy - National Standards to Protect the Privacy of Personal Health Information (http://www.hhs.gov/ocr/hipaa/finalreg.html)*

BIBLIOGRAPHY

Agency for Healthcare Research and Quality. *Diagnosis and Management of Specific Breast Abnormalities.* Evidence Report/Technology Assessment 33. AHRQ Publication No. 01-E-046. Rockville, MD: AHRQ, 2001.

Albert TJ, Landon MB, Wheller JJ. Prenatal detection of fetal anomalies in pregnancies complicated by insulin-dependent diabetes mellitus. *Am J Obstet Gynecol* 1996;174:1424–1428.

American College of Obstetricians and Gynecologists (ACOG) Committee Opinion Number 219: Scheduled Cesarean Delivery and the Prevention of Vertical Transmission of HIV Infection. 2000 Compendium of Selected Publications. Washington, DC: ACOG, 2000. pp. 233–5.

Anne-Marie L, Beth P. Diagnosis and management of ectopic pregnancy. *Am Fam Physician* 2005;72: 1707–1714.

Bacon JL. Prepubertal labial adhesions: evaluation of a referral population. *Am J Obstet Gynecol* 2002;187(2):327–331.

Barakat RR. Tamoxifen and the endometrium. *Cancer Treat Res* 1998;94:195–207.

Barbieri RL. Osteoporosis. *ACOG Educ Bulletin* number 246, 1998.

Becker AE, Grinspoon SK, Klibanski A, et al. Eating disorders. *N Engl J Med* 1999;340:1092–1098.

Beckmann CRB, Ling FW, Laube DW, et al. *Obstetrics and Gynecology*, 4th ed. Baltimore, MD: Lippincot Williams & Wilkins, 2002.

Buttram VD, Reiter RC. Uterine leiomyomata: etiology, symptomatology, and management. *Fertil Steril* 1981;36:433–445.

Candiani M, Vasile C, Sgherzi MR, et al. Contemporary treatment of borderline ovarian tumors. *Cancer Invest* 1999;17(3):206–210.

Centers for Disease Control: www.cdc.gov/mmwr/ preview/mmwrhtml/rr5106a1.htm.

Coates KW, Harris RL, Cundiff GW, et al. Uroflowmetry in women with urinary incontinence and pelvic organ prolapse. *Br J Urol* 1997;80:217–221.

Corfman RS, Davis J, Bryant BJ. Ovarian surgery. In: Gershenson DM, DeCherney AH, et al. *Operative Gynecology*, 2nd ed. Philadelphia, PA: W.B. Saunders, 2001, pp. 676–677.

Cunningham FG, Gant NF, Leveno KJ, et al. *Williams Obstetrics*, 21st ed. New York, NY: McGraw-Hill, 2001.

Czeizel AE, Dudas I. Prevention of the first occurrence of neural tube defects by periconceptional vitamin supplementation. *N Engl J Med* 1992;327: 1832–1835.

Estrogen replacement therapy and endometrial cancer. American College of Obstetricians and Gynecologists (ACOG) Committee Opinion: Committee on Gynecologic Practice Number 126—August 1993. *Int J Gynaecol Obstet.* 1993 Oct;43(1):89.

Gabbe SG, Niebyl JR, Simpson JL. *Obstetrics: Normal and Problem Pregnancies*, 4th ed. New York, NY: Churchill Livingstone, 2002.

Gold LH. Postpartum disorders in primary care. *Prim Care Clin Office Pract* 2002;29(2):27–41.

Good AE. Diagnostic options for assessment of postmenopausal bleeding. *Mayo Clin Proc* 1997;72:345–349.

Gross TP, Schlesselman JJ. The estimated effect of oral contraceptive use on the cumulative risk of epithelial ovarian cancer. *Obstet Gynecol* 1994;83:419–425.

Hillard PA. Benign diseases of the female reproductive tract: symptoms and signs. In: Berek JS, ed. *Novak's Gynecology*, 12th ed. Baltimore, MD: Lippincott Williams & Wilkins, 1996, pp. 331–397.

Irvin W, Andersen W, Taylor P, et al. Minimizing the risk of neurologic injury in gynecologic surgery. *Obstet Gynecol* 2004;103(2):374–382.

Koetsawang S. The effects of contraceptive methods on the quality and quantity of breast milk. *Int J Gynaecol Obstet* 1987;25(Suppl):115–127.

Lindhout D, Schmidt D. In utero exposure to valproate in neural tube effects. *Lancet* 1986;2:1392–1393.

Lister D, Evans AJ, Burrell HC, et al. The accuracy of breast ultrasound in the valuation of clinically benign discrete, symptomatic breast lumps. *Clin Radiol* 1998;53:490–492.

Lucius H, Gahlenbeck H, Kleine H, et al. Respiratory functions, buffer system, electrolyte concentration of blood during human pregnancy. *Respir Physiol* 1970;9:311–317.

Marsden DE, Hacker NF. Contemporary management of primary carcinoma of the vulva. *Surg Clin North Am* 2001;81(4):799–813.

Marx JA, Hockberger RS, Walls RM, eds. *Rosen's Emergency Medicine: Concepts and Clinical Practice*, 6th ed. St. Louis, MO: Mosby, 2006, Chap. 205.

McIntosh DG. Pap smear screening after hysterectomy. *Compr Ther* 1998;24:14–18.

Montella JM. Management of overactive bladder. In: Bent AE, Ostergard DR, et al *Ostergard's Urogynecology and Pelvic Floor Dysfunction*, 5th ed. Philadelphia, PA: Lippincott Williams & Wilkins, 2003, pp. 293–306.

Morrow CP, Curtin JP. *Gynecologic Cancer Surgery.* New York, NY: Churchill Livingstone, 1996.

Mutch DG. Surgical management of ovarian cancer. *Semin Oncol* 2002;29(Suppl 1):3–8.

Nader S. Thyroid disease and other endocrine disorders in pregnancy. *Obstet Gynecol Clin* 2004;31(2): 257–285.

Neale D, Burrow G. Thyroid Disease in Pregnancy Obstet Gynecol Clin North Am 2004;31(2):893–905.

Nonacs R, Cohen LS. Assessment and treatment of depression during pregnancy: an update. *Psychiatr Clin North Am* 2003;26(3):547–562.

Nulman I, Scolnik D, Chitayat D, et al. Findings in children exposed in utero to phenytoin and carbamazepine monotherapy: independent effects of epilepsy and medications. *Am J Med Genet* 1997;68:18–24.

Ozols RF. Paclitaxel (Taxol)/carboplatin combination chemotherapy in the treatment of advanced ovarian cancer. *Semin Oncol* 2000;27:3–7.

Piper JM, Ray WA, Rosa FW, et al. Pregnancy outcome following exposure to angiotensin converting enzyme inhibitors. *Obstet Gynecol* 1992;80:429–432.

Reese EA, Hobbins JC. Diabetic embryopathy: pathogenesis prenatal diagnosis and prevention. *Obstet Gynecol Surv* 1986;41:325–335.

Roesser KA. Understanding hereditary breast and ovarian cancer. *Clin J Oncol Nurs* 2003;7(5):591–594.

Savitz DA, Terry JW, Dole N, et al. Comparison of pregnancy dating by last menstrual period, ultrasound scanning and their combination. *Am J Obstet Gynecol* 2002;187(6):1660–1666.

Schnitzer T, Bone HG, Crepaldi G, et al. Therapeutic equivalence of alendronate 70 mg once weekly and alendronate 10 mg daily in the treatment of osteoporosis. *Aging (Milano)* 2000;12:1–12.

Speroff L, Glass RH, Kase NG. *Clinical Gynecologic Endocrinology and Infertility*, 6th ed. Baltimore, MD: Lippincot Williams & Wilkins, 1999.

Stenchever M, Droegemueller W, Herbst AL, et al. *Comprehensive Gynecology*, 4th ed. St. Louis, MO: Mosby, 2001.

Stovall TG, Muneyyirci-Delale O, Summitt RL Jr, et al. GnRH agonist and iron versus placebo and iron in the anemic patient before surgery for leiomyomas: a randomized controlled trial. *Obstet Gynecol* 1995;86:65–71.

Strohbehn K, Hackford A, Aronson M. Surgical treatment of anal incontinence and rectovaginal fistulas. In: Gershenson DM, DeCherney AH, et al. *Operative Gynecology,* 2nd ed. Philadelphia, PA: W.B. Saunders, 2001, pp. 429–438.

The American College of Obstetricians and Gynecologists. Prolog. Gynecologic Oncology and Surgery, 4th ed. Washington, D.C.: ACOG, 2001.

Thomsen AC, Espersen T, Maigaard S. Course and treatment of milk stasis, noninfectious inflammation of the breast, and infectious mastitis in nursing women. *Am J Obstet Gynecol* 1984;149:492–495.

Tyring SK. Vulvar squamous cell carcinoma: guidelines for early diagnosis and treatment. *Am J Obstet Gynecol* 2003;189(Suppl 3):S17–S23.

Ullom-Minnich P. Prevention of osteoporosis and fractures. *Am Fam Physician* 1999;60:194–202.

Vasen HFA, Wijnen JT, Menko FH, et al. Cancer risk in families with hereditary nonpolyposis colorectal cancer diagnosed by mutation analysis. *Gastroenterology* 1996;110:1020–1027.

Weinberger M. Differential diagnosis of urinary incontinence. In: Bent AE, Ostergard DR, et al. *Ostergard's Urogynecology and Pelvic Floor Dysfunction*, 5th ed. Philadelphia, PA: Lippincott Williams & Wilkins, 2003, pp. 64–65.

Wharton JT, Tortolero-Luna G, Linares AC, et al. Vaginal intraepithelial neoplasia and vaginal cancer. *Obstet Gynecol Clin North Am* 1996;23:325–345.

Wilson JG, Fraser FC, eds. *Handbook of Teratology.* New York, NY: Plenum Press, 1979.

Winter R. Conservative surgery for microinvasive carcinoma of the cervix. *J Obstet Gynaecol Res* 1998;24:433–436.

Witlin AG, Sibai BM. Magnesium sulfate therapy in preeclampsia and eclampsia. *Obstet Gynecol* 1998;92:883–889.

Wright TC, Cox JT, Massas LS, et al. *2001 Consensus Guidelines for the Management of Women with Cervical Cytological Abnormalities*. JAMA 2002; 287:2120–2129.

Wright VC, Chapman W. Intraepithelial neoplasia of the lower female genital tract: etiology, investigation, and management. *Semin Surg Oncol* 1992;8:180–190.

Zaleznik DF, Kasper DL. Intraabdominal Infections and Abscesses in Braunwald E, Fauci AS, Kasper DL, et al. *Harrison's Principles of Internal Medicine*, 15th ed. New York, NY: McGraw-Hill, 2001, pp. 831–2.

CHAPTER 5

Psychiatry
Questions

Questions 1 and 2

A 29-year-old woman presents to the primary care clinic complaining of frequent headaches for several months. During the interview she appears tearful and withdrawn, with minimal eye contact and reluctance to answer questions. With further encouragement and support, she is able to describe intense feelings of sadness, along with significant insomnia, poor concentration, fatigue, anhedonia, and little appetite with a 20-lb weight loss.

1. Before she leaves the office, what is the most important question to ask her?

   (A) "Have you been drinking alcohol or using illicit drugs recently?"
   (B) "Have you been taking any over-the-counter medications?"
   (C) "Have you been treated for any medical conditions?"
   (D) "Have you ever felt like this before?"
   (E) "Have you had thoughts of hurting yourself?"

2. It is decided to begin treatment for her depressive symptoms with pharmacotherapy. Regarding the selection of the specific class of medication, a family history of what would be crucial?

   (A) allergies
   (B) depressive symptoms
   (C) manic symptoms
   (D) medical illnesses
   (E) substance abuse

Questions 3 and 4

The patient is a 28-year-old divorced female who presents in the emergency room complaining of insomnia. Further history reveals that she has been depressed since the divorce settlement 3 months ago. She also has anergia, poor concentration, decreased appetite with a 15-lb weight loss, anhedonia, and guilt surrounding her "failed marriage." She reluctantly admits to pervasive thoughts of killing herself, with a plan to overdose on two bottles of Tylenol as "I heard it can kill you." She has purchased the medicine and written a suicide note. She asks to leave to go home, and when discussion of admission is brought up, she becomes angry and demands to be discharged from the emergency room.

3. What is the next most appropriate course of action?

   (A) admit her to the hospital involuntarily
   (B) admit her to the hospital voluntarily
   (C) discharge her against medical advice
   (D) discharge her with instructions to return in the morning
   (E) prescribe a selective serotonin reuptake inhibitor (SSRI) and provide outpatient follow-up

4. The above decision is based on which of the following ethical principles?

   (A) autonomy
   (B) beneficence
   (C) confidentiality
   (D) justice
   (E) nonmaleficence

Questions 5 and 6

A 40-year-old male is returning to the office for a follow-up visit. He is told about his blood work results, which are consistent with leukemia. He is informed that he should receive a bone marrow biopsy for further clarification. While being presented with this information, he remains silent, peering, and staring intensely. When finished, he comments, "Doctors think they are so smart!" He then explains that he has been mistreated by physicians in the past and, in fact, has several malpractice suits pending. He feels that the biopsy was recommended only "because you want to use me in order to publish and further your career."

5. Based on the above, what is his most likely diagnosis?

   (A) antisocial personality disorder
   (B) narcissistic personality disorder
   (C) paranoid personality disorder
   (D) schizoid personality disorder
   (E) schizotypal personality disorder

6. When interacting with this patient, which of the following approaches would be most effective?

   (A) defend the recommendation by citing professional credentials
   (B) encourage him to speak with a psychiatrist to provide added support
   (C) interpret his anger as a defense against his fears of having leukemia
   (D) provide detailed information regarding his differential diagnosis
   (E) refer him to a colleague to avoid litigation

Questions 7 and 8

A 38-year-old married female is brought in to the primary care clinic by her husband. She is minimally responsive to questioning, head bowed, and staring at the floor. Most of the history is obtained from her spouse. He denies any known personal or family history of mental illness, but he claims for the past several months his wife has become increasingly depressed and withdrawn. Instead of taking part in her usual hobbies, she is lying around the house. "She tosses and turns" throughout the night. Her husband ensures that she eats a limited amount of food, but she has lost a significant amount of weight. She has been ruminating about guilty feelings regarding a number of issues and recently has been speaking about suicide, although she has no plan or intent. She has refused to come in to see a doctor. Her husband insisted that she come today, as she informed him that the devil has possessed her and told her she will "go to hell."

7. What is her most likely diagnosis?

   (A) bipolar disorder, depressed, with psychotic features
   (B) delusional disorder, somatic type
   (C) major depressive disorder with psychotic features
   (D) schizoaffective disorder, depressed type
   (E) schizophrenia, paranoid type

8. What is the most effective pharmacologic treatment for this patient?

   (A) antidepressant alone
   (B) antidepressant and antipsychotic
   (C) antipsychotic alone
   (D) mood stabilizer alone
   (E) mood stabilizer and antipsychotic

Questions 9 and 10

A 16-year-old girl is brought into the family practice clinic for her yearly health maintenance examination. Her height is average and her weight is above average. When this is mentioned to her, she blushes and quickly states that she is trying to lose weight. When asked further about her dieting habits, she eventually admits to routinely eating large amounts of food at one sitting, such as two pizzas, a large sandwich, and a gallon of ice cream. She also confides that she frequently will self-induce vomiting in order to compensate but denies laxative use. She realizes that her behavior is unhealthy, but she feels "out of control."

9. Routine blood work would most likely demonstrate which of the following?

   (A) acidosis
   (B) hyperchloremia

(C) hypernatremia

(D) hypokalemia

(E) leukopenia

10. After discussion of her condition with her parents, it is decided to begin her on psychotropic medication and refer her to an eating disorder program. What class of pharmacotherapy would be the most efficacious in this patient?

(A) anticonvulsants

(B) antipsychotics

(C) benzodiazepines

(D) mood stabilizers

(E) SSRIs

Questions 11 and 12

A 4-year-old boy is brought into the emergency room by his mother for evaluation. When the child is asked regarding specific complaints, he looks anxiously away and states, "It hurts when I go pee-pee." His mother confidently adds, "He has another urinary tract infection (UTI)." She lists the antibiotics that he has been treated with in the past and then demands that he be admitted for a workup. On examination, his vitals signs are unremarkable except for a temperature of 102°F. His physical examination is notable for suprapubic tenderness and some evidence of recent urethral trauma. His urinalysis is consistent with a UTI. Further review of his medical chart reveals multiple emergency room visits for various physical complaints including similar presentations for recurrent UTIs. Prior inpatient and outpatient assessments have not been able to adequately account for any underlying etiologies.

11. What is the most appropriate next step in the management of this patient?

(A) admit to inpatient and notify child protective services

(B) confront the mother regarding the suspicions

(C) consult with a psychiatrist to speak with the mother

(D) refer the patient to a urologist

(E) treat the patient for a UTI and send home

12. What is the most likely explanation for the mother's behavior?

(A) conscious production of symptoms to assume the sick role

(B) conscious production of symptoms to obtain secondary gain

(C) expectable reaction from a concerned parent

(D) hysterical reaction from an overly concerned parent

(E) unconscious production of symptoms due to unconscious conflict

Questions 13 and 14

A 40-year-old single male with chronic schizophrenia is seen for a routine primary care clinic appointment for diabetes management. He is currently taking glyburide 5 mg bid and aripiprazole (Abilify) 20 mg daily. He claims to be compliant with his medications but appears poorly groomed with noticeable body odor. He is reluctant to talk, being somewhat guarded, but he eventually confides that he has been programmed by the government to kill his landlord, who he is convinced is working for Al Qaeda. His orders have been transmitted through his apartment walls to a receiver in his brain. He has been informed that if he does not comply, he will be sent to hell, so he has recently purchased several knives and plans to carry out "my mission" as soon as possible. When the subject of voluntary admission is brought up, he adamantly refuses.

13. What is the most appropriate next step in his management?

(A) admit the patient involuntarily

(B) call the landlord and warn him

(C) continue current medications with close follow-up

(D) discuss the potential legal issues with the patient

(E) switch the patient to another atypical antipsychotic

14. After consultation with a psychiatrist, the decision is made to admit the patient involuntarily. This course of action is in compliance with which of the following forensic psychiatry provisions?

(A) Durham rule
(B) M'Naghten rule
(C) Tarasoff I
(D) Tarasoff II
(E) Testamentary capacity

Questions 15 and 16

A 19-year-old newly married female presents to the emergency room, accompanied by her spouse. She states that she awoke this morning to find that she could not move her legs. She denies any pain but claims that she is unable to feel anything below her abdomen. She denies any trauma or past medical history. She is 24 weeks' pregnant, has had an uneventful pregnancy, and only takes prenatal vitamins. She is concerned if her symptoms will get better and wonders whether the "baby is pulling on my spinal cord." Her neurologic examination is remarkable for 0/5 motor strength in her lower extremities bilaterally, with decreased sensation to light touch and pinprick below the level of her umbilicus. Her cranial nerves and reflexes are normal, and she does not display any upper motor neuron signs. A STAT MRI performed is read as normal.

15. Which of the following is the most likely explanation for her current symptoms?

(A) conscious production of symptoms to assume the sick role
(B) conscious production of symptoms to obtain secondary gain
(C) pathology involving the central nervous system
(D) pathology involving the peripheral nervous system
(E) unconscious production of symptoms due to unconscious conflict

16. Which of the following is the most appropriate approach for this patient?

(A) administer intravenous fluids, informing her it will cure her symptoms
(B) admit her to the inpatient neurologic unit for further tests
(C) confront the patient regarding the nature of her symptoms
(D) obtain consultation with a psychiatrist in the emergency room
(E) reassure her and suggest that her symptoms will improve

17. A 30-year-old woman with a prior history of depression is attending her postpartum follow-up appointment after the birth of her first child. She has no physical complaints and her examination demonstrates no significant problems. She appears anxious. When asked, she describes intrusive thoughts of wanting to harm her baby but quickly states, "I'm not like that. I would never do anything to hurt him."

Which of the following is the most appropriate next step in her management?

(A) assess further for symptoms of psychosis and support system
(B) begin immediate treatment with an antidepressant
(C) call child protective services in order to have the child removed
(D) hospitalize the woman immediately for further evaluation
(E) reassure her that these thoughts are normal

Questions 18 and 19

An 80-year-old woman is admitted to the medical service for treatment of a UTI. While she is hospitalized, she is evaluated for confusion. On her mental status examination (MSE), she appears somnolent at times, fluctuating with an alert state. She is not cooperative, is hostile, and clearly is hallucinating at times. Her insight and memory are poor. The differential diagnosis includes both delirium and dementia.

18. Which of the following signs/symptoms is the most specific for delirium?

    (A) aggressiveness
    (B) fluctuating consciousness
    (C) poor memory
    (D) psychosis
    (E) uncooperativeness

19. Which of the following is the most appropriate pharmacotherapy for her behavioral management?

    (A) low-dose diphenhydramine (Benadryl)
    (B) low-dose donepezil (Aricept)
    (C) low-dose haloperidol (Haldol)
    (D) low-dose lorazepam (Ativan)
    (E) low-dose risperidone (Risperdal)

Questions 20 and 21

A young White female, age unknown, is brought into the emergency room after being found unresponsive at the bus station. She is obtunded and her vitals signs are temperature 97.8°F, blood pressure (BP) 94/60, pulse 55, and respirations 8. Her physical examination is notable for a markedly underweight, poorly groomed woman. She appears pale with cold, dry skin and mucous membranes. She is uncooperative with the examination. Her pupils are pinpoint and minimally reactive to light. Her cardiac examination demonstrates bradycardia without murmurs or rubs. Her lungs are clear with shallow breathing. Her abdomen appears to be slightly distended.

20. Intake of which of the following substances would most likely account for her presentation?

    (A) alcohol
    (B) anticholinergic
    (C) benzodiazepine
    (D) heroin
    (E) phencyclidine (PCP)

21. Administration of which of the following would be most appropriate?

    (A) disulfiram (Antabuse)
    (B) flumazenil (Romazicon)
    (C) naloxone (Narcan)
    (D) physostigmine
    (E) thiamine

Questions 22 and 23

A 30-year-old married male with a history of depression presents to the family medicine clinic. He appears embarrassed and somewhat anxious during his appointment. He denies significant sadness or crying spells. He is sleeping adequately and eating well, without recent changes in his weight. His energy and concentration are normal, and he denies any suicidal or homicidal ideation. He claims to be compliant with his citalopram (Celexa), which he is taking for his depression, but he complains of "problems with sex."

22. Which of the following symptoms would this patient most likely exhibit?

    (A) decreased libido
    (B) painful intercourse
    (C) premature ejaculation
    (D) priapism
    (E) retrograde ejaculation

23. Consideration is given to switching the patient to another antidepressant in order to minimize his side effects. Which of the following would be the most appropriate medication to choose?

    (A) desipramine (Norpramin)
    (B) fluoxetine (Prozac)
    (C) mirtazepine (Remeron)
    (D) phenelzine (Nardil)
    (E) venlafaxine (Effexor)

Questions 24 and 25

An 86-year-old woman is brought to the emergency room by her daughter. The patient is a poor historian with limited insight. Her daughter understands that she has a history of high BP and is treated with an unknown medication. The patient has been living by herself in a retirement community. The daughter became concerned a year prior, when she noticed that her mother seemed more confused. She had attributed this to "old age," but 2 weeks ago she noticed an abrupt worsening in her condition. Her mother now has difficulty recognizing close relatives and remembering information. For the past 2 weeks, she has been getting lost, forgetting to turn off the stove, and has been unable to bathe herself. The daughter is concerned that she may inadvertently harm herself.

24. An MRI of the brain would most likely demonstrate which of the following findings?

(A) caudate nucleus atrophy
(B) dilated ventricles without atrophy
(C) frontotemporal atrophy
(D) generalized atrophy
(E) white matter infarcts

25. Which of the following will be the most likely course of her illness?

(A) gradual improvement
(B) rapid decline
(C) stable course
(D) steady worsening
(E) stepwise deterioration

Questions 26 and 27

A 67-year-old man is seen in the clinic for a scheduled visit. He complains of walking difficulties that have progressively worsened over many months. He also has noticed "shaking" of his hands, resulting in his dropping objects occasionally. He is greatly upset by these problems and admits to frequent crying spells. His only chronic medical illnesses are gastroesophageal reflux disease and hyperlipidemia. He is currently prescribed a proton pump inhibitor and cholesterol-lowering agent. His MSE is notable for little expression or range of affect. His vitals signs are within normal

limits. On physical examination, there is a noticeable coarse tremor of his hands, left greater than right. His gait is slow moving and broad-based.

26. Which of the following brain structures is most likely affected in this man's condition?

(A) caudal raphe nuclei
(B) hippocampus
(C) locus ceruleus
(D) nucleus basalis of Meynert
(E) substantia nigra

27. Some time after initiation of treatment with the proper medication, he becomes agitated and is noted to be hallucinating. Which of the following medications would be the most appropriate to treat these new symptoms?

(A) clozapine (Clozaril)
(B) haloperidol (Haldol)
(C) risperidone (Risperdal)
(D) quetiapine (Seroquel)
(E) thioridazine (Mellaril)

28. A 32 year-old male presents to the primary care clinic with recurrent episodes of bronchitis. He is otherwise healthy but admits to a 14 pack-year history of cigarette smoking. He is prescribed another trial of appropriate antibiotics, but he has "had enough" of smoking and wants to quit. Use of which of the following modalities would most likely give him the best chance of quitting?

(A) bupropion
(B) nicotine gum
(C) nicotine inhaler
(D) nicotine nasal spray
(E) nicotine patch plus behavioral therapy

Questions 29 and 30

The patient is a 28-year-old female medical student who is referred to the Office of Student Affairs due to receiving an incomplete on her surgery clerkship. Upon questioning, she admits to "sneaking out" of the operating room in order to avoid participating in surgeries. When confronted with her unprofessional behavior and expectations of the rotation, she claims to have significant anxiety revolving around the operating room. She states, "It's not that I mind the surgery itself, just the blood." She proceeds to reveal numerous instances of feeling dizzy, lightheaded, and even fainting when seeing blood. As a result, she has been unable to donate blood while in college or medical school and has, thus far, been able to "work around" drawing blood in other clerkships.

29. Which of the following is her most likely diagnosis?

    (A) agoraphobia
    (B) generalized anxiety disorder (GAD)
    (C) panic disorder
    (D) social phobia
    (E) specific phobia

30. Which of the following treatment modalities would be the most effective for this individual?

    (A) beta-blocker
    (B) exposure therapy
    (C) insight-oriented therapy
    (D) SSRI
    (E) supportive therapy

31. A 48-year-old man with no prior psychiatric history is seen in the acute care clinic because of concerns over having a sexually transmitted disease. He denies any dysuria, penile discharge, or lesions. His physical examination is unremarkable. When informed of this information, he insists on being tested. When inquiries are made regarding his sexual history, he claims to be monogamous with his wife, who happens to be Senator Hilary Clinton. When confronted with the fact that she is already married to someone else and living in another state, he states that he married her 2 years ago in a "secret" ceremony. He adds that she flies in on weekends to have "conjugal visits," but he is afraid that she has been unfaithful to him and has given him a venereal disease. He has no medical problems and is not taking any medications

currently. Further history reveals that he holds a steady job as a security guard. He lives alone in an apartment. He denies alcohol or illicit drug use. On MSE, he appears well-dressed and groomed. He is cooperative overall. His mood and affect are anxious. His thoughts are logical. He denies any suicidal or homicidal ideation, or any perceptual disturbances.

Which of the following is his most likely diagnosis?

(A) bipolar disorder, manic
(B) delusional disorder
(C) paranoid personality disorder
(D) schizoaffective disorder
(E) schizophrenia

Questions 32 and 33

The patient is a 7-year-old boy brought in for evaluation by his father. He has been concerned with his son's behavior. At school conferences, he has been told that his son will not stay in place and moves around the room despite being informed about the rules. He neither listens at home nor at school when given feedback. For example, he continues to have difficulty waiting in line, completing his homework, and cleaning up his toys, regardless of numerous consequences. In department stores, he will run around and grab at items, and this has resulted in his breaking merchandise on many occasions. The father states that his son has been this way "since he could walk" and is worried about his son's future.

32. Which of the following is his most likely diagnosis?

    (A) attention deficit/hyperactivity disorder (ADHD)
    (B) autistic disorder
    (C) conduct disorder
    (D) obsessive-compulsive disorder (OCD)
    (E) oppositional defiant disorder

33. After further history is obtained and consultation with the school is initiated, a definitive diagnosis is made. The recommendation to begin a stimulant is presented to the father, but he has concerns regarding that treatment choice. How should he be counseled regarding the use of this medication?

(A) It may cause paradoxical sedation.

(B) It only improves behavior and not school performance.

(C) It requires regular BP monitoring.

(D) It should be taken daily, throughout the year.

(E) It will increase the risk of future addiction.

Questions 34 through 36

The patient is a 9-year-old girl brought into the urgent care clinic by both of her parents. Over the past 18 months, they have noticed emerging "habits" including repetitive squinting and grimacing, along with associated clearing of her throat and grunting noises. These behaviors occur almost every day and frequently occur together. She has gotten increasingly teased because of her peculiarities and her anxiety has only worsened her symptoms. She has no major illnesses and is not taking any medications. Her physical examination is within normal limits with the exception of the above stereotypes.

34. Further history would most likely reveal which of the following comorbid diagnoses?

(A) autistic disorder

(B) major depressive disorder

(C) OCD

(D) panic disorder

(E) conduct disorder

35. Which of the following would be the most effective pharmacotherapy for her presenting illness?

(A) clonidine

(B) haloperidol (Haldol)

(C) lorazepam (Ativan)

(D) methylphenidate (Ritalin)

(E) paroxetine (Paxil)

36. A history of infection with which of the following organisms would be most likely in this patient?

(A) herpes simplex virus

(B) HIV

(C) influenza virus

(D) *Staphylococcus*

(E) *Streptococcus*

Questions 37 and 38

The patient is a 26-year-old male graduate student presenting to his health maintenance organization. He is having ongoing difficulty completing his thesis. When he is working on the computer, he finds it necessary to print out and save every draft of his paper. Even though he realizes that it is unnecessary to do so, he feels compelled to read and reread all of his versions in case he made a mistake. As a result, he has been unable to move forward with his dissertation. He is consumed with doubts about his thesis, but at the same time he cannot throw away discarded sections. In fact, his apartment contains stacks of paper spread throughout his rooms. He understands that these thoughts and behaviors are "not rational," and he is greatly distressed by them and the problems they have caused.

37. Which of the following would be the most appropriate pharmacotherapy for his condition?

(A) alprazolam (Xanax)

(B) bupropion (Wellbutrin)

(C) citalopram (Celexa)

(D) desipramine (Norpramin)

(E) olanzapine (Zyprexa)

38. The patient does not wish to take medication but is interested in psychotherapy. Which of the following would be the most efficacious in reducing his symptoms?

(A) behavioral therapy

(B) eye movement desensitization and reprocessing (EMDR)

(C) psychoanalysis

(D) psychodynamic psychotherapy

(E) supportive therapy

Questions 39 and 40

A 29-year-old married male is seen in the emergency room with the chief complaint of, "I'm afraid I'm having a heart attack." He states a 2-month history of experiencing recurrent episodes of chest pain and shortness of breath that last 10–20 minutes. He also describes associated tachypnea, lightheadedness, tingling in his extremities, nausea, diaphoresis, anxiety, and fears that he may die. These symptoms are now occurring almost daily but are not provoked by any situations or activities such as exertion or exercise. He is significantly worried about having future episodes and is genuinely concerned that he will suffer a myocardial infarction. He denies having any medical illnesses or taking any medications. He drinks three beers on the weekends only and does not use illicit drugs. His physical examination reveals a slightly elevated BP and pulse. An ECG demonstrates sinus tachycardia.

39. Which of the following medications would be most appropriate in the acute management of this patient's symptoms?

   (A) bupropion (Wellbutrin)

   (B) buspirone (Buspar)

   (C) imipramine (Tofranil)

   (D) lorazepam (Ativan)

   (E) paroxetine (Paxil)

40. Which of the following medications would be most appropriate in the long-term management of this patient's symptoms?

   (A) bupropion

   (B) buspirone

   (C) imipramine

   (D) lorazepam

   (E) paroxetine

41. A 55-year-old lawyer without past psychiatric history presents to her internist with complaints of insomnia. Since her husband suddenly passed away 5 weeks ago, she has had difficulty sleeping, frequently awakening throughout the evening. She subsequently finds herself tired during the day. When asked about her mood, she states that she is "sad" and will often break down in tears when thinking about

her husband. Although she feels that her job occupies her mind, she describes being distracted and making minor mistakes at work. Her appetite has diminished, but her weight has not changed. While she feels "lost" and that her life is not enjoyable without him, she denies any suicidal ideation. She reluctantly admits to occasionally hearing her husband calling her name at nighttime. She understands that it is not real but still finds it comforting for her.

Which of the following is the most appropriate next step in the management of this patient?

   (A) hospitalize her for further evaluation and treatment

   (B) initiate treatment with an antidepressant alone

   (C) initiate treatment with an antidepressant and antipsychotic

   (D) monitor her symptoms over the next several weeks

   (E) refer her to a psychiatrist for medication management

Questions 42 and 43

A 30-year-old separated female with borderline personality disorder is brought in by her roommate after she admitted to feeling suicidal and taking several handfuls of "an old prescription" some hours ago. Her vitals demonstrate a slight fever, elevated BP, and tachycardia. On physical examination, her pupils are dilated, she has a tremor, and she complains of "seeing scary faces." She also has noticeably dry mucous membranes.

42. Which of the following medications did this patient most likely ingest?

   (A) alprazolam

   (B) amitryptyline

   (C) oxycodone

   (D) risperidone

   (E) tranylcypromine

43. Which of the following medications should be immediately administered in the above case?

(A) benztropine
(B) flumazenil
(C) naloxone
(D) phentolamine
(E) physostigmine

Questions 44 and 45

The patient is a 70-year-old man brought to the primary care clinic by his family over concerns that he has Alzheimer's disease. They have noticed a worsening of his memory over the past 6 months. He does not seem to want to get out of bed, and he appears to have difficulty providing for his basic needs such as cleaning, dressing, and cooking for himself. He is hesitant when talking, but it is unclear whether he is unable or unmotivated to speak. His family has also noticed that he appears depressed and is often seen crying. A MSE of the patient is performed to help determine whether he is suffering from a dementing illness or a depressive illness (pseudodementia).

44. Which of the following characteristics on MSE is most consistent with pseudodementia?

(A) appears unconcerned during examination
(B) attends poorly to questions on MSE
(C) displays poor insight into symptoms
(D) gives "don't know" answers to questions
(E) consistently performs poorly to tasks

45. Further history, cognitive examinations, physical examination, and laboratory/radiographic studies are obtained. The results are consistent with Alzheimer's dementia. While the family had been able to take care of him initially, they have since returned to the clinic stating that they can no longer keep him at home. They feel that he is becoming much more agitated. He is staying up at night. Lately he has been rearranging the furniture, claiming to look for "the little people who are teasing me." They have noticed that he has difficulty walking, often moving slowly and dropping items. The family has pursued nursing home placement,

but they wish to have something prescribed in order to help him sleep and keep him calm.

Which of the following medications should be avoided in this patient?

(A) buspirone (Buspar)
(B) donepezil (Aricept)
(C) lorazepam (Ativan)
(D) trazodone (Desyrel)
(E) risperidone (Risperdal)

Questions 46 and 47

A 12-year-old boy is brought into the office by his mother, who states, "I can't deal with this anymore!" She appears exasperated, claiming that her son has been getting into more and more trouble over the past 15 months since the finalization of a particularly long and difficult divorce. He has been leaving the house at night without notifying his mother or telling her of his whereabouts. She suspects that he is responsible for the increased vandalism in the neighborhood. He has recently been caught shoplifting at a nearby store. His grades have always been poor, but he has just been suspended for missing classes and skipping school over the past year. He has often come home with evidence of having been in fights. She suspects that he may be hanging out with gang members. She is afraid of his ending up in jail and "becoming like his father."

46. A history of which of the following premorbid diagnoses would most likely be found in this patient?

(A) antisocial personality disorder
(B) ADHD
(C) autistic disorder
(D) childhood schizophrenia
(E) mental retardation

47. If untreated, which of the following diagnoses is most likely to transpire in this patient?

(A) alcohol dependence
(B) oppositional defiant disorder
(C) panic disorder
(D) schizoid personality disorder
(E) schizophrenia

Questions 48 and 49

A 19-year-old male United States Army veteran presents to the outpatient clinic. He recently returned from combat in Iraq where he was assigned to the infantry. While on patrol 1 month ago, he witnessed several friends killed by a road-side bomb. Since that time he has had difficulty sleeping, with frequent awakenings after recurrent nightmares about the event. He finds himself "jumpy" at times, especially with loud noises. He stayed in his parents' house around the July 4th holiday, and he became acutely anxious when hearing firecrackers. He has not spent time with friends or family. He refuses to watch any television or listen to the radio for fear of hearing news of more casualties. He complains of a sense of "numbness" and gets easily distracted. He denies suicidal ideation but sometimes feels that "my life ended over [in Iraq]."

48. What is his likelihood of a complete recovery in 1 year if *not* treated?

    (A) 0–20%
    (B) 20–40%
    (C) 40–60%
    (D) 60–80%
    (E) 80–100%

49. Which of the following medications as monotherapy is most likely to be effective in treating his symptoms?

    (A) amobarbital (Amytal)
    (B) haloperidol (Haldol)
    (C) lorazepam (Ativan)
    (D) sertraline (Zoloft)
    (E) trazodone (Desyrel)

50. An 18-month-old boy is brought into the urgent care clinic by his mother who complains that he is "eating weird stuff." For the past few months since being able to walk, he has been found chewing and swallowing odd substances, such as hair, paper, and string. She has been more concerned since she recently noticed him eating clay from around the foundation of their apartment in the projects. His appetite has been affected because of this, and she is worried that he will become sick as a result.

Determination of which of the following blood levels would be the most appropriate next step in the workup and management of this patient?

    (A) folate
    (B) iron
    (C) lead
    (D) manganese
    (E) zinc

51. A 14-month-old girl is brought into the primary care clinic by her parents. Her prior well-baby checks have been normal, but her parents have noticed that while she used to be "outgoing," she has now become shyer and less responsive. Whereas she had been beginning to walk, she has recently been falling more and unable to even stand up. Her mother noticed that she has been flapping her hands and that her sun hats have become too big for her.

    Which of the following is the most likely diagnosis for this patient?

    (A) Asperger disorder
    (B) autistic disorder
    (C) childhood disintegrative disorder
    (D) fragile X syndrome
    (E) Rett's disorder

Questions 52 and 53

A 60-year-old male with a history of chronic schizophrenia and multiple hospitalizations checks into the emergency room with complaints of "funny movements." He has been compliant with risperidone (Risperdal) 3 mg bid, and he has been taking that dose for the last 6 years while living at a group home. He appears overweight but with adequate hygiene. His thoughts are somewhat tangential but not grossly disorganized. He denies any paranoia, ideas of reference, or delusions. He denies perceptual disturbances or suicidal/homicidal ideation. His physical examination is unremarkable except for occasional involuntary blinking and grimacing, as well as rotation of his left ankle. He is greatly distressed about these "habits" and wishes something to be done about them.

52. Which of the following would be the most appropriate management for this patient?

(A) add benztropine to the risperidone
(B) continue the current dose of risperidone
(C) decrease the dose of risperidone
(D) discontinue the risperidone
(E) increase the dose of risperidone

53. The same patient is brought back to the emergency room via ambulance 1 month later due to "catatonia." According to his chart, he was maintained on his current dose of risperidone by his outpatient psychiatrist. On examination, he is unresponsive to questions. His vital signs demonstrate a temperature of 103.5°F, BP of 180/95, pulse of 105, and respirations of 20. His physical examination is notable for significant diaphoresis, muscular rigidity, and lack of cooperation with much of the examination.

Which of the following would be the most appropriate management for this patient?

(A) add benztropine (Cogentin) to the risperidone
(B) continue the current dose of risperidone
(C) decrease the dose of risperidone
(D) discontinue the risperidone
(E) increase the dose of risperidone

54. A 22-year-old male is brought into the emergency room by the police as he was found yelling in the middle of the street, naked. In the quiet room, he is unpredictable during the examination. He displays extreme lability, alternating between agitation with kicking the bed and listlessness. He is observed responding to internal stimuli and appears paranoid. A limited physical examination demonstrates mildly elevated BP and heart rate, nystagmus, ataxia, and muscle rigidity.

Intoxication with which of the following substances is most likely in this patient?

(A) alcohol
(B) cannabis
(C) heroin

(D) lysergic acid diethylamide (LSD)
(E) PCP

Questions 55 and 56

A 25-year-old male presents to his psychiatrist for follow-up after a lengthy psychiatric hospitalization. He was diagnosed with schizophrenia and discharged on risperidone 6 mg daily. He has no known medical problems and is without physical complaints. He continues to have some paranoia and ideas of reference regarding CNN, but he is not overtly delusional. He denies hallucinations as well. Although he feels "depressed" regarding his illness, he denies suicidal or homicidal ideation.

55. Which of the following should be routinely monitored in this patient?

(A) body mass index (BMI)
(B) BP
(C) complete blood count (CBC)
(D) electrocardiogram (ECG)
(E) liver function tests (LFTs)

56. The above patient continues to be compliant with his medication and remains asymptomatic. He returns 6 months later with complaints of urinary frequency and weight gain. A fasting glucose is 200. Consideration is given to switching to another antipsychotic. Which of the following medications would be the most appropriate?

(A) aripiprazole (Abilify)
(B) clozapine (Clozaril)
(C) olanzapine (Zyprexa)
(D) quetiapine (Seroquel)
(E) thioridazine (Mellaril)

57. A 55-year-old woman with recurrent major depressive episodes presents for medical clearance prior to receiving electroconvulsive therapy (ECT) as she is deemed to be treatment refractory. She complains of pervasive depressive feelings and neurovegetative symptoms as well as suicidal ideation. She denies any physical complaints but is taking felodipine 5 mg daily for her hypertension, which has been well-controlled. Despite receiving a detailed explanation of the procedure, she remains "nervous" about receiving ECT and its potential complications. What should she be told is the most likely side effect from ECT?

(A) broken teeth
(B) fractures
(C) hypertension
(D) memory loss
(E) vomiting

Questions 58 and 59

A 68-year-old widow presents to the primary care clinic for a routine appointment. Her current medical problems include hypertension, obesity, and chronic obstructive pulmonary disease. She has no significant psychiatric history, although she saw a psychologist for eight sessions after her husband died. She does not drink alcohol or use illicit drugs. She has smoked one-and-a-half to two packs of cigarettes per day for the past 45 years and she wishes to quit. She has heard about some of the options but is unsure which would be the most effective.

58. Which of the following strategies is most likely to succeed in helping her to quit smoking?

(A) abrupt cessation
(B) behavior therapy
(C) education
(D) medications such as nicotine replacement
(E) medications with group therapy

59. After being informed of the various choices, she decides to proceed with medication. Which of the following medications is most useful for tobacco cessation?

(A) bupropion (Wellbutrin)
(B) fluoxetine (Prozac)
(C) mirtazepine (Remeron)
(D) trazodone (Desyrel)
(E) venlafaxine (Effexor)

Questions 60 and 61

A 32-year-old female presents to the outpatient clinic with complaints of ongoing headaches. For the past

8 months, she has had recurrent headaches which she describes as bilateral, occipital, with a tight/squeezing pain, lasting for several hours and relieved with non-steroidal anti-inflammatory medication (NSAIDs). Further questioning reveals chronic feelings of fatigue and poor concentration. She admits to "constantly worrying" about her job performance as well as issues involving her relationship with a live-in boyfriend. In fact, her focusing on these concerns interferes with her sleep. As a result, she has on more than one occasion awakened with extreme panic, tremors, diaphoresis, nausea, and palpitations. Her medical problems include gastroesophageal reflux disease that is treated with famotidine. She drinks an occasional glass of wine and denies drug use.

60. Which of the following is her most likely diagnosis?

(A) GAD
(B) major depressive disorder
(C) OCD
(D) panic disorder
(E) social phobia

61. Which of the following medications would be the most appropriate in the long-term treatment of this patient's symptoms?

(A) alprazolam (Xanax)
(B) atenolol
(C) bupropion (Wellbutrin)
(D) lithium
(E) venlafaxine (Effexor)

Questions 62 and 63

The patient is an 18-year-old male brought into the emergency room in the early morning by his friends after attending a dance party. He is agitated, pacing the hallway but unsteady. Despite this, he claims that he feels "wonderful" and states, "Everything will be all right." He also seems focused on seeing many colored flashes and hearing "all conversations at once." He has no known medical problems and is not taking any medication. He does admit to ingesting something early on, which he was told would help him "party all night." On physical examination, he has an elevated BP and pulse, dilated pupils, and significant diaphoresis.

62. Which of the following is the most likely pharmacologic effect of the substance taken?

(A) blockade of dopamine reuptake
(B) blockade of glutamate receptors
(C) increased activity of serotonin receptors
(D) release of dopamine
(E) release of dopamine and serotonin

63. This same patient is eventually admitted for detox and successfully completes a drug treatment program. He is attending college and performing well. He returns to the urgent care clinic with complaints of reoccurring experiences similar to those he had when he was "high," such as flashing lights, intensified sounds, and halos. He is greatly upset about these and feels that they interfere with his studying. A complete physical examination and blood work (including toxicology screen) are negative.

Administration of which of the following medications may worsen his symptoms?

(A) carbamazepine (Tegretol)
(B) clonazepam (Klonopin)
(C) fluoxetine (Prozac)
(D) haloperidol (Haldol)
(E) valproic acid (Depakene)

Questions 64 and 65

The patient is a 48-year-old Marine veteran who has self-referred to the emergency room. He complains of feeling "depressed" and suicidal for the past several days. He admits to using "crack" cocaine daily for the past 3 weeks, but he is vague regarding how he obtains and affords his drugs. He also drinks several 40 oz beers three to four times per week and smokes marijuana "on occasion." He has been homeless, staying with "friends" and in shelters. He last used cocaine this morning and wishes to be admitted for detoxification.

64. Which of the following is most likely to be a comorbid diagnosis in this individual?

(A) antisocial personality disorder
(B) bipolar disorder
(C) GAD

(D) major depressive disorder
(E) schizophrenia

65. He is subsequently admitted to the mental health unit but the next day is evaluated for complaints of withdrawal symptoms. He complains of insomnia, listlessness, irritability, and worsening dysphoria. Which of the following would be the most appropriate treatment strategy for his current condition?

(A) antidepressant treatment
(B) benzodiazepine taper
(C) education and reassurance
(D) methadone detox
(E) phenobarbital detox

Questions 66 and 67

A 6-year-old girl is brought in to the primary care clinic for evaluation by her foster parents, who are concerned that "something is wrong with her." They have noticed odd behavior, with repetitive words and phrases, and difficulty following directions. Her vital signs are normal. Her physical examination is remarkable for a head circumference greater than the 90th percentile but a height less than the 30th percentile, large-appearing ears, and significant flexibility in the joints.

66. Which of the following chromosomes is most likely abnormal in this patient?

(A) 5
(B) 15
(C) 18
(D) 21
(E) X

67. Which of the following is the most likely comorbid diagnosis in this patient?

(A) anorexia nervosa
(B) ADHD
(C) OCD
(D) oppositional defiant disorder
(E) Tourette disorder

Questions 68 and 69

A 17-year-old boy is reluctantly taken to the family medicine clinic by his mother, who is upset as "he is hanging out with the wrong crowd." She strongly believes that he has been smoking marijuana every day after school and on weekends with his friends. The patient appears irritated about the appointment but denies using any drugs or alcohol. His mother would like him to be counseled about the potential dangers of "smoking pot."

68. Which of the following physical effects would be most consistent with cannabis intoxication?

   (A) decreased respiration
   (B) increased salivation
   (C) decreased appetite
   (D) normal motor function
   (E) tachycardia

69. Which of the following would be the most serious potential long-term consequence of smoking cannabis in this individual?

   (A) amotivational syndrome
   (B) cerebral atrophy
   (C) chromosomal damage
   (D) lung cancer
   (E) seizures

Questions 70 and 71

A 38-year-old married woman presents to her urgent care clinic complaining of "crying spells" for several weeks since the termination of her employment. She admits to feeling "down all the time." She also has difficulty falling asleep, poor energy, decreased appetite, and is "not able to enjoy anything." She fears that her condition will never improve. She has begun to feel that "it wouldn't matter if I died," but she denies any suicidal plan or intent. She drinks one to two mixed drinks per week and denies any drug use. It is decided to begin antidepressant therapy with paroxetine (Paxil) 20 mg at bedtime.

70. If there is no significant improvement in her symptoms, but the medication is tolerated, after what length of time should a dosage increase be considered?

   (A) 4 days
   (B) 1 week
   (C) 2 weeks
   (D) 4 weeks
   (E) 7 weeks

71. Which of the following side effects would be most likely to emerge after several months of treatment?

   (A) headache
   (B) inhibited orgasm
   (C) loose stools
   (D) nausea
   (E) vivid dreams

Questions 72 and 73

An 8-year-old boy is brought in for evaluation by his parents, who are worried about his behavior in school. Recently, he has become increasingly upset about attending school. Whereas he had always enjoyed being read to as a small child, he has appeared easily frustrated when reading or being asked to write. During those times, he will often disrupt the class, and this has led to his parents being asked to remove him from the school.

72. Which of the following tests would be the most useful in the evaluation of this child?

   (A) Bender Visual Motor Gestalt Test
   (B) Children's Apperception Test
   (C) Reitan-Indiana Neuropsychological Test
   (D) Rorschach Inkblots Test
   (E) Wechsler Intelligence Scale for Children

73. Which of the following additional diagnoses most likely would be present in this patient?

   (A) ADHD
   (B) autistic disorder
   (C) major depressive disorder
   (D) mental retardation
   (E) tic disorder

Questions 74 and 75

The patient is a 52-year-old male presenting to the emergency room with complaints of severe leg pain. The patient states he has had ongoing left knee pain of 6 months' duration, unrelieved by NSAIDs but improved with vicodin. He denies any trauma but claims to have arthritis. His vital signs are stable. Physical examination of his knee demonstrates no significant findings except for decreased range of motion but with little effort. There is no swelling, erythema, or signs of trauma. An x-ray is obtained which is read as "normal," without evidence of arthritis. He asks for narcotic analgesics, but when he is offered a trial of NSAIDs and a referral to a specialty clinic, he becomes angry and walks out of the emergency room.

74. Which of the following is the most likely motivation for this patient's presentation?

    (A) conscious production of symptoms to assume the sick role
    (B) conscious production of symptoms to obtain secondary gain
    (C) false belief that he has arthritis
    (D) fear that he is suffering from a serious disease
    (E) unconscious production of symptoms due to unconscious conflict

75. Which of the following would be the most appropriate management should this patient return?

    (A) accusation regarding drug-seeking behavior
    (B) admission to a psychiatric facility
    (C) confrontation and further evaluation
    (D) notification of the police
    (E) referral to a psychiatrist

Questions 76 and 77

A 54-year-old woman is triaged in the emergency room for nausea and vomiting. Upon examination, she appears somewhat disheveled and anxious, smelling of alcohol. Her sclerae are injected, and she has moderate tenderness to palpation over her upper abdomen, without rebound or guarding.

Although she initially denies alcohol use, she eventually concedes that she drinks daily, her last drink being "late last night."

76. Which of the following signs or symptoms would most likely occur first in this patient?

    (A) delirium
    (B) delusions
    (C) hallucinations
    (D) seizures
    (E) tremulousness

77. Which of the following medications would be most helpful in decreasing her future cravings for alcohol?

    (A) disulfiram (Antabuse)
    (B) fluoxetine (Prozac)
    (C) lithium
    (D) naltrexone (ReVia)
    (E) risperidone (Risperdal)

78. A 26-year-old man is brought into the emergency room via ambulance, minimally responsive to questioning or examination. According to his girlfriend, he has a history of major depressive disorder as well as alcohol dependence. He was found unconscious with a suicide note and many empty beer bottles. She also believes that he had taken "some other drug" that he purchased from a local drug dealer.

    Which of the following substances found in urine toxicology would be the most dangerous in this patient?

    (A) barbiturate
    (B) cannabis
    (C) cocaine
    (D) opiate
    (E) PCP

Questions 79 and 80

A 26-year-old divorced woman is brought into the emergency room after being found wandering the streets aimlessly. She is a relatively good historian but gives few spontaneous answers to questions. She describes a 1-year history of the belief that she is being followed by "agents" of the Vatican, who watch her closely to "see if I'm a good Catholic." While they monitor her, they also use radio signals to tell her she is a "whore" and a "slut." Due to these experiences, she has been unable to work. She is afraid to associate with others for fears of being "judged." She denies any medical problems and takes no medications. Her parents were divorced when she was an infant. She does not know anything about her father, but her mother has "manic-depression" and is taking lithium. Her MSE is notable for significant psychomotor slowing, paucity of speech, and a flat affect.

79. Which of the above symptoms or signs is **necessary** in order to make a diagnosis of schizophrenia?

   (A) belief of being followed by the Vatican
   (B) inability to work and social dysfunction
   (C) psychomotor slowing and paucity of speech
   (D) radio signals transmitting curses
   (E) wandering in the streets

80. She is hospitalized and eventually stabilized on quetiapine 400 mg twice daily. As she nears discharge, she asks about her prognosis *if she maintains medication compliance*. What should she be told about her likelihood of leading a moderately well-functioning life?

   (A) 0–20%
   (B) 20–40%
   (C) 40–60%
   (D) 60–80%
   (E) 80–100%

81. A 25-year-old woman returns for her well-baby check 1 week after delivery. The baby has been gaining weight adequately and awakens several times per night to breast feed. Although the mother claims she enjoys being a mom overall, she looks sad and does reluctantly admit to feeling "down" quite a bit. While she feels a great deal of support by her husband, she finds herself crying when alone. Her sleep is erratic, and she often feels tired, but she is eating adequately. She denies significant guilt or any

thoughts of suicide or infanticide. What is the appropriate treatment approach for this patient?

   (A) antidepressant
   (B) hospitalization
   (C) mood stabilizer
   (D) psychotherapy
   (E) reassurance

82. A 74 year-old widowed man presents for evaluation to his physician. He has a history of several episodes of major depression, with one prior hospitalization many years ago although he cannot remember the medication he was prescribed. He complains of 3 months of depression, crying spells, terminal insomnia, poor appetite with weight loss, anhedonia, and passive suicidal ideation without plan. His medical history is significant for hypertension, peripheral vascular disease, hypercholesterolemia, and unstable angina. He is currently prescribed diltiazem, aspirin, metoprolol, and simvastatin. Which of the following antidepressants would be the most appropriate treatment option?

   (A) amitriptyline (Elavil)
   (B) citalopram (Celexa)
   (C) fluoxetine (Prozac)
   (D) paroxetine (Paxil)
   (E) phenelzine (Parnate)

Questions 83 and 84

A 30-year-old man is seen in the primary care clinic. He complains of 3 months of "feeling down" that began soon after his job loss 6 months ago. His appetite has decreased, and he has noticed his clothes are baggy on him. He has felt extremely distracted and fatigued. He attributes this to waking up at approximately 3:00 a.m. every day and then not falling back to sleep. While he has felt "lower than I've ever been," he denies any suicidal ideation. He does not have any past psychiatric history or current medical problems. He is prescribed mirtazepine (Remeron) 15 mg at bedtime, but he asks, "how long does the medication take to work"?

83. Which of the following symptoms should he be told will most likely improve last?

(A) anergia
(B) hopelessness
(C) insomnia
(D) low concentration
(E) poor appetite

84. His illness is successfully treated and remits for 1 year. He returns to the clinic wishing to stop the medications. He asks whether he needs to take the medications "for the rest of my life." What should he be counseled regarding his approximate risk of recurrence if he discontinues the medication?

(A) 0–10%
(B) 10–30%
(C) 30–50%
(D) 50–80%
(E) 80–100%

Questions 85 and 86

The patient is a 25-year-old woman recently released from the hospital after her first manic episode. She is currently taking lithium 1200 mg/day, and her lithium level is 1.1 meq/L. She has a slight, but tolerable, tremor and has gained 5 lbs, but she is otherwise tolerating the medication. She claims her mood is "pretty good." She is sleeping approximately 7 hours per night. Her energy and concentration are adequate, and she denies racing thoughts, talkativeness, or increased activity. She has no major medical problems, and her only other medication is birth control pills. She does not consume alcohol or drugs. She wonders, "How long will I have to take medications for this problem?"

85. How long should she be recommended to continue on maintenance therapy?

(A) 6 months
(B) 1 year
(C) 2 years
(D) 5 years
(E) lifelong

86. This patient returns to the clinic 6 months later. She has continued to take the lithium and her level remains at 1.2 meq/L. She states that for the past several weeks, she has become increasingly sad. She is now sleeping over 10 hours per night but still feels tired. She is having difficulty focusing on her schoolwork, and she doesn't eat more than one meal a day. She has not enjoyed pursuing her usual hobbies and feels that "life is not worth living," although she denies any suicidal plan or intent.

Which of the following would be the most appropriate next step in the management of this patient?

(A) add lamotrigine (Lamictal)
(B) add sertraline (Zoloft)
(C) add valproate (Depacon)
(D) decrease lithium
(E) increase lithium

Questions 87 through 89

A 68-year-old retired male is accompanied by his son and daughter to a family medicine clinic. They are concerned about their father's health, as they have noticed him becoming gradually more "confused" over the past year. While he had always been capable of managing to live alone, he has not been keeping up with his bills. The patient explains that he needs his bifocals, but both of his children quickly interrupt, stating that he has glasses but misplaces them frequently. He also frequently loses his keys and forgets to shut his door. The management of the condominium has complained because they recently found him wandering around the lobby and pool in the middle of the night while dressed in his underwear. He has no medical problems and takes only an aspirin daily. His MSE is significant for defensiveness to questioning with some irritability. His Mini-Mental State Examination is 19/30, with notable memory deficits and word-finding difficulties.

87. A definitive diagnosis of this patient's most likely condition would require which of the following?

   (A) cerebrospinal fluid tests
   (B) genetic testing
   (C) MRI
   (D) neuropathologic examination
   (E) neuropsychological testing

88. An MRI performed would most likely demonstrate which of the following findings?

   (A) atrophy of frontal and temporal lobes
   (B) caudate nucleus atrophy with cortical atrophy
   (C) diffuse cortical atrophy with dilatation of ventricles
   (D) dilatation of cerebral ventricles without cortical atrophy
   (E) subcortical white matter infarcts

89. Which of the following will be the most likely course of his illness?

   (A) gradual progression
   (B) no worsening
   (C) rapid progression
   (D) steady improvement
   (E) stepwise progression

Questions 90 through 92

An 82-year-old woman is admitted to the surgical ward after suffering a fracture of her right hip due to a fall down her stairs. Her surgery and recovery are uneventful, but 3 days later, the nurses are frustrated when she does not let them take her vitals or draw blood. On interview, she exhibits drowsiness with occasional agitation. She is unable to answer questions well and is oriented only to person. She also picks at the empty air and begins yelling and swinging at the nurse who is present.

90. An electroencephalogram (EEG) performed on this patient would most likely show which of the following?

   (A) diffuse slowing
   (B) localized spikes
   (C) low-voltage fast activity
   (D) random activity
   (E) triphasic delta waves

91. Which of the following is the most important in managing this patient?

   (A) haloperidol (Haldol) to decrease agitation
   (B) lorazepam (Ativan) to regulate sleep
   (C) soft restraints to prevent injury
   (D) techniques to promote orientation
   (E) treatment of underlying condition

92. Which of the following most likely represents her mortality rate in 6 months after discharge?

   (A) 0–20%
   (B) 20–40%
   (C) 40–60%
   (D) 60–80%
   (E) 80–100%

93. A 14-year-old girl is admitted to the medical unit due to dehydration. She is found to be severely underweight, at 75% of expected weight. She has no significant medical problems, but she stopped menstruating 9 months ago after having regular periods since age 12. She has no prior psychiatric history and is a very successful student and athlete at school. She denies feeling depressed but does admit to feeling tired. When confronted about her weight loss, she does not appear concerned, stating, "I was very fat and still have more weight to lose." Which of the following treatment modalities is the most effective for her gaining weight?

   (A) amitriptyline (Elavil)
   (B) behavioral therapy
   (C) fluoxetine (Prozac)
   (D) growth hormone
   (E) lithium

Answers and Explanations

1. **(E)**

2. **(C)**

Explanations 1 and 2

This woman likely suffers from a major depressive episode. While asking about substance abuse, current medications, medical problems, and a past history of depression are very important in a complete psychiatric evaluation, assessment of suicidality is essential. The risk of suicide in patients with major depressive disorder is about 20 times higher than those without the illness. The estimated lifetime risk of suicide is approximately 15% in those individuals with major depressive disorder.

The choice of a specific antidepressant may be influenced by many factors, including prior response in the patient or a family member and comorbid medical problems or substance abuse in the family (and, therefore, potentially the patient). If a patient or family member has a history of manic symptoms or bipolar disorder, consideration should be given to beginning a mood stabilizer prior to initiating antidepressant therapy, as antidepressants can cause a switch into mania in those individuals. *(Guideline Watch: Practice Guideline for the Treatment of Patients with Major Depressive Disorder, 2nd ed., 2005, APA; Practice Guideline for the Assessment and Treatment of Patients with Suicidal Behaviors, 2003, APA; Practice Guideline for the Treatment of Patients with Major Depressive Disorder, 2000, APA)*

3. **(A)**

4. **(B)**

Explanations 3 and 4

This patient appears to be suffering from a major depressive episode and is exhibiting

acute suicidal ideation with a definitive plan and intent to overdose on a potentially lethal substance. She clearly poses an increased risk of self-harm and requires immediate hospitalization. As she refuses a voluntary admission, involuntary admission (commitment) is warranted.

Autonomy is the right of a patient to self-determination. Confidentiality is not a core ethical principle. Nonmaleficence is the duty to "first, do no harm." The concept of justice involves social, political, legal, and religious considerations. The important code of beneficence (preventing harm) is illustrated in the above case, where an immediately suicidal patient is admitted *involuntarily*. *(Synopsis, pp. 1357, 1365, 1368).*

5. **(C)**

6. **(D)**

Explanations 5 and 6

This patient clearly presents with a paranoid stance, although he is not overtly psychotic. Individuals with antisocial personality disorder are usually more dishonest, aggressive, and exploitative in their attitudes. Narcissistic patients may become easily offended by interactions when not feeling as though they are being treated as "special," but they do not display as much overt mistrust. Patients with schizoid and schizotypal personality disorders appear indifferent or odd, usually with a detached attitude. Patients with paranoid personality disorder display a pervasive suspiciousness toward others, continuously feeling slighted and bearing grudges, not unusually in the form of litigiousness *(Diagnostic and Statistical Manual of Mental Disorders [DSM IV-TR]).*

Becoming defensive will likely only serve to "confirm" the patient's suspicions. A referral to a psychiatrist, while theoretically helpful, is usually not beneficial given the primitive and inflexible defenses (projection, denial, and so on) seen in these individuals. While the patient may have worsening paranoia as a consequence of his fears of having cancer, presenting him with this while he is upset may make matters worse. In fact, the patient may then feel even more accused and become angrier. Referral to a colleague would be indicated for a second opinion to further cultivate trust, but doing so in order to solely avoid a lawsuit may also be seen as defensive and "having something to hide." Individuals with paranoid personality disorder respond best to an empathic, not overly friendly and very professional attitude. Answering all questions with full disclosure of information pertaining to diagnosis, treatment, and prognosis can serve to strengthen the therapeutic alliance in these patients.

7. (C)

8. (B)

Explanations 7 and 8

While patients with bipolar depression do present with psychotic features, this individual does not give any history of manic episodes, making the diagnosis difficult at this time. The bizarre delusions (those that cannot possibly exist in life) and auditory hallucinations that this patient has are not consistent with delusional disorder. Schizoaffective disorder, depressed type, includes both psychotic as well as depressive symptoms. However, the psychotic symptoms must last at least 1 month and occur in the absence of a depressed mood. The diagnosis of schizophrenia also requires at least 1 month of active psychosis but a total of 6 months of attenuated or residual symptoms. Although a depressed mood is very commonly seen in schizophrenia, the total duration of depression is brief overall compared to the psychotic symptoms. This patient presents with major depression with psychotic features, consisting of a depressed mood with neurovegetative symptoms for at least 2 weeks,

as well as psychotic symptoms, which are only present along with the mood symptoms (DSM IV-TR).

Mood stabilizers alone or with antipsychotic medications are not the first-line treatments for major depression with psychotic features, but rather for mania with or without psychotic features. Studies have demonstrated that the combination of antidepressants and antipsychotics is more effective in treating major depression with psychotic features than either pharmacotherapy alone. *(Guideline Watch: Practice Guideline for the Treatment of Patients with Major Depressive Disorder, 2nd ed., 2005, APA; Practice Guideline for the Treatment of Patients with Major Depressive Disorder, 2000, APA)*

9. (D)

10. (E)

Explanations 9 and 10

This patient is suffering from bulimia nervosa, categorized by recurrent episodes of binge eating associated with compensatory behaviors including self-induced emesis, diuretic, or laxative abuse. Because of the repeated vomiting of gastric fluids, patients are prone to develop various electrolyte abnormalities, such as hypochloremic alkalosis or hypokalemia. Hypernatremia and leukopenia are not commonly seen.

Anticonvulsants, such as valproic acid and carbamazepine, as well as mood stabilizers such as lithium, may be helpful for treating comorbid bipolar disorder but are not in and of themselves efficacious in the treatment of bulimia nervosa. Similarly, antipsychotics and benzodiazepines may be used in co-occurring psychotic or anxiety disorders, but do not help with binging or purging. Antidepressants, especially the SSRIs, have been shown to be successful in decreasing both the binging and purging behaviors. *(Synopsis, pp. 748, 750)*

11. (A)

12. (A)

Explanations 11 and 12

The child's mother demonstrates factitious disorder by proxy, categorized by a parent or caretaker intentionally inducing an illness in someone under their care. Confronting the mother in the emergency room setting would likely lead to defensiveness, denial, and anger. The mother could possibly leave abruptly with the child. Having a psychiatrist present in this situation may also create a similar result. While a referral to urology and treatment of the infection may be indicated and appropriate, it does not address the immediate concern, which is the mother's abuse of her son. As factitious disorder by proxy is considered a form of child abuse, the physician has the legal obligation to notify child protective services. Admitting the boy to the hospital will both enable treatment of his medical illness and provide time for the proper authorities to intervene if necessary.

The conscious production of symptoms for secondary gain (e.g., avoidance of work, school, jail, military service) is the rationale behind malingering. Although the mother's apparent concern for her child may appear expectable, her elaborate methods of abusing her son demonstrate significant pathology. The unconscious production of symptoms or signs due to unconscious conflict is the classic drive in conversion disorder. The motivation for factitious disorder is believed to be the purposeful production of an illness in order to assume the sick role *(DSM IV-TR)*.

13. (A)

14. (D)

Explanations 13 and 14

The patient has chronic schizophrenia with an acute exacerbation consisting of disorganization, paranoia, persecutory delusions, and command hallucinations to kill his landlord. Although all of the choices may be indicated, this patient appears to be at significant risk of harm to others, namely his landlord. Therefore, only admission to the hospital for treatment (either voluntary or involuntary) would adequately protect the landlord.

The Durham rule refers to criminal responsibility, that one is not criminally responsible if the illegal act was a product of a mental disease or defect. The M'Naghten rule was established by the British courts and posits that one is not guilty by reason of insanity if, due to a mental disease, one was unaware of the nature of the act or was incapable of realizing the act was wrong. Testamentary capacity refers to one's competence to make a will. The Tarasoff I and Tarasoff II rulings refer to the duty to *warn* others of danger and duty to *protect* others from danger, respectively. *(Synopsis, pp. 1354–1357, 1360, 1362)*

15. (E)

16. (E)

Explanations 15 and 16

This young woman would be diagnosed with conversion disorder. The conscious production of symptoms to assume the sick role is the motivation underlying factitious disorder. Malingering is not a diagnosable mental illness but is the conscious inventing or exaggerating of physical or psychiatric symptoms in order to obtain secondary gain, such as disability benefits, or avoidance of work or a prison sentence. Given her unremarkable MRI, normal reflexes, absence of pathologic reflexes, and hemianesthesia along her umbilicus, her presentation is not consistent with either central or peripheral nervous system pathology. The apparent stressors of a new marriage and pregnancy are likely related to the genesis of her symptoms. Conversion symptoms are created through the unconscious production of neurologic symptoms due to unconscious conflict.

While administering a "placebo," such as intravenous saline, may resolve her symptoms, it is both dishonest and unethical. Admission to neurology is unnecessary unless there is a concern regarding an actual underlying or comorbid disease. It may also serve to reinforce the somatization of her conflict. Confronting a patient with conversion disorder often results in a subsequent worsening of symptomatology. Consultation with a psychiatrist may be useful in helping the patient cope with the stress of her dysfunction but, in the emergency room, may also lead to feelings of not being believed and an increase in symptoms. Many cases of conversion disorder spontaneously remit, but recovery may be significantly facilitated through support, reassurance, and actual suggestion that improvement will occur. *(Synopsis, p. 650)*

17. **(A)** Although antidepressant treatment may be appropriate if the patient is suffering from a depressive illness, further questioning would have to be made prior to that determination. Postpartum depressive symptoms are not uncommon and they may not require treatment. If there is felt to be immediate danger to the child, calling child protective services would certainly be indicated. Having intrusive thoughts does not equate with acting on the thoughts, and thoughts similar to those in this case are not unusual given the stress of a newborn. Again, more information would need to be obtained. On the other hand, premature reassurance regarding the thoughts of harm without knowing additional facts might be dangerous if the patient is harboring a plan or intent to harm her child. Hospitalization may be necessary if the patient is suffering from postpartum psychosis or is suicidal. Only by gathering further history and symptoms, especially focusing on a support system and possible psychotic symptoms, can the clinician determine if there is significant cause for concern. Postpartum psychosis is considered a psychiatric emergency because of the risk of harm to the infant and usually requires immediate hospitalization *(DSM IV-TR).*

18. **(B)**

19. **(E)**

Explanations 18 and 19

This case demonstrates a classic presentation for delirium. Delirium can present with many symptoms, including aggressiveness, hostility, memory impairment, psychotic symptoms (especially visual hallucinations), and overall uncooperativeness, such as pulling out IVs and getting out of bed. While these symptoms are common in delirious patients, they are not specific for delirium and can be seen in many psychiatric illnesses, including dementias, psychotic disorders, substance use disorders, personality disorders, and others. The hallmark of delirium is a fluctuating level of consciousness over time, ranging from sedation to agitation.

Diphenhydramine can be sedating but, due to its anticholinergic side effects, can also worsen delirium and cause urinary retention and constipation, especially in the elderly. Anticholinesterase inhibitors such as donepezil may be indicated for mild-to-moderate dementias, especially Alzheimer dementia. It is not indicated for the treatment of delirium and it would be difficult to diagnose a dementing illness in the context of a delirious state. Giving benzodiazepines such as lorazepam may be useful for agitation caused by a delirium, but they can also disinhibit a patient and cause further agitation, especially in older individuals. A benzodiazepine would be the preferred treatment of alcohol withdrawal delirium (delirium tremens [DTs]), however. A low dose of antipsychotic would be the best choice to decrease the agitation in a delirious patient. While a high-potency medication such as haloperidol can be used, it is more likely to cause extrapyramidal side effects than a second-generation (or atypical) antipsychotic such as risperidone. *(Guideline Watch: Practice Guideline for the Treatment of Patients with Delirium, 2004, APA; Practice Guideline for the Treatment of Patients with Delirium, 1999, APA)*

20. **(D)**

21. **(C)**

Explanations 20 and 21

Alcohol and benzodiazepine intoxication commonly present with disinhibited behavior, slurred speech, poor coordination, and nystagmus, but not typically with dry mucous membranes or constricted pupils. Patients with anticholinergic overdose classically demonstrate psychotic symptoms and dry skin, similar to the above case. However, physical examination usually shows dilated pupils, warm skin, and tachycardia. PCP intoxication also manifests itself with vertical or horizontal nystagmus, dysarthria, and even coma, but it will usually cause hypertension or tachycardia (DSM IV-TR). This case is a typical presentation of opiate (such as heroin) overdose. The clinical triad is coma/unresponsiveness, pinpoint pupils, and respiratory depression. Other signs may include hypothermia, hypotension, and bradycardia.

Disulfiram is an oral, nonemergent medication that blocks aldehyde dehydrogenase to cause a noxious reaction in those who consume alcohol while taking it. It is useful as a deterrent to drinking alcohol but not indicated for alcohol or opiate overdose. Flumazenil is a benzodiazepine receptor antagonist used to reverse the symptoms of overdose with benzodiazepines, especially the sedation and respiratory depression. It would have no effect on overdose on opiates unless benzodiazepines have been ingested concurrently. Intravenous thiamine is indicated for the treatment of Wernicke's encephalopathy, due to the thiamine deficiency seen in alcoholics. The classic triad seen in Wernicke encephalopathy consists of oculomotor disturbances, ataxia, and delirium. Although individuals with chronic opiate dependence are often malnourished, thiamine would not prevent complications seen with overdose. Physostigmine is an anticholinesterase inhibitor used in the emergent treatment of anticholinergic toxicity, but it could be dangerous in opiate overdose since it can cause further hypotension. Intravenous naloxone, an opiate antagonist, is the treatment of choice for the urgent management of heroin overdose, as it rapidly reverses the sedation, respiratory depression, hypotension, and bradycardia seen in cases similar to the patient above. (*Synopsis, pp. 454, 908, 1014, 1046*)

22. **(A)**

23. **(C)**

Explanations 22 and 23

Many psychotropic medications, including most of the antidepressants, cause a variety of sexual dysfunction symptoms. Both painful intercourse and retrograde ejaculation are not seen with antidepressant therapy. These are usually caused by other classes of medications, medical conditions, or surgical procedures. Premature ejaculation is not caused by antidepressants and, in fact, may actually be helped by antidepressants, especially SSRIs. Priapism is an uncommon side effect seen in patients treated with trazodone and even more rarely with the other antidepressants. Decreased libido is a frequent sexual side effect seen in individuals taking antidepressants, especially SSRIs. Other sexual problems caused by these medications include decreased erection and delayed ejaculation.

Almost all of the antidepressants, including the tricyclic antidepressants such as desipramine and the monoamine oxidase inhibitors such as phenelzine, can cause sexual dysfunction. Fluoxetine is a SSRI that commonly causes sexual dysfunction. Venlafaxine is a serotonin and norepinephrine reuptake inhibitor that has also been shown to cause similar problems with sexual performance. Mirtazapine, a novel antidepressant which blocks serotonin and noradrenergic receptors, causes little to no sexual dysfunction. Bupropion has likely dopaminergic properties, and it not only causes little sexual dysfunction, but it also is used to help treat antidepressant-induced sexual dysfunction in some patients. (*Synopsis, pp. 707, 709, 711, 1029, 1075*).

24. **(E)**

25. **(E)**

Explanations 24 and 25

This is a case of dementia, vascular type (multi-infarct dementia), caused by poorly controlled hypertension. Atrophy of the caudate nucleus is seen in Huntington chorea, which accounts for the movement disorder and dementia that are seen in that illness. Dilated ventricles without atrophy are characteristic of normal pressure hydrocephalus (NPH), one of the potentially reversible causes of dementia. The triad seen in NPH consists of dementia, gait disturbance, and urinary incontinence. Pick's disease is a gradually progressing dementia, displaying marked but preferential atrophy of the frontal and temporal lobes of the brain. Generalized atrophy can often be seen with neuroimaging in Alzheimer dementia. Vascular dementia classically will show lacunar infarcts of the white matter on MRI.

With the exception of reversible causes (e.g., NPH, metabolic causes, or heavy metal toxicity), improvement is unusual in dementing illnesses. A rapid decline is common in dementias due to prion infection, such as Creutzfeldt-Jakob disease. Stable dementias are also unusual, most notably seen in dementia due to a head injury. Both Alzheimer's and Pick's dementias demonstrate a steady worsening of the illness over many years. The multiple small infarcts causing vascular dementia correspond to a stepwise deterioration in functioning of the patient. (*Guideline Watch: Practice Guideline for the Treatment of Patients with Alzheimer's Disease and Other Dementias of Late Life, 2006, APA; Practice Guideline for the Treatment of Patients with Alzheimer's Disease and Other Dementias of Late Life, 1997, APA*)

26. (E)

27. (D)

Explanations 26 and 27

This patient suffers from Parkinson's disease, a disorder involving decreased dopaminergic transmission. The nigrostriatal system originates in the substantia nigra. It is the primary dopaminergic tract in the central nervous system and is significantly affected in Parkinson's disease. The caudal raphe nuclei are the origin of the serotonergic system in the brain. The hippocampus is responsible for emotional and memory processing. The locus ceruleus is the location of the norepinephrine cell bodies. The nucleus basalis of Meynert is where the neurotransmitter acetylcholine originates.

The concern with treating agitation and psychosis in patients with Parkinson's disease is that antipsychotics block certain dopamine receptors, which can subsequently worsen the Parkinson's symptoms. While clozapine has minimal extrapyramidal symptoms (EPS), its risk of agranulocytosis and need for regular blood monitoring make it less practical as a first-line agent. Haloperidol is a high potency neuroleptic. It is efficacious in treating psychotic symptoms and reducing agitation, but its potency also presents a significant risk of worsening the Parkinson's disease. Risperidone is an atypical, or second-generation, antipsychotic. Although the risk of EPS at low doses is less than with haloperidol, risperidone tends to still be more of a problem when compared with other atypical medications. Thioridazine is another older antipsychotic. While its lower potency creates less EPS and, therefore, less likelihood of worsening Parkinson symptoms, it has significant anticholinergic side effects that may worsen the confusion. A more concerning risk is prolongation of the QTc interval on ECG, potentially causing a ventricular arrhythmia. Quetiapine is a second-generation antipsychotic medication with essentially no EPS. This gives it a unique advantage in treating the psychosis and/or agitation in Parkinson's patients without also worsening the movement disorder. (*Katzung, pp. 252–255, 260–263*)

28. (E) Any of the nicotine replacement therapies (gum, patch, or inhaler) have been found to double cessation rates. Bupropion has also been shown to double quit rates. Several studies have demonstrated that the combination of nicotine replacement and behavior therapy increases quit rates over either alone. (*Synopsis, pp. 447–448*)

29. (E)

30. (B)

Explanations 29 and 30

Agoraphobia is characterized by anxiety about being in places where escape might be difficult or help might not be available in the event that a panic attack occurs (e.g., crowds, bridges, standing in lines). GAD involves excessive worry about a number of events for at least 6 months. Panic disorder is diagnosed if there are recurrent, *unexpected* panic attacks along with concerns about having further attacks or about the consequences of having an attack (e.g., heart attack, losing control). Social phobia is characterized by a persistent dread of social or performance situations due to fears of acting in an embarrassing or humiliating way. This woman experiences symptoms consistent with a specific phobia, blood-injection-injury type (DSM IV-TR).

Due to the sympathetic discharge, individuals with certain phobias, most notably social phobia, can sometimes be managed with the use of beta-blockers. This is particularly useful when a known exposure will occur. Beta-blockers could worsen the symptoms of blood-injury phobia, however, given the vasovagal nature of the response. Insight-oriented and supportive therapies are not particularly helpful with treating phobias, as phobias usually require specific behavioral techniques. SSRIs can be efficacious in certain anxiety disorders, such as social phobia, panic disorder, and GAD; however, they are not useful for phobias such as blood-injury type. Exposure therapy is considered to be the optimal treatment for phobias in general, especially specific phobias. In this therapy, the patient is exposed to particular phobic stimuli of an increasingly anxiety-provoking nature, and certain relaxation techniques are introduced.

31.   **(B)** Bipolar disorder usually has its onset in late adolescence or early adulthood. A manic episode consists of symptoms such as decreased need for sleep, increased energy, talkativeness, and an elevated or irritable mood. Individuals with paranoid personality disorder are chronically mistrustful and suspicious. Although they can distort reality, they are not overtly delusional as in the above case. Both schizoaffective disorder and schizophrenia display overt psychotic symptoms, including delusions, hallucinations, and disorganization. Patients with schizoaffective disorder additionally have either a major depressive or manic episode, while patients with schizophrenia require significant social or occupational impairment. Neither of these criteria is present in the above case. The patient demonstrates delusional disorder, which consists of a nonbizarre delusion (i.e., one that could actually exist) without significantly impaired function, odd behavior, or the presence of a major mood disorder. The age of onset for delusional disorder is commonly during middle age, whereas evidence of the other disorders is generally present at a much earlier age *(DSM IV-TR)*.

32.   **(A)**

33.   **(C)**

Explanations 32 and 33

This patient suffers from ADHD as evidenced by numerous inattentive and hyperactive/impulsive symptoms and signs. Autistic disorder is a pervasive developmental disorder (PDD) consisting of impairments in social interaction and communication, in addition to stereotyped behaviors. Conduct disorder is a disruptive behavior disorder characterized by aggression and violation of the rights of others. While oppositional defiant disorder is also a disruptive behavior disorder, it is not as severe as conduct disorder, occurring at an earlier age and demonstrating a pattern of negativistic and defiant behaviors. OCD is an anxiety disorder not uncommonly seen in children, diagnosed by the presence of recurrent, distressing obsessions and/or compulsions.

Stimulants are the first-line treatment for ADHD. However, there are many misconceptions regarding their use, which may necessitate the use of more detailed psychoeducation. It was previously believed that stimulants exert their clinical effect through sedation, but this is no longer considered to be true. Stimulants not only improve behavior, but there is evidence that they actually "normalize" school performance as well. The use of drug holidays, such as weekends and during the summer, is recommended in order to make up for any growth suppression. The use of stimulants has not been shown to increase the risk of further substance abuse; on the contrary, treatment of ADHD with stimulants may actually lower the risk. The American Academy of Child and Adolescent Psychiatry recommends baseline and, thereafter, regular monitoring of height, weight, pulse, and BP in children and adolescents treated with stimulants. *(Synopsis, pp. 1208, 1225, 1227–1229, 1232, 1234)*

34. (C)

35. (B)

36. (E)

Explanations 34 through 36

This patient has Tourette disorder, characterized by the existence of both motor and vocal tics which have been present for 1 year. There is not a significantly increased comorbidity for autistic disorder, major depressive disorder, panic disorder, or conduct disorder. There is a very high comorbidity, however, for both ADHD and OCD in individuals with Tourette's disorder.

Lorazepam, a benzodiazepine, may be useful in the short-term management of the anxiety associated with Tourette's disorder, but it is not indicated for the treatment of the tics themselves. Methylphenidate, a stimulant, may be used if there is associated ADHD along with the tic disorder, but it may increase the frequency of tics. Paroxetine, a SSRI, is used in treating both depressive disorders and OCD, but it is not indicated for treatment of Tourette disorder. Clonidine, an alpha-2 adrenergic agonist, can be somewhat helpful in reducing some symptoms of Tourette's disorder. The most efficacious, and first-line, treatment for Tourette's disorder is the use of dopamine antagonists such as antipsychotics (e.g., haloperidol).

The etiology of several disorders, among them Tourette's and OCD, may be related to an autoimmune process. It is believed that infection with certain microorganisms, specifically streptococcal infections, may act synergistically with a genetic vulnerability to cause those mental illnesses. The full significance of

this in terms of diagnosis, prevention, and treatment of these conditions has yet to be determined. *(Synopsis, p. 1247)*

37. (C)

38. (A)

Explanations 37 and 38

This patient has OCD. Benzodiazepines such as alprazolam may be helpful for the acute anxiety associated with OCD, but they are not a first-line medication to reduce the obsessions or compulsions. Although antipsychotics such as olanzapine are sometimes used in conjunction with other psychotropics in patients with severe, intractable OCD, they are not recommended as monotherapy given their significant side effects. Antidepressants that mostly affect norepinephrine, such as bupropion and desipramine, are not particularly effective in treating OCD. Serotonergic drugs, such as citalopram and the tricyclic clomipramine, have been proven to improve both obsessions and compulsions. Because of this fact, OCD is thought to involve the serotonergic system.

EMDR is a treatment used specifically for posttraumatic stress disorder (PTSD). Although psychoanalysis and psychodynamic (or insight-oriented) psychotherapies may be beneficial for some individuals with OCD, there have not been enough studies to document their effectiveness. Supportive psychotherapy can be useful in helping the patients to cope with their severe anxiety and limitations, but it does not particularly address the obsessions and compulsions themselves. Behavioral therapy has consistently demonstrated success in treating OCD, and studies have shown it to be as efficacious as pharmacotherapy. *(Synopsis, p. 623)*

39. (D)

40. (E)

Explanations 39 and 40

This patient is most likely experiencing panic attacks as part of panic disorder. Dopaminergic antidepressants such as bupropion have not demonstrated significant efficacy in panic disorder. Buspirone is approved in the treatment of GAD but is not useful in panic disorder. While tricyclic antidepressants, such as imipramine, and SSRIs, such as paroxetine, are both effective in the treatment of panic disorder, therapeutic benefit for both may require several weeks. Benzodiazepines, such as lorazepam and alprazolam, have been shown to be effective in the treatment of panic disorder. Their more rapid onset of action (hours to days) make them ideally suited for the immediate and acute management of panic attacks.

Neither bupropion nor buspirone are considered to be first-line treatments for panic disorder. Imipramine and other tricyclic antidepressants have demonstrated their efficacy in panic disorder. The disadvantages are several: the need to increase up to a therapeutic dose over time, a significant side effect profile, and lethality in overdose. While benzodiazepines such as alprazolam are also effective in the long-term treatment of panic disorder, their potential for abuse and withdrawal if/when tapered make them less than ideal overall. It is not unusual to initiate a benzodiazepine for more immediate relief of anxiety along with another agent that will require a longer time period until its benefits become apparent. Given their proven efficacy, reduced side effects, lack of abuse potential and safety in overdose, SSRIs such as paroxetine are the most suitable choice for the long-term pharmacotherapy of panic disorder. *(Guideline Watch: Practice Guideline for the Treatment of Patients with Panic Disorder, 2006, APA; Practice Guideline for the Treatment of Patients with Panic Disorder, 1998, APA)*

41. **(D)** This is a woman who is suffering from bereavement, which is not a diagnosable mental illness. Bereavement is considered to be a normal grief reaction to the death of a loved one. Hospitalization would only be indicated if the patient were imminently dangerous to herself (or others) or if she were unable to take care of herself. As she is not suicidal and is functioning adequately at work, hospitalization would be neither necessary nor helpful. Beginning an antidepressant would be appropriate if treating major depressive disorder. While she exhibits some symptoms consistent with MDD, it has been less than 2 months since the sudden death of her spouse and her complaints are not as pervasive as those seen in MDD (DSM IV-TR). Another factor favoring bereavement over major depressive disorder in this patient is the lack of a prior history of depression or current suicidality. Pharmacotherapy with both an antidepressant plus antipsychotic would be the treatment of choice if she were suffering from major depressive disorder with psychotic features. Although she does have occasional perceptual disturbances, this phenomenon is not unusual in uncomplicated bereavement. Her insight and lack of other psychotic symptoms, such as delusions or disorganization, are not consistent with a major psychotic illness. Individuals with bereavement do not usually require referral to a psychiatrist unless there is another existing mental disorder or complicating problem. Given the time-limited nature of bereavement, monitoring her symptoms over time is the most appropriate approach for this patient. Referral to grief therapy, either individual or group, may also be helpful. If the patient's symptoms worsen, persist for more than 8 weeks, impair her ability to function, or cause her to be dangerous, then referral to a psychiatrist or hospitalization may be warranted.

42. **(B)**

43. **(E)**

Explanations 42 and 43

Overdose of benzodiazepines such as alprazolam would cause depressed rather than elevated vitals, as well as somnolence and ataxia. Opiates such as oxycodone, taken in large amounts, cause the classic triad of miosis, respiratory depression, and coma. Risperidone may cause excess sedation or orthostasis, but in high doses it may also cause extra-pyramidal symptoms including dystonic reactions. Monoamine oxidase inhibitors (MAOIs) such as tranylcypromine, when taken with tyramine-rich foods, are likely to cause a hypertensive crisis consisting of hypertension, headache, stiff neck, sweating, and nausea/vomiting. Tricyclic antidepressants such as amitryptyline have significant anticholinergic toxicity which can cause dry skin, dry mucous membranes, hyperpyrexia, tachycardia, mydriasis, restlessness, and psychotic symptoms such as hallucinations.

Benztropine is indicated for the treatment of extra-pyramidal symptoms, such as acute dystonia. Flumazenil is used in benzodiazepine intoxication. Naloxone is the treatment of choice for opiate overdose. Phentolamine or other alpha-adrenergic blockers are employed to treat hypertensive crisis. Physostigmine is considered the treatment of choice for anticholinergic toxicity. *(Synopsis, pp. 908–909)*

44. (D)

45. (E)

Explanations 44 and 45

Older patients with cognitive decline due to depression, sometimes called pseudodementia, display characteristic findings on MSE. They usually are greatly concerned about their problems, even emphasizing their difficulties when compared with demented patients, who attempt to hide or minimize their deficits and appear unconcerned. Patients with pseudodementia are able to attend well to tasks despite their cognitive complaints. Individuals with dementias, however, have significant difficulty with attention and concentration. Patients with depression are more likely to demonstrate good insight into their presumed memory loss than those with dementia, who will commonly deny that there is anything wrong with them. On tests of cognition, those individuals with pseudodementia will show inconsistent results, performing better at some times and worse at others. Patients with dementia, however, will consistently perform poorly on various tests that address the same function.

This patient displays characteristics of Lewy body disease, a dementia which may be related to Alzheimer's dementia. The classic triad of Lewy body dementia is a fluctuating course, peduncular hallucinations (visual hallucinations of small people, animals, or objects), and parkinsonian features. These patients tend to be very sensitive to extrapyramidal side effects and, therefore, antipsychotics such as risperidone should be avoided or sparingly used. *(Synopsis, pp. 333, 340)*

46. (B)

47. (A)

Explanations 46 and 47

This patient exhibits the criteria for conduct disorder. Antisocial personality disorder can only be diagnosed in a person who is over age 18. In fact, the diagnosis of antisocial personality disorder requires evidence of conduct disorder prior to age 15 (DSM IV-TR). Children with autism, schizophrenia, and mental retardation may display aggressive or disruptive behavior, but these illnesses do not necessarily predict future conduct disorder. Patients with ADHD and learning disorders are at an increased risk of developing conduct disorder as they get older.

It is not uncommon for patients with conduct disorder to have a history of oppositional defiant disorder as a younger child. Indeed, the disorders are often thought of as being on a spectrum, with oppositional defiant disorder early on, followed by conduct disorder and eventually antisocial personality disorder. Having conduct disorder does not by itself predict panic disorder, schizoid personality disorder, or the development of schizophrenia. If left untreated, there is a significantly increased risk of developing a substance use disorder, which also predicts a worse prognosis. *(Synopsis, p. 1237)*

48. (B)

49. (D)

Explanations 48 and 49

The patient is experiencing symptoms consistent with PTSD. Untreated, only approximately 30% of patients completely recover, 60% continue to have mild-to-moderate symptoms, and 10% remain unchanged or worsen. A rapid onset, short duration of symptoms, good premorbid functioning, strong social supports, and absence of other psychiatric or medical illnesses predict a better prognosis.

Sertraline, and the other SSRIs, are very effective and well-tolerated treatments for PTSD. SSRIs have been shown to improve all of the symptom clusters of PTSD (i.e., re-experiencing symptoms, avoidance of stimuli, and increased arousal). Based on their efficacy, tolerability, lack of abuse potential, and safety in overdose, they are considered to be first-line agents for treating PTSD. Administering amobarbital, or an amytal interview, has been used sometimes in conjunction with psychotherapy to help individuals work through their traumatic event. It has not been used as a treatment alone, however, given its addicting potential and lethality in overdose. Antipsychotics such as haloperidol have little evidence supporting their use in treating PTSD symptoms, but they may be used acutely to manage agitation or violence. Lorazepam can also be used in a similar manner, but given the high comorbidity of substance abuse in patients with PTSD, this is not recommended as a solo treatment. Trazodone, in lower doses, can be used to help treat insomnia in these individuals. Treatment of the PTSD symptoms, however, would likely require a full antidepressant dose, which carries significant side effects, such as daytime sedation and orthostasis. *(Synopsis, p. 630)*

50. **(E)** This toddler has developed pica, the eating of nonnutritive substances. Decreased levels of folate may be associated with depression and dementia in adults but is not seen in cases of pica. Iron deficiency, a potential cause of pica, may present with eating of dirt. A lead level would be necessary to determine if the child were eating lead-based paint. Manganese levels have not been shown to be abnormal in pica. As zinc deficiency is another cause of pica, assessment of a zinc level is essential in children who consume clay (as is being done by the child in this case) *(Synopsis, pp. 1241–1242)*.

51. **(E)** Asperger disorder is a pervasive developmental disorder manifested with impairments in social interaction and stereotyped behaviors, without the additional language abnormalities seen in autism. Childhood disintegrative disorder is also a pervasive developmental disorder characterized by normal development until age 2, followed by a rapid decline in the use of language, motor skills, and social interaction. Fragile X syndrome is a genetic syndrome displaying mental retardation, characteristic physical features, and a high rate of pervasive developmental disorder. The above patient displays a history consistent with Rett's disorder, a progressively worsening pervasive developmental disorder seen only in females. Rett's patients routinely demonstrate normal development until at least 5 months of age, with subsequent head deceleration, stereotyped hand movements, loss of social engagement, gait difficulties, and impaired language *(DSM IV-TR)*.

52. **(C)**

53. **(D)**

Explanations 52 and 53

The patient has likely developed tardive dyskinesia (TD), a late-occurring movement disorder associated with chronic antipsychotic use. Adding an anticholinergic agent like benztropine would be indicated for treating an acute dystonia but is not effective for TD. Continuing the current dose of his antipsychotic will not lessen his movements, and increasing it will more than likely worsen them over time. Discontinuing his psychotropic will not reduce his dyskinesia, and it will provide a high risk for relapse of his psychosis. Once an individual has TD, reducing the dose (if clinically indicated) may minimize the progression or even improve the abnormal movements.

The patient displays features consistent with neuroleptic malignant syndrome (NMS), a life-threatening condition associated with antipsychotic therapy. Adding benztropine will not treat NMS. Immediate discontinuation of the antipsychotic is recommended. Initiation of dantrolene, a muscle relaxant, as well as bromocriptine, a dopamine receptor agonist, may also be used to manage the patient. *(Synopsis, pp. 1059–1060)*.

54. (E) This patient presents with agitation and psychosis, likely caused by intoxication with a substance of abuse. While intoxication with alcohol can cause unsteadiness and belligerence, it does not present with hypertension and tachycardia. Cannabis can cause tachycardia and feelings of paranoia but, by itself, does not usually spur violence or grossly disorganized behavior. Intoxication with heroin or other opiates more often presents with drowsiness or apathy rather than the overt psychotic symptoms and sympathetic discharge seen in the above case. While LSD and other hallucinogens obviously cause psychotic symptoms, the nystagmus and muscular rigidity are not as common. Patients are not characteristically as hostile as in the case example. PCP use classically presents with the unpredictability, paranoia, and aggressiveness similar to the above case. It is not uncommonly mistaken for schizophrenia. Physical findings may include nystagmus, hypertension, tachycardia, ataxia, and muscular rigidity *(DSM IV-TR)*.

55. (A)

56. (A)

Explanations 55 and 56

Routine vital signs, ECG, and blood work such as CBC or LFTs are not required for ongoing use of second-generation (atypical) antipsychotics in healthy patients. Due to the risk of weight gain, hyperlipidemia, and diabetes ("metabolic syndrome"), regular monitoring for these is recommended. Due to variations in height, calculating a BMI is preferred when monitoring for weight gain in these patients.

This patient has developed new-onset diabetes, presumably from the risperidone. Although all of the second-generation antipsychotics have Food and Drug Administration (FDA) warnings about causing metabolic syndrome, studies have demonstrated that they have varying rates of causing or exacerbating this: clozapine > olanzapine > quetiapine ≥ risperidone > aripiprazole ≥ ziprazidone. Therefore, assuming there is no contraindication

to using one of the listed agents, aripiprazole would be the most appropriate choice based on its likely minimal risk of causing or exacerbating diabetes. *(American Diabetes Association, American Psychiatry Association, American Association of Clinical Endocrinologists: Consensus development conference on antipsychotic drugs and obesity and diabetes. J Clin Psychiatry 2004; 65:267–272; Lieberman et al., 2005)*

57. (D) ECT is considered a very safe procedure overall. The mortality rate is comparable to general anesthesia and childbirth. Unlike in years past, the routine use of muscle relaxants makes broken teeth and fractures unlikely. ECT should not raise BP appreciably in a patient with controlled hypertension. Nausea and vomiting are uncommon and can be minimized with antiemetics given during the ECT sessions. By far, the most common side effect is memory loss, which almost always resolves. *(Synopsis, pp. 1143–1144)*

58. (E)

59. (A)

Explanations 58 and 59

The quit rates for abrupt cessation and education/advice are quite low when used alone. The rates increase significantly with behavioral interventions or the use of medications such as nicotine replacement. The highest quit rates are likely seen with the combination of medications plus behavioral therapy such as group therapy. *(Synopsis, p. 446)*

The reinforcing aspects of nicotine addiction are thought to involve the dopaminergic system in the central nervous system. This may be one reason why bupropion, which likely increases dopamine activity, is very effective in helping patients to quit smoking. The other antidepressants listed have not demonstrated efficacy for nicotine dependence.

60. (A)

61. (E)

Explanations 60 and 61

The patient does not complain of significant depression, anhedonia, problems with appetite, or guilt consistent with major depressive disorder. She also does not complain of specific obsessions or compulsions necessary for OCD, such as fears of dirt, hurting individuals, or the need for symmetry. While she does have panic attacks, they are not unexpected as they relate to her worries about aspects of her life. She also does not have the ongoing fear of having more attacks characteristic of panic disorder. Social phobia consists of fears of acting in an embarrassing or humiliating way in public, which are not apparent in the above case. She complains of excessive anxiety and worry about a number of activities associated with other cognitive and physical symptoms. This case fits the criteria for GAD *(DSM IV-TR)*.

GAD tends to be chronic, often requiring lifelong treatment. Although benzodiazepines such as alprazolam are effective, they should not be prescribed indefinitely given their side effects (sedation, disinhibition) and potential for tolerance, withdrawal, and abuse. They are not infrequently used in conjunction with another medication, often in the short-term, until the primary psychotropic medication takes effect. Atenolol or other beta-blockers can be useful in situational anxiety, such as social phobia (social anxiety disorder) or specific phobia. Beta-blockers treat the somatic manifestations of anxiety more than the cognitive and affective components. As bupropion is thought to block the reuptake of dopamine and/or norepinephrine, it tends to cause activation and is not considered to be a first-line treatment for GAD. Lithium is a mood stabilizer that is also used in cases of refractory depression. It is inappropriate for use in the treatment of GAD. Venlafaxine, which blocks the reuptake of both serotonin and norepinephrine, and other SSRIs are effective and well tolerated in patients suffering with GAD. Their safety and efficacy make them appropriate first-line and maintenance therapies for GAD. *(Synopsis, pp. 635–636)*

62. (E)

63. (D)

Explanations 62 and 63

This patient most likely ingested MDMA (3, 4-methylenedioxymethamphetamine, *ecstasy*) at a rave. Cocaine likely causes its effects through blockade of dopamine reuptake, which is responsible for its reinforcing and, therefore, highly addicting nature. PCP intoxicated individuals can often be agitated, but they typically will also display nystagmus and, not infrequently, violent behavior. PCP works through blockade of glutamate receptors. Hallucinogens are thought to increase the activity of the serotonin system, and they do not necessarily cause the feeling of euphoria seen in the above case. Amphetamine intoxication, by causing the release of dopamine, can appear similar to the above case, but florid perceptual disturbances are not as frequent. Ecstasy, classically taken at raves, acts as an amphetamine and a hallucinogen, thereby creating feelings of well-being or euphoria as well as causing hallucinations. Its dual nature is likely due to its neurophysiologic effects of releasing both dopamine and serotonin in the brain.

This patient gives a history consistent with hallucinogen persisting perception disorder (flashbacks), characterized by the re-experiencing of perceptual disturbances after cessation of use. Although there is no medication which definitively treats the flashbacks, various drugs may be helpful. These include anticonvulsants, such as carbamazepine and valproic acid, or benzodiazepines such as clonazepam. Antidepressants such as fluoxetine would be indicated if the patient displayed a depressive disorder in addition. Antipsychotics such as haloperidol are to be avoided as they have been shown to actually worsen the symptoms of flashbacks. *(Synopsis, pp. 414, 440)*

64. (A)

65. (C)

Explanations 64 and 65

There frequently are comorbid diagnoses in individuals with cocaine dependence. Affective disorders (including bipolar and major depression) as well as anxiety disorders are not uncommonly seen in cocaine-addicted patients. Schizophrenia is not appreciably increased in this patient population. Antisocial personality disorder is the most likely associated diagnosis in patients with cocaine dependence.

Antidepressant treatment may be indicated if there is a comorbid depressive illness, but it will not specifically alleviate any withdrawal symptoms. A benzodiazepine taper would be necessary if this patient were displaying significant alcohol withdrawal symptoms. A methadone detox is often used for patients who are having severe opiate withdrawal but is not appropriate for cocaine withdrawal. A phenobarbital detox can be used to prevent withdrawal from benzodiazepines and can also be used (less frequently) for alcohol withdrawal. Unlike alcohol, benzodiazepine, or barbiturate withdrawal, withdrawal from cocaine is not life threatening and does not require pharmacologic intervention. Education about cocaine addiction and withdrawal, as well as reassurance regarding the likely short duration of symptoms, are all that are needed. *(Synopsis, p. 429)*

66. (E)

67. (B)

Explanations 66 and 67

This patient displays the classic phenotype for fragile X syndrome: a large, long head, long ears, short stature, hyperextensible joints, and macro-orchidism (in males). Cri du chat syndrome involves a deletion affecting chromosome 5 and is characterized by microcephaly, low-set ears, and severe mental retardation. Chromosome 21 is involved in Down syndrome, the most common single cause of mental retardation. Patients with Down syndrome exhibit slanted eyes, epicanthal folds, and a flat nose. Fragile X syndrome results from a mutation on the X chromosome.

Fragile X syndrome is the second most common single cause of mental retardation, with affected individuals having mild-to-severe mental retardation. It is also associated with various comorbid diagnoses, including learning disorders, autism, and approximately a 75% rate of ADHD. *(Synopsis, pp. 1163, 1165)*

68. (E)

69. (D)

Explanations 68 and 69

Cannabis is one of the few substances of abuse that does not affect the respiratory rate. Consuming marijuana classically produces symptoms of a dry mouth and increased appetite (*the munchies*). Contrary to what is sometimes claimed, intoxication with cannabis does significantly impair motor function and, therefore, interferes with driving ability. It also can cause tachycardia (DSM IV-TR).

Amotivational syndrome is a potential, but controversial, long-term effect of heavy cannabis use. It is characterized by apathy and boredom. Cerebral atrophy, chromosomal damage, and seizures have also been reported, but not confirmed, in individuals with chronic cannabis use. The most concerning medical consequences of smoking cannabis over the long term are similar to those from smoking tobacco, such as lung cancer and respiratory disease. *(Synopsis, p. 425)*

70. (D)

71. (B)

Explanations 70 and 71

This woman likely suffers from major depressive disorder. Treatment with a SSRI is considered to be first-line therapy. Although the neurovegetative symptoms of depression (e.g., insomnia, change in appetite, anergia, poor concentration) can sometimes improve after several days of initiating pharmacotherapy, the feelings of depression and hopelessness may take up to 4–6 weeks to significantly improve.

As long as she is tolerating the SSRI, the urge to quickly increase the dose should be avoided so as to minimize side effects. Upon initiation of a SSRI, education and reassurance should be provided to the patient regarding the expected time until remission.

Although there are characteristic side effects, most patients tolerate treatment with SSRIs. Many of these side effects, such as headaches, gastrointestinal disturbances, and vivid dreams, transpire at the start of treatment and may resolve over days to weeks. Sexual dysfunction, such as impotence or inhibited orgasm, not uncommonly occurs after several weeks to months of treatment with SSRIs and can continue with ongoing treatment. *(Katzung, pp. 269–273)*

72. (E)

73. (A)

Explanations 72 and 73

This child may have reading disorder, a type of learning disorder characterized by reading achievement below expected given measured intelligence and age (DSM IV-TR). The Bender Visual Motor Gestalt Test is not a diagnostic test, but it may be used to identify perceptual performance difficulties. Projective psychological tests, such as the Children's Apperception Test and the Rorschach, are not useful for intelligence testing. The Reitan-Indiana Neuro-psychological Test is helpful for children with suspected brain damage. In diagnosing learning disorders, it is essential to measure intelligence in order to compare the results with any discrepancies in achievement. The Wechsler Intelligence Scale for Children is one of the most widely used for this purpose.

Many patients with learning disorders, such as reading disorder, have comorbid axis I disorders. It is not uncommon to find other learning disorders, such as mathematics disorder, present as well. Conditions such as autistic disorder and mental retardation make it difficult to diagnose a learning disorder. If another deficit in functioning is present, the learning difficulties must be in excess of those

associated with it (DSM IV-TR). Depressive symptoms are not unusual in individuals with learning disorders, given the problems with school performance and peer relationships. Tic disorders are not significantly increased in those with reading disorder. There is a high level of correlation between ADHD and reading disorder, with figures up to 25%; there may also be a relationship between the etiologies associated with each. *(Synopsis, pp. 1158–1159, 1181)*

74. (B)

75. (C)

Explanations 74 and 75

This case is a characteristic presentation for malingering. Consciously producing symptoms in order to assume the sick role is the motivation behind factitious disorder. There is no evidence of psychotic symptoms as would be seen in delusional disorder. Hypochondriasis involves the preoccupation with fears of having a serious illness rather than the focus on complaints of pain. The unconscious production of symptoms due to unconscious conflict is the hallmark of conversion disorder, which presents with a neurologic deficit. Malingering, which is not considered a mental illness, is defined as the intentional production of symptoms motivated by external incentives. These incentives may include such things as avoidance of work, military duty, and jail, or the acquisition of drugs (which is seen in the above case) *(DSM IV-TR)*.

In cases of suspected malingering, accusations or law enforcement involvement will likely result in further hostility and harm to any therapeutic alliance. Referral for admission to a mental health facility or to a psychiatrist may also have the same effect and is not warranted unless another mental illness or safety concerns are present. While limit setting is absolutely necessary with these individuals, a professional demeanor must be maintained. Gentle confrontation coupled with a focus on understanding their underlying problems (leading to their feigning illness) are the most helpful approaches. A more complete evaluation may be necessary to determine whether or not there is an additional mental illness or substance dependence that will need to be treated.

76. (E)

77. (D)

Explanations 76 and 77

This patient is at risk for alcohol withdrawal. Although the progression of withdrawal may vary, tremors are generally the first signs seen. These usually begin 6–8 hours after cessation of drinking. Psychotic symptoms, such as delusions or hallucinations, typically develop 8–12 hours after cessation. Seizures typically occur between 12 and 24 hours, and DTs takes place within 72 hours. (*Synopsis, p. 403*)

Disulfiram is used in individuals with alcohol dependence. As it inhibits acetaldehyde dehydrogenase, thereby causing a deleterious reaction when combined with alcohol, it is used as a deterrent and not for cravings. Antidepressants, lithium, and antipsychotics have not been shown to reduce cravings. Naltrexone, an opiate antagonist, has shown small but positive results in promoting abstinence, reducing heavy drinking days, and blunting cravings. The presumed mechanism involves the blockade of opiate receptors, thereby interfering with the euphoric and rewarding effects of alcohol. (*Practice Guideline for the Treatment of Patients with Substance Use Disorders, 2006, APA*)

78. (A) Even large amounts of cannabis do not cause death. Cocaine, PCP, and opiates can certainly be lethal in overdose, particularly when combined with alcohol. However, because of their similar effects on the GABA (gamma-aminobutyric acid) receptors in the brain, barbiturates (and benzodiazepines) are especially deadly when added to alcohol in an overdose. (*Katzung, pp. 288–292*)

79. (B)

80. (B)

Explanations 79 and 80

This patient likely suffers from schizophrenia. While the paranoid and persecutory delusions, auditory hallucinations, disorganization, and negative symptoms (e.g., alogia) are all commonly seen in schizophrenia, none of these alone is necessary. Her occupational and social dysfunction, however, are necessary criteria when making the diagnosis of schizophrenia (*DSM IV-TR*).

Even with appropriate antipsychotic treatment, the likelihood of maintaining a high level of functioning is low. Studies indicate that with treatment, approximately 50% of patients will still exhibit significant symptomatology and display poor functioning. Only 20–40% of patients with schizophrenia will be able to lead somewhat unimpaired lives. (*Synopsis, p. 497*)

81. (E) This woman is likely suffering from "baby blues," which is considered a normal reaction to the stress of the postpartum period. It occurs in up to 50% of women after delivery, usually beginning within several days. It is very important to distinguish this from a major depressive episode, postpartum onset, which requires antidepressant treatment and/or psychotherapy. Hospitalization would be indicated only if there were concerns over suicide, or, in cases of "postpartum psychosis," where psychotic symptoms put the infant in immediate danger. Mood stabilizers would be appropriate if the mood disorder were considered to be a bipolar illness. Baby blues are usually self-limiting and respond to reassurance and support. (*Synopsis, p. 870*)

82. (B) This patient is having a recurrence of his major depression. While all of the listed antidepressants are equally efficacious, the tricyclics such as amitriptyline and monoamine oxidase inhibitors such as phenelzine are not considered to be first-line treatments. This is especially true in the elderly considering medication side effects, dietary restrictions, drug interactions, and lethality in overdose. The remaining listed serotonin-specific reuptake inhibitors are also equally efficacious, but they inhibit the liver cytochrome P450 enzymes 2D6 and 3A4 to varying degrees. This is especially concerning in this elderly patient who is on a beta-blocker and calcium channel blocker, both of which are metabolized by these hepatic enzymes; therefore, blood levels of each can increase appreciably and cause or exacerbate side effects. Fluoxetine inhibits both cytochrome P450 2D6 and 3A4, while paroxetine primarily inhibits cytochrome P450 2D6. Citalopram and sertraline are *not* believed to considerably inhibit P450 enzymes, so in this patient with polypharmacy, either would be appropriate first choices. (*Synopsis, pp. 1329–1330*)

83. (B)

84. (D)

Explanations 83 and 84

This patient presents with a major depressive episode. He is appropriately begun on an antidepressant, namely mirtazepine. With all antidepressants, the first symptoms to improve over days to weeks will be the neurovegetative symptoms such as insomnia, anergia, appetite, and concentration. Unfortunately, the depressed mood and hopelessness are often the last symptoms of depression to remit.

Like many other psychiatric as well as medical illnesses, MDD tends to be a recurrent illness. While individual episodes are very treatable, there is a high risk of recurrence without continued treatment. After having a single episode of depression, studies indicate approximately 50–85% of individuals will develop subsequent episodes of major depression. (*Practice Guideline for the Treatment of Patients with Major Depressive Disorder, 2000, APA*)

85. (E)

86. (A)

Explanations 85 and 86

This woman has bipolar disorder, most recent episode manic, and she has been stabilized on lithium. Bipolar disorder is a chronic mental illness, with a high number of future episodes (mania and depression) likely. Because of this, after one episode of mania, it is generally recommended to continue on maintenance

treatment indefinitely in order to minimize the risk of future recurrences.

This woman has now developed an episode of bipolar disorder, depressed. While adding an antidepressant such as sertraline may help the depression, there is always a risk of provoking a manic episode. Adding another mood stabilizer in order to treat the depression has little data to support it. Decreasing the lithium will not help her depression, and it may make her more vulnerable to a switch into mania. As her lithium level is therapeutic, increasing the dose will likely only add to her side effects and may lead to toxicity. Lamotrigine has been found to be beneficial in treating bipolar depression and does not appear to increase the likelihood of causing a manic episode, as other antidepressants do. It is recommended as a first-line treatment for depressive episodes in bipolar patients. In fact, it has been shown to be useful in maintenance treatment of bipolar disorder by decreasing the likelihood that a patient experiences a depressive, manic, or mixed episode. (*Guideline Watch: Practice Guideline for the Treatment of Patients with Bipolar Disorder, 2005, APA; Practice Guideline for the Treatment of Patients with Bipolar Disorder, APA*)

87. (D)

88. (C)

89. (A)

Explanations 87 through 89

This patient presents with a dementia, most likely Alzheimer's type. Although some cases have been found to have a genetic component, genetic testing is not routinely performed. Neuropsychological testing may be used to specify or confirm the presence of cognitive deficits. Cerebrospinal fluid and MRI may be used to rule-out other causes of dementia but are not necessarily used to diagnose Alzheimer's disease. Although dementia of the Alzheimer's type is a clinical diagnosis, the final diagnosis can only be made by a neuropathologic examination, which classically demonstrates senile plaques, neurofibrillary tangles, and neuronal loss. *(Synopsis, p. 331)*

Preferential atrophy of the frontotemporal regions is consistent with Pick's disease, which may present similarly to Alzheimer's disease. Huntington's disease, another cause of dementia, is characterized by a severe movement disorder. It demonstrates striking atrophy of the caudate nucleus along with possible cerebral atrophy. Dilatation of the ventricles without atrophy is the hallmark of NPH, one of the few potentially reversible causes of dementia. The classic triad of NPH is dementia, gait disturbance, and urinary incontinence. The second most common cause of dementia is vascular dementia, which is often caused by uncontrolled hypertension. It results in multiple small infarcts of the white matter surrounding the ventricles. Alzheimer's dementia, the most common cause of dementia, is characterized by diffuse cerebral atrophy and dilatation of the ventricles.

Stable dementias without progression are unusual. They are seen sometimes in patients after head trauma. Rapid deterioration of functioning is seen commonly in prion diseases, such as Creutzfeldt-Jakob disease. A steady improvement is only possible in reversible causes, such as metabolic etiologies. Stepwise progression is classically observed in vascular dementia, thought to be caused by lacunar infarcts. Most dementias, including Alzheimer's, display a gradual but steady deterioration in cognition and overall functioning. *(Guideline Watch: Practice Guideline for the Treatment of Patients with Alzheimer's Disease and Other Dementias of Late Life, 2006, APA; Practice Guideline for the Treatment of Patients with Alzheimer's Disease and Other Dementias of Late Life, 1997, APA)*

90. (A)

91. (E)

92. (B)

Explanations 90 through 92

This patient exhibits signs and symptoms of delirium. An EEG is very sensitive for delirium.

Localized spikes would be seen in a patient with seizure activity. Random activity is characteristic of the normal, awake state. Low-voltage fast activity is very specific to delirium secondary to alcohol or sedative/hypnotic withdrawal. Triphasic delta waves are characteristic of delirious states caused by hepatic failure. All other causes of delirium, however, demonstrate diffuse slowing on EEG.

Medications, such as antipsychotics and benzodiazepines, may be helpful in reducing the agitation often seen in delirium. Soft restraints may also be necessary to permit the treatment team to perform appropriate examinations, tests, or procedures and to prevent the pulling out of intravenous access, feeding tubes, and so on. Behavioral interventions may be employed to reinforce orientation to person, place, and time. Some of these interventions may include the use of pictures, lights, clocks, or calendars. The primary and essential approach in the management of patients with delirium, however, is to determine and treat the underlying cause.

The presence of a delirium is a poor prognostic sign. The mortality rate for 1 year after a delirium is approximately 50%. The mortality rate for 6 months after an episode of delirium is approximately 25%. *(Synopsis, p. 324)*

93. (B) This girl meets criteria for anorexia nervosa, restricting type. The efficacy for tricyclic antidepressants such as amitriptyline in anorexia nervosa is quite limited. While some studies have demonstrated benefit with SSRIs such as fluoxetine in anorexia *after* adequate weight has been restored, the evidence for gains in weight *restoration* is lacking. Neither growth hormone injections nor lithium have promoted weight gain in anorexic patients. The best evidence for the short-term treatment of anorexia nervosa lies with behavioral interventions while the patient is in a structured inpatient or partial hospital setting; the treatment modalities often include individual (cognitive-behavioral), group, and family therapies. *(Practice Guideline for the Treatment of Patients with Eating Disorders, 3rd ed., 2006, APA)*

BIBLIOGRAPHY

American Diabetes Association, American Psychiatry Association, American Association of Clinical Endocrinologists: Consensus development conference on antipsychotic drugs and obesity and diabetes. *J Clin Psychiatry* 2004;65:267–272.

American Psychiatric Association. *Practice Guideline for the Treatment of Patients with Alzheimer's Disease and Other Dementias of Late Life.* Washington, DC: American Psychiatric Association, 1997.

American Psychiatric Association. *Practice Guideline for the Treatment of Patients with Panic Disorder.* Washington, DC: American Psychiatric Association, 1998.

American Psychiatric Association. *Practice Guideline for the Treatment of Patients with Delirium.* Washington, DC: American Psychiatric Association, 1999.

American Psychiatric Association. *Diagnostic and Statistical Manual of Mental Disorders*, 4th ed., Text Revision. Washington, DC: American Psychiatric Association, 2000.

American Psychiatric Association. *Practice Guideline for the Treatment of Patients with Major Depressive Disorder*, 2nd ed. Washington, DC: American Psychiatric Association, 2000.

American Psychiatric Association. *Practice Guideline for the Treatment of Patients with Borderline Personality Disorder.* Washington, DC: American Psychiatric Association, 2001.

American Psychiatric Association. *Practice Guideline for the Treatment of Patients with Bipolar Disorder*, 2nd ed. Washington, DC: American Psychiatric Association, 2002.

American Psychiatric Association. *Practice Guideline for the Assessment and Treatment of Patients with Suicidal Behaviors.* Washington, DC: American Psychiatric Association, 2003.

American Psychiatric Association. *Guideline Watch: Practice Guideline for the Treatment of Patients with Delirium.* Washington, DC: American Psychiatric Association, 2004.

American Psychiatric Association. *Guideline Watch: Practice Guideline for the Treatment of Patients with Bipolar Disorder*, 2nd ed. Washington, DC: American Psychiatric Association, 2005.

American Psychiatric Association. *Guideline Watch: Practice Guideline for the Treatment of Patients with Borderline Personality Disorder.* Washington, DC: American Psychiatric Association, 2005.

American Psychiatric Association. *Guideline Watch: Practice Guideline for the Treatment of Patients with Major Depressive Disorder*, 2nd ed. Washington, DC: American Psychiatric Association, 2005.

American Psychiatric Association. *Guideline Watch: Practice Guideline for the Treatment of Patients with Alzheimer's Disease and Other Dementias of Late Life.* Washington, DC: American Psychiatric Association, 2006.

American Psychiatric Association. *Guideline Watch: Practice Guideline for the Treatment of Patients with Panic Disorder.* Washington, DC: American Psychiatric Association, 2006.

American Psychiatric Association. *Practice Guideline for the Treatment of Patients with Eating Disorders*, 3rd ed. Washington, DC: American Psychiatric Association, 2006.

Lieberman JA, Stroup TS, McEvoy JP, et al. Effectiveness of antipsychotic drugs in patients with chronic schizophrenia. *N Engl J Med* 2005;353:1209–1223.

Sadock BJ, Sadock VA. *Kaplan and Sadock's Synopsis of Psychiatry*, 9th ed. Philadelphia, PA: Lippincott Williams & Wilkins, 2003.

Trevor AJ, Katzung BG. *Katzung and Trevor's Pharmacology: Examination and Board Review*, 6th ed. New York, NY: McGraw-Hill, 2002.

CHAPTER 6

Preventive Medicine and Ethics
Questions

Questions 1 through 3

A 50-year-old male presents to your office for a routine annual physical examination. He has no specific complaints for this visit other than wanting to be checked for all the usual stuff. His last visit with you was a year ago for a physical examination. At that time his examination was normal. You performed blood work that was within normal limits and included a total cholesterol of 172 with a high-density lipoprotein (HDL) of 45 and low-density lipoprotein (LDL) of 100. He reports that he had a tetanus shot 5 years ago.

Past medical history:	Unremarkable
Past surgical history:	1. Appendectomy at age 17
	2. Vasectomy at age 43
Medications:	Daily multivitamin
Allergies:	NKDA (no known drug allergies)
Family history:	Father died at age 78 of a heart attack
	Mother is alive at age 76. She has hypertension and osteoarthritis
	Brother aged 48 without known chronic medical condition
	Children aged 16, 14, and 8—no known chronic medical illness
Social history:	Married, employed as an accountant; college graduate
	Denies tobacco or recreational drug use
	Drinks one alcoholic drink (either beer or wine) a day
	Does not exercise on a regular basis

1. Which of the following office examinations would be recommended for this patient?

   (A) measurement of his blood pressure
   (B) abdominal palpation to screen for abdominal aortic aneurysm
   (C) testicular examination to screen for testicular cancer
   (D) whole body skin examination to screen for skin cancer
   (E) palpation of the thyroid gland to screen for thyroid cancer

2. Which of the following tests would be recommended for this patient?

   (A) fasting lipid panel
   (B) chest x-ray
   (C) electrocardiogram (ECG)
   (D) glaucoma screening by measurement of intraocular pressure
   (E) fecal occult blood test

3. Which of the following interventions would be recommended for this patient?

   (A) pneumococcal vaccine
   (B) tetanus toxoid vaccine
   (C) complete cessation of all alcohol intake
   (D) beta-carotene supplementation to prevent cancer and heart disease
   (E) screening for depression with a patient-completed questionnaire

Questions 4 through 6

A 65-year-old White female presents to the office for her annual gynecologic examination. She has been a patient of yours for many years. She also sees you on a routine basis for treatment of hypertension and hypothyroidism. Her last pap smear was 5 years ago and she has never had an abnormal pap smear. She had a mammogram 1 year ago that was normal. She does not perform self-breast examination. She is without complaint today.

Past medical history:	1. Hypertension for 15 years 2. Graves' disease, treated with radioactive iodine thyroid ablation at age 50
OB/GYN history:	1. Menarche at age 14 2. Four term pregnancies with vaginal deliveries (at age 22, 25, 27, and 32) 3. Total abdominal hysterectomy and bilateral salpingo-oophorectomy (TAH/BSO) age 47 for fibroids 4. On estrogen replacement therapy from age 47 to 55
Past surgical history:	1. Appendectomy at age 16 2. TAH/BSO as noted above
Medications:	1. Hydrochlorothiazide 25 mg daily 2. Levothyroxine 0.1 mg daily 3. Potassium chloride 20 meq daily
Allergies:	None
Family history:	Parents, siblings unknown as patient was adopted Children are alive and well without known chronic medical conditions
Social history:	Widowed for 5 years, has not been involved in a sexual relationship since the death of her husband; retired school teacher; college educated; does not smoke cigarettes, drink alcohol, or use drugs; walks 30–45 min a day for exercise

4. At this visit you should do which of the following?

   (A) perform a pap smear
   (B) recommend that she restart estrogen replacement therapy
   (C) tell her that she can reduce her risk of dying of breast cancer by performing self-breast examinations monthly
   (D) order a bone density test to screen for osteoporosis
   (E) send a urine culture as a screening test for asymptomatic bacteruria

5. Which of the following conditions results in the most deaths of American women over the age of 65?

   (A) breast cancer
   (B) ovarian cancer
   (C) lung cancer
   (D) cardiovascular disease
   (E) pneumonia

6. Which of the following vaccinations would be routinely recommended for this patient?

   (A) hepatitis B vaccine
   (B) measles, mumps, rubella (MMR) if patient does not recall having the measles
   (C) pneumococcal conjugate vaccine (PCV-7)
   (D) pneumococcal polysaccharide vaccine (PPV-23)
   (E) hepatitis A vaccine

Questions 7 through 9

A 40-year-old male comes to your office as a new patient to get established for care, as he recently moved into your city from another state. He has been on medical therapy for type 2 diabetes mellitus for 3 years and has had good glycemic control. He takes metformin 500 mg bid and reports having fasting glucose levels of less than 100 on home monitoring. He has records from his previous physician that show that he had a dilated eye examination 6 months ago that was normal and a hemoglobin A1C (HgbA1C) level of 6.2 that was taken 3 months ago. He has no known history of coronary artery disease. His last fasting lipid measurement was 14 months ago. You order a fasting lipid panel today and get the following results:

Total cholesterol: 235 mg/dL
Triglycerides: 210 mg/dL
HDL cholesterol: 45mg/dL
LDL cholesterol: 162 mg/dL

7. Your management today should include which of the following?

   (A) institution of a low-carbohydrate diet
   (B) increasing his dosage of metformin
   (C) starting the patient on insulin therapy
   (D) continuing his current care without change
   (E) starting the patient on a hydroxymethylglutaryl-coenzyme A (HMG-CoA) reductase inhibitor (statin)

8. The patient follows up in 2 months and has been compliant with your recommendations. Results of a repeat fasting lipid panel are as follows:

   Total cholesterol: 160 mg/dL
   Triglycerides: 140 mg/dL
   HDL cholesterol: 48 mg/dL
   LDL cholesterol: 98 mg/dL

   Your recommendations for today include which of the following?

   (A) continue his current regimen without change
   (B) add nicotinic acid
   (C) add a fibric acid
   (D) refer the patient to a dietician for counseling
   (E) increase the dosage of his HMG-CoA reductase inhibitor

9. He states that he has not had any immunizations in "longer than I can remember." Which of the following would be recommended for him?

   (A) hepatitis A and hepatitis B vaccines
   (B) herpes zoster vaccine (Zostavax)
   (C) tetanus, diphtheria, and acellular pertussis (Tdap) vaccine
   (D) tetanus and diphtheria (Td) vaccine
   (E) Tdap and PPV-23

Questions 10 through 13

A 42-year-old male presents to the office for a refill of the nasal steroid medication that he uses every spring to control his allergies. You notice on the vital signs taken by the nurse that his blood pressure is 150/95. Except for some sneezing and nasal congestion, the patient has no symptoms. He has no other medical history and his only medication is a nasal steroid. He does not smoke cigarettes, does not drink alcohol, and does not exercise. His body mass index is 24 kg/m².

10. Initial management at this time should include which of the following?

    (A) institution of therapy with a beta-blocker or thiazide diuretic
    (B) repeat blood pressure in each arm after he sits quietly for 5 minutes
    (C) recommendation to start taking a baby aspirin a day
    (D) a treadmill exercise stress test to stratify his risk for coronary artery disease
    (E) discontinuation of his nasal steroid

11. The patient returns for a follow-up visit and his blood pressure is 165/105 mmHg. You diagnose him with which of the following?

    (A) elevated blood pressure without hypertension
    (B) prehypertension
    (C) stage 1 hypertension
    (D) stage 2 hypertension
    (E) stage 3 hypertension

12. Further evaluation at this point should include which of these?

    (A) 24-hour urine collection for protein and creatinine clearance
    (B) renal artery Doppler studies to evaluate for renal artery stenosis
    (C) an ECG
    (D) an echocardiogram to evaluate for ventricular hypertrophy
    (E) a serum measurement of thyroid-stimulating hormone (TSH)

13. Of the options listed, which would be the most appropriate management at this point?

    (A) recommendation of a low salt diet and follow-up in 9–12 months
    (B) increasing the dosage of the previously started antihypertensive medication
    (C) initiating therapy with a calcium channel blocker
    (D) initiating therapy with a thiazide diuretic
    (E) initiating therapy with a thiazide diuretic and an angiotensin-converting enzyme (ACE) inhibitor

Questions 14 through 17

A recent study compared two drugs—exemestane and tamoxifen—for the treatment of estrogen-receptor positive breast cancer in postmenopausal women. At the end of the study, 91.5% of the women treated with the drug exemestane and 86.8% of the women treated with tamoxifen were disease free ($P < 0.001$).

14. What is the relative risk of developing recurrent breast cancer in a woman treated with exemestane compared to a woman treated with tamoxifen?

    (A) 90%
    (B) 72%
    (C) 64%
    (D) 36%
    (E) 4.7%

15. What is the relative risk reduction for the development of recurrent breast cancer for women taking exemestane compared to women taking tamoxifen?

    (A) 95.3%
    (B) 72%
    (C) 64%
    (D) 36%
    (E) 4.7%

16. What is the absolute risk reduction (ARR) for the development of recurrent breast cancer for women taking exemestane compared to women taking tamoxifen?

    (A) 95.3%
    (B) 72%
    (C) 64%
    (D) 36%
    (E) 4.7%

17. What is the number needed to treat (NNT) with exemestane compared to tamoxifen to prevent one breast cancer recurrence?

    (A) 79
    (B) 50
    (C) 36
    (D) 21
    (E) 14

Questions 18 through 21

You are evaluating a journal article describing a test for the diagnosis of congestive heart failure (CHF). In the study described, 250 consecutive patients were given the test. Of the 250 subjects, 106 tested positive for CHF and 144 tested negative. All 250 subjects were then evaluated by expert cardiologists who were blinded to the results of the experimental test. These cardiologists determined that of the 106 persons who tested positive, 95 actually had CHF. Further, the cardiologists found that of the 144 who tested negative, 2 truly had CHF.

18. What is the sensitivity of this test for the diagnosis of CHF?

    (A) 98%
    (B) 93%
    (C) 75%
    (D) 61%
    (E) 39%

19. What is the specificity of this test for the diagnosis of CHF?

    (A) 39%
    (B) 61%
    (C) 75%
    (D) 93%
    (E) 98%

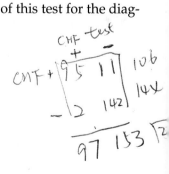

20. What is the positive predictive value (PPV) of this test for the diagnosis of CHF?

   (A) 99%
   (B) 93%
   (C) 90%
   (D) 85%
   (E) 77%

21. What is the negative predictive value (NPV) of this test for the diagnosis of CHF?

   (A) 99%
   (B) 93%
   (C) 90%
   (D) 85%
   (E) 77%

142/144

Questions 22 through 25

In your role as a physician in a community health center, you agree to perform sports preparticipation examinations on students from the local high school. You have several scheduled for today.

Your first appointment is with a 16-year-old male who is planning to run on the cross-country team in the Fall and play baseball in the Spring. He reports that one time he "blacked out" while running, but he has never had chest pain while exercising and he is one of the top runners on the team. He has no known medical history, denies alcohol, tobacco, recreational drug, or performance-enhancing drug use. He has a cousin who died at the age of 21 of "some kind of heart disease," although your patient is not sure of any details. On examination, he is healthy appearing and has normal vital signs, with a pulse rate of 72 and a blood pressure of 100/65. Auscultation of his heart reveals no cardiac murmur while he is lying down, a soft systolic murmur when he stands which increases on having the patient perform a Valsalva maneuver. The remainder of his examination is normal.

22. At this point, what is your most appropriate management option?

   (A) allow unrestricted participation in sports
   (B) allow participation in noncontact sports

   (C) allow him to play baseball but not run cross-country
   (D) restrict him from all athletic participation until he is evaluated by a cardiologist
   (E) restrict him from competitive athletics but allow him to participate in gym class

23. Your next appointment is with a 15-year-old female who plans to play basketball and volleyball. She has no significant medical history, denies a family history of premature cardiac deaths, and denies tobacco, alcohol, recreational drug, or performance-enhancing drug use. She reports having regular menstrual cycles. On examination, she is 72 in. tall, weighs 150 lbs, and has an arm-span of 77 in. Her vital signs are normal. She has a high-arched palate, pectus excavatum, and long, slender fingers. Her cardiac, pulmonary, abdominal, and dermatologic examinations are normal.

Your management at this point should include further evaluation for the possible diagnosis of which of the following?

   (A) Turner syndrome
   (B) Marfan syndrome
   (C) the female athlete's triad
   (D) type 1 diabetes mellitus
   (E) atlantoaxial instability

24. Appropriate diagnostic testing would include which of the following?

   (A) chromosomal analysis
   (B) echocardiography
   (C) serum calcium measurement
   (D) fasting plasma glucose
   (E) cervical spine x-rays with flexion and extension views

25. Your last patient of the day is a 16-year-old male who plans to play on the football team. He has no complaints today, no significant medical history, and no concerning family history. He denies the use of tobacco, alcohol, or any kinds of drugs. His physical examination is entirely normal. Review of his vaccinations reveals that he had a Td vaccination 3 years ago, a varicella vaccination at age 17 months, and 2 MMR vaccinations at age 17 months and 5 years.

Appropriate management at this time would include which of the following?

(A) MMR vaccine

(B) Td vaccine

(C) varicella vaccine

(D) screening ECG

(E) urinalysis

26. Of the following conditions, which results in the most deaths each year in the United States?

(A) acquired immunodeficiency syndrome (AIDS)

(B) breast cancer

(C) motor vehicle accidents

(D) occupational injuries

(E) medical errors

Questions 27 and 28

A meta-analysis of randomized-controlled trials was published comparing two methods of managing postterm pregnancies. The question studied was whether the routine induction of labor at 41 weeks' gestation would result in improved maternal or fetal outcomes compared with expectant management. The authors reported that the odds ratio for caesarian delivery rate in the induction group compared to the expectant management group was 0.88 with a 95% confidence interval (CI) of 0.78–0.99. A second outcome studied was perinatal mortality. For this outcome, the odds ratio for the induction group compared to the expectant management group was 0.41 with a 95% CI of 0.14–1.18.

27. Which of the following statements is true?

(A) There was a statistically significant reduction in the number of caesarian deliveries in the induction group compared to the expectant management group.

(B) There was a statistically significant reduction in perinatal mortality in the induction group.

(C) There was no statistically significant difference for either outcome.

(D) There was a statistically significant increase in the number of caesarian deliveries in the induction group compared to the expectant management group.

(E) There was a statistically significant decrease in both the number of caesarian deliveries and perinatal mortality in the induction group.

28. The authors assessed the study as being underpowered for the outcome of perinatal mortality. Possible ways to increase the statistical power of a study include which of the following?

(A) using P-value to determine statistical significance in place of 95% CI

(B) performing a "case-control" study in place of a meta-analysis of randomized-controlled trials

(C) reporting the results as a relative risk in place of an odds ratio

(D) performing a subgroup analysis

(E) increasing the number of subjects enrolled in a study

Questions 29 through 31

While you are working in the community health center, a 40-year-old male presents to you as a referral from the dental clinic. The patient reported on the intake history form at the dental office that he had rheumatic fever at the age of 7. The dentist refused to allow him to have a dental examination and cleaning until he was cleared by a medical doctor. Other than rheumatic fever, the patient has no medical history and does not take any medications. He denies chest pain, palpitations, dyspnea, or any other symptoms. On examination, he has normal vital signs and a normal general examination. On auscultation of his heart, you hear a 2/6 systolic ejection murmur at the left upper sternal border without radiation. Review of his chart shows that he had an echocardiogram approximately 9 months ago that revealed mild mitral valve prolapse without evidence of mitral regurgitation, but otherwise normal valves and cardiac function.

29. Which of the following would be the most appropriate management at this time?

(A) Proceed with the dental work.

(B) Give the patient a 2 g dose of oral amoxicillin and then perform the dental cleaning an hour later.

(C) Delay the dental work until the patient can undergo a repeat echocardiogram.

(D) Delay the dental work until the patient is cleared by a cardiologist.

(E) Allow the patient to undergo the dental cleaning now, but caution that he will need antibiotic prophylaxis if he requires any fillings.

30. For which of the following cardiac conditions is bacterial endocarditis prophylaxis recommended?

(A) cardiac pacemaker

(B) isolated secundum atrial septal defect

(C) previous coronary artery bypass graft

(D) bicuspid aortic valve

(E) the presence of any cardiac murmur

31. In patients in whom it is required, for which of the following dental procedures is bacterial endocarditis prophylaxis recommended?

(A) fluoride treatments

(B) taking of oral impressions

(C) taking of dental x-rays

(D) dental extractions

(E) adjustment of orthodontic appliances

Questions 32 and 33

A 13-year-old boy is brought into the emergency room with a laceration of his right arm. According to his parents, he received the injury when he fell on the ground while playing at the family farm about 1 hour ago. He has no known history of any medical problems. His parents say that they haven't brought him to the doctor in years. On questioning, they report that he only received one of his "baby shots" and they are not sure which one that was. On examination, he is healthy appearing. He is appropriately apprehensive but calm and consolable. His right arm has a 5 cm linear laceration with visible soil particles in and about the wound. The remainder of his examination is unremarkable. You carefully clean and irrigate the wound and then primarily repair the laceration with sutures.

32. What immediate tetanus prophylaxis would be optimal in this case?

(A) IM injection of adult Td vaccine only

(B) IM injection of both adult Td vaccine and tetanus immune globulin (TIG)

(C) IM injection of Tdap only

(D) IM injection of TIG only

(E) IM injection of both Tdap and TIG

33. After the treatment given above, what would be the recommended "catch-up" immunization schedule to protect against tetanus?

(A) Td every 5 years

(B) Td in 6 months then booster every 10 years

(C) Td in 4 weeks and 6–12 months then booster every 10 years

(D) Td in 2 months, 4 months, 15–18 months, and 5 years and then booster every 10 years

(E) TIG IM every 5–10 years

34. Which of the following statements regarding vaccinations of pregnant women is true?

    (A) Women who will be beyond the first trimester of pregnancy during flu season should routinely receive the inactivated influenza vaccine.

    (B) Pregnancy is an absolute contraindication to the hepatitis B vaccine.

    (C) Women who test negative for rubella at their initial prenatal visit should routinely receive a rubella vaccine during their second trimester of pregnancy.

    (D) Pregnant women who have not completed a Td primary series should start this series in the immediate postpartum period.

    (E) Women who receive a rubella vaccination within 4 weeks of becoming pregnant should be advised of the high risk having a baby with congenital rubella syndrome.

Questions 35 and 36

A 50-year-old male presents to your office after reading an article on the Internet stating that a recent study showed that the drug finasteride can prevent prostate cancer. He asks you to prescribe this medication for him. You review the article and find the following information: a randomized-controlled trial of men over the age of 55 with normal prostate-specific antigen (PSA) readings was performed comparing finasteride and a placebo. At the end of the study, 18% of the men in the finasteride group and 24% of the men in the placebo group had developed prostate cancer.

35. How many men need to be treated with finasteride to prevent one case of prostate cancer (NNT)?

    $\frac{100}{6} = 1$

    (A) 6
    (B) 10
    (C) 17
    (D) 24
    (E) 32

36. Further review of the article reveals that 6.4% $\frac{100}{1.3} =$ of the men in the finasteride group and 5.1% in

the placebo group developed high-grade prostate cancers.

How many men need to take finasteride in order to have one excess case of high-grade prostate cancer (number needed to harm [NNH])?

    (A) 1.3
    (B) 12
    (C) 37
    (D) 77
    (E) 94

Questions 37 and 38

A 65-year-old White woman presents to your office and requests to have a screening test for osteoporosis. She has been menopausal for 15 years. She never took hormone replacement therapy (HRT). She currently takes 500 mg of calcium a day and walks 2 miles a day. She has no history of fractures.

37. Which of the following tests would be the most appropriate screening test to perform?

    (A) lateral thoracic spine x-ray

    (B) dual energy x-ray absorptiometry (DEXA) of the lumbar spine and proximal femur

    (C) quantitative ultrasound of the phalanges of the hand

    (D) peripheral quantitative computed tomography (CT) of the distal radius

    (E) single energy x-ray absorptiometry (SXA) of the calcaneus

38. The result of the test that you ordered shows the patient's bone mineral density to be 2.5 standard deviations below the mean bone density of a 25-year-old woman. What is the most appropriate management at this point?

    (A) start therapy with an oral bisphosphonate

    (B) increase her calcium supplement to 1000 mg/day

    (C) suggest diet and exercise changes then recheck her bone density in 6 months

(D) add vitamin D and continue her current calcium supplement

(E) no intervention as her bone density is considered normal for her age

Questions 39 through 41

A 34-year-old woman with a history of type 1 diabetes mellitus presents to your office for a routine follow-up visit. She is feeling well and has no complaints. Her fasting blood sugars usually run 140–160 and her HgbA1C was recently measured at 8.2. She tells you that she would like to become pregnant but wants to know if there are any risks for her and a baby due to her diabetes.

39. Which of the following statements about the risk to offspring of diabetic mothers is true?

(A) Approximately 20% of children of diabetic mothers will develop type 1 diabetes.

(B) Diabetes is associated with an increased risk of stillbirth.

(C) Diabetes is associated with an increased risk of chromosomal anomalies.

(D) The incidence of preterm birth is the same in both diabetics and nondiabetics.

(E) Maternal diabetes delays the development of fetal lung maturity.

40. Which of the following statements regarding the risk of pregnancy to the diabetic mother is true?

(A) Pregnancy significantly exacerbates diabetic nephropathy.

(B) Most diabetic women will develop neuropathic symptoms while pregnant.

(C) About 10% of diabetic women will develop ketoacidosis during pregnancy.

(D) Most diabetic women develop at least one infection during pregnancy.

(E) The occurrence of preeclampsia is directly related to diabetic control.

41. Which of the following preconception counseling statements is true?

(A) All diabetics planning to become pregnant should be placed on ACE inhibitors for renal protection.

(B) Diabetic women should not take folic acid because all commercially available supplements contain sugar.

(C) The goal HgbA1C level during her pregnancy is approximately 9%.

(D) Insulin pump treatment is contraindicated during pregnancy.

(E) Women with good preconception diabetic control have infants with a lower incidence of congenital malformations than women with poor preconception diabetic control.

Questions 42 through 44

42. You would like to design a study to evaluate the prevalence of a certain disease in your patient population. Which study design would be the most appropriate?

(A) case-control study

(B) cohort study

(C) prospective, randomized-controlled trial

(D) cross-sectional study

(E) meta-analysis

43. You find that the specific disease that you are studying is very rare in your patient population. You are interested in determining which risk factors may contribute to the development of this disease.

Which study design would be the most appropriate to further pursue this question?

(A) case-control study

(B) cohort study

(C) prospective, randomized-controlled trial

(D) cross-sectional study

(E) meta-analysis

44. The results of your study in question 43 find two risk factors associated with the development of the disease that you are studying. Risk factor "X" was found to have an odds ratio for the development of the disease of 2.5 (95% CI: 1.3–4.0). Risk factor "Y" had an odds ratio of 1.9 (95% CI: 1.1–3.3).

Which of the following statements is true?

(A) Both risk factors X and Y are now proven to cause the disease.

(B) Persons with risk factor X will have a worse prognosis than those with risk factor Y.

(C) Risk factor X was more common in your study population than risk factor Y.

(D) Both risk factors occurred more commonly in persons with the disease than in persons who did not have the disease.

(E) For every 100 people with the disease, 25 will have risk factor X and 19 will have risk factor Y.

Questions 45 through 47

45. One of your responsibilities at the community health center is to serve as director of the tuberculosis (TB) screening and prevention program. Which of the following statements about testing for TB is true?

(A) Multiple puncture (Tine) testing is recommended for children.

(B) Previous recipients of the BCG (Bacille Calmette-Guérin) vaccine should not receive TB skin testing because they almost always will test positive for the rest of their lives.

(C) If a patient has a positive skin test, the next test is collection of sputum for acid-fast bacilli (AFB).

(D) Any patient with 10 mm induration at the site of injection 72 hours after skin test placement should have a chest x-ray.

(E) Repeat skin testing 2 weeks after a negative purified protein derivative (PPD) can increase the sensitivity of the test.

46. Which of the following test results would be considered positive?

(A) 10 mm redness and 3 mm induration in a man with HIV

(B) 10 mm redness and 10 mm induration in a nursing home resident

(C) 20 mm redness and 8 mm induration in a person with no known risk factors

(D) 5 mm redness and 5 mm induration in a physician having a routine, annual screening

(E) 10 mm redness and 5 mm induration in an immigrant from Southeast Asia

47. Which of the following statements regarding the management of an asymptomatic person with a positive TB skin test is true?

(A) Because of the development of resistant TB strains, recent converters both with and without symptoms should be treated with four drug therapy.

(B) A pregnant woman with a positive skin test should not have a chest x-ray until after she delivers because of the risk of radiation exposure to the fetus.

(C) A positive reaction in a person who has previously received a BCG vaccine should be considered a false positive and ignored.

(D) Isoniazid should not be given to an asymptomatic person over the age of 50 because the risk of the medication is higher than the risk of developing active TB.

(E) Isoniazid daily for 9 months is the preferred treatment for most asymptomatic persons with positive TB skin tests.

48. You see a 2-week-old child for a routine well-baby check-up. The mother is feeding him formula that she prepares by mixing powdered formula with her home tap water that comes from a well. The local health department considers the water to be nonfluoridated. Which of the following suggestions would be appropriate?

(A) She should start giving her baby a fluoride supplement now.

(B) Powdered infant formula contains an adequate amount of fluoride, so a supplement will not be required as long as she continues formula feeding.

(C) A fluoride supplement would be recommended starting at age 6 months.

(D) She should take a fluoride supplement during subsequent pregnancies for the benefit of the fetus.

(E) There is no risk to fluoride supplementation, so any dosage may be used.

Questions 49 and 50

A 19-year-old woman comes in for a routine obstetrical follow-up visit at 24 weeks' gestation. She is here with her boyfriend, who is the father of the baby. She is wearing dark sunglasses in the examination room. When you ask her to remove the glasses, you see that she has a bruise around her left eye. Her boyfriend quickly states that she accidentally bumped into a door and she quietly nods in agreement.

49. Which of the following statements about domestic violence is true?

(A) All states require that physicians report partner violence to the police.

(B) Domestic violence is rare in same sex couples.

(C) A woman cannot make a sexual assault claim against her husband.

(D) Domestic violence is less likely when one partner is ill or disabled.

(E) Psychological intimidation without violence is considered a form of abuse.

50. Which of the following would be the most appropriate intervention at this time?

(A) Provide the woman with information about domestic violence, including the phone number of shelters and counseling services.

(B) Confront the boyfriend with your concerns regarding physical abuse.

(C) No intervention is necessary, as partner violence usually stops while a woman is pregnant.

(D) Encourage the woman to have ready access to a weapon to defend herself at home.

(E) Report the boyfriend to Child Protective Services at the time of delivery of the baby, so that they can intervene before child abuse occurs.

Questions 51 through 53

A husband and wife, both aged 30, come to the community health center for advice and evaluation prior to a month-long mission trip to central Africa. Both are in good health. She takes oral contraceptive pills and he is on no prescription medication. Review of their records shows that they have had all of the appropriate vaccinations for their ages, have completed a three-dose hepatitis B series and had dT boosters 2 years ago. Their mission will involve building a school and health clinic in a rural area of Cameroon.

51. Which of the following immunizations would be recommended prior to the trip?

(A) MMR booster
(B) dT booster
(C) hepatitis B booster
(D) injectable polio vaccine
(E) smallpox vaccine

52. What advice would be the most appropriate to provide?

(A) Swimming in freshwater lakes would be a recommended type of exercise in the hot African climate.

(B) The mosquito that transmits malaria is most active in the middle of the day.

(C) The risk of motor vehicle related injuries is much lower because there are fewer cars on the road.

(D) Due to its potential toxicity, N, N diethyl-m-toluamide (DEET)-containing insect repellents should be avoided.

(E) Medication for malaria prophylaxis should be started before their trip and continued after they return home.

53. How would you advise them regarding food safety?

    (A) Carbonated soft drinks served with ice cubes are considered safe to drink.

    (B) Locally grown oranges and bananas are safe to eat.

    (C) Water is safe to drink after filtering through an absolute 1 μm filter.

    (D) Brushing teeth with untreated water is safe as long as it is not swallowed.

    (E) Salads are generally safer to eat than cooked meats.

Questions 54 and 55

A 6-month-old boy is brought to the office for a routine check-up by his mother. They have recently moved to the area and are new to your practice. He is the product of an uncomplicated term pregnancy, has grown and developed appropriately for his age, and is up-to-date on his immunizations. He has had two cases of otitis media in his life. Neither of his parents has been diagnosed with any chronic medical conditions. Both of his parents smoke cigarettes, but "not in the same room" as the child.

54. What information about secondhand smoke could you provide to the parents?

    (A) The health risks of secondhand smoke are lower because it has a significantly different chemical composition than directly inhaled tobacco smoke.

    (B) Secondhand smoke exposure has been associated with the sudden infant death syndrome (SIDS).

    (C) Smoking in another room of the home eliminates the exposure to secondhand smoke.

    (D) The amount of carcinogens absorbed by household contacts of smokers is clinically insignificant.

    (E) When a cigarette is smoked, most of the smoke is inhaled and very little is released into the environment.

55. Which of the following statements is true?

    (A) Children of parents who smoke become smokers less often than children of nonsmokers.

    (B) Chemicals from cigarette smoke do not get into breast milk.

    (C) More than 95% of the smoke from a cigarette is out of a room within 30 minutes of smoking cessation.

    (D) The United States Environmental Protection Agency (EPA) does not consider secondhand smoke to be a carcinogen.

    (E) Parental smoking may be considered as a factor in assessing the "best interest" of a child in child custody hearings.

Questions 56 through 58

A 39-year-old woman presents to the office for the evaluation of a mole on her left arm. It has been present and enlarging over the past 6 months. It itches and occasionally bleeds.

56. Which of the following attributes would be considered high risk for skin cancer?

    (A) diameter of greater than 6 mm

    (B) a sharply demarcated, regular border

    (C) a uniform coloration

    (D) a symmetric, circular shape

    (E) a flat lesion

57. Which of the following statements regarding skin cancer is true?

    (A) Skin types III and IV are more prone to developing melanoma.

    (B) Squamous cell carcinoma only occurs in sun-exposed areas.

    (C) Basal cell carcinomas do not occur in persons of African descent.

    (D) Squamous cell carcinomas of the skin have a higher metastatic potential than basal cell carcinomas.

    (E) A shave biopsy is recommended for the evaluation of suspicious pigmented lesions.

58. How would you advise this patient regarding sun exposure?

(A) A cotton T-shirt worn while swimming provides adequate protection from the sun for the chest and back.

(B) Melanomas are more highly associated with intermittent sunburns than cumulative sun exposure.

(C) Tanning booths are recommended for persons desiring a suntan, as they are not associated with an increased risk of skin cancer.

(D) To protect against skin cancer, a sunscreen needs to inhibit only UV-B rays.

(E) Waterproof sunscreen does not need to be reapplied after swimming.

Questions 59 through 61

A 26-year-old G_2P_1 female comes to your office for her initial obstetric visit. The first day of her last menstrual period was 6 weeks ago. Other than some mild morning sickness, she is feeling fine. Her first pregnancy was 40 weeks in gestation and uncomplicated. She has no significant medical history.

59. Which of the following tests is recommended for the initial obstetric visit?

(A) TSH

(B) blood glucose measurement 1 hour after a 50 g glucose load

(C) urine culture

(D) vaginal culture for group B *Streptococcus*

(E) basic metabolic panel (Chem-7)

60. Which of the following tests is recommended as screening for hepatitis B in pregnancy?

(A) hepatitis B surface antibody

(B) hepatitis B surface antigen

(C) hepatitis B core antibody

(D) hepatitis B e antigen

(E) hepatitis B e antibody

61. The result of the test that you ordered in question 60 is positive. What would be appropriate management for the neonate to reduce the risk of perinatal transmission of the hepatitis B virus?

(A) hepatitis B vaccine within 2 days of birth

(B) hepatitis B immune globulin within 2 days of birth

(C) hepatitis B immune globulin and hepatitis B vaccine within 12 hours of birth

(D) deliver the baby by scheduled caesarian section

(E) advise the mother not to breast feed

Questions 62 and 63

A 50-year old male presents to the office for prostate cancer screening because he saw a TV show recommending that men get tested. He has no significant medical history, takes no medications, and has no genitourinary symptoms. There is no family history of prostate cancer.

62. What can you tell him about prostate cancer and the PSA test?

(A) PSA testing has been proven to reduce all-cause mortality in men over 50.

(B) In spite of PSA testing, the disease-specific mortality from prostate cancer has not changed in the past 30 years.

(C) Prostate cancer is the only condition that causes an elevated PSA level.

(D) PSA testing can prevent the development of prostate cancer.

(E) PSA testing can increase the chances of detecting prostate cancer.

63. How would you advise him regarding prostate cancer screening?

(A) All men over the age of 50 should have a PSA test every year.

(B) As blood tests are very safe, there is no harm associated with PSA screening.

(C) Only men with symptoms of prostate enlargement should have PSA screening.

(D) A PSA level of less than 4.0 ng/mL rules out the diagnosis of prostate cancer.

(E) Certain medications may alter PSA level.

Questions 64 through 67

A 49-year-old male postal worker presents to your office for the evaluation of a lesion on his left arm. The lesion started about a week ago as a red pustule but has grown and now has a thick black scab. The lesion is painless. A coworker showed the patient a similar appearing lesion that she developed on her arm for which her doctor prescribed an oral antibiotic. Examination reveals a 5 cm circular black eschar with some surrounding vesicles. A Gram stain of fluid drained from a vesicle reveals chains of gram-positive bacilli.

64. What organism is most likely responsible for this lesion?

(A) methicillin-resistant *Staphylococcus aureus*

(B) smallpox virus

(C) *Clostridium tetani*

(D) *Bacillus anthracis*

(E) group A beta-hemolytic *Streptococcus*

65. What is the most appropriate management at this point?

(A) topical mupirocin ointment tid for 10 days

(B) oral cephalexin 500 mg qid for a week

(C) oral clindamycin 300 mg tid for 10 days

(D) urgent quarantine of patient's coworkers and family contacts

(E) immediate notification of Public Health Authorities

66. The patient asks how he contracted this infection. Which of the following do you tell him?

(A) from direct contact with the coworker who had the similar appearing lesion

(B) ingestion of contaminated food in the postal facility cafeteria

(C) a small skin cut or sore was directly contaminated with spores

(D) inhalation of bacteria from a contaminated ventilation system

(E) exposure to respiratory droplets from an infected person

67. Which of the following is characteristic of Varicella (chickenpox) but not smallpox?

(A) The mortality rate is high.

(B) The lesions are commonly on the palms of the hands and soles of the feet.

(C) The pox lesions evolve synchronously.

(D) There is typically a 2- to 4-day prodrome of fever, malaise, headache, and backache before the development of the rash.

(E) The vesicles typically occur on an erythematous base (described as *dewdrops on a rose petal*)

Questions 68 and 69

A 60-year-old woman presents to your office to discuss her ongoing treatment with HRT that she takes for menopausal symptoms. She was started on estrogen and progesterone replacement at the age of 51 and has been on them since that time. She has read several articles in newspapers and on the Internet stating that hormone therapy is dangerous. You briefly review the results of the Women's Health Initiative study, a randomized-controlled trial comparing health outcomes in women taking combined estrogen-progestin therapy (HRT) versus a placebo. The results are as follows:

Condition	Hazard ratio for women taking HRT	95% CI
Coronary heart disease (CHD)	1.29	1.02–1.63
Breast cancer	1.26	1.00–1.59
Stroke	1.41	1.07–1.85
Pulmonary embolus	2.13	1.39–3.25
Colorectal cancer	0.63	0.43–0.92
Endometrial cancer	0.83	0.47–1.47
Hip fracture	0.66	0.45–0.98
Deaths from other causes	0.92	0.74–1.14

68. Based on the results listed, what can you tell your patient about women taking HRT?

(A) They have no difference in endometrial cancer risk.

(B) They have no difference in CHD risk.

(C) They have no difference in pulmonary embolus risk.

(D) They have no difference in stroke risk.

(E) They have no difference in hip fracture risk.

69. The authors provided composite data on total cardiovascular disease, cancer, fracture, and mortality risks, which are summarized in the chart.

Composite outcome	Hazard ratio for women taking HRT	95% CI
Cardiovascular disease	1.22	1.09–1.36
Total cancer	1.03	0.90–1.17
Combined fractures	0.76	0.69–0.85
Total mortality	0.98	0.82–1.18

Based on the data presented, which of the following statements is true?

(A) There is an increase in total cancer risk for women on HRT.

(B) There is an increase in cardiovascular disease risk for women on HRT.

(C) There is an increase in combined fracture risk for women on HRT.

(D) There is a reduction in total mortality for women on HRT.

(E) There is an overall detriment to the quality of life of women on HRT.

70. A 1-year-old boy is brought to the office for a well-child examination. Your office nurse has plotted his growth on the following chart (see Figure 6-1). The most appropriate initial management of this abnormality is which of the following?

FIG. 6-1

(A) Order a CT scan of the head.

(B) Repeat the measurement.

(C) Recommend that the mother cut down on the child's caloric intake.

(D) Review the growth chart of the child's older sibling to look for a similar pattern.

(E) Ask the mother to bring the child back to the office at monthly intervals to follow his growth more closely.

Questions 71 and 72

The modern history of the protection of human research subjects began in the twentieth century in response to human experimentation which occurred during World War II. The Nuremberg Military Tribunal set forth initial basic standards for the conduct of research which ultimately became known as the Nuremberg Code (1947/1948). In subsequent years, these recommendations have been modified and expanded to reflect various aspects of medical ethics in biomedical and behavioral research. These international ethical guidelines include the Declaration of Helsinki (1964), the Belmont Report (1979), CIOMS (1982), and the Common Rule (1991).

71. The concept of beneficence in the Belmont Report emphasizes the importance of which of the following?

    (A) establishing institutional research boards (IRBs)
    (B) maximizing benefits and minimizing harms to research subjects
    (C) ensuring independent ethical review of research
    (D) ensuring scientific validity of research
    (E) including patient advocates on scientific advisory boards

72. The concept of justice as described in the Belmont Report means which of the following?

    (A) ensuring that risks to research subjects are minimized
    (B) ensuring the protection of privacy
    (C) maintaining confidentiality
    (D) ensuring informed consent
    (E) ensuring the equitable distribution of research burdens and benefits

Questions 73 and 74

Mr. Jones is a 34-year-old married businessman. He and his wife are both patients in your practice. As part of his annual physical, you screen for high-risk behaviors and he admits to receiving confidential treatment at a public health clinic for gonorrhea and genital herpes. He has not revealed this information to his wife even though they are planning to have a baby. He did not return for the results of HIV screening at the public health clinic. On physical examination, you note that he has cervical and axillary lymphadenopathy, oral thrush, and seborrheic dermatitis.

73. What is the best step in his clinical management?

    (A) Prescribe Mycelex troches.
    (B) Schedule a lymph node biopsy.
    (C) Prescribe Lotrisone (betamethasone/clotrimazole) cream.
    (D) Repeat HIV serologic testing.
    (E) Contact his wife for sexually transmitted disease (STD) screening.

74. Mr. Jones returns to your office for a follow-up visit. He adamantly refuses to discuss his HIV status with his wife and threatens to sue if you reveal the test results. What is your role as a physician?

    (A) Respect Mr. Jones' patient autonomy.
    (B) Protect Mr. Jones' confidentiality.
    (C) Contact Mrs. Jones and ask her to come in for an annual examination.
    (D) Advise Mr. Jones you have a responsibility to notify his wife.
    (E) Refer Mr. Jones to an HIV specialist.

Questions 75 and 76

As an intern on a medical consultation service, you are providing a cardiology consultation for a patient who developed a myocardial infarction while undergoing an elective cholecystectomy. Although not described in the medical record, the cardiology consultant attending stated the patient experienced the myocardial infarction because of prolonged general anesthesia. The surgical attending did not make the initial incision until the patient had been sedated for more than 1 hour. As you review the medical record, you realize the patient is the father of your college roommate. When you walk in the room, the family is very happy to see you and asks, "What happened? What went wrong?"

75. What is your ethical responsibility?

(A) disclosure of your knowledge of the clinical circumstances to the patient

(B) disclosure of your knowledge of the clinical circumstances to your college roommate

(C) disclosure of the family's questions to the attending physician

(D) documentation in the medical record of your assessment of the iatrogenic patient injury

(E) request a random drug test of the surgeon

76. Which of the following is a commonly used mechanism for reducing medical errors in hospitals?

(A) confidential peer review

(B) national hospital accreditation

(C) departmental grand rounds

(D) longer work shifts for employees to promote continuity of patient care

(E) random drug testing

77. You are contacted by the regional Federal Bureau of Investigations (FBI) field office to evaluate a prisoner in custody. The prisoner has confessed to crimes for which he could receive the death penalty. The FBI believes that he has information that could lead to the arrest of multiple co-conspirators and end an on-going criminal enterprise. For which of the following actions is physician participation ethical?

(A) providing medical clearance for verbal interrogation

(B) providing medical treatment for sustained physical interrogation

(C) starting intravenous access and administering medications to sedate a prisoner prior to execution

(D) certifying the death of an executed prisoner

(E) continuing medical treatment based only on medical record documentation

78. The practice of confidentiality has roots in the Hippocratic Oath. However, the increasing use of health information technology has increased the efficiency of acquisition, manipulation, and dissemination of this potentially sensitive data. Federal laws have been adopted to safeguard health information privacy. Under the Health Insurance Portability and Accountability Act (HIPAA), which of the following is allowed?

(A) conducting teaching rounds at a table in the hospital cafeteria, as long as patient names are not used

(B) sharing a patient's diagnosis with any family member who requests the information

(C) discussing patient information with a consulting physician

(D) leaving an electronic medical record page with patient information open on a computer in the hallway of the ICU, to allow the nurse to have more rapid access to information

(E) sharing health information about a patient with his or her employer if the employer is paying for the patient's health insurance

79. You have been the geriatrician for a 79-year-old patient with a 10-year history of Alzheimer's disease, diabetes mellitus, and coronary artery disease. His 75-year-old wife has been his caretaker in the home. In the last 3 months, he has become progressively more combative and violent toward his wife. He was recently discharged from the hospital after intravenous antibiotic therapy for pneumococcal pneumonia but had to be readmitted to the intensive care unit with resistant, pneumococcal bacteremia, altered mental status, renal insufficiency, hypotension, CHF, and hypoxemia. When he was first aware of his early loss of memory, he told a family friend and his wife he would not want to be kept alive under such conditions. However, he did not execute an advanced directive. He does not have any surviving blood relatives and has no children. His wife refuses to sign the consent form to intubate her husband.

Which of the following is the most appropriate action to take at this time?

(A) Continue antibiotic therapy but don't intubate the patient.
(B) Send the wife home because of her emotional exhaustion.
(C) Intubate the patient.
(D) Request that a judge appoint a legal decision maker for the patient.
(E) Write a Do Not Attempt Resuscitation (DNR) order.

80. One of your long-time patients, a 17-year-old with cystic fibrosis, after experiencing several hospital admissions in respiratory crisis requiring intubation, requests that she not be intubated again in the event of future respiratory crisis. She requests comfort care only. The patient lives with her mother, who is mildly mentally retarded and unable to understand or participate in her daughter's health decisions. Her father is deceased. After numerous discussions over several visits, you assist her in filling out an outpatient DNR form and request a bracelet with DNR instructions. Several weeks later, the young girl is at a friend's house and stops breathing. She is not wearing the DNR bracelet and the friends know nothing of

her wishes. The ambulance is called and she is intubated en route to the hospital. You are called to the emergency room where she is being stabilized for transfer to pediatric intensive care unit (PICU).

What is the most ethically justified next step in this case?

(A) Wait to see if the patient regains consciousness before extubating.
(B) Assist in the extubation of the patient per her request.
(C) Seek a consultation from the ethics committee.
(D) Approve the transfer to the PICU and proceed with stabilization.
(E) Write a DNR order.

81. A third-year medicine resident has taken a trip to Guatemala to assist in a medical clinic for 2 weeks. After returning to work at the hospital, she faints during her grand rounds presentation of a case and is admitted to the teaching hospital where she works. She has a high temperature that cycles every few hours. The attending physician, a professor in her program, works her up for Dengue Fever and Malaria. Blood and urine laboratory tests are drawn and she receives many visitors from her concerned colleagues and coworkers. A fellow resident in her program, who is not directly involved in her care, reviews her chart and sees that her urine test came back positive for a pregnancy. Another resident sees him with the chart and asks, "So does she have Dengue or Malaria?"

How should he respond to this request for information?

(A) Order another pregnancy test to confirm.
(B) Talk to the patient before sharing any information.
(C) Refrain from sharing the test results with the other resident.
(D) Share the information with the other resident in confidence.
(E) Only share the information with the attending physician.

Answers and Explanations

1. **(A)**

2. **(E)**

3. **(E)**

Explanations 1 through 3

The United States Preventative Services Task Force (USPSTF) is an independent panel of experts in primary care and prevention that systematically reviews the evidence of effectiveness and develops recommendations for clinical preventative services. By carefully and systematically reviewing the available literature, the USPSTF makes recommendations on the effectiveness of screening, counseling, immunization, and chemoprevention using the following rating system:

A. The USPSTF strongly recommends that clinicians provide the service to eligible patients.
B. The USPSTF recommends that clinicians provide this service to eligible patients.
C. The USPSTF makes no recommendation for or against routine provision of the service.
D. The USPSTF recommends against routinely providing the service to asymptomatic patients.
I. The USPSTF concludes that the evidence is insufficient to recommend for or against routinely providing the service.

All of the recommendations of the USPSTF are available free of charge at their web site www.preventiveservices.ahrq.gov.

In a 50-year-old male who is generally healthy and does not present any apparent high-risk personal or family history, the USPSTF gives a level A recommendation to blood pressure measurement as a screening tool for hypertension in adults over the age of 18, as there is good evidence that screening for, and treating, hypertension can reduce the incidence of cardiovascular disease. There is insufficient evidence to recommend for or against screening for abdominal aortic aneurysm by abdominal palpation or for screening for skin cancer by a whole body skin examination (level I recommendation). This suggests that the evidence is lacking that performing these interventions will reduce the morbidity or mortality associated with these conditions. The USPSTF gives level D recommendations to screening for thyroid cancer by palpation and for screening for testicular cancer by palpation.

Fecal occult blood testing using three self-collected stool cards as a screening test for colon cancer has been given a level A recommendation, with good data to support reduction in colon cancer mortality from periodic screening. There is also evidence to support screening for colon cancer by flexible sigmoidoscopy or colonoscopy, with double-contrast barium enema as a possible alternative as well. Screening for lipid disorders in men over the age of 35 and women over the age of 45 also receives a level A recommendation. In general, the interval for repeat screening for an otherwise low-risk patient with lipid levels within the goal range, based on the National Cholesterol Education Project's Consensus opinion statement, would be 5 years. As this patient had lipid levels within the goal range 1 year ago, it would not be necessary to repeat this blood test at this visit. Screening for cardiovascular disease by the routine use of electrocardiography in asymptomatic, low-risk patients has been given a D recommendation, as there is an absence of evidence of improved health outcomes from this intervention. Screening for lung cancer by chest x-ray and for glaucoma by measurement of intraocular pressure are level I recommendations, with insufficient evidence to recommend for or against these interventions.

Screening for depression, either by a patient-completed questionnaire or physician interview, is a level B recommendation, as there is good evidence that screening improves the identification of depressed patients and treatment results in reduced morbidity. Beta-carotene supplementation to prevent cardiovascular disease or cancer is a level D recommendation, with no evidence of benefit in middle age or older adults and some evidence of increased risk of harm in certain populations (e.g., heavy smokers). Routine pneumococcal vaccination in adults without high-risk comorbidity, such as diabetes mellitus, is recommended at the age of 65 or older. Tetanus vaccination is recommended at 10-year intervals, in the absence of other risks such as a potentially contaminated wound. Multiple studies have shown that the intake of one to two alcoholic drinks a day in men does not increase morbidity or mortality and may, in fact, lower the risk of cardiovascular disease. (USPSTF: www.preventiveservices.ahrq.gov)

4. (D)

5. (D)

6. (D)

Explanations 4 through 6

Screening for osteoporosis in women 65 years old or older is a level B recommendation of the USPSTF, as detection and treatment of osteoporosis may reduce fracture risk. In women who have had a hysterectomy (with removal of the cervix) for reasons other than cervical cancer, pap smear screening of the vaginal cuff is not recommended and cytologic screening can be discontinued. Therapy with either estrogen alone (in women who do not have a uterus) or combined estrogen and progesterone (in women who have a uterus) in postmenopausal women is controversial. Based on findings of the Women's Health Initiative and other studies, the USPSTF gives a level D recommendation to the use of combined estrogen and

progesterone therapy and level I recommendation for estrogen therapy alone for the prevention of chronic conditions. Screening for asymptomatic bacteruria in all populations other than pregnant women is given a level D recommendation. No benefit from the intervention has been found and overtreatment with antibiotics may produce harm. While mammography for breast cancer screening has been given a level B recommendation, both self-breast examination and clinical breast examination are level I recommendations, with insufficient evidence to show any benefit in morbidity or mortality. (USPSTF: www.preventiveservices.ahrq.gov)

According to the Centers for Disease Control, diseases of the heart make up the most common cause of death in women in this age group. Heart disease is responsible for approximately one-third of all deaths in women aged 65 and older. Malignant neoplasms make up the next largest cause of death, followed by cerebrovascular diseases and chronic lower respiratory diseases. (Centers for Disease Control, 2003)

PPV-23 is recommended for all adults over the age of 65 and at younger ages for individuals at high risk for pneumonia or complications of pneumonia. These include persons with diabetes mellitus, chronic obstructive pulmonary disease, coronary artery disease, and those who have had a splenectomy or are functionally asplenic. The PCV-7 is recommended for the routine vaccination of children. Hepatitis B vaccine is recommended universally for children and for adults who are at high risk for the disease based on profession or lifestyle. Hepatitis A vaccine is recommended for children who live in certain areas of the United States in which the disease is prevalent and may be offered electively to persons traveling to endemic areas. The MMR vaccine is recommended to all children but is not indicated in adults. Rubella vaccination is recommended for women of childbearing age who may become pregnant and who do not have immunity to rubella, in an effort to reduce the risk of congenital rubella infection. (Centers for Disease Control: www.cdc.gov)

7. **(E)**

8. **(A)**

9. **(E)**

Explanations 7 through 9

The Third Report of the National Cholesterol Education Program Expert Panel on the Detection, Evaluation, and Treatment of High Blood Cholesterol in Adults (ATP III) was published in May 2001 by the National Heart, Lung, and Blood Institute of the National Institutes of Health. It is available on-line at: www.nhlbi.nih.gov/guidelines/cholesterol/atp3xsum.pdf. This evidence-based report provides guidelines for the evaluation and management of blood lipid levels for the primary and secondary prevention of heart disease. The basis of the recommendations for management is an overall evaluation of an individual's risk factors for developing cardiovascular disease. Persons at the highest risk for future cardiac events are those with already established coronary artery disease or "coronary artery disease equivalents," which include diabetes mellitus, other forms of atherosclerotic disease, or multiple risk factors that confer a 10-year CHD risk of greater than 20%. Multiple studies have shown that elevated LDL cholesterol levels are a risk for coronary artery disease and that lowering LDL levels can reduce the risk of events. ATP III goals are targeted at LDL levels. For persons with LDL levels above this goal, the options for lowering LDL can include therapeutic lifestyle changes, lipid-lowering medications, or a combination of both. In a patient with coronary artery disease, diabetes mellitus, or other CHD equivalents, the LDL goal level is 100 mg/dL. In this population, therapeutic lifestyle changes alone would be recommended for those with LDL levels of 100–130 and medication could be started concomitantly with lifestyle changes for those with LDL above 130, as most persons would require medication to achieve the recommended goal. For the patient in this question with an LDL of 160 mg/dL, therapy with an HMG-CoA reductase inhibitor would be recommended first-line therapy to try to get his LDL to goal. Therapeutic lifestyle changes alone would be very unlikely to reduce his LDL to less than 100 mg/dL, but are still an important part of his overall lipid management program and should be recommended along with medication therapy. Neither increasing his dosage of metformin nor adding insulin would be recommended as they would not be expected to improve his dyslipidemia significantly and because his diabetic control is appropriate. At his follow-up visit, the patient's lipid levels have met the recommended guidelines; therefore, the recommendation would be to continue with his current therapy. Increasing the dosage of his statin, adding a fibric acid, nicotinic acid, or referring the patient to a dietician would all be appropriate considerations in someone who had not successfully reached his goal lipid levels.

A recent addition to the ATP III provides an option for changing the target LDL goal for those at the highest of risk for coronary events. For persons with known coronary artery disease, or CAD equivalent, and multiple risk factors, such as diabetes or continued smoking, one could consider using an LDL of 70 as a goal. For this patient, with diabetes but no history of CAD or equivalent, the recommended goal would remain an LDL of 100 or less.

Immunizations should be a routine part of the adult health maintenance evaluation. All patients with diabetes are recommended to be vaccinated with the pneumococcal vaccine (PPV-23) both because of the incidence of pneumonia in diabetics and the increased risk of complications should infection occur. A recent recommendation for all adults is to provide a single dose of Tdap vaccine in place of one booster dose of Td. The rationale for this is to attempt to reduce the incidence of pertussis in the population, as pertussis has been recurring in the United States in spite of routine childhood vaccination. Hepatitis A and B are routine vaccinations for children. The current recommendation for adult immunizations against these diseases is to target high-risk adults. Diabetes is not considered a high risk for these infections. Herpes zoster vaccine is recommended for adults over the age of 60. *(Centers for Disease Control: www.cdc.gov)*

10. (B)

11. (D)

12. (C)

13. (E)

Explanations 10 through 13

The Seventh Report of the Joint National Committee on the Prevention, Detection, Evaluation, and Treatment of High Blood Pressure (JNC 7) was released in May, 2003 and is available on-line at: www.nhlbi.nih.gov/guidelines/hypertension/express.pdf. It provides evidence-based guidelines for the detection, evaluation, and treatment of hypertension, the most common primary diagnosis in the United States. One of the key guidelines presented in this report is the classification of blood pressure for adults. The classification is based on the average of two or more properly measured, seated, blood pressure readings on each of two or more office visits. The proper measurement of blood pressure is critical. Blood pressure should be measured using a properly calibrated instrument in a patient who has been seated quietly in a chair for at least 5 minutes, with his feet on the floor and arm supported at heart level. The blood pressure cuff should encircle at least 80% of the arm. The systolic blood pressure is the point at which the first of two or more sounds is heard and the diastolic blood pressure is the point before the sounds disappear. In question 10, where an incidentally noted elevated blood pressure reading is found, it is then necessary to perform blood pressure measurements following the JNC 7 guidelines—two or more readings after the patient has been seated quietly in a chair for 5 or more minutes. Institution of antihypertensive medications would be inappropriate based on one blood pressure reading in this range, as the patient has not been diagnosed as hypertensive as of yet. Aspirin therapy is recommended for most persons over the age of 50 for the primary prevention of CHD events and would be recommended for others at high risk of heart disease. In persons with hypertension, it is recommended to start aspirin after their blood pressure is controlled because the risk of hemorrhagic stroke is increased in uncontrolled hypertension. Risk stratification with an exercise stress test at this point is not supported by evidence showing a reduction of morbidity or mortality and is likely to have many false positive results. Discontinuation of his nasal steroid is unnecessary as it is unlikely to be affecting his blood pressure adversely and should provide good symptomatic relief of his seasonal allergy symptoms.

The blood pressure classifications from the JNC 7 report are as follows:

Blood pressure classification	Systolic BP in mmHg	Diastolic BP in mmHg
Normal	<120	and <80
Prehypertension	120–139	or 80–89
Stage 1 hypertension	140–159	or 90–99
Stage 2 hypertension	≥160	or ≥100

This classification regimen represents a change from previous JNC guidelines with the designation of a prehypertension classification and the combination of the previous stage 2 and stage 3 into a single stage 2 category. By this categorization, the patient in this question has stage 2 hypertension. Recommended evaluation of patients with hypertension includes an ECG, measurement of blood glucose, hematocrit, serum potassium, creatinine and calcium, urinalysis, and a fasting lipid profile. Other testing is not indicated unless suggested by the presence of symptoms or if blood pressure control cannot be achieved.

The management of hypertension involves the institution of lifestyle recommendations and, frequently, the use of antihypertensive medications. Lifestyle modifications can lower blood pressure, enhance the effectiveness of medications, and reduce cardiovascular risks. A low salt diet by itself may lower systolic blood pressure by 2–8 mmHg and is not likely to bring this patient to a goal blood pressure if that is the only modification made. Other lifestyle modifications, including the DASH (dietary approaches to stop hypertension) eating plan and increasing physical activity, could be beneficial as well. When the decision is made to institute pharmacotherapy, the weight of the evidence suggests that thiazide diuretics should be the first-line therapy for most individuals, in the absence of other compelling indications, such as a diabetic patient with nephropathy or a postmyocardial infarction patient. For patients whose blood pressure is more than 20 mmHg above the desired goal, the recommendation is to start the patient on two drug therapy, as lifestyle modifications and single drug therapy alone are unlikely to bring the patient to goal. When starting multidrug therapy, it is recommended that a thiazide be included as one of the components. *(www.nhlbi.nih.gov/ guidelines/hypertension/express.pdf)*

14. (C)

15. (D)

16. (E)

17. (D)

Explanations 14 through 17

Relative risk is the percentage of subjects who achieve an outcome in one experimental group divided by the percentage of subjects who achieve the same outcome in another group. This statistic is used frequently in placebo-controlled trials, where the comparison occurs between the experimental group and the control group. In the study referenced in this set of questions, the comparison is between two groups who were given two different active medications—exemestane and tamoxifen. The outcome studied here is the development of recurrent breast cancer. The data presented state that after the course of treatment, 91.5% of the women in the exemestane group and 86.8% of the women in the tamoxifen group were disease free. Therefore, 8.5% in the exemestane group and 13.2% in the tamoxifen group developed the outcome of recurrent breast cancer. The relative risk is then calculated as 0.085/0.132 = 0.64 = 64%.

The relative risk reduction is the percentage by which the risk in one group has been reduced when compared to the other group. In other words, if the rate of an outcome in one group is 100%, the relative risk reduction is the difference between 100% and the measured relative risk. It is calculated by the formula:

Relative risk reduction = 1 − relative risk

In this example, the relative risk reduction is 1 − 0.64 = 0.36 = 36%.

The ARR, also known as the risk difference, is calculated by subtracting the percentage of subjects who achieve an outcome in one group from the percentage who achieve the outcome in another. In this study, the ARR for those in the exemestane group compared to those in the tamoxifen group is 13.2% − 8.5% = 4.7%.

The NNT is the number of subjects who need to receive an intervention (such as a medication) in order for one of them to have a beneficial outcome. In this study, the beneficial outcome would be one less case of recurrent breast cancer. The NNT is calculated as 1/ARR. In this case, the NNT = 1/0.047 = 21. In other words, 21 women need to be treated with exemestane in order for there to be one fewer case of recurrent breast cancer compared to women treated with tamoxifen. *(Coombes et al., 2004, pp. 1081–1092)*

18. (A)

19. (D)

20. (C)

21. (A)

Explanations 18 through 21

Understanding the concepts of sensitivity, specificity, PPV, and NPV is crucial to interpreting diagnostic test results. Sensitivity is defined as the percentage of people who have a disease who test positive for that disease. Specificity is defined as the percentage of people who are free of a disease who test negative. These two concepts are considered characteristics of the specific test in question and are independent of the prevalence of the disease in the population. The PPVs and NPVs of a test are the test's clinical characteristics and these concepts are directly related to the prevalence of the disease in the population. The PPV is the percentage of people who have a positive test result who actually have the disease. Similarly, the NPV is the percentage of people who have a negative test result who don't have the disease. While the definitions may seem subtly different, the implications are significant.

The usual way to calculate sensitivity, specificity, PPV, and NPV is with the 2×2 table, using the following definitions:

Disease

		+	−
Test	+	True positive $\quad$ a	B $\quad$ False positive
	−	c $\quad$ False negative	d $\quad$ True negative

The definitions of sensitivity, specificity, PPV, and NPV would then be:

Sensitivity = $a/(a + c)$

Specificity = $d/(d + b)$

PPV = $a/(a + b)$

NPV = $d/(d + c)$

The specific information in this question comes from an article describing a study of B-type natriuretic peptide (BNP) for the diagnosis of CHF. The data presented show that 106 persons tested positive using the BNP test. After comparison with the "gold standard," in this case, a review by expert cardiologists, 95 of these 106 were determined to truly have CHF. Therefore, 11 of the 106 were false positives and 95 were true positives. Similarly, 144 persons tested negative using the BNP test. Of these, 142 were confirmed as true negatives and 2 were determined to be false negatives. Putting these numbers into a 2×2 table reveals:

CHF

		+	−
BNP	+	True positive $\quad$ 95 $\quad$ a	b $\quad$ 11 $\quad$ False positive
	−	2 $\quad$ c $\quad$ False negative	d $\quad$ 142 $\quad$ True negative

The calculations then become:

Sensitivity = $a/(a + c) = 95/(95 + 2) = 98\%$

Specificity = $d/(d + b) = 142/(142 + 11) = 93\%$

PPV = $a/(a + b) = 95/(95 + 11) = 90\%$

NPV = $d/(d + c) = 142/(142 + 2) = 99\%$

(Dao et al., 2001, pp. 379–385; Slawson and Shaughnessy, 2003)

22. **(D)**

23. **(B)**

24. **(B)**

25. **(C)**

Explanations 22 through 25

Primary care physicians are frequently called on to perform preparticipation examinations on young athletes. These types of encounters can be used to serve a number of purposes, including attempting to identify conditions that may adversely affect the athlete during participation, identify conditions that may predispose the athlete to injury, provide anticipatory guidance on high-risk behaviors common to the age group being addressed, and fulfill legal conditions of the institution involved. Fortunately, the rate of sudden death in young athletes is low.

In those under the age of 35, the most common cause of sudden death is congenital cardiac anomalies. Hypertrophic cardiomyopathy (HCM) is responsible for about one-third of these deaths. Unfortunately, sudden death may be the presenting symptom of HCM. A personal or family history of congenital heart disease, symptoms of chest pain or tightness, palpitations, dyspnea, syncope or near-syncope are important. A family history of HCM or unexplained sudden death in someone under the age of 50 is significant as well. The murmur of HCM may not be present in all persons with this disorder. To identify the murmur, dynamic auscultation is often necessary. The heart should be auscultated while the patient is lying and then standing. As this murmur is accentuated by maneuvers which reduce cardiac preload, the murmur will get louder when the patient stands or performs a Valsalva maneuver and will diminish as the patient lies or squats. As the patient in question 22 has the concerning historical point of exertional syncope and a family history of an unexplained, early death along with a characteristic murmur on examination, further evaluation is warranted. In the 26th Bethesda Conference report, the American College of Cardiology recommends that persons with HCM should be restricted from all, except possibly for the least strenuous, athletic activity. In this case, restriction of all athletic activity until the patient can be further evaluated by a cardiologist—preferably one with experience in dealing with the evaluation of athletes—would be the most appropriate option of the choices given.

Marfan syndrome is a connective tissue disorder that typically affects the eyes, skeletal system, and cardiovascular system. Persons with Marfan syndrome are typically tall and have arm spans that are greater than their height. Signs include long, slender digits, high-arched palates, and pectus deformities of the chest. Lens dislocations in the eye are common. Detecting Marfan syndrome during a preparticipation examination is important because of the occurrence of aortic root dilation and the risk of sudden death caused by aortic rupture. The patient in questions 23 and 24 has multiple signs of Marfan syndrome and further evaluation would be indicated. Of the options given, an echocardiogram to evaluate the aortic root and to look for other valvular abnormalities would be indicated. These persons usually require referral to an ophthalmologist as well for a dilated eye examination to evaluate for lens dislocations. Turner syndrome is a syndrome of gonadal dysgenesis, associated with a 45, X karyotype (or another defect of the X chromosome). This syndrome is typically associated with a short stature and multiple anomalies including a webbed neck and "shield" chest. The female athlete triad is a syndrome of disordered eating, amenorrhea, and osteoporosis. It is seen most often in participants in activities that emphasize low body weights,

such as gymnastics or ballet. The presence of regular menstrual cycles makes this diagnosis unlikely. Atlantoaxial instability can be associated with Down syndrome. Physicians performing preparticipation examinations on someone with Down syndrome must consider performing lateral cervical spine x-rays with flexion and extension views. This patient does not have any of the classic findings of Down syndrome. Similarly, she does not exhibit any of the classic symptoms of type 1 diabetes—polydipsia, polyphagia, and polyuria. Performing serum glucose testing would therefore not be indicated.

The patient in question 25 is the most typical type of patient who presents for a preparticipation examination—the healthy adolescent. This may be the only encounter that a physician will have with an adolescent, especially an adolescent male. It is in this population where a physician can use this encounter to address other age appropriate health maintenance issues. As the patient had a Td booster 3 years ago, another one at this point would not be indicated (although consideration could be given to providing a Tdap). Other vaccinations to consider would be hepatitis B and MMR, if he has not previously been adequately immunized. As he has had two MMR vaccines, he has completed the recommended series. There is no history given regarding hepatitis B vaccination and this would be something to address clinically. A nonjudgmental discussion of sexual behaviors, drug use, alcohol use, and other high-risk behaviors would also be appropriate. Screening athletes who have neither concerning symptoms nor signs with ECGs is not recommended because of the poor predictive values and significant costs involved with mass screening. ECGs should be performed without hesitation in any athlete who has a history, examination finding, or preexisting diagnosis of a potentially high-risk condition. Although some localities may require a urinalysis as part of a preparticipation examination, there is no evidence to recommend universal screening.

A recent recommendation from the Advisory Committee for Immunization Practices is to provide a varicella booster at age 4–6 years for all children and to provide a booster vaccine to all children and adolescents who have only had a single dose. This is recommended because recent studies have shown a waning effect to the protection provided by the single varicella vaccine regimen, with a resultant shift to the development of varicella disease in older children, adolescents, and adults. The rate of complications resulting from varicella infection is higher in older ages. For these reasons, a booster dose is now recommended. *(McKeag and Sallis, 2000, pp. 2617–2618; Kurowski and Chandran, 2000, pp. 2683–2690, 2696–2698)*

26. **(E)** The landmark 1999 Institute of Medicine report, *To Err is Human: Building a Safer Health System*, estimated that between 44,000 and 98,000 Americans died each year in hospitals as a result of medical errors. Even using the lower number, this represents more deaths than breast cancer, motor vehicle accidents, and AIDS. About 7000 deaths are attributable to medication errors. This number alone is greater than the number of deaths in work-related injuries. Errors in diagnosis, treatment, prevention, communication, equipment failure, and other system failures result not only in significant morbidity and mortality, but also an estimated 17–29 billion dollars in costs. Further, there is a significant loss in trust in the health system by patients and loss in satisfaction by patients, their families, and health care providers. Unfortunately, many of these errors that occurred, and continue to occur, are preventable. Many hospitals, health care organizations, and oversight agencies, including the Quality Interagency Coordination Task Force of the Federal Government, are actively pursuing mechanisms of quality improvement to reduce this epidemic. *(Institute of Medicine: www.iom.edu/Object.File/Master/4/117/0.pdf)*

27. **(A)**

28. **(E)**

Explanations 27 and 28

The odds ratio is a frequently published statistic. The odds of an event occurring are the number of times an event occurred divided by the number of times that it did not. In medical studies, it is calculated by dividing the number of subjects who achieved a certain outcome by the number of subjects who did not. An odds ratio is calculated by dividing the odds of an event in one group by the odds of the same event in another group. This is frequently an experimental group and a control group.

In the study presented in this question, the "experimental" group is the induction of labor group and the control is the expectant management group. An odds ratio of less than one means that the outcome in question occurred less often in the experimental group than in the control group. Conversely, an odds ratio of greater than one reveals that the outcome occurred more often in the experimental group than the control group. In the study presented, the odds ratios for both the outcomes of caesarian delivery and perinatal mortality are less than one, suggesting that these outcomes occurred less often in the group of women treated with induction of labor at 41 weeks' gestation compared to those treated with expectant management.

A CI is a range within which the "true" result is likely to be found. A 95% CI states that there is a 95% probability that the true answer exists within these bounds. For statistics, such as odds ratios or relative risks, a 95% CI that includes the number 1 within its bounds is considered not statistically significant. This is because an odds ratio of 1 means that there is no difference in the odds of an event occurring in either group. For the outcome of caesarian delivery, the odds ratio is 0.88 with a 95% CI that does not include 1. Therefore, one can say that there is a statistically significant reduction in the number of caesarian deliveries in the induction group compared to the expectant management group. For the outcome of perinatal mortality, the odds ratio is 0.41 but the 95% CI extends up to 1.18. This result cannot be considered statistically significant. The answer to question 27 is therefore A.

Statistical power is the ability of a study to determine a difference between two groups if a difference truly exists. It is a function of the magnitude of the difference between the two groups and the number of subjects in the study. For the result of perinatal mortality, the odds ratio is low at 0.41, suggesting that a difference may exist between the two groups. However, the presence of wide CIs around this result suggests that the study is underpowered to detect this difference. For this particular study, it is because the outcome in question—perinatal mortality—occurred (fortunately) rarely. The only realistic way to increase the power of a study is to increase the number of subjects enrolled. (n.b.: This particular meta-analysis had approximately 6000 subjects. The authors estimate that approximately 16,000 would be needed to achieve adequate power to find a statistically significant difference in perinatal mortality.) *(Sanchez-Ramos et al., 2003, pp. 1312–1318)*

29. (A)

30. (D)

31. (D)

Explanations 29 through 31

Bacterial endocarditis is a rare, but life-threatening, disease. It occurs primarily in persons with underlying structural heart defects who develop bacteremia with organisms that are likely to cause endocarditis. Most cases of endocarditis are not a complication of invasive medical or dental procedures. Because of the risks associated with the disease, efforts should be made to prevent bacterial endocarditis when appropriate. The American Heart Association has published updated, evidence-based recommendations on the prevention of bacterial endocarditis. These guidelines are available at the American Heart Association web site (www.americanheart.org). These guidelines outline conditions for which endocarditis prophylaxis is appropriate, procedures for which endocarditis prophylaxis is necessary, and antibiotic regimens that are recommended. Cardiac conditions are stratified into high-risk, moderate-risk, and negligible risk. Negligible risk conditions are those in which, although endocarditis may develop, the risk is no greater than in the general population.

This patient has a history of rheumatic fever, which can potentially result in high-risk valvular damage. However, his echocardiogram did not reveal any such condition. Mitral valve prolapse without a regurgitant jet (which is not a complication of rheumatic fever) is considered a negligible risk condition, so the proposed dental work can proceed without delay. Of the conditions listed in question 30, only bicuspid aortic valve would require antibiotic prophylaxis, as it is a moderate-risk congenital cardiac malformation. All of the other conditions listed are considered to be of negligible risk.

Procedures which require antibiotic prophylaxis are those which produce a significant bacteremia with organisms commonly causing endocarditis. For dental procedures, those that tend to cause significant bleeding from hard or soft tissues would necessitate prophylaxis. Of the procedures listed, only dental extraction is likely to do this. During the course of other procedures, if unexpected significant bleeding occurs, antibiotics within 2 hours following the procedure would be recommended. *(American Heart Association, 2004: www.americanheart.org/presenter.jhtml?identifier=4436)*

32. (E)

33. (C)

Explanations 32 and 33

The disease tetanus is caused by an exotoxin produced by the anaerobic, gram-positive bacterium *C. tetani*. The spores of *C. tetani* are endemic in soil, particularly in agricultural areas. They can also be found in the intestines and feces of many animals. Human infection usually is the result of the introduction of the spores through a wound, such as a puncture or laceration. The spores can then germinate and toxins are released. Tetanus is characterized by unopposed muscle contractions and spasms. Autonomic nervous system manifestations, seizures, and difficulty swallowing may occur. Recovery may take months, but the disease is often fatal. In the developed world, most cases of tetanus occur in those who either were never vaccinated or who completed a primary vaccine series but have not had a booster in the preceding 10 years. The currently available vaccine is a toxoid which consists of a formaldehyde-treated toxin. It is available as a single antigen vaccine, combined with diphtheria (pediatric DT or adult Td) or combined with both diphtheria and acellular pertussis vaccine (DTaP). Whenever possible, tetanus toxoid should be given in combination with diphtheria toxoid to provide periodic boosting for both antigens. There is little reason to use single antigen tetanus toxoid alone.

Management of a potentially contaminated wound initially involves local wound care. Necrotic tissue should be debrided, foreign material removed, and the wound irrigated. The need for active and/or passive immunization against tetanus depends on the wound and the patient's history of immunization. A person who has completed a primary series of three or more doses of tetanus toxoid vaccine will not require passive immunization with TIG, but may require a booster of dT or Tdap. For a clean, minor wound, a Td or Tdap booster would be indicated if it has been more than 10 years since the patient's most recent booster. For all other wounds, a booster would be indicated if it has been 5 years since the most recent booster. In a person who has not completed a primary series, who is completely unimmunized, or in whom the vaccine status is unknown, initiating passive immunization with Td or Tdap is indicated for all wounds. If the wound is clean and minor then TIG would not be recommended. For all other wounds, both Td and TIG would be indicated, as the initial doses of Td/Tdap may not produce immunity and TIG can provide immediate, temporary immunity. Antibiotic prophylaxis against tetanus is not useful. As noted in explanation 9 (above), Tdap is recommended as a substitute for a single Td dose in order to address the increasing rates of pertussis being encountered in the population. As the patient in question 32 has no history of having completed a primary vaccine series and has a contaminated wound, the optimal management would be to provide both Tdap and TIG. If Tdap were not available, then utilizing Td and TIG would be an acceptable substitute, with a

dose of Tdap to be given as part of his "catch-up" series in the future.

Following the initial management in the emergency room, efforts should be made to ensure that an appropriate primary series of tetanus vaccination is completed. For adults and for children age 7 or older with no history of having received a primary series, the recommended Td schedule is to provide a three-dose primary series with an initial dose, a second dose in 4 weeks, and a third dose in 6–12 months. Following completion of the primary series, a booster would be recommended every 10 years. Options A and B in question 33 do not provide for an adequate primary series. Option D is the recommended, routine vaccination schedule for infants. Option E is not indicated as TIG provides only temporary immunity and should only be used in the prophylaxis of wounds in those who are under-immunized or in the treatment of persons with tetanus disease. (*Centers for Disease Control: www.cdc.gov/nip/publications/pink/tetanus.pdf*)

34. **(A)** There is an increased risk of influenza-related complications in pregnant women who contract influenza, therefore the influenza vaccine is recommended for all pregnant women who will be beyond the first trimester during influenza season. The live, attenuated influenza vaccine is contraindicated during pregnancy but the inactivated influenza vaccine is recommended. The hepatitis B vaccine contains only noninfectious hepatitis B surface antigen particles and poses no real or theoretical risk of fetal infection, whereas the disease hepatitis B may cause severe illness for the pregnant woman and chronic disease for the newborn. For these reasons, neither pregnancy nor lactation is a contraindication to vaccination with hepatitis B vaccine. All pregnant women should routinely be tested for immunity to the rubella virus and should be immunized postpartum if they have no measurable immunity. The rubella vaccine, like other live-virus vaccines, is contraindicated during pregnancy due to the theoretical risk of causing fetal infection. In reality, studies of women who were pregnant or soon became pregnant after receiving rubella vaccination showed that the risk is extremely

small. A registry of 226 susceptible women who received the rubella vaccine between 3 months before and 3 months after conception showed no evidence of congenital rubella syndrome. Women who inadvertently receive this vaccine should be counseled about the theoretical risk involved, however this would not be considered a reason to terminate a pregnancy. Finally, Td toxoid is routinely indicated for pregnant women. A woman with no documented booster within 10 years should receive one and a woman with no documented primary series should start or complete her primary series. Some authorities do recommend waiting until the second trimester to administer a Td in order to minimize any theoretical concerns regarding teratogenicity. (*Centers for Disease Control: www.cdc. gov/nip/publications/preg_guide.htm*)

35. (C)

36. (D)

Explanations 35 and 36

The NNT is calculated by first determining the ARR for a specific outcome between two groups in a study. The ARR, or risk difference, is calculated by subtracting the percentage of subjects who develop an outcome in the treatment group from the percentage who develop the outcome in the control group. In question 35, the outcome considered is the development of prostate cancer. This occurred in 24% of the control group and 18% of the finasteride group. The ARR is calculated as 24% − 18% = 6% or 0.06. The NNT is calculated as: NNT = 1/ARR. In this example, the NNT = 1/0.06 = 16.67, approximately 17. This suggests that for every 17 men who took finasteride there was one fewer case of prostate cancer.

The NNH is calculated in exactly the same manner as the NNT. The only difference is that the outcome is adverse. In this study, high-grade prostate cancers occurred more often in the finasteride group than the placebo group; 6.4% of men who took finasteride and 5.1% who took a placebo developed high-grade prostate cancer. The risk difference, in this case an absolute risk increase, is 6.4% − 5.1% = 1.3%

or 0.013. The NNH = 1/absolute risk increase = 1/0.013 = 77. (*Thompson et al., 2003, pp. 215–224*)

37. (B)

38. (A)

Explanations 37 and 38

DEXA is the most widely used test for the screening and diagnosis of osteoporosis. It is sensitive for the loss of bone density, exposes the patient to a relatively low dose of radiation, and is widely available at a reasonable cost. It is the mode of evaluation that has been used in most of the studies of the evaluation and management of osteoporosis. The American College of Radiology Guidelines state that DEXA of the lumbar spine and proximal femur is the most appropriate screening test for osteoporosis in postmenopausal women who are not on any therapy. Quantitative CT scanning is also highly sensitive but is less widely available, more expensive, and exposes the subject to higher radiation doses. Lateral thoracic spine radiographs can diagnose or confirm the presence of osteoporotic fractures but are not appropriate as a screening test for bone density. Quantitative ultrasonography, usually of the calcaneus or digits, is becoming more widely available at low costs, but has the disadvantage of being unable to directly evaluate the areas where most ostoporotic fractures are likely to occur— hip, spine, and radius. SXA has not correlated as well to fracture risk as dual energy techniques and is, therefore, less appropriate than DEXA.

The T score is a comparison of the subjects' bone density to that of the mean bone density of a 25-year-old woman, when bone density is predicted to be at or near its maximum. The T score represents the number of standard deviations away from the mean value that a specific bone density represents. The World Health Organization defines osteoporosis as a T score of less than −2.5; that is to say, a bone density of 2.5 standard deviations less than that of the mean bone density of a 25-year-old woman. Osteopenia is defined as a T score of between −1 and −2.5, and a T score greater than −1 is considered normal. Of the options listed in question 38, treatment with a bisphosphonate, which has been shown both to increase bone density and reduce fracture incidence, would be indicated as we are treating a patient with established osteoporosis. Increasing the intake of both calcium and vitamin D are also important but not adequate as sole interventions. Most authorities recommend 1200–1500 mg calcium intake per day for postmenopausal women. Exercise, particularly weight-bearing exercise, is also important in the management of patients with osteoporosis both to maintain bone density but also to improve strength, coordination, and balance in an effort to reduce fall risk. It should be part of an overall management plan. When osteoporosis is treated, most authorities recommend waiting approximately 2 years for repeat bone density testing. (*American College of Radiology (ACR), 2001, p. 17; ACR Appropriateness Criteria, 2002*)

39. (B)

40. (D)

41. (E)

Explanations 39 through 41

Pregestational diabetes is associated with numerous risks to both the mother and the fetus. Stillbirths are more common in pregnancies to diabetic women and stillbirths without an identifiable cause, called "unexplained" stillbirths, are a well-described phenomenon. Similarly, preterm births are more common in diabetics than nondiabetics. While congenital malformations are more common in pregnancies to diabetic women, fetal chromosomal abnormalities are not more common. Children of women with diabetes have an approximately 1–3% incidence of developing type 1 diabetes. While earlier obstetrical teaching suggested that maternal diabetes delayed fetal lung maturation, more recent studies do not support this. Gestational age is likely the most significant factor in the development of respiratory distress.

While there are significant maternal risks from the interaction of diabetes and pregnancy, with the possible exception of diabetic retinopathy, the long-term course of diabetes does not appear to be affected by pregnancy. Pregnancy neither exacerbates nor modifies diabetic nephropathy and the development of diabetic peripheral neuropathy during pregnancy is uncommon. While preeclampsia is a significant risk and the perinatal mortality rate is 20 times higher in preeclamptic diabetic women compared to normotensive women, the occurrence of preeclampsia does not appear to be related to diabetic control. Diabetic ketoacidosis is a serious complication with an approximately 20% rate of fetal loss. However, it is estimated to occur in 1% of pregnancies of diabetic women. Infections occur in approximately 80% of pregnancies in insulin-dependent diabetics, with candida vaginitis, urinary tract infections, and respiratory infections being common.

Preconception counseling in diabetic women who desire to become pregnant is a critical issue that often is best served by a team that includes the obstetrician, primary care physician, endocrinologist, and diabetic educators. When possible, attempts should be made to attain optimal diabetic control. Women with good diabetic control have been shown in observational studies to have a lower rate of having infants with congenital anomalies than women with poorer diabetic control. Optimal diabetic control has been defined as glycated hemoglobin levels within or near the upper limit of the normal range. This can be obtained with multiple daily insulin injections or, in selected patients, a continuous infusion via an insulin pump. All women—diabetic or not—should be counseled to take folic acid prior to conception in order to lower the rate of neural tube defects. ACE inhibitors are contraindicated during pregnancy and should, whenever possible, be discontinued prior to conception. (*Cunningham et al., 2001, pp. 1367–1376*)

42. (D)

43. (A)

44. (D)

Explanations 42 through 44

All types of study designs have potential benefits and drawbacks and it is important to understand this when designing research or reviewing research reports. A cross-sectional study is one in which information is gathered from a certain population at one point in time with no follow-up period. This type of study is very useful for the determination of the prevalence of a disease or risk factor in a population at a certain point in time. Cross-sectional studies cannot determine cause and effect because there are no interventions being made and there is no follow-up. A case-control study is very useful and efficient at studying diseases that occur rarely. In a case-control study, persons with a disease are identified and then information is determined by looking back in time (i.e., retrospective review). A population of those without the disease (controls) is also defined and studied in the same way. The prevalence of a risk factor in the cases and controls can then be determined and compared. A case-control study cannot prove cause and effect, but it can be a powerful tool to determine risk factors that can generate hypotheses for further study. A cohort study is one in which a population is defined and then followed over time. A cohort study may be either prospective or retrospective. Cohort studies can be used to describe the incidence of diseases over time or to determine associations between predictors and outcomes. Cohort studies are inefficient for the study of rare outcomes, as a very large sample size would be required in order to find a few events. A prospective, randomized-controlled trial is the gold standard study for determining the effect of a treatment or intervention. It is not the type of study that would be used to determine the prevalence of a disease in a population or to determine what risk factors are associated with the development of a disease. A meta-analysis is a systematic review of completed research studies. By evaluating similarly done studies, the meta-analysis technique can allow for an evaluation of a body of literature and can be used to increase the overall statistical power by creating a larger sample by combining studies.

The odds ratios given in question 44 show that both risk factors X and Y occurred more often in those with the disease (cases) than they did in those without the disease (controls). Neither of the CIs given cross 1, therefore, these are statistically significant findings. We cannot use this type of study to definitively prove cause and effect, therefore option A is false. While risk factor X had a higher odds ratio for the development of the disease than risk factor Y, no prognostic data are supplied and none can be inferred from the information given, therefore B is false. The odds ratios as given in this case compare the prevalence of a risk factor in the case group with the control group, not the prevalence of one risk factor compared to another. For this reason, we cannot say which risk factor is more common in the population and option C is false. No absolute numbers are presented in this question and therefore we cannot determine how often each of the risk factors occurs in our population, so E is false as well. *(Hulley et al., 2001)*

45. **(E)**

46. **(B)**

47. **(E)**

Explanations 45 through 47

Current guidelines for TB control emphasize testing of those who are at high risk for the development of TB and who would benefit from the treatment of a latent TB infection, if detected. Based on that principle, testing is encouraged in those who are at high risk and discouraged among those who are at low risk. Further, anyone who is at high risk for the development of TB and who tests positive should be offered treatment, regardless of age. The preferred testing modality for asymptomatic persons of all ages is the intradermal (Mantoux) method of testing with PPD. Multiple puncture tests (e.g., Tine) are not sufficiently accurate and should not be used. The test should be read at 48–72 hours and the diameter of induration, not redness, should be measured and recorded. Previous BCG vaccination is not a contraindication to skin testing and a positive skin reaction should be used as an indication of TB infection when the tested person is at increased risk for infection or has medical conditions that increase the risk of the disease. Delayed-type hypersensitivity reactions may wane over time. This is especially a problem in older individuals. Repeating a PPD placement may result in a "booster" phenomenon, in which a person who initially tests negative develops a positive reaction. This increases the overall sensitivity of the testing process.

Three cutoff points for the determination of a positive test are currently in use: ≥5 mm of induration is used for those who are at the highest risk of disease, such as those immunosuppressed from HIV or medications, or those recently exposed to TB; ≥10 mm induration is used as a positive result for persons who have an increased probability of infection (such as immigrants from endemic areas), who have clinical conditions that increase the risk for TB (such as injection drug users) or who are residents or employees in high-risk settings (nursing homes, hospitals, prisons, and so on); ≥15 mm is used as a cutoff for those who have no known risk factors. In question 46, ignoring the amount of redness and using only induration as the criteria for positive or negative, the nursing home resident (option B) is the only one with a positive test.

All persons who test positive by a skin test should then have a chest x-ray to evaluate for evidence of pulmonary TB. In an asymptomatic person, sputum studies are not necessary to determine the need for treatment. Pregnant women should still get a chest x-ray, with appropriate abdominal shielding, as soon as feasible. As stated above, a history of BCG vaccination should not deter from the need for further evaluation and treatment of a positive test result. Age should also not be a determining factor in treating someone who is at risk for the development of TB. Currently, there are four acceptable treatment recommendations for latent TB infections. Daily isoniazid for 9 months is the most widely used regimen and has the highest level of recommendation because of its effectiveness, relative safety, ease of administration, and low cost. Twice-weekly

isoniazid may also be used but should only be given as directly observed therapy, due to the fact that a missed dose of this regimen represents a substantial risk of undertreatment. Rifampin alone or rifampin plus pyrazinamide are alternative regimens for use in certain, specified situations. *(Centers for Disease Control: www.cdc.gov/mmwr/PDF/rr/rr4906.pdf)*

48. **(C)** The widespread use of fluoride has been a major factor in the decline in the prevalence and severity of tooth decay in the United States. In most communities public water supplies are fluoridated. Supplementation is recommended by the Centers for Disease Control, American Academy of Pediatrics, American Academy of Family Physicians, and other authorities, for those who do not have access to fluoridated water. Fluoride supplementation can occur from both ingestion and from topical supplementation, such as in fluoride-containing toothpaste. Current guidelines recommend no supplementation until 6 months of age and then a dietary fluoride supplement of 0.25 mg/day from the age of 6 months to 3 years, 0.5 mg/day for ages 3–6 years, and 1.0 mg/day for ages 6–16 years for those persons who do not have access to fluoridated water. Current powdered infant formulas do not provide a significant amount of fluoride because of the risk of a child receiving too much fluoride if the formula is mixed with fluoridated water. The chronic ingestion of high levels of fluoride can result in fluorosis, a state of hypomineralization of tooth enamel. Studies have shown that fluoride supplements taken by pregnant women do not benefit their offspring. *(Centers for Disease Control: www.cdc.gov/mmwr/PDF/RR/RR5014.pdf)*

49. **(E)**

50. **(A)**

Explanations 49 and 50

Domestic violence is an abuse of power in a relationship in which a more powerful person exerts inappropriate control or domination over a less powerful person. Abuse is not only physical, but also can be emotional, sexual, or economic. Intimidation and psychological abuse also occur and are used sometimes by batterers in place of physical violence. Domestic, or partner, violence occurs in all types of relationships, regardless of the gender of the partners. The risk of violence increases in many situations, which exaggerate the disparity in power in the relationship, such as illness or disability in one of the partners. Pregnancy, especially unintended pregnancy, may also increase the risk of battery. Laws regarding the reporting of domestic violence vary from state to state. Many states do not require the reporting of domestic violence when the abused is a competent adult. Marriage, in and of itself, does not prevent a partner from making a sexual abuse charge against the other partner.

Management in the setting of partner violence can be difficult. Providing information and referrals to appropriate shelters and services is critical. Assisting with the development of emergency plans may be of benefit as well. Asking about the availability of weapons in the home is important, as up to half of female murder victims are killed by a current male partner or ex-partner. At this time, reporting to the Child Protective Services is inappropriate, as they cannot intervene. After the baby is born, however, any sign of child abuse should be immediately reported. *(Eyler and Cohen, 1999, pp. 2569–2576)*

51. **(D)**

52. **(E)**

53. **(B)**

Explanations 51 through 53

Encounters with persons traveling to other countries are common in primary care or community health settings. The advice and interventions provided are dependent on where the person is going, what he or she will be doing, and for how long he or she will be there. The most accessible and up-to-date source of this information in the United States is at the Centers for Disease Control web site, which provides detailed recommendations on vaccinations, health, and safety risks involved in overseas travel. In this series of questions, the travelers are going to the region of central Africa and, more specifically, to a rural area of Cameroon. This is an area of the world where polio remains a risk. As most Americans have not been vaccinated against polio since childhood, booster immunization against polio is recommended. The injectable polio vaccine is recommended as it does not carry with it the risk of vaccine-induced disease that the oral (live virus) vaccine does. Smallpox has been eliminated as a naturally occurring disease, although it remains of importance in bioterrorism discussions. The smallpox vaccine is not necessary for travel to any part of the world, but is used by the military or medical first-responders who may be exposed in the event of a biowarfare attack. The traveling couple is up-to-date on their dT status with boosters within the past 2 years. They have completed a series of both MMR and hepatitis B, which is felt to confer lifetime immunity.

Malaria prevention is an important consideration for travel to many areas of the developing world. Different regimens may be used depending on the area to which the travel will occur. All regimens, however, require the institution of prophylaxis prior to travel and the continuation of prophylaxis for up to 4 weeks after completion of travel. This is due to the life cycle of organisms that cause the disease. Prevention of malaria also involves attempts to reduce one's risk of exposure to the *Ixodes* mosquito which can transmit the disease. This mosquito tends to be more active early in the morning and at dusk, and less active in the middle of the day. Wearing long sleeved clothing, using mosquito nets, and insect repellent is important. DEET-containing insect repellents are recommended as the most effective products available and are safe when used appropriately. The most common cause of injury during travel is motor vehicle accidents. The risk of injury is higher in many developing countries than in the United States due to poor roads, poor vehicle maintenance, lack of seat belts, and other issues. Very cautious driving and avoidance of driving after dark may help to reduce the risk somewhat. While swimming is an ideal exercise in such hot climates as central Africa, freshwater lake swimming should be avoided due to the risk of exposure to schistosomiasis. The *Schistosoma* species that cause this disease are endemic in standing freshwater bodies. Swimming or bathing in salt water or chlorinated swimming pools is safer.

Traveler's diarrhea and exposure to foodborne pathogens is a common cause of illness during travel to developing countries. The guideline with food is to cook it, peel it, purify it, or forget it. Fruits that can be peeled, such as oranges or bananas, are generally safe to eat. Carbonated beverages are also safe. However, ice cubes made from local water supplies are a common, and sometimes ignored, source of infection. Water purification can be accomplished by boiling or by filtering through an absolute 1 μm filter and then purifying with iodine. Filtering alone does not provide adequate protection. Salads that are not made of carefully cleaned vegetables should be avoided and salad dressings may also be contaminated. Meats that are well cooked and served hot would be considered less likely to transmit an infection. Finally, brushing one's teeth with unpurified water carries a significant risk of transmission of waterborne illness and should be avoided. Purified water or bottled water should be used instead. *(Centers for Disease Control: www.cdc.gov)*

54. (B)

55. (E)

Explanations 54 and 55

Environmental tobacco smoke, or "secondhand smoke," consists of both "mainstream smoke" which is exhaled by the smoker and "sidestream smoke" which comes from the burning cigarette between puffs. About half of the smoke from a cigarette is sidestream smoke, which consists of the same chemicals as the mainstream smoke that is inhaled by the user. Nonsmokers exposed to secondhand smoke absorb nicotine, carcinogens, and other chemicals from the smoke just as the smoker does.

While the concentration of the chemicals absorbed is less than in a smoker, the levels absorbed increase as exposure increases and there are significant health risks involved. The EPA considers secondhand smoke to be a class A carcinogen—a substance that causes cancer in humans. Among the health risks are increased incidences of asthma, respiratory infections, otitis media, and SIDS in children exposed to secondhand smoke. Nursing mothers can pass harmful chemicals from cigarette smoke in breast milk.

While separating smokers and nonsmokers in the same airspace may reduce the exposure to secondhand smoke, the exposure is not eliminated. It is estimated to take 3 hours to remove 95% of the cigarette smoke from a room once smoking is completed, so there is still significant risk for exposure even though the nonsmoker is not in the same room. Courts in the United States and Canada have considered the smoking behaviors of parents as factors in determining the "best interests" of a child during custody hearings. Finally, parental smoking is an important predictor of the smoking behaviors of their children as they become adolescents. *(American Academy of Pediatrics: www.aap.org/advocacy/chmhets.htm; National Cancer Institute: cis.nci.nih.gov/fact/3_9.htm)*

56. (A)

57. (D)

58. (B)

Explanations 56 through 58

The mnemonic "ABCDE" is often used to remember some of the attributes of skin lesions that would make them more suspicious for being malignancies. "A" is for asymmetry; "B" for border that is irregular or indistinct from the surrounding skin; "C" for color such as dark black or variations in colors within the same lesion; "D" for diameter greater than 6 mm, or larger than the size of a pencil eraser; "E" for elevation of lesion with surface irregularity. Of the choices in question 56, the presence of a diameter of greater than 6 mm would be considered a higher-risk attribute.

Primary skin malignancies are divided into three major categories—basal cell carcinoma, squamous cell carcinoma, and melanoma. Basal cell carcinomas may grow large and be locally destructive, but they have the lowest metastatic potential of the three types of skin cancer. Basal cell carcinomas are more common in persons with fair complexions but they occur in all skin types and colors. Squamous carcinomas of the skin have a metastatic potential greater than basal cell carcinomas and less than malignant melanomas. Squamous carcinomas most commonly occur in sun-exposed areas but are also associated with other etiologies, such as human papilloma virus (HPV), and can occur anywhere on the body.

Malignant melanoma has the highest metastatic potential of the primary skin malignancies. Melanoma can occur in any skin type, but is more common in skin types I and II (fair skin). Obtaining a tissue sample for pathologic studies of suspicious skin lesions is critical for diagnosis and planning of appropriate treatment of melanoma. The thickness of the lesion is an important factor in these decisions. Therefore, shave biopsy would be inappropriate for the evaluation of a pigmented lesion. Complete excisional biopsy would be preferable, or, when that is not possible, full-thickness punch biopsy is an acceptable alternative. While sun exposure is an important risk factor for all types of skin cancers, for melanomas there is some evidence that intermittent, intense sun exposure and sunburning is more of a risk than cumulative sun exposure.

Actinic keratoses are sun-induced skin lesions that are considered risks for the development of squamous carcinomas. They can be treated with local destructive methods, such as cryosurgery or the topical chemotherapeutic agent 5-fluorouracil. Protection of susceptible skin from excessive sun exposure from childhood is important in reducing the risk of developing skin cancer. Precautions such as wearing broad-brimmed hats, long sleeved clothing, and avoidance of intense midday sunlight are helpful. Using chemical sunscreens with SPF of greater than 15 with frequent reapplication is also beneficial. Even "waterproof" sunscreens need to be reapplied after bathing or swimming. A wet cotton T-shirt provides very little, if any, protection from ultraviolet light exposure. Both the UV-A and UV-B rays play roles in skin damage from the sun and it is important to use sun protection products, which block both types of rays. Sun tanning booths are also considered risks for the induction of skin damage and skin cancer as they expose skin to potentially damaging ultraviolet rays. (*Wolff et al., 2005*)

59. (C)

60. (B)

61. (C)

Explanations 59 through 61

At the initial prenatal visit, a complete history and physical examination is performed along with a panel of laboratory studies. Routinely, a complete blood count, blood type, and Rh group with antibody screen, rubella antibody, rapid plasma reagin (RPR), HIV, pap smear, cervical swab for gonorrhea and chlamydia, urinalysis, and urine culture are performed. Pregnancy is one of the few conditions in which treatment of asymptomatic bacteruria would be recommended. Neither a basic metabolic panel nor a TSH measurement would be indicated unless the patient had an underlying medical condition that warranted further evaluation. Screening for gestational diabetes with a glucose measurement after ingestion of 50 g of glucose is performed in many pregnancies, but not until 24–28 weeks' gestation. Routine screening for vaginal or rectal colonization with group B *Streptococcus* is also performed, but not until 34 weeks of gestation or later.

It is recommended that all pregnant women be screened for hepatitis B at their initial prenatal visit by obtaining a hepatitis B surface antigen. This helps to determine if the woman has hepatitis B that could put her baby at risk for the infection. Hepatitis B surface antibody may be a sign of previous infection or of previous vaccination with the hepatitis B vaccine. The presence of core antibody and e antibody may be signs of previous infection.

Testing for the e antigen is not useful for initial screening purposes but may be warranted if the patient were found to have chronic hepatitis B infection.

If the mother tests positive for hepatitis B surface antigen during her pregnancy then the neonate should receive both hepatitis B immune globulin and the initial dose of the hepatitis B vaccine series. This combination has been shown to reduce risk of perinatal transmission from approximately 10% if the woman is surface antigen positive to less than 3%. There are currently no data to show that delivering a baby by caesarian section will reduce the risk of perinatal transmission of the infection. Breastfeeding has not been shown to increase the rate of transmission of infection to a nursing infant. *(Lin and Kirchner, 2004, pp. 75–82, 86)*

62.   (E)

63.   (E)

Explanations 62 and 63

Screening for prostate cancer with the PSA test is a controversial area. Some advocate routine screening of most men over the age of 50 while others recommend selective screening or no routine screening at all. The USPSTF gives prostate cancer screening an "I" recommendation, stating that there is insufficient evidence to recommend for or against this intervention. Prostate cancer is the second most common cause of cancer death in men (behind lung cancer). PSA screening does not help to prevent prostate cancer but it does increase the likelihood of detection of prostate cancer. However, many prostate cancers are slow growing and many with prostate cancer die of other causes. PSA screening has not been shown to reduce all cause mortality. While the mortality from prostate cancer has been decreasing over the years, the reason for this is not yet clear. PSA screening may play a role in this but improvements in the treatment of prostate cancer may also be responsible. The PSA also has significant rates of false positive and false negative readings. Benign conditions such as prostatic hyperplasia or prostatitis can

elevate PSA readings and prostate cancer can exist in men with normal PSA readings.

Another factor that can interfere with PSA readings is the presence of medications. Finasteride and dutasteride, which are widely used in the treatment of benign prostatic hyperplasia, can lower PSA readings, even in the presence of prostate cancer. If PSA screening is chosen by the patient and his physician, selection of appropriate patients for screening is important. The presence of symptoms related to the prostate may influence one's decision to perform a PSA test. However, many prostate cancers are asymptomatic, so the absence of symptoms may not be a reason to withhold testing. Most authorities would not recommend the routine screening of men with significant comorbidities that would result in them having a life expectancy of fewer than 10 years. One of the reasons for the controversy surrounding PSA screening is the risk of harm of testing. Elevated PSA levels frequently result in further—sometimes invasive—testing and may result in the detection of cancers that may or may not have become clinically significant. The treatment of these cancers with surgery, radiation, medical therapy, or combinations, does have significant risks, side effects, and potential harms. Further studies are currently underway to help us to be better able to address the controversies involved in PSA testing. *(USPSTF: www.preventiveservices.ahrq.gov)*

64.   (D)

65.   (E)

66.   (C)

67.   (E)

Explanations 64 through 67

B. anthracis causes three diseases in humans: cutaneous, inhalation, and gastrointestinal anthrax. Cutaneous anthrax is the most common of the naturally occurring anthrax diseases. The spores of the gram-positive bacillus can survive for years in soil. The disease cutaneous anthrax occurs when the spores contaminate a wound on the skin of the victim and then start to grow. This disease occurs most commonly in agricultural areas where the soil becomes contaminated by the presence of animals. Initially a painless papule develops, followed by vesicles which then ulcerate and a black eschar forms. In the setting of cutaneous anthrax in a postal worker who has a coworker with an apparently similar disease, bioterrorism must be suspected. This type of attack occurred in the Fall of 2001, when anthrax spores were sent through the U.S. Postal system and over 20 persons were infected. In this setting, the most appropriate initial management is to immediately contact the appropriate Public Health Authorities, usually the local or state health department. Appropriate treatment will also need to be instituted, under the guidance of the public health specialists, as untreated cutaneous anthrax may carry a 20% mortality rate. Antibiotic therapy would usually be with ciprofloxacin, penicillin, or doxycycline. Anthrax does not spread from person to person, so quarantine is not necessary. Inhalation anthrax is caused by the direct inhalation of spores into the lungs and gastrointestinal anthrax, the least common of the anthrax syndromes, is caused by ingestion.

Smallpox does not occur naturally anywhere in the world. Therefore, any suspicion of smallpox must be assumed to be a bioterror event and must be reported immediately to public health officials. Physicians should be able to recognize the signs and symptoms of smallpox and be able to distinguish them from the common occurrence of chickenpox. Chickenpox lesions tend to occur in clusters and evolve asynchronously. They are often described as "dew drops on a rose petal" as they are vesicles occurring on an erythematous base. The lesions tend to start on the trunk and rapidly spread outward. The rash will be associated with a fever but there are usually few to no prodromal symptoms. Because of the asynchronous growth and outbreaks, a patient will typically have lesions in different stages of evolution. In contrast, smallpox lesions tend to occur synchronously and the lesions tend to be uniform. The rash frequently occurs on the palms and soles. It typically starts on the face and arms and then spreads to the trunk and legs. The development of the rash tends to be slower than that of chickenpox. There is often a dramatic prodrome of high fever, malaise, headache, and backache for 2–4 days prior to the onset of the rash. Smallpox carries an approximately 30% mortality, while mortality associated with chickenpox is very low. *(O'Brien et al., 2003, pp. 1927–1934)*

68. (A)

69. (B)

Explanations 68 and 69

The hazard ratio statistic as presented is a comparison of the rate of development of an outcome in the treatment group divided by the rate of development of the same outcome in the control group. It is a "hazard" ratio because all of the outcomes measured are adverse. A hazard ratio of 1.00 means that there is no difference in the rate of development of the outcome between the two groups. Further, if the 95% CI crosses 1.00 then there is no statistically significant difference between the two groups. From the data presented, the hazard ratio for the development of endometrial cancer is 0.83, suggesting that there may be a reduction in the risk of endometrial cancer for women on HRT. However, the 95% CI crosses 1, therefore we cannot consider this result to be statistically significant. For the other outcomes listed, the 95% CIs do not cross 1.00, thus representing statistically significant increases in the risk of CHD, pulmonary embolism, and stroke and a statistically significant reduction in the risk of hip fracture.

In question 69, the data reveal statistically significant rates of combined cardiovascular disease and fracture risk between the two groups. The risk of cardiovascular disease is increased but the combined fracture risk is reduced in women on HRT. The combined cancer risk and total mortality do not reach the level of statistical significance. There are no data presented on quality of life in the chart, so we cannot state that option E is true. *(Women's Health Initiative Investigators, 2002, pp. 321–333)*

70. (B) The most common reason for an unusual or unexpected finding on a pediatric growth chart is erroneous measurement. Whenever such an occurrence is noted, the first intervention should be to repeat and confirm the measurement. All of the other options may be appropriate for further evaluation and management if the abnormality noted is confirmed to be real.

71. (B)

72. (E)

Explanations 71 and 72

On September 30, 1978, the National Commission for the Protection of Human Subjects of Biomedical and Behavioral Research submitted the report "Ethical Principles and Guidelines for the Protection of Human Subjects of Research," named after the Belmont Conference Center in the Smithsonian Institution. The three ethical principles emphasized in this report include justice, beneficence, and respect for persons.

Justice is the equitable distribution of research burdens and benefits. Beneficence is the mechanism to maximize benefits and minimize harm to research subjects. Respect for persons is the ethical principle which prioritizes the respect for individual autonomy and the protection of individuals with reduced autonomy. The principle of respect emphasizes the protection of subjects' privacy, maintenance of confidentiality, informed consent, and the utilization of additional safeguards for the protection of vulnerable populations.

Health and Human Service (HHS) regulations delineate additional mechanisms to protect human subjects, which include (1) institutional assurances of compliance, (2) Institutional Review Board (IRB) review, and (3) informed consent. An institutional assurance of compliance is documentation that the institution will follow HHS regulations for the protection of human subjects. An IRB is a committee that has been established to protect human subjects involved in research activities. These committees must have at least five members of varying backgrounds who possess the professional competence to review research activities.

Informed consent is the voluntary choice of an individual to participate in research activities.

To be truly informed consent, the individual must have a clear and accurate understanding of the purpose of the research, the risks involved, the potential benefits, the procedures to be performed and the alternative modalities of treatment available. Typically, these are in a written consent form. The legal arguments for informed consent emphasize the right of self-determination. This is in contrast to the ethical basis of individual autonomy. Therefore, a mere signature by the individual participant does not fulfill the ethical requirements of the informed consent process.

Any research study must have scientific validity, a fair selection of individual subjects for populations, protection of vulnerable populations, fair access to the benefits of medical research, acceptable risk-benefit ratios, appropriate informed consent, and independent review of the study. In addition, Data Safety Monitoring Boards are being utilized to further monitor the safety of research protocols and participation. *(Ethical Principles and Guidelines for the Protection of Human Subjects of Research, www.hhs.gov/ohrp/belmontarchive.html, accessed December 12, 2006; HHS Regulations and Institutional Responsibilities, http://ohrp-ed. od.nih.gov/CBTs/ assurance, accessed December 12, 2006)*

73. (D)

74. (D)

Explanations 73 and 74

Although Mycelex troches would be appropriate in the management of his oral candidiasis and the Lotrisone would treat his seborrheic dermatitis, the patient has previously described risk factors for HIV infection and physical symptoms of immunodeficiency. Accurate knowledge of his HIV status is essential in the appropriate long-term management of this patient. In fact, his current physical examination suggests long-standing HIV infection. A lymph node biopsy is not warranted. His wife will eventually need screening for STDs since active STDs increase her risk of cotransmission of HIV.

The patient's refusal to discuss his situation with his wife raises many controversial issues with no simple solution. There are multiple arguments which support the ethical guidelines for supporting patient confidentiality. These include:

- An appeal to consequences (potential patient discrimination secondary to health information; importance of trust)
- Appeal to virtue (physician fidelity)
- Respect (awareness and compassion for patient vulnerability)
- Do no harm (breach of medical information may lead to discrimination)

Respect for patient autonomy incorporates the patient in the treatment process and is based on mutual trust. Referring Mr. Jones to another physician doesn't address the concerns involved in the care of Mrs. Jones.

The Tarasoff case (1976) established the following precedent: Patient confidentiality must be upheld as part of the protected clinician-patient relationship but the physician has a duty to warn specific, innocent third parties of potential harm threatened or posed by the patient. In fact, failure to warn by the physician may constitute negligence.

This is not the law in all states. Some states interpret the standard as a strict duty to warn; other states permit physicians to warn affected third parties but not require it. If the physician unilaterally discloses the HIV status, it would represent a breach of confidentiality. However, their marital status may allow this disclosure.

Even if the patient is adamant in his refusal, the physician needs to determine the reasons for his reticence. As his physician, you can provide additional information about HIV prevention and treatment. It would be highly unusual for Mr. Jones to ultimately refuse notification of his spouse once he has been urged to do so by his physician.

The mechanism for how these complex issues are addressed has potential ramifications for his future trust of physicians, consent to HAART (highly active antiretroviral therapy) treatment, and medication compliance. If these barriers to disclosure cannot be addressed within the physician-patient relationship, the health department can provide a mechanism for contact testing.

Although you could ask Mrs. Jones to come in for a physical examination, she might refuse to have STD tests performed, especially if she perceives herself to be at minimal risk. Ideally, this assessment should be performed prior to a pregnancy. If she is currently HIV negative, then protective measures against future infection can be introduced. *(Tarasoff v. Regents of the University of California (17 Cal.3d 425 (1976))*

75. (C)

76. (A)

Explanations 75 and 76

Disclosure of unanticipated outcomes is one of the most challenging communications that can occur in the physician-patient relationship. Determining which events require disclosure and the appropriate mechanism to provide this information is part of the professional behavior inherent in our roles as physicians. Concepts for effective disclosure include:

- Accurate information
- Appropriate timing
- Effective communication skills
- Determining the patient's perspective
- Documentation of the interactions
- Mechanisms for follow-up communication

Many institutions have already developed policies and mechanisms to provide this communication.

The attending physician is the most appropriate person to lead this process. Your knowledge of the clinical circumstances is hearsay. It is not appropriate for you to provide unsubstantiated information to the patient or to the friend. Appropriate documentation in the medical record provides the facts surrounding the primary event. It is inappropriate to document opinions, accusations, or arguments.

Medical errors are responsible for more than 98,000 excessive patient deaths per year. In order for medical errors to be reduced, there need to be mechanisms for accountability which occur within a supportive environment. Peer review, morbidity and mortality rounds, shorter work weeks, and root cause analysis are all mechanisms to prevent future errors from fatigue, impaired system processes, and inadequate knowledge. Frequently when medical errors occur, the families want to know what is being done to prevent this from happening again. Although the peer review process is confidential and not subject to subpoena, it provides an effective mechanism to honestly evaluate our colleagues and enforce necessary discipline to improve patient safety. Random drug testing is not a systemic solution. *(Gallagher et al., 2003, pp. 1001–1007; Kohn et al., 2000; Wusthoff, 2001, pp. 1080–1081)*

77. **(D)** The United Nations *Standard Minimum Rules for the Treatment of Prisoners* offers ethical guidelines for physicians working with prisoners. Physicians must not participate in the use of torture, cruel, or unusual punishment, disciplinary activities, or abuse of human rights. This includes medicating individuals to facilitate interrogation or providing supportive medical services in order to facilitate additional torture. Physicians have the ethical responsibility to provide independent medical judgments and must act as advocates for their individual care. Incarceration does not change a patient's ethical right to health care or permit a physician to ignore these rights. Under no circumstances are physicians to be used as an instrument of governments, even in legally sanctioned death penalty scenarios. They can, however, certify death. Furthermore, when completing a death certificate in military environments, the physician cannot leave out the role of torture (if applicable). Even if these concepts are not adopted by incarceration facilities or in the field of war, noncompliance with these standards has significant consequences for physicians, patients, and society. *(Snyder and Leffler, 2005, pp. 558–560)*

78. **(C)** In 1996, the U.S. Congress recognized the need for comprehensive national health information privacy standards, which required full compliance by April 14, 2004. This rule provided the first systematic privacy protection for health information and is grounded in the principle of protecting the confidentiality of information about patients while protecting the legitimate interests of third parties (e.g., proxy and surrogate decision makers, health care providers, health care institutions, teaching situations). This legislation provides mechanisms to release information for payment of health care services, and consumer access to medical records.

HIPAA does not restrict the normal exchange of clinical information between consulting physicians or nurses on the patient's case. However, this normal exchange of information must occur in a medical context, not in elevators, public hallways, or the cafeteria. Health care providers must obtain the individual's written consent prior to disclosure of health information except in the management of emergencies or if the consent can be inferred from a patient with impaired communication. Procedures must be developed to prevent open access to patient information via computers or documents which can be easily accessed, including paper medical records. The privacy legislation also protects the release of medical information to an employer without the patient's consent. *(Gostin, 2001, pp. 3015–3021)*

79. **(E)** Medical care of the critically ill is focused on those individuals who, despite therapeutic interventions, may either recover with significant morbidity or die from their underlying illness. Part of the care of terminally ill patients is to ameliorate suffering, prevent disability, or recognize the finitude of life. The SUPPORT study provides physicians with accurate predictive information on the functional ability of patients and survival probability for end-of-life care. This study revealed that care provided to critically ill patients was often inconsistent with their preferences. Nearly half of the DNR orders were written in the last 2 days of life.

In this clinical situation, the patient has multiple organ system failure with sepsis, acute respiratory failure, CHF, and altered mental status (coma). Although the physician could provide any of the medical interventions, he is aware of the patient's preferences as expressed by an appropriate proxy decision maker (wife).

Ethical justifications for DNR orders include:

- Further treatment would cause more harm than benefit.
- Further treatment is reliably judged as medically futile.
- Further treatment would violate the expressed wishes of the patient and violate his/her right to choose how to live and die.

These decisions require cultural sensitivity and awareness of the variety of beliefs surrounding death among patients, their families, physicians, hospital systems, and society. Although physicians are best qualified to identify possible outcomes, it is patients and their families who determine the significance of these outcomes. (*Society of Critical Care Medicine Ethics Committee, 1994, pp. 1200–1203; The Support Principal Investigators, 1995, pp. 1591–1598*)

80. **(B)** Part of the care of terminally ill patients is to ameliorate suffering, prevent disability, or recognize the finitude of life. The SUPPORT study provides physicians with accurate predictive information on the functional ability of patients and survival probability for end-of-life care. This study revealed care provided to critically ill patients was often inconsistent with their preferences. Nearly half of the DNRs were written in the last 2 days of life.

In this clinical situation, the patient makes an informed decision about her future treatment and clinical interventions. Despite her age, she exhibits maturity of thought and demonstrates sufficient capacity to make informed decisions. Such capacity can be assessed by the primary physician. If there are serious concerns about capacity, a psychiatric consultation can help determine ability to consent or refuse treatment. If she has sufficient capacity she may refuse even life-saving treatment. In early discussions about the Out-of-Hospital DNR, it would be important to inquire whether the patient's father is involved in her care and her life. In this case, the father was no longer alive and mother did not have sufficient capacity to understand even minor decisions regarding her daughter's care. She

would qualify as a mature minor under most state statutes in the United States.

Although the physician could support intubation, he is aware of the patient's preferences as documented in the DNR. Failure to extubate represents a violation of her clearly expressed wishes. The fact that intubation was started does not change the fact that intubation was an initial violation of the patient's wishes. Failure to extubate would further that violation. The sometimes asserted distinction between not starting an intervention and continuing the intervention once started is not appropriate in situations where the patient's wishes were clearly not to have the intervention in the first place.

Ethical justifications for DNR orders include:

- Further treatment would cause more harm than benefit.
- Further treatment is reliably judged as medically futile.
- Further treatment would violate the expressed wishes of the patient and violate his/her right to choose how to live and die.

These decisions require cultural sensitivity and awareness of the variety of beliefs surround death among patients, their families, physicians, hospital systems, and society. Although physicians are best qualified to identify possible outcomes, it is patients and their families who determine the significance of these outcomes. (*The Support Principal Investigators, 1995, pp. 1591–1598*)

81. **(C)** The actions of the resident who reviewed the patient's chart were unethical. He is not involved in the case and the fact that he is a physician and colleague of the patient does not free him of the requirements that protect patient confidentiality, backed by federal regulations (see discussion of HIPAA above). He should not have pulled her chart. He would only be making matters worse by further violating the patient's right to confidentiality in sharing her results with the other resident. The attending clinicians involved in the case are the only people who should have privileged access to the patient's sensitive health information.

BIBLIOGRAPHY

ACR Appropriateness Criteria. *Osteoporosis: Prevention and Treatment*. Ann Arbor, MI: University of Michigan Health System, 2002.

American Academy of Pediatrics: www.aap.org/advocacy/chmhets.htm.

American College of Radiology (ACR). Expert Panel on Musculoskeletal Imaging. *Osteoporosis and Bone Mineral Density*. Reston, VA: American College of Radiology (ACR), 2001, p. 17.

American Heart Association, 2004: www.americanheart.org/presenter.jhtml?identifier=4436.

Centers for Disease Control: www.cdc.gov.

Centers for Disease Control: www.cdc.gov/mmwr/PDF/rr/rr4906.pdf.

Centers for Disease Control: www.cdc.gov/mmwr/PDF/RR/RR5014.pdf.

Centers for Disease Control: www.cdc.gov/nip/publications/pink/tetanus.pdf.

Centers for Disease Control: www.cdc.gov/nip/publications/preg_guide.htm.

Centers for Disease Control. National Vital Statistics Reports, Vol. 7, No. 9, 2003.

Coombes RC, Hall E, Gibson LJ, et al. A randomized trial of exemestane after two to three years of tamoxifen therapy in postmenopausal women with primary breast cancer. *N Engl J Med* 2004; 350:1081–1092.

Cunningham FG, Gant NF, Leveno KJ, et al. *Williams Obstetrics*, 21st ed. New York, NY: McGraw-Hill, 2001, pp. 1367–1376.

Dao Q, Krishnaswamy P, Kazanegra R, et al. Utility of B-type natriuretic peptide in the diagnosis of congestive heart failure in an urgent-care setting. *J Am Coll Cardiol* 2001;37:379–385.

Eyler AE, Cohen M. Case studies in partner violence. *Am Fam Physician* 1999;60:2569–2576.

Gallagher TH, Waterman AD, Ebers AG, et al. Patients' and physicians' attitudes regarding the disclosure of medical errors. *JAMA* 2003;289(8): 1001–1007.

Gostin LO. National Health Information Privacy Regulations Under the Health Insurance Portability and Accountability Act. *JAMA* 2001;285: 3015–3021.

Hulley SB, Cummings SR, Browner WS, et al. *Designing Clinical Research*, 2nd ed. Philadelphia, PA: Lippincott Willams & Wilkins, 2001.

Institute of Medicine. *To Err is Human: Building a Safer Health System*. Report available online at: www.iom.edu/Object.File/Master/4/117/0.pdf.

Kohn LT, Corrigan JM, Donaldson MS. *To Err is Human: Building a Safer Health System*. Washington, DC: National Academy Press, 2000.

Kurowski K, Chandran S. The preparticipation athletic evaluation. *Am Fam Physician* 2000;61: 2683–2690, 2696–2698.

Lin KW, Kirchner JT. Hepatitis B. *Am Fam Physician* 2004;69:75–82, 86.

McKeag DB, Sallis RE. Factors at play in the athletic preparticipation examination. *Am Fam Physician* 2000;61:2617.

National Cancer Institute: cis.nci.nih.gov/fact/3_9.htm.

National Commission for the Protection of Human Subjects of Biomedical and Behavioral Research. The Belmont Report: Ethical Principals for the Protection of Human Subjects of Research. Department of Health, Education and Welfare Publication, 1978. Available at http://www.hhs.gov/ohrp/humansubjects/guidance/belmont.htm

O'Brien KK, Higdon ML, Halverson JJ. Recognition and management of bioterrorism infections. *Am Fam Physician* 2003;67:1927–1934.

Sanchez-Ramos L, Oliver F, Delke I, et al. Labor induction versus expectant management for post-term pregnancies: a systematic review with meta-analysis. *Obstet Gynecol* 2003;101:1312–1318.

Slawson D, Shaughnessy A. *Becoming an Information Master*. Course materials, 2003.

Snyder L, Leffler C. Ethics manual. *Ann Intern Med* 2005;142(7):558–560.

Society of Critical Care Medicine Ethics Committee. Consensus statement on the triage of critically ill patients. *JAMA* 1994;271:1200–1203.

The Support Principal Investigators. A controlled trial to improve care for seriously ill hospitalized patients: The Study to Understand Prognoses and

Preferences for Outcomes and Risks of Treatments (SUPPORT). *JAMA* 1995;274:1591–1598.

Thompson IM, Goodman PJ, Tangen CM, et al. The influence of finasteride on the development of prostate cancer. *N Engl J Med* 2003;349:215–224.

USPSTF: www.preventiveservices.ahrq.gov.

Vitaly Tarasoff, et al, v the Regents of the University of California, et al. Supreme Court of California. 17 Cal 3d 425; 551 P.2d 334; 131 Cal Rptr. 14. July 1, 1976.

Wolff K, Johnson RA, Suurmond D. *Fitzpatrick's Color Atlas and Synopsis of Clinical Dermatology*, 5th ed. New York, NY: McGraw-Hill, 2005.

Women's Health Initiative Investigators. Risks and benefits of estrogen plus progestin in healthy post-menopausal women. *JAMA* 2002;288:321–333.

Wusthoff CJ. MSJAMA: medical mistakes and disclosure: the role of the medical student. *JAMA* 2001;286(9):1080–1081.

CHAPTER 7

Pathology
Questions

Questions 1 through 3

A full-term baby boy was noted in the immediate neonatal period to fail to pass meconium. Progressive abdominal distention was noted. Multiple laboratory and clinical tests lead to a decision to perform a rectal biopsy.

1. What is the most important histologic finding that you expect to see in the rectal biopsy?

   (A) ischemic necrosis of the bowel mucosa
   (B) acute ulcerative colitis
   (C) granulomatous inflammation
   (D) absence of ganglion cells in the rectal mucosa and submucosa
   (E) a malignant tumor

2. What special stains would you use that would be helpful to confirm the finding of ganglion cells?

   (A) periodic acid-Schiff (PAS)
   (B) mucicarmine
   (C) elastic stain
   (D) trichrome stain
   (E) acetylcholinesterase

3. The treatment of choice for Hirschsprung disease is which of the following?

   (A) laxatives
   (B) colonoscopy with relief of the obstruction
   (C) surgical therapy
   (D) antiperistaltic drugs
   (E) chemotherapy

Questions 4 through 6

A $3^1/_2$-year-old female presented with a left upper quadrant abdominal mass. The child had no previous history of medical illnesses. An ultrasound examination revealed a markedly deformed left kidney with 12 cm nonhomogenous soft tissue mass arising from the upper pole. Medial displacement of the bowel loops was also noted.

4. What would be the most likely diagnosis in this case?

   (A) hydronephrotic kidney
   (B) Wilms tumor
   (C) tuberculosis
   (D) congenital malformation
   (E) papillary transitional cell carcinoma of the renal pelvis

5. Characteristically, Wilms tumors are histologically recognizable for which of the following?

   (A) classic triphasic combination of blastema, stromal, and epithelial cells
   (B) epithelial elements alone
   (C) blastemic elements
   (D) focal keratinization
   (E) glandular formation

6. What is the survival rate of this tumor with chemotherapy, radiation therapy, and surgery?

(A) 10%

(B) 30%

(C) 60%

(D) 90%

(E) no long-term survival can be achieved with this tumor

Questions 7 and 8

A 23-year-old female sought medical help because of a painless asymmetrical enlargement of the lower neck. The patient had no history of dyspnea, dysphagia, hoarseness, or previous radiation exposure. On physical examination, besides the enlarged asymmetrical thyroid gland, there was also a palpable lymphadenopathy. A lymph node biopsy (see Figure 7-1) was performed. Hematoxilin and eosin (H&E) stained slide shows the lesion.

FIG. 7-1 (*Courtesy of Edison Catalano, MD.*)

7. What is the most appropriate diagnosis?

(A) medullary carcinoma of the thyroid

(B) follicular carcinoma

(C) papillary carcinoma

(D) anaplastic carcinoma

(E) small cell anaplastic carcinoma

8. What are the typical nuclear findings of this tumor?

(A) ground glass appearance with intranuclear inclusions

(B) abnormal mitosis

(C) scant cytoplasm

(D) glandular formations

(E) squamous metaplasia

9. A 60-year-old male is evaluated following a pathologic fracture of his humerus. As part of the workup, a bone biopsy is performed and the photomicrograph is shown in Figure 7-2. Which of the following is the most likely diagnosis?

FIG. 7-2

(A) benign neoplasm

(B) cellular hyperplasia

(C) osteogenic sarcoma

(D) metastatic lesion

(E) chronic leukemia

10. An autopsy was performed following the death of a 72-year-old man. The kidney is shown in Figure 7-3. Which of the following clinical scenarios is most likely to explain the changes seen in this kidney?

FIG. 7-3

(A) complete urinary outflow obstruction from an enlarged prostate

(B) renal infarct from an embolism originating in the atrium of the heart due to atrial fibrillation

(C) long-standing hypertension

(D) renal cell carcinoma

(E) chronic abuse of analgesics and nonsteroidal anti-inflammatory drugs

11. A middle-aged female presents with a painless enlargement of the lower aspect of the neck. With appropriate testing this is proven to be thyroid enlargement. Thyroid function tests were normal. A surgical intervention was performed for diagnostic purposes. Figure 7-4

FIG. 7-4 (Courtesy of Edison Catalano, MD.)

depicts a representative area of how most of the thyroid gland histologic features were seen. What are the clinical thyroid function test characteristics of the last stages of this disease?

(A) thyrotoxicosis

(B) normal thyroid function tests

(C) some degree of hypothyroidism

(D) invasion of the recurrent laryngeal nerve

(E) hoarseness

12. Polyarteritis nodosa (PAN) typically involves which of the following?

(A) large elastic arteries

(B) small- or medium-sized muscular arteries

(C) arterioles

(D) capillaries

(E) venules

13. The most likely cause of the pathologic findings in the spleen shown in Figure 7-5 is which of the following?

FIG. 7-5

(A) amyloidosis

(B) metastatic carcinoma

(C) septic infarct

(D) Hodgkin disease

(E) traumatic rupture

Questions 14 through 16

A 72-year-old male presented with nonspecific symptoms of easy fatigability, weight loss, and anorexia. On physical examination, generalized lymphadenopathy and hepatosplenomegaly were present. On the peripheral blood, he was found to have a marked lymphocytosis and in the serum, a small monoclonal spike was present.

14. What would be the most likely histology seen in a lymph node biopsy?

    (A) reactive germinal centers
    (B) diffuse effacement of the normal architecture by a small lymphocytic population
    (C) diffuse architecture effacement with large cells with prominent nucleoli
    (D) a pleomorphic background composed of eosinophils, plasma cells, and small lymphocytes
    (E) a total replacement of the node by plasma cells

15. This disease is most prevalent in which age group?

    (A) teenagers
    (B) 20–30 age group
    (C) 30–40 age group
    (D) over 50 years
    (E) it may appear at any age

16. The clinical behavior of this disease can best be described by which of the following?

    (A) rapidly progressive
    (B) never relapses
    (C) can be completely eradicated by chemotherapy
    (D) the median survival is 4–6 years
    (E) never responds to chemotherapeutic agents

17. An autopsy is performed on an 82-year-old female diagnosed with Alzheimer disease. Which of the following is most likely to be found on evaluation of her brain?

    (A) fibrosis
    (B) necrosis
    (C) senile plaques
    (D) calcifications
    (E) neuronal vacuolization

18. You are following up in your office with a patient who had a magnetic resonance imaging (MRI) of his head for evaluation of persistent headaches. The MRI report reveals a mass suspicious for malignancy. While explaining the need for ongoing testing to determine the etiology, the patient's spouse asks you, "What is the most common tumor in the brain?" Which of the following would be the correct response to this question?

    (A) glioblastoma multiforme
    (B) metastatic tumors
    (C) medulloblastoma
    (D) oligodendroglioma
    (E) ependymoma

19. A 60-year-old male presents to the office with a growth on the inside of his lower lip. It has been present for several months and is slowly growing. He is a nonsmoker but has a long history of chewing tobacco. Which of the following is the most likely to be found on biopsy of the lesion?

    (A) adenocarcinoma
    (B) lymphoma
    (C) basal cell carcinoma
    (D) carcinoid tumor
    (E) squamous cell carcinoma

20. A 25-year-old female presents for evaluation of a breast mass and tenderness. She describes the breast soreness as varying with her menstrual cycles. On examination, you feel a firm, movable, irregular 2 cm mass. Her breast tissue is diffusely dense bilaterally. Of the options listed, which is the most likely?

    (A) lipoma
    (B) fibroadenoma
    (C) hemangioma

(D) intraductal papilloma

(E) phylloides tumor, benign

Questions 21 and 22

A 45-year-old woman presents with a slowly growing mass near the right jaw. You palpate a firm nodule in the parotid gland but find no adenopathy and no other abnormality on examination. A biopsy reveals both epithelial and stromal elements.

21. What is this patient's diagnosis?
(A) pleomorphic adenoma (mixed tumor)
(B) Whartin tumor
(C) monomorphic adenoma
(D) basal cell adenoma
(E) oxyphilic adenoma

22. What is the appropriate treatment for this lesion?
(A) observation, as this is a benign lesion
(B) external beam radiation therapy
(C) excision with narrow margins
(D) excision with a wide margin of normal tissue
(E) chemotherapy

Questions 23 through 25

A 67-year-old female was admitted to the hospital because of chronic fatigue and low back pain. An x-ray of the vertebral column showed diffuse osteoporosis and compression fractures of L1 and L2 vertebral bodies. The complete blood count (CBC) was within normal limits. The peripheral blood smear showed rouleaux formation. The immunoelectrophoresis showed a monoclonal spike of more than 3 g. A bone marrow biopsy was performed and showed an increase of more than 20% in plasma cells (see Figure 7-6).

FIG. 7-6 *(Courtesy of Edison Catalano, MD.)*

23. Radiographs of the bone and skeletal system in multiple myeloma will more characteristically show which of the following?

(A) fractures
(B) osteoblastic lesions
(C) destructive bone lesions throughout the skeletal system
(D) the skeletal system will remain intact
(E) changes that resemble Paget disease

24. In this particular patient what would be the electrophoretical characteristic changes?

(A) increases levels of IgG and light chains in the urine
(B) IgM spike
(C) IgA elevation
(D) increase in albumin
(E) polyclonal electrophoretic pattern

25. Microscopically, the bone marrow examination will reveal which of the following?

(A) normocellular marrow with normal hematopoiesis
(B) an increase in myeloid elements
(C) increase in megakaryocytes
(D) increase in mature lymphocytes
(E) increase in plasma cells, usually more than 30% of the total cells

26. A 17-year-old male is evaluated for a painless neck mass. You assess the mass as lymphadenopathy and arrange for a biopsy. The pathology report subsequently notes the presence of Reed-Sternberg cells. Which of the following is the most likely diagnosis?

    (A) Hodgkin lymphoma
    (B) non-Hodgkin lymphoma
    (C) metastatic testicular cancer
    (D) acute lymphocytic leukemia
    (E) papillary carcinoma of the thyroid

27. A 54-year-old woman has a dilation and curettage procedure for the evaluation of postmenopausal bleeding. Which of the following pathologic diagnoses would carry the most favorable prognosis for the patient?

    (A) well-differentiated adenocarcinoma with a squamous differentiation
    (B) serous carcinoma
    (C) clear cell adenocarcinoma
    (D) carcinosarcoma
    (E) carcinosarcoma with heterologous elements

28. A 52-year-old woman has biopsy of a breast lesion which confirms the mass as malignant. She is also found to clinically have a palpable ipsilateral axillary lymph node. Which of the following would be the most likely pathologic finding in this node?

    (A) acute lymphadenitis
    (B) follicular hyperplasia
    (C) paracortical hyperplasia
    (D) granulomatous inflammation
    (E) sinus histiocytosis

29. Of the following, which is the best indicator of response to treatment or progression of disease in monitoring patients being treated for prostate cancer?

    (A) digital rectal examination
    (B) serum prostate-specific antigen (PSA)

    (C) computed tomography (CT) scans
    (D) MRI
    (E) positron emission tomography (PET) scans

30. A 62-year-old male, who has been smoking two packs of cigarettes a day for the past 35 years, was found to have a 2.5 cm peripheral solitary nodule in the left upper lobe of lung. Thoracotomy with biopsy was performed and a picture of the biopsy findings is depicted in Figure 7-7. With the clinical information and the biopsy findings what would be the most likely diagnosis?

FIG. 7-7 (Courtesy of Edison Catalano, MD.)

    (A) pulmonary infarct
    (B) adenocarcinoma
    (C) small cell anaplastic carcinoma
    (D) tuberculosis
    (E) granulomatous inflammation.

31. A 32-year-old female was seen by her family physician because of an enlarged and pigmented lesion of her back. On examination, the lesion measures 2 × 1.5 cm and it is variegated by hues of brown, black, and pink areas. The central area appears to ulcerate. A biopsy of the area was performed. What would be the most likely diagnosis?

    (A) malignant melanoma
    (B) keratoacanthoma
    (C) drug eruption
    (D) squamous cell carcinoma
    (E) dermatofibroma

Questions 32 and 33

32. A 65-year-old postmenopausal woman relates a complaint of being excessively tired for 6 months. Her laboratory results were remarkable for a microcytic anemia. A colonoscopy followed by a biopsy revealed a mass of the right colon. After the initial biopsy, a right colectomy was performed (see Figure 7-8). What would be the most likely diagnosis?

FIG. 7-8 *(Courtesy of Edison Catalano, MD.)*

(A) adenomatous polyp
(B) lipoma of the cecal valve
(C) adenocarcinoma of the right colon
(D) ischemic colitis
(E) Crohn's disease

33. A history of which of the following conditions would result in the greatest increase in the likelihood of developing colon cancer?

(A) Crohn's disease
(B) diverticulosis
(C) hamartomatous polyp
(D) pseudomembranous colitis
(E) ulcerative colitis

34. Which of the following is the most common characteristic of a serous cystadenocarcinoma of the ovary?

(A) It causes pseudomyxoma peritonei.
(B) It is composed of transitional epithelial cells.
(C) It is frequently bilateral.
(D) It is most common in children and young adults.
(E) It often metastasizes to the brain.

35. A 28-year-old female shows clinical manifestations related to secretion of excess androgenic hormones and persistent anovulation. What would be the most likely finding in the ovary?

(A) endometriosis
(B) polycystic ovary
(C) endometrioid carcinoma of the ovary
(D) granulosa cell tumor of the ovary
(E) mature cystic teratoma

36. A small area of abnormality is noted on the lateral wall of the urinary bladder during a cystoscopy on a patient being evaluated for asymptomatic microscopic hematuria. Biopsy of the lesion is most likely to reveal which of the following?

(A) adenocarcinoma
(B) neuroendocrine carcinoma
(C) rhabdomyosarcoma
(D) squamous cell carcinoma
(E) papillary transitional cell carcinoma

37. A 60-year-old male developed painless hematuria. On further clinical evaluation, a CT scan showed a 7 cm mass on the lower pole of the right kidney. What would be your most likely diagnosis in this case?

(A) neuroblastoma
(B) medullary fibroma
(C) Wilms tumor
(D) transitional cell carcinoma
(E) renal cell carcinoma

38. A 28-year-old male undergoes an orchiectomy because of a suspicious testicular mass. The pathologic evaluation reveals the tumor to have gross and microscopic hemorrhage and necrosis. The tumor is noted to be composed mostly of cytotrophoblastic and syncytiotrophoblastic cells. What is this patient's diagnosis?

(A) embryonal carcinoma

(B) seminoma

(C) teratoma

(D) choriocarcinoma

(E) yolk sac tumor

39. An 18-year-old male developed chills, fever, and a painful swollen knee. What test would be most appropriate in order to help in making the diagnosis?

(A) culture of joint fluid from the affected knee

(B) Lyme disease test

(C) MRI

(D) serum protein electrophoresis

(E) study of crystals in the synovium

40. Which factor is most directly related to prognosis in a patient with the diagnosis of squamous cell carcinoma of the esophagus?

(A) degree of differentiation

(B) duration of the symptoms

(C) method of treatment

(D) stage at the time of diagnosis

(E) type of symptoms

41. Which of the following patients is most likely to progress to develop cirrhosis?

(A) a man with chronic liver disease due to cytomegalovirus infection

(B) a man with chronic liver disease due to hepatitis B

(C) a man with chronic liver disease due to hepatitis C

(D) a man chronic with liver disease due to hepatitis D

(E) a man with chronic liver disease due to human immunodeficiency virus

42. A 14-year-old male is evaluated for thigh pain. He has no history of injury. An x-ray of the leg shows a mass in the distal femur that extends into the soft tissue. A biopsy is performed and cytogenetic studies show translocation of chromosomes 11 and 22. What is this patient's diagnosis?

(A) osteosarcoma

(B) osteoblastoma

(C) metastatic carcinoma

(D) multiple myeloma

(E) Ewing sarcoma

43. A 49-year-old female noticed that, in the morning, the small joints of her hands are swollen, painful, and stiff. Her rheumatoid factor is reportedly strongly positive. Citruline tests (cyclic citrullinated peptide [CCP]) are also positive. What disease does the patient most likely have?

(A) degenerative joint disease

(B) rheumatoid arthritis

(C) spondyloarthritis

(D) tennis elbow

(E) septic arthritis

44. A 28-year-old man presents with vague complaints of fatigue, nausea, and dyspnea. He has had occasional episodes of hemoptysis and some burning with urination. Laboratory studies reveal a mild anemia and an elevation of both blood urea nitrogen (BUN) and creatinine. Urinalysis reveals the presence of blood, protein, and red cell casts. Antibodies against which of the following is the cause of this condition?

(A) platelet surface antigens

(B) basement membrane

(C) parietal cell antigens

(D) colonic mucosal cells

(E) macrophage receptors

45. A 20-year-old man undergoes a colonoscopy for abdominal pain, weight loss, and diarrhea. Pathologic evaluation reveals transmural chronic inflammation with often noncaseating granulomas. What is the most likely diagnosis?

(A) ulcerative colitis
(B) ischemic colitis
(C) pseudomembranous colitis
(D) Crohn's disease
(E) celiac sprue

46. Routine screening is advocated by numerous authorities for many different types of cancer. These screening programs have resulted in various degrees of success in terms of reduction in mortality. Cytologic screening for cancer of which of the following organs has successfully produced a marked reduction in mortality?

(A) breast
(B) lung
(C) uterine cervix
(D) pancreas
(E) prostate

47. The specimen shown in Figure 7-9 was removed during an exploratory laparotomy of a 22-year-old male who went to surgery because of an intestinal obstruction. What is the most likely diagnosis for the lesion shown in this image?

FIG. 7-9 *(Courtesy of Roland Schwarting, MD.)* (Also see color insert.)

(A) intestinal infarction
(B) ulcerative colitis
(C) Crohn's disease
(D) intestinal tuberculosis
(E) small bowel carcinoma

Answers and Explanations

1. (D)

2. (E)

3. (C)

4. (B)

5. (A)

6. (D)

Explanations 1 through 3

Hirschsprung disease usually manifests in the immediate neonatal period by failure to pass meconium, followed by obstructive constipation. Abdominal distention develops and, in general, a large segment of the colon is involved and distended. The incidence of Hirschsprung disease is 1 in 5000 live births, with an 80% male predominance in nonfamilial cases. There is no apparent difference in occurrence among races. A number of abnormalities have been associated with Hirschsprung disease, including Down syndrome (2–3% of the cases), congenital heart disease, colonic atresia, and malrotation. The tissue diagnosis is made on the basis of an absence of ganglion cells in the submucosa and the myenteric plexus on a full-thickness rectal biopsy. Some surgeons prefer suction biopsy to full-thickness biopsy because it is easy to obtain the specimen and they can avoid scarring and fibrosis in the area. The other four choices are not applicable and can be ruled out on the basis of clinical history and an extremely low incidence of other pathologic conditions at the perinatal age.

When suction biopsies are performed, the tissue sample for acetylcholinesterase stain should be frozen as soon as possible. All of the other stains would not be helpful to identify ganglion cells. As soon as the diagnosis is confirmed with the rectal biopsy, a surgical procedure should be undertaken that consists of a resection of the aganglionic section of colon. All the other options are not the treatment of choice for this disease. (Cotran et al., 1999, pp. 805–806)

Explanations 4 through 6

Wilms tumor is the most common primary renal tumor in childhood, usually diagnosed between the ages of 2 and 5. The risk of Wilms tumor is increased in association with at least three recognizable groups of congenital malformations exhibiting alteration in at least two distinct chromosomal loci. A few familial cases of Wilms tumor not associated with identifiable lesions or mutations involving either the WT-1 or the WT-2 gene suggest that there may be another locus that plays a role in some tumors, but that still remains unknown. Wilms tumor presents as a large solitary mass and in 10% of cases may be bilateral. Microscopically, the Wilms tumor is characterized by recognizable attempts to recapitulate different stages of nephrogenesis. The classic triphasic combination of blastemic, stromal, and epithelial cell types is observed in the majority of the lesions. Occasional skeletal muscle differentiation can be seen, as well as squamous, mucinous epithelium, cartilage, or bone. The combined therapy of chemo, radiation, and surgery has dramatically improved the results of long-term survival in these patients, up to 90%. (Cotran et al., 1999, pp. 487–489)

7. (C)

8. (A)

Explanations 7 and 8

Papillary carcinoma of the thyroid is the most common form of thyroid cancer. Most cases are seen between the second and third decade of life and are associated with previous radiation therapy. Many times the first manifestation is a metastasis to the regional neck nodes. The histologic characteristics of papillary carcinoma are branching papillae with single or multiple layers of cuboidal to columnar cells. The characteristic appearance of the nucleus is rather clear, ground-glass (orphan Annie) nuclei. Characteristic intracytoplasmic inclusions, and occasional grooves, are seen. Psammoma bodies are often present in the papillae. The most common variant of papillary carcinoma is the follicular variant, in which the tumor cells form follicular architecture; however, the nuclear changes, as well as focal areas of papillary structures, are enough to make the differential diagnosis from follicular carcinoma. (*Cotran et al., 1999, pp. 1143–1144*)

9. **(D)** The photomicrograph accompanying the question shows bone marrow spaces replaced by a well-differentiated adenocarcinoma. The bone spicules are normal. The glandular structures replacing the interspicular spaces and replacing the marrow elements are diagnostic of metastatic adenocarcinoma. (*Cotran et al., 1994, pp. 268–271*)

10. **(A)** The photograph that accompanies the question demonstrates severe hydronephrosis, which is due to obstruction of the flow of urine. The obstruction may be located at any site along the urinary outflow tract and may be partial or total, unilateral or bilateral. Because glomerular filtration may continue for some time after the development of the obstruction, the renal pelvis and calices become dilated by continued urine production. The resultant backpressure produces atrophy of the renal parenchyma with obliteration of the pyramids. The degree of hydronephrosis depends on the extent and rapidity of the obstructive process. (*Cotran et al., 1994, p. 988*)

11. **(C)** Hashimoto thyroiditis is a very common cause of hypothyroidism in the parts of the world where iodine levels are insufficient. The clinical picture is characterized by a gradual enlargement of the thyroid gland with autoimmune destruction. There is a great female to male predominance, with ratio of 10–20:1. Clusters of families are seen which are associated with HLA-DR5 on the major histocompatibility complex (MHC). A few cases are also characterized by HLA-DR3. The pathogenesis is attributed to cellular and humoral immunity which produces thyroid tissue injury. The morphology of the thyroid gland is characterized by typical destruction of the thyroid parenchyma with dense lymphocytic infiltrate and many secondary germinal centers. Occasional scattered Hurthle cells are also seen. Depending on the stage of the disease, extensive areas of fibrosis may also be present. The clinical course of Hashimoto thyroiditis is usually an initial period of time in which the patient may be euthyroid followed by hypothyroidism. (*Cotran et al., 1999, pp. 1134–1135*)

12. **(B)** PAN typically involves small- to medium-sized muscular arteries. In contrast, large arteries and the aorta are involved in Takayasu arteritis. Small arteries and arterioles are involved in a number of other diseases, including systemic lupus erythematosus. Active lesions in PAN demonstrate a neutrophilic infiltration of the involved vessel wall with thrombosis and segmental, fibrinoid necrosis. Intermittent healing produces fibrosis of the arterial wall and intimal thickening, which may lead to obstruction and infarction. Aneurysmal dilations may arise as a result of asymmetrical involvement. Although the lesions in PAN resemble other immune-mediated vascular lesions, the exact etiology of the disorder has not been elucidated. PAN generally affects middle-aged men and has a poor prognosis, although steroids may be beneficial. (*Cotran et al., 1994, pp. 520–521*)

13. **(A)** Amyloidosis is caused by the deposition of an abnormal proteinaceous material between cells. The majority of the cases are idiopathic, but a small percentage is secondary to chronic infection or inflammation, plasma cell dyscrasias, or immune diseases. One of the characteristic presentations of amyloidosis is splenic infiltration and splenomegaly caused by deposition of amyloid in the follicular regions. Grossly, the spleen has a diffuse, pink, glassy, waxy appearance with obliteration of

the white pulp. Amyloid infiltration can also affect the kidneys, liver, and heart. Clinical symptoms are usually due to functional impairment of the diseased organ. The diagnosis of amyloidosis is made by tissue biopsy or, more recently, by fat-pad biopsy looking for amyloid deposits. With Congo red stain, amyloid appears red; with polarization, it shows an apple-green birefringence, which is diagnostic of amyloid. *(Cotran et al., 1994, pp. 251–257)*

14. (B)

15. (D)

16. (D)

Explanations 14 through 16

Chronic lymphocytic leukemia is a disease that presents generally over the age of 50 with a male predominance. For a long time many of these patients remain asymptomatic and, when they do present, the symptomatology is nonspecific, with generalized lymphadenopathy and hepatosplenomegaly. The peripheral lymphocyte count is generally high and composed of small lymphocytes. A low percentage of patients develop autoantibodies directed against red cells or platelets, which produces autoimmune hemolytic anemia or thrombocytopenia. Although the disease progresses and relapses in spite of the chemotherapy treatment, the overall median survival is 4–6 years, but this appears to be very variable. Some patients may survive longer than 10 years. All of the parameters for a worse prognosis have to be measured before a final statement of prognosis can be made. The lymph node architecture is diffusely effaced by a population of small lymphocytes, which contain nondiscernible cytoplasm and inconspicuous nucleoli. Mitotic activity is rare, focal proliferation centers with an increase in the number of mitotic activity cells are seen. *(Cotran et al., 1999, pp. 658–659)*

17. (C) Senile plaques are the most conspicuous histologic lesion also known as neuritic plaque, constitute a spherical deposit of A β fragments (amyloid beta fragments) of variant degree

length. They are surrounded by reactive astrocytes, microglia, and display alpha-synuclein immunoreactive neuronal process. *(Rubin and Strayer, 2007, p. 1218)*

18. (B) Metastatic tumors reach the intracranial compartment through the blood stream, generally in patients with advanced cancer. Tumors of different organs vary in their incidences of intracranial metastasis. For example, a patient with disseminated melanoma has a greater than 50% likelihood of acquiring intracranial metastasis, whereas the incidences of such metastasis in carcinoma of the breast and lungs is 35%. Certain carcinomas such as those of the prostate, liver, and adrenals and sarcomas of all types rarely establish intracranial metastasis. A metastasis contrast with the primary glioma in its discrete appearance, globoid shape, and prominent halo of edema. *(Rubin and Strayer, 2007, p. 1235)*

19. (E) Squamous cell carcinoma is the most common malignant tumor of the oral mucosa and may occur at any site. It most frequently involves the tongue, followed in descending order by the floor of the mouth, alveolar mucosa, palate, and buccal mucosa. The male to female ratio is 2:1 for the gum, but 10:1 for the lip. There are substantial variations in the geographical distribution of the oral cancer. For example, it is the single most common cancer of men in India. *(Rubin and Strayer, 2007, p. 1061)*

20. (B) Fibroadenoma is the most common benign neoplasm of the breast and is composed of two types of tissues. A mesenchymal element most commonly composed of edematous or collagenized fibrous tissue and an epithelial component, which consists of compressed, and sometimes hyperplastic, irregular ductal lumens. They are usually found in young women and may be hormonally reactive during pregnancy or menopause. *(Cotran et al., 1999, pp. 1102–1103)*

21. (A)

22. (D)

Explanations 21 and 22

Pleomorphic adenoma (mixed tumor) is the most common tumor of the salivary glands. Pleomorphic adenoma is a benign neoplasm characterized by a mixture of epithelium and stromal elements. Two-thirds of all tumors of the major salivary glands and about half of those in the minor ones are pleomorphic adenomas. The tumor is nine times more frequent in the parotid than in the submandibular gland and usually arises in the superficial lobe of the parotid. It occurs most often in the middle-aged people and shows a female preponderance. While it is a benign tumor, the recommended treatment is removal, as it will continue to grow and cause symptoms. Most authorities recommend wide local excisions, in an effort to reduce the risk of recurrence. (*Rubin and Strayer, 2007, p. 1075*)

23. **(C)**

24. **(A)**

25. **(E)**

Explanations 23 through 25

Multiple myeloma is a plasma cell dyscrasia that is characterized by involvement of the skeleton in multiple sites. The characteristic x-ray shows punched-out bone lesions that are very easily seen in the calvarium. Extension of the disease to lymph nodes and extranodal sites, such as skin, can be seen. The bone marrow biopsy and smears reveal an increased number of plasma cells, which usually constitute greater than 20% of all of the cells. The cells either diffusely infiltrate and replace the marrow elements or can be seen scattered throughout the hematopoietic elements. The neoplastic plasma cells have a perinuclear hof and an eccentrically placed nucleus which allows the recognition. In 99% of patients with multiple myeloma, electrophoretic analysis reveals increased levels of IgG in the blood, light chains (Bence-Jones proteins) in the urine, or both. The monoclonal IgG produces a high spike when seen in the serum or in the urine, subject to electrophoresis. In general, the quantitative analysis of the monoclonal IgG is more than 3 g. The clinicopathologic diagnosis of multiple myeloma rests on radiographic and laboratory findings. Marrow examination may reveal increased plasma cells or sheet-like aggregates that may completely replace the normal elements. The prognosis for this condition is variable, but generally poor. (*Cotran et al., 1999, pp. 664–666*)

26. **(A)** The Reed-Sternberg cell can be classified as the classic type, the mononuclear variant, the lymphocytic histiocytic variant, lacunar and pleomorphic variant. The classic Reed-Sternberg cell is a binucleated cell that contains an ovoid-shaped nucleus with regular contours and prominent eosinophilic nucleoli. Cytoplasm is abundant and eosinophilic. On cytogenetic studies, the Reed-Sternberg cells are either aneuploid or frequently hypertetraploid. The classic Reed-Sternberg cell is thought to be an end-stage cell that does not divide. The mononuclear variants of the Reed-Sternberg cells (so-called Hodgkin cells) could be identified in any type of Hodgkin disease, but they are not diagnostic of Hodgkin's. (*Cotran et al., 1999, pp. 670–675*)

27. **(A)** One-third of all endometrial adenocarcinomas contain squamous cells, in addition to glandular elements. If the squamous element is well differentiated with no more than minimal atypia, the tumor is called well-differentiated adenocarcinoma with squamous differentiation. These tumors enjoy a better prognosis stage-by-stage compared with all of the others listed in the question. These tumors are less common and they show an aggressive behavior. The histologic grading, therefore, is not of clinical value. These aggressive tumors are serous carcinoma, clear cell adenocarcinoma, carcinosarcoma. (*Rubin and Strayer, 2007, p. 810*)

28. **(E)** Sinus histiocytosis represents hyperplasia of the endothelial lining of the sinusoids, which become dilated and contain many histiocytes. This reaction, which is also called reticular hyperplasia, becomes very prominent in lymph nodes when they are draining a cancerous process. This is particularly common in the

axillary nodes when cancer of the breast has been detected. It is thought to represent an immune response to the host against the tumor products. *(Cotran et al., 1999, p. 650)*

29. **(B)** At present, we have widespread screening programs for prostatic cancer using the digital rectal examination in combination with the serum PSA. These detect most of the malignant processes in the prostate. Patients with elevated serum PSA are further evaluated with needle biopsies. Preoperative PSA levels are correlated with the cancer volume. Serum PSA levels are a useful monitor for response to treatment and progression or recurrence of disease following therapy. *(Rubin and Strayer, 2007, p. 779)*

30. **(B)** The incidence of adenocarcinoma of the lung has increased significantly in the last two decades and is now the most common form of lung cancer in women and, in some studies, also in men. There may be mixtures of histologic patterns in the same cancers and, therefore, the finding of squamous cell carcinoma is not infrequent. A recent classification that is more common for clinical use has been developed in response to the necessity for the different therapies. These two large groups are divided into small cell versus nonsmall cell carcinomas. On histologic examination, the adenocarcinomas can be divided into bronchial-derived adenocarcinoma and bronchioloalveolar carcinoma. This classification is based on histologic findings alone. The lesions, in general, are peripherally located and tend to be smaller. Adenocarcinoma, including the bronchioloalveolar variant, is the least frequently associated with a history of cigarette smoking. Special stains for mucin are frequently positive. *(Cotran et al., 1999, pp. 743–744)*

31. **(A)** Malignant melanoma is a malignant neoplasm of the melanocyte. Most melanomas arise in the basal layer of the epidermis and remain confined to the epidermis in a radial growth phase for sometime. Later in the tumor development, it will grow down into the dermis (vertical growth phase) and gain access to the lymphatics. Clinically, most melanomas display a variegated brown, tan, pink, or black appearance. Irregular edges, enlargement, and central nodular ulceration may be noted. The microscopic appearance is characterized by nests of cells and single cells with eccentrically located nuclei and prominent eosinophilic macronucleoli. Melanin is present in the cytoplasm. Squamous cell carcinomas are not pigmented and they are rare on the back. Basal cell carcinomas can sometimes be confused with the melanomas when they are the pigmented variety. (This was not a selection given.) Generally, those happen in the sun-exposed areas. The prognosis of melanoma is related to the depth of invasion measured by either the Clark level or Breslow thickness. Deeply invading tumor and thicker tumors are associated with poor prognosis. *(Cotran et al., 1999, pp. 1177–1179)*

32. **(C)**

33. **(E)**

Explanations 32 and 33

Adenocarcinoma of the colon is the most common type of malignancy arising in the large intestine. Iron deficiency and microcytic anemia may be the presenting symptoms due to the bleeding from the tumor's ulceration. Alternatively, the tumor may be suspected by detention of occult fecal blood test, bowel obstruction, or through the development of hepatic enlargement secondary to metastasis. The gross appearance of this tumor is usually polypoid and ulcerated. Many ulcerating tumors involve the full circumference of the bowel and appear radiologically as an "apple core" lesion. The microscopic appearance is that of gland-forming malignant cells and usually mucin production is present. The prognosis is related to the stage of the disease.

Ulcerative colitis is an inflammatory disease of uncertain etiology that has a relapsing course. Patients with ulcerative colitis have a higher than normal incidence of developing colon carcinoma, approximately 10%.

Carcinoid tumors originate in the neuroendocrine cells throughout the intestinal tract. The appendix is most frequently involved, followed by the terminal ileum. On histologic examination, carcinoids are composed of uniform, round cells forming small nests or cords without encapsulation. Special stains performed show neurosecretory granules in the cytoplasm, which are positive for chromogranin, neuron-specific enolase, and other staining. *(Cotran et al., 1999, pp. 833–836)*

34. **(C)** Serous cystadenocarcinoma of the ovary is the most common malignant ovarian tumor and is frequently bilateral. Microscopically, they show a variegated appearance with papillary pattern. Different degrees of anaplasia of the cuboidal to columnar cells cover the papilla and occasional calcified concretions (Psammoma bodies) are present. These tumors almost never metastasize to the brain and they are not seen in children or young adults. *(Cotran et al., 1999, pp. 1069–1070)*

35. **(B)** Polycystic ovary syndrome is characterized by clinical manifestations related to the secretions of excess of androgen hormones. There is usually a persistent anovulation, resulting clinically in irregular or absent menstruation. The ovaries are moderately enlarged and contain many small cysts located in the cortex. *(Cotran et al., 1999, p. 1066)*

36. **(E)** Papillary cancer arises most frequently from the lateral and posterior bladder walls. At cystoscopy, tumors may be small, delicate, low-grade papillary lesions limited to the mucosal surface or larger high grade, solid, and invasive which are often ulcerated. Papillary and exophitic cancers tend to be better differentiated. Infiltrating tumors are usually more anaplastic.

   Nonurothelial forms of bladder cancer are squamous cell carcinomas, adenocarcinomas, neuroendocrine carcinomas, and rhabdomyosarcomas. The frequency of these tumors is much lower. *(Rubin and Strayer, 2007, p. 757)*

37. **(E)** The most important and frequent cause of painless hematuria is renal cell carcinoma. This symptom is usually associated with a palpable mass on the flank, as well as costovertebral pain. Occasionally, renal cell carcinomas are associated with a paraneoplastic syndrome, which includes polycythemia, hypercalcemia,

hypertension, feminization or masculinization, Cushing syndrome, and so on. The other answers listed are mostly seen in children. Transitional cell carcinoma is rarer than renal cell carcinoma and medullary fibroma is a benign tumor. *(Cotran et al., 1999, pp. 991–994)*

38. **(D)** Choriocarcinoma is a rare tumor of the testicles, but it is characterized by hemorrhage and necrosis. This tumor comprises only 1% of the malignant germ cell tumors and is rarely seen in a pure form. In general, they are small (no larger than 5 cm in diameter) and human chorionic gonadotropin (hCG) can be readily demonstrated in the blood. The cells seen in the hemorrhagic areas are cytotrophoblastic, as well as syncytiotrophoblastic, cells. *(Cotran et al., 1999, pp. 1021–1022)*

39. **(A)** Because we suspect that this patient has suppurative arthritis, the test to be ordered would be a culture of the joint fluid from the affected knee to ascertain which organism is involved and, with further identification and sensitivity, to determine which would be the antibiotic of choice. It would also be important to determine whether this is a hematogenous spread, secondary to osteomyelitis or contamination of the joint by a wound. *(Cotran et al., 1999, p. 1253)*

40. **(D)** Carcinoma of the esophagus is a highly lethal tumor and is a disease of the elderly. Etiology factors include alcoholism, cigarette smoking, hot drinks, aflatoxins, and smoked fish. The overall prognosis is very poor with 70% of the patients dying within 1 year after diagnosis of the disease. The most important parameter of the prognosis is the stage at the time of diagnosis, because over 80% 5-year survival is present in the tumors detected during the surveillance of Barrett esophagus. *(Catalano and Gwent, 2003, p. 238)*

41. **(C)** Hepatitis C which is caused by a single-stranded RNA virus is responsible for over 90% of the cases of hepatitis associated with transfusion of blood and blood products in the United States. The disease also occurs in drug abusers and transplant recipients, as well as

renal dialysis patients. It is associated with a higher incidence of chronic hepatitis, which occurs in 50% of those affected and cirrhosis complicates 20% of the cases. *(Catalano and Gwent, 2003, p. 242)*

42. **(E)** Ewing sarcoma is a malignant neoplasm of the bone that originates in the medullary canal and is composed of small uniform round cells. This tumor belongs to the primitive neuroectodermal tumors (PNET) of childhood. Approximately, 85% of these tumors show the C-MYC oncogene expression and there is a reciprocal transformation of chromosomes 11 and 22. *(Cotran et al., 1999, pp. 1244–1245)*

43. **(B)** In this case, the patient most likely has rheumatoid arthritis, an autoimmune chronic relapsing disorder that mostly affects the joints. The disease is usually seen in Western European and North American White females between the ages of 30 and 50. The clinical hallmark of the disease is symmetric swelling of the small joints of the hands and feet, particularly the proximal and interphalangeal joints. Swelling, pain, and stiffness are most severe in the morning. Pathologically, a pannus, or hypertrophic inflamed synovium, is produced that may eventually erode into the articular cartilage, with subsequent fibrosis, restriction of movements, and deformity. *(Cotran et al., 1999, pp. 1248–1251)*

44. **(B)** Goodpasture syndrome is characterized by antibasement antibodies, with the lungs and

kidneys bearing the brunt of the damage. Antibodies against platelet surface antigens, parietal cells, antigens, receptors, and colonic mucosal cells are seen in autoimmune thrombocytopenia, pernicious anemia, myasthenia gravis, and ulcerative colitis, respectively. *(Cotran et al., 1999, pp. 943–945)*

45. **(D)** Crohn's disease is a chronic inflammatory disorder of unknown etiology that has the potential to involve the different portions of the gastrointestinal (GI) tract from the mouth to the anus. It is characterized by a transmural inflammation with skipped areas in which the intestinal wall is not affected. Frequently, the presence of noncaseating epithelioid granulomas is seen. *(Catalano and Gwent, 2003, p. 240)*

46. **(C)** Mortality from cervical carcinoma has been considerably falling throughout the years and that is secondary to multiple factors, such as cytologic screenings (pap smears), early detection, and treatment of dysplasia. *(Catalano and Gwent, 2003, p. 174)*

47. **(C)** This image shows the typical segmental involvement of the terminal ileum seen in Crohn's disease. There is no evidence for hemorrhagic infarction. Ulcerative colitis may involve the terminal ileum, but is less likely as are intestinal tuberculosis and small bowel carcinoma. *(Rubin and Strayer, 2007, pp. 593–595)*

BIBLIOGRAPHY

Catalano E, Gwent M. *Appleton and Lange's Review of General Pathology*. New York, NY: McGraw-Hill, 2003.

Cotran RS, Kumar V, Collins T. *Robbins Pathologic Basis of Disease*, 6th ed. Philadelphia, PA: W.B. Saunders, 1999.

Cotran RS, Kumar V, Robbins SL. *Robbins Pathologic Basis of Disease*, 5th ed. Philadelphia, PA: W.B. Saunders, 1994.

Rubin R, Strayer DS. *Rubin's Pathology: Clinicopathologic Foundations of Medicine*, 5th ed. Philadelphia, PA: Lippincott Williams & Wilkins, 2007.

CHAPTER 8

Practice Test 1
Questions

Read each question carefully and in the order in which it is presented. Then select the one best response option of the choices offered. More than one option may be partially correct. You must select ONE BEST answer. You have 60 minutes to complete this test.

Setting I: Office/Health Center

You see patients in two locations: at your office suite, which is adjacent to a hospital, and at a community-based health center. Your office practice is a primary care generalist group. Most of the patients you see are from your own practice and are appearing for regularly scheduled return visits. Occasionally, you will encounter a patient whose primary care is managed by one of your associates. Reference may be made to the patient's medical records. Known patients may be managed by the telephone. You may have to respond to questions about information appearing in the public media, which will require interpretation of the medical literature. The laboratory and radiology departments have a full range of services available.

Questions 1 through 3

1. On a routine school physical you note that an 11-year-old female has some freckles in her axillae. This is new since last year and there are no other new skin marks noted. She is doing well in school. The only other change is that there has been some increase in her scoliosis. Which condition does she likely have?

(A) Sturge-Weber syndrome
(B) neurofibromatosis, type 1 (NF-1, von Recklinghausen's disease)
(C) tuberous sclerosis
(D) CHARGE Association
(E) Beckwith-Wiedemann syndrome

2. Which of the following physical findings would be expected on closer physical examination?

(A) port-wine stain in the V1 distribution
(B) subungual hamartomas
(C) Lisch nodules on the iris
(D) Hutchinson's teeth
(E) kinky brittle scalp hair

3. After she has been diagnosed, you spend time counseling her about future complications. These would include which of the following?

(A) increased risk of glaucoma
(B) increased risk of melanoma
(C) decreased fertility in females due to ovarian failure
(D) increased risk of blindness due to optic gliomas
(E) short final height due to hypothyroidism

Questions 4 through 6

A 62-year-old woman presents to the office with diarrhea. She is well known to you, as you recently discharged her from the hospital after a 4-day admission for pneumonia. She has completed a course of a macrolide antibiotic. She is now having about 10 watery bowel movements a day. She has mild abdominal cramps and fever, but denies vomiting or blood in her stool. On examination, she is mildly ill appearing. Her temperature is 101°F and otherwise normal vital signs. Her abdominal examination is notable for hyperactive bowel sounds and diffuse, mild tenderness without rebound or guarding. A stool occult blood test is negative.

4. Which of the following tests is most likely to yield a diagnosis?

   (A) fecal leukocytes
   (B) stool culture
   (C) stool for ova and parasites
   (D) Gram stain of fresh stool specimen
   (E) stool for *Clostridium difficile* toxin

5. What would be the most appropriate management at this time?

   (A) oral rehydration only
   (B) antidiarrheal agent only
   (C) oral ciprofloxacin
   (D) oral metronidazole
   (E) oral vancomycin

6. The patient calls you on the phone 3 days later stating that she continues to have 10 watery stools a day and is still running a low-grade fever. Since you saw her in the office, the diagnostic test that you ordered initially came back with a positive result, confirming your suspicion. Which of the following would be the best intervention at this time?

   (A) increase the dose of the oral antibiotic you initially started
   (B) start oral vancomycin
   (C) start intravenous metronidazole
   (D) start intravenous vancomycin
   (E) perform a colonoscopy to confirm diagnosis

Questions 7 and 8

A 33-year-old married male is seen in the office for a routine visit. He comes to the appointment with his wife but enters the examination room alone. He quickly becomes tearful and, with further questioning, admits that he has been feeling "down" for the past several months. He feels fatigued and has lost 10 lbs. He casually mentions that "my life is not worth living." Consideration is given to hospitalizing this individual.

7. What is the most appropriate approach for this patient?

   (A) Ask him directly if he has thoughts of suicide.
   (B) Immediately call in his wife and ask about suicide.
   (C) Inform him that his wife will not be told if he is suicidal.
   (D) Reassure him that his life is worth living.
   (E) Wait for him to bring up the subject of suicide.

8. The patient reveals that he has a plan to shoot himself with a gun that he keeps at home. He is unable to agree to come in for a further appointment. He insists on going home but does not wish to inform his wife of his suicidality. What is the next most appropriate step?

   (A) Begin treatment with an antidepressant and make a follow-up appointment.
   (B) Inform his wife and ask her about hospitalizing her husband.
   (C) Inform the wife and ask her to remove the gun when her husband returns home.
   (D) Recommend admission, notify his wife, and certify him if he is involuntary.
   (E) Recommend a follow-up appointment and inform him of emergency numbers.

9. A better control of cervical carcinoma has been attributed to which of the following?

   (A) early radical hysterectomy
   (B) external beam radiation therapy

(C) treatment of precursor lesion after detection by cytology screening

(D) development of multiagent chemotherapeutic regimes

(E) public awareness of the risk factors for cervical cancer

Questions 10 and 11

A 45-year-old businessman with no significant medical history presents to your office for a routine physical examination. He feels fine and has no complaints. Review of systems reveals that he may have had an elevated cholesterol level in the past but otherwise is negative. He says that there is no family history of significant disease and that all of his relatives die of "old age." He is a nonsmoker, drinks one alcoholic beverage three times per week in the evenings with clients during business meetings and exercises two or three times a week. He does not take any recreational drugs, prescriptions, over-the-counter (OTC) medications, herbs, or other supplements. His vital signs and examination are entirely normal. You order a lipid panel, fasting blood sugar, and liver function tests (LFTs). The lipid panel and blood sugar results came back within normal limits. The LFTs were essentially normal except for aspartate aminotransferase (AST) of 56 U/L and alanine aminotransferase (ALT) of 75 U/L.

10. What would be the initial management of this patient?

(A) ultrasound of the liver

(B) drug screen

(C) repeat LFTs after refraining from alcohol use for 1 month

(D) hepatitis panel

(E) order a GGT (gamma glutamyl transpeptidase) level

11. The patient has been compliant with your recommendations and has followed up regularly with you. Subsequent blood tests reveal that his AST and ALT remain essentially unchanged. What do you recommend at this time?

(A) observation and repeat of LFTs every 6 months, as long as they do not go any higher

(B) ultrasound of the liver

(C) antinuclear antibody (ANA), ceruloplasmin levels, and antismooth muscle Ab

(D) hepatitis panel and iron studies

(E) referral to a hepatologist for a liver biopsy

12. Which of the following statements regarding gastric lymphoma is true?

(A) It is the second most common site of primary intestinal lymphoma (small bowel is first).

(B) Chemotherapy is the treatment of choice.

(C) Gastrointestinal bleeding is the most common presenting symptom.

(D) Stage III disease is usually cured after resection alone.

(E) In most cases, radiation therapy provides a long-standing remission that may be equal to that of resection.

Questions 13 through 16

A 36-year-old African American male presents to your clinic for a well adult examination. He has no significant medical history. His only medication is prn loratadine (Claritin) for occasional allergic rhinitis symptoms. His family history is positive for hypertension and coronary artery disease in his father, who died of a heart attack at age 81. His brother was diagnosed with prostate cancer at age 62 but is cancer free now. Mother is alive at age 80 with Alzheimer's disease and osteoarthritis. He has two healthy children aged 15 and 12. He denies tobacco or recreational drug use. He drinks a "couple of beers" on weekends. His vital signs in the clinic showed blood pressure (BP) 134/80, heart rate (HR) 76, respiratory rate (RR) 18, temperature 97.9°F, and a body mass index (BMI) of 30.

13. Which of the following tests would be recommended at this visit?

   (A) a baseline electrocardiogram (ECG)
   (B) colonoscopy for colon cancer screening
   (C) rectal examination and prostate-specific antigen (PSA) level for prostate cancer screening
   (D) complete blood count (CBC)
   (E) total cholesterol and high-density lipoprotein (HDL) cholesterol

14. He asks you if he needs any vaccinations at this time. What do you recommend?

   (A) hepatitis A vaccine (HAV)
   (B) hepatitis B vaccine (HBV)
   (C) measles, mumps, rubella (MMR) booster every 10 years
   (D) diphtheria-tetanus (dT) booster every 10 years
   (E) pneumococcal vaccine

15. Two weeks later, the patient returns with the following results of a fasting lipid panel from a health fair at work: total cholesterol 234 mg/dL, triglyceride 158 mg/dL, LDL 153 mg/dL, HDL 38 mg/dL.

   This patient's recommended low-density lipoprotein (LDL) goal is less than which of the following?

   (A) 160 mg/dL
   (B) 130 mg/dL
   (C) 120 mg/dL
   (D) 100 mg/dL
   (E) 90 mg/dL

16. To achieve this goal, what do you recommend?

   (A) continuation of his current diet and activity level as he is at his goal
   (B) a prescription for cholestyramine
   (C) therapeutic lifestyle changes in diet and exercise
   (D) a prescription for a hydroxymethylglutaryl-coenzyme A (HMG-CoA) reductase inhibitor (statin)
   (E) supplementation with OTC niacin

Questions 17 and 18

A 26-year-old woman is a new referral to the primary care clinic. Review of her medical chart reveals numerous outpatient and urgent care visits over the past 12 months for different complaints relating to her concerns about having cancer. She has had extensive past workups, which were unrevealing of any significant major illness. On this visit, she presents with "gas pains" and is focused on obtaining an abdominal computed tomography (CT) to diagnose her presumed stomach cancer. When educated about the low likelihood and her prior negative findings she states, "I know it's unlikely, but I can't stop feeling that I probably have stomach cancer." On further interview, she denies any past history of depression or substantial anxiety, except relating to her fears of developing a malignancy.

17. Which of the following is her most likely diagnosis?

   (A) body dysmorphic disorder
   (B) conversion disorder
   (C) delusional disorder, somatic type
   (D) hypochondriasis
   (E) somatization disorder

18. Which of the following would be the most beneficial approach in treating this patient?

   (A) confrontation regarding the lack of basis for her concerns
   (B) extensive evaluation to provide reassurance
   (C) initiation of a serotonin-specific reuptake inhibitor (SSRI)
   (D) referral to a psychiatrist for management
   (E) regularly scheduled medical appointments

19. A 54-year-old man with hypertension, 30 pack-year history of smoking, and a family history of premature coronary artery disease has a fasting lipid profile with total cholesterol 247 mg/dL, triglycerides 210 mg/dL, HDL cholesterol 35 mg/dL, and LDL cholesterol 177 mg/dL. The patient has been maintaining a low fat, low cholesterol diet. His physician decides to place him on a statin. What is the most appropriate next step?

(A) The physician should write a prescription for a statin stating that it will lower the patient's cholesterol but with no further explanation.

(B) If the physician is of the opinion that the statin is the best therapy for the patient, there is no need to suggest any other options.

(C) The physician should explain that blood tests may need to be checked periodically to be sure the patient is tolerating the medication.

(D) The physician should not inform the patient of potential liver or muscle toxicity so as not to unduly alarm the patient.

(E) Since statins are commonly advertised and used, it is not necessary for the physician to determine if the patient has any questions about taking the new medication.

20. At what age should an evaluation for primary amenorrhea be initiated if a female adolescent has had normal linear growth (height) and normal breast and pubic hair development?

(A) 13
(B) 14
(C) 15
(D) 16
(E) 18

Questions 21 and 22

You are asked by the health department to evaluate the prevalence of lung cancer in your hometown.

21. What would be the most appropriate study design to accomplish this?

(A) randomized-controlled study
(B) case-control study
(C) cross-sectional study
(D) prospective cohort study
(E) case series

Your study reveals the following:

- The prevalence of lung cancer in the eastern half of the city is 5/1000 adults.
- The prevalence of lung cancer in the western half of the city is 2/1000 adults.

Further investigations reveal that the prevalence of smoking is the same throughout the city, but that the eastern part of the city has several chemical factories.

22. Which of the following statements is true?

(A) If the average age of the population is higher on the east side of town, the study confirms that the cumulative use of cigarettes for more years increases the rate of lung cancer.

(B) If the population of the two halves of town is equal then more people have lung cancer in the eastern part of the city than the western part.

(C) More people will die from lung cancer in the eastern half of the city.

(D) If the prevalence of cigarette smoking is the same in both sides of town, then the chemical factories are responsible for the development of the lung cancer.

(E) A person could reduce his risk of getting lung cancer by moving from the eastern side of town to the western.

Questions 23 and 24

A 30-year-old gravida 2, para 2 female uses an intrauterine device (IUD) for contraception. Over the last 6 months, she complains of feeling extremely irritable around the time of her menstrual period.

23. In order to meet diagnostic criteria for premenstrual syndrome (PMS), which of the following must be true?

    (A) A patient must report being irritable and bloated in the follicular phase of her menstrual cycle.

    (B) A patient must admit to feeling hopeless and suicidal before her menses.

    (C) A patient must complain of constipation and hot flashes with the onset of her menstrual cycle.

    (D) A patient must report at least one affective symptom (e.g., irritability, anxiety, social withdrawal) and one somatic symptom (e.g., mastalgia, bloating, headache) during the 5 days before menses for at least three prior consecutive menstrual cycles as documented on a symptom calendar.

    (E) A patient must admit to feeling increasingly fatigued 1 week before her menstrual period.

24. Which of the following recommendations are based on consistent scientific evidence for the treatment of PMS?

    (A) primrose oil

    (B) vitamin B_6

    (C) SSRIs

    (D) natural progesterone

    (E) avoidance of caffeine

25. A 74-year-old White female presents to your office with a 4-month history of abdominal distention, bloating, satiety, and associated shortness of breath. She reports an involuntary weight loss of 15 lbs, with associated lethargy and malaise. Her physical examination suggests mild cachexia, fluid wave, and a palpable abdominal mass. Her pelvic examination is unremarkable

with the exception of thickened nodularity appreciated within the posterior cul de sac.

What is the appropriate diagnostic test to order at this point?

    (A) pelvic ultrasound

    (B) endoscopic retrograde cholangiopancreatography (ERCP)

    (C) pelvic MRI

    (D) abdominal/pelvic CT scan

    (E) abdominal plain films

Setting II: Emergency Department and Inpatient Facilities

You encounter patients in the emergency department and inpatient facilities, including the hospital, the adjacent nursing home/extended-care facility, and detoxification unit. Most patients in the emergency department are new to you and are seeking urgent care, but occasionally, you arrange to meet there with a known patient who has telephoned you. You have general admitting privileges to the hospital, including to the children's and women's services. On occasion you see patients in the critical care unit. Postoperative patients are usually seen in their rooms unless the recovery room is specified. You may also be called to see patients in the psychiatric unit. There is a short-stay unit where you may see patients undergoing same-day operations or being held for observation. Also available to you are a full range of social services, including rape crisis intervention, family support, and security assistance backed up by local police.

26. A 41-year-old patient with a 20 pack-year history of smoking is admitted with weight loss, nausea, fatigue, and hypertension. There is no history of diabetes, drugs, medications, arthritis, or travel. The patient reports noticing foamy urine. On physical examination, the patient is afebrile and her blood pressure is 194/106. The patient is thin. The fundi are normal. The remainder of the examination was unremarkable. Laboratory examination reveals the WBC to be 3000, hemoglobin (Hgb) 7.0 mg/dL, platelet count 110,000. The blood urea nitrogen

(BUN) is 84, Cr 5.8, albumin 2.1. The urinalysis has no RBCs or WBCs but has 4+ protein. Twenty-four hour urine protein is 5.4 g/24 h.

Which of the following is the most appropriate next step to diagnose this patient's illness?

(A) a bone marrow examination to evaluate the leukopenia and anemia

(B) a chest x-ray to rule out lung cancer

(C) complement levels to evaluate for systemic lupus erythematosus

(D) an antibody to human immunodeficiency virus (HIV) by enzyme-linked immunosorbent assay (ELISA)

(E) a monospot test

27. During prolonged starvation, the central nervous system will use which of the following as its primary fuel source?

(A) glucose

(B) fatty acids

(C) protein

(D) glycogen

(E) ketones

28. A 32-year-old woman presents at 18 weeks estimated gestational age for a prenatal assessment. The fundal height measures 14 cm. A sonogram is obtained that reveals a nonviable intrauterine pregnancy. A D&C is performed that reveals a small fetus and associated hydropic swelling in some of the placental tissue. The appropriate diagnosis to explain these findings is which of the following?

(A) spontaneous miscarriage

(B) cervical incompetence

(C) partial mole

(D) luteal phase defect

(E) intrauterine growth retardation

29. You are assisting in the nursery and are the first to examine a newborn. On your examination you find a palpable abdominal mass. Which of the following is the most likely diagnosis?

(A) hydronephrosis

(B) neuroblastoma

(C) Wilms tumor

(D) hepatoma

(E) diaphragmatic hernia

Questions 30 and 31

A 22-year-old presents with a 2-week history of fever. The patient initially had sore throat and rash, then headache and nausea. On physical examination, the patient's oral temperature is 100°F, RR is 16, BP is 110/70, and pulse is 84. There is nuchal rigidity, the throat is red, there is cervical lymphadenopathy, and a faint macular rash (see Figure 8-1). You perform a lumbar puncture (LP) with the following results: opening pressure 8 cm of water, glucose 78, protein 30, WBC 25 with 76% lymphocytes, RBC 2, CSF VDRL is negative.

FIG. 8-1

30. What is the next most appropriate step?

(A) perform a monospot

(B) perform a rapid strep screen

(C) perform an HIV antibody test

(D) perform cultures for *Neisseria gonorrhea*

(E) perform an HIV RNA qualitative viral load

31. After getting the results of the LP, what is the next most appropriate step?

(A) treat with empiric therapy for tuberculosis

(B) treat for *Haemophilus influenzae* meningitis

(C) perform an MRI scan of the head to rule out a brain tumor or lymphoma

(D) send serum antibody tests for West Nile virus

(E) consider repeating the LP in 2 days to see if there has been a change

32. Two days following a repair of an abdominal aortic aneurysm, a 57-year-old male develops episodes of bloody diarrhea. Which of the following is the most important intervention?

(A) immediate operative exploration

(B) serial hemoglobin evaluation and blood transfusion as indicated

(C) proctosigmoidoscopy

(D) arteriogram

(E) CT scan

33. A 6-year-old child with Down syndrome is noted to have a recent onset of bleeding gums and petechia on the upper torso. On CBC, the white count was found to be markedly elevated due to a monomorphic population of immature lymphoid cells (100,000). What would be the most likely diagnosis in this case?

(A) infectious mononucleosis

(B) acute bacterial infection

(C) septicemia

(D) lymphoblastic leukemia

(E) reactive lymphocytosis

Questions 34 and 35

A 6-month-old female infant is brought to the emergency room with vomiting and fever of 2 days' duration. On examination, the infant is lethargic and appears dehydrated but has no other focal findings. Her WBC is elevated, a chest x-ray is clear, and a cath urine specimen shows WBCs and bacteria.

34. What organism is most likely to be responsible for this infection?

(A) group B *Streptococcus* (GBS)

(B) herpes simplex virus

(C) *Chlamydia trachomatis*

(D) *Pseudomonas aerogenosa*

(E) *Escherichia coli*

35. The parents report that she has not had any prior infections. What would be the best way to evaluate this infant?

(A) both a voiding cystourethrogram (VCUG) and a renal ultrasound

(B) VCUG only

(C) renal ultrasound and subsequent VCUG if the ultrasound is abnormal

(D) nuclear medicine reflux scan

(E) intravenous pyelogram (IVP)

Questions 36 through 40

A 23-year-old White male, with a history of insulin-dependent diabetes mellitus and medical noncompliance, is brought into the emergency room by his girlfriend for decreased responsiveness. The girlfriend states that he ran out of his insulin 1 week ago. Moreover, he has been urinating frequently and recently started complaining of nausea, vomiting, and abdominal pain. His physical examination shows an oral temperature of 99.5°F, BP of 95/40, HR of 125 bpm, and RR of 28. In general, he is tachypneic, lethargic, and unable to follow any commands. His mucus membranes are dry with very poor skin turgor. Cardiac examination reveals a tachycardic rate with a regular rhythm and no gallop. His lungs are clear. His abdominal examination is significant for mild diffuse tenderness but normoactive bowel sounds. His extremities are negative for edema. The laboratory results are as follows:

	Blood	Urine
Sodium	128	Specific gravity: 1.012
Potassium	6.5	Protein: trace
Chloride	92	RBCs: 1–3
CO_2	12	WBCs: 0–3
BUN	65	Ketones: 2+
Creatinine	2.0	No cellular casts
Glucose	900	

Glycosylated Hgb: 9.5
ECG: sinus tachycardia, no ST/T wave abnormalities
Serum ketones: 3+
Arterial blood gas: pH: 7.38/pCO_2: 21/pO_2: 95
WBC: 11,300
Hgb: 16.5
Hematocrit (HCT): 49.2
Platelets (PLT): 400

36. What is this patient's "corrected" serum sodium level?

(A) 120
(B) 115
(C) 141
(D) 152
(E) 156

$128 + 1.7 \times 800$
=

37. What is this patient's acid-base status?

(A) primary anion-gap metabolic acidosis
(B) anion-gap and nonanion-gap metabolic acidosis
(C) anion-gap metabolic acidosis and respiratory acidosis
(D) anion-gap metabolic acidosis and respiratory alkalosis
(E) anion-gap metabolic acidosis, nonanion-gap metabolic acidosis, respiratory alkalosis

38. In addition to volume replacement, which of the following statements is correct with regard to managing this patient?

(A) His acidosis should be treated with IV sodium bicarbonate.
(B) He should be started on subcutaneous 70/30 insulin until his blood glucose is below 200.
(C) You should stop the intravenous insulin drip when his blood glucose is normalized.

(D) You should start a dextrose-containing IV fluid when his blood glucose approaches 280.
(E) You should immediately administer 60 g of kayexalate orally.

39. Four hours after the initiation of therapy, the patient complains of severe muscle weakness. Which electrolyte disturbance is most likely responsible for these symptoms?

(A) hyperkalemia
(B) hypocalcemia
(C) hypophosphatemia
(D) hypomagnesemia
(E) hyponatremia

40. Toxic ingestion of which of the following could cause a similar acid-base disturbance?

(A) isopropyl (rubbing) alcohol
(B) lithium
(C) ethylene glycol (antifreeze)
(D) methanol
(E) salicylate

41. Which of the following is the most likely cause of hypotension and tachycardia in an unconscious patient with an apparent isolated head injury following a high-speed motor vehicle collision?

(A) neurogenic in origin
(B) low plasma volume
(C) cardiogenic in origin
(D) herniation of the brain stem
(E) subdural hematoma

Questions 42 and 43

A 20-year-old male is brought into the emergency room by the police after a disruption at the local college campus. According to his medical chart, he has been treated for a depressive episode in the past. He describes his mood as "great" but claims to have been awake for 4 days due to working on several inventions. He admits to rapid thoughts and believes that God has chosen him to be the next Messiah. In fact, angels have commanded him to steal from the student union in order to begin a new church.

42. Urine toxicology performed in order to rule out a substance of abuse as a cause of his symptoms would most likely reveal which substance?

   (A) alcohol
   (B) benzodiazepines
   (C) cannabis
   (D) cocaine
   (E) opiates

43. The toxicology screen is negative, and the patient is admitted to the hospital. Which of the following medications would be the most appropriate for the immediate management of his symptoms?

   (A) divalproex sodium
   (B) lamotrigine
   (C) lithium
   (D) lorazepam
   (E) mirtazapine

44. A 45-year-old male sustains a stab wound to the left upper chest. In the emergency department, he develops hypotension along with elevated jugular venous distention. His vital signs include a BP of 90/65 and a HR of 135 bpm. A chest x-ray is obtained and shown in Figure 8-2. Which of the following is the most appropriate intervention?

FIG. 8-2 (Reproduced, with permission, from Schwartz DT, Reisdorff EJ. Emergency Radiology. New York, NY: McGraw-Hill, 2000, p. 558.)

   (A) bedside echocardiogram
   (B) placement of a left chest tube
   (C) placement of a three quarter occlusive dressing over the stab wound entrance site
   (D) needle pericardiocentesis
   (E) emergency room thoracotomy

Questions 45 and 46

45. A 12-year-old boy is rushed to the emergency room after ingesting a caustic material. Following initial resuscitation and stabilization, what is the next most important intervention?

   (A) induction of emesis
   (B) oral ingestion of activated charcoal
   (C) steroid therapy
   (D) barium swallow
   (E) esophagoscopy

46. Which of the following is a potential delayed complication that he may develop?

   (A) diffuse esophageal spasm
   (B) esophageal carcinoma
   (C) Barrett esophagus
   (D) achalasia
   (E) Zenker diverticulum

Questions 47 and 48

A 48-year-old male presents to the emergency room with fever, chest pain, and cough for the past 2 days. His symptoms started abruptly. He describes the pain as a "sharp" pain in his left chest when he takes a deep breath or cough. His cough is productive of rusty-appearing sputum. He has a medical history of hypertension, for which he takes an angiotensin-converting enzyme (ACE) inhibitor. He does not smoke cigarettes. On examination, he is ill, but not toxic appearing. His temperature is 38.5°C, pulse is 115, RR is 26, and BP is 110/70. His oxygen saturation is 93% on room air. His pulmonary examination reveals rhonchi and rales in the left hemithorax. His heart is tachycardic but regular. He has no physical examination signs of hypoxia. His chest x-ray is shown in Figures 8-3A and B.

A   B

FIG. 8-3 *(Reproduced, with permission, from Chen MYM, Pope TL Jr, Ott DJ.* Basic Radiology. *New York, NY: McGraw-Hill, 2004, p. 83.)*

47. His history, examination, and radiographs are most consistent with which of the following?

    (A) aspiration pneumonia caused by enteric anaerobic organisms
    (B) pulmonary tuberculosis
    (C) *Pneumocystis carinii* pneumonia
    (D) community-acquired pneumonia caused by *Streptococcus pneumoniae*
    (E) pulmonary embolism

48. Which of the following is the most appropriate management of this patient?

    (A) hospitalization on the general medical floor for IV antibiotics
    (B) hospitalization in the intensive care unit for antibiotics, oxygen, and close monitoring
    (C) 23-hour observation in the hospital with oral antibiotics; admission to the general medical floor for IV antibiotics if not improved at the end of the observation time
    (D) outpatient management with oral antibiotics and close follow-up
    (E) inpatient admission to the general medical floor for oxygen, IV heparin, and institution of oral warfarin

Answers and Explanations

1. **(B)**

2. **(C)**

3. **(D)**

Explanations 1 through 3

Axillary freckling (also called the Crowe sign) is highly associated with NF-1. Café au lait spots and hypermelanotic macules in the axillae make up two major criteria in the diagnosis of NF-1. Having both of these would fulfill the National Institutes of Health (NIH) consensus criteria for the diagnosis of NF-1. Children with NF-1 may develop Lisch nodules, which are hamartomas on the iris. Lisch nodules do not affect vision and do not have any malignant potential. They are usually not present in early childhood, but appear during adolescence. *(Jones, 1997, pp. 508–509)*

The finding listed which is most consistent with NF-1 is Lisch nodules on the iris. These nodules are benign hamatromas of the iris. The sentinel physical finding of Sturge-Weber is a port-wine stain of the trigeminal V1 or V2 distribution. Subungual hamartomas are a common finding in tuberous sclerosis. Hutchinson's teeth are associated with congenital syphilis. Kinky brittle scalp hair is seen in Menke Kinky hair syndrome.

It is recommended that yearly visual acuity be followed in children with NF-1 due to the increased risk of optic nerve gliomas. These benign tumors can result in blindness. The other findings listed are unrelated to the diagnosis of NF-1. *(Committee on Genetics, 1995, pp. 368–372)*

4. **(E)**

5. **(D)**

6. **(B)**

Explanations 4 through 6

Toxin-producing strains of *C. difficile* are the only identified cause of colitis induced by antibiotic use. The diagnosis of this type of colitis requires that the onset of symptoms occur during or within 4 weeks of administration of the antibiotic and that there be no other identifiable cause of the symptoms. The diagnosis is confirmed most often by an ELISA assay for *C. difficile* toxin A. The ELISA has comparable specificity and only slightly less sensitivity than a tissue culture assay, which requires more time, specialized facilities, trained technicians, and higher costs. Fecal leukocyte testing is likely to be positive, but is not specific for the cause of this patient's diarrhea. Neither stool ova and parasites nor Gram stain would play a role in the diagnosis of antibiotic-induced colitis.

The preferred initial treatment for *C. difficile* colitis is oral metronidazole. It is preferred to vancomycin because they have similar efficacy, while metronidazole is significantly less expensive and has not been associated with the development of vancomycin-resistant enterococci. When a patient continues to have diarrhea and signs of systemic toxicity after 48 hours of treatment with metronidazole, changing to oral vancomycin would be a reasonable intervention. IV metronidazole could be used for a hospitalized patient or someone who could not take oral medication, but vancomycin must be given orally to be effective. *(Braunwald et al., 2001, pp. 922–927)*

7. **(A)**

8. **(D)**

Explanations 7 and 8

This individual is likely suffering from a major depressive disorder. He is expressing thoughts of death and may be having active suicidal ideation. Calling in his wife prior to notifying the patient or asking him further about suicidal ideation may frighten and anger him, damaging feelings of trust. Assuring him about confidentiality, when a voluntary or involuntary hospitalization may be necessary, might be inaccurate and may also hurt the therapeutic alliance in the future. Reassuring an individual who is in the midst of a depressive illness and who may be contemplating suicide is not beneficial and may inadvertently promote further guilty feelings, conversely increasing suicidal intent. Often, patients who are having thoughts of committing suicide do feel guilty or embarrassed and, if not directly questioned, may not bring up the subject. Indeed, directly inquiring about suicidal ideation in a nonjudgmental way may help to comfort the patient and enable further discussion about the subject.

The rate of completed suicide is approximately 12 out of 100,000 persons in the United States. There are numerous factors that increase the risk of suicide. The presence of concurrent anxiety symptoms is one factor that increases the risk. Previous suicide attempts are actually the best indicator that a patient is at an increased risk to commit suicide. Asking about a specific plan for suicide is essential in a thorough risk assessment. It can demonstrate concern for patient and enhance the therapeutic alliance. Seriously suicidal individuals are often suffering from a severe depressive illness and can respond significantly to antidepressant therapy. A family history of suicide is another factor that increases the risk of attempted suicide.

This patient has a clear plan and access to a lethal method for suicide. While beginning treatment with an antidepressant appears appropriate, he has indicated he will not follow up as an outpatient. Notifying the wife in order to obtain further history, assess his support system, and remove the firearms may also be appropriate; however, this patient requires more immediate intervention, namely immediate psychiatric hospitalization. While his wife's agreement with hospitalization is important and helpful, it is *not* necessary. In this case, it is warranted to certify the patient if he does not agree to be voluntarily

admitted to the hospital. *(Sadock and Sadock, 2003, p. 913, 917)*

9. **(C)** With the introduction of screening tests for cytologic evaluation of cervical cells, a dramatic decrease in mortality from invasive cervical carcinoma has occurred. This has been accomplished because of early detection of intraepithelial neoplasia of different degrees that may lead, if untreated, to carcinoma. Mild, moderate, and severe dysplasia can be diagnosed with regular pap smears and, more recently, with a different technique (ThinPrep). In cases of high-grade dysplasia, further adequate early treatment can be achieved before progressing into an invasive carcinoma. *(Cotran et al., 1999, pp. 1048–1052)*

10. **(C)**

11. **(D)**

Explanations 10 and 11

LFTs have now become part of many standard chemistry panels. They are often ordered for a variety of conditions or to follow for medication side effects. Because of the frequency with which they are ordered, abnormalities in asymptomatic persons are often found.

Abnormal liver enzymes may be benign and transient or may be due to alcohol use, viral hepatitis, and drug or herbal medication use. They may also be the initial finding of a more serious underlying problem. A practical and methodological approach to the evaluation of abnormal LFTs should be followed both to avoid misdiagnosis and to prevent unwarranted studies and interventions.

According to the American Gastroenterology Association (AGA), 1–4 % of the asymptomatic population may have abnormal LFTs. ALT and AST are fairly reliable markers of hepatocellular injury or necrosis. These values can be elevated in a multitude of hepatic disorders. ALT is usually more specific for hepatic injury, as it is mostly present in the liver. AST is present in the liver, heart, skeletal muscle, kidneys, brain, pancreas, lungs, WBCs, and RBCs. It is important to note that ALT and AST levels can be normal in the presence of significant liver disease.

The ratio of AST to ALT can be useful to suggest an etiology but may also have limitations. Traditionally, an AST/ALT of greater than 2 is suggestive of alcoholic hepatitis, whereas the opposite may suggest viral hepatitis. Nonalcoholic steatohepatitis (NASH) can also result in mildly elevated AST and ALT levels. Wilson's disease, although a rare problem, can also lead to elevated transaminases. Muscle injury, hyperthyroidism, and even genetic or racial influences can cause elevations of the AST/ALT. Some studies have reported diurnal variations in LFTs and increases from exercise.

Routine screening of LFTs in asymptomatic patients is not warranted or recommended. The AGA has developed guidelines for the workup of abnormal LFTs in an asymptomatic patient. The initial approach should be a thorough history and physical to help discern the etiology and assess for risk factors. Specific inquiries about family history, drug and alcohol use, exercise regimen, and the use of herbs and OTC medications/vitamins/supplements should be made.

For mildly elevated AST/ALT levels (less than five times normal) in asymptomatic individuals in whom the history and physical is inconclusive, the first step in the approach should be to repeat the liver function studies. If the patient is using alcohol, drugs, medications, or herbs/supplements that may alter the LFTs, they should be advised to refrain from these products for several weeks prior to repeating the study. If the abnormality persists, a CBC, comprehensive metabolic panel (electrolytes, BUN, creatinine, LFTs, albumin), prothrombin time (PT), hepatitis panel, and iron studies should be ordered. These studies are to look for evidence suggestive of viral hepatitis, liver function (PT, albumin), renal function, Wilson's disease, and hemachromatosis. If these results are normal and the patient remains asymptomatic, then the LFTs should be repeated in 6 months. If these are normal, observation is justified.

If the repeat is abnormal, further testing with ultrasound should be initiated. If the ultrasound does not suggest an etiology,

additional serologic studies are warranted: ANA and antismooth muscle antibody (r/o autoimmune hepatitis), ceruloplasmin (Wilson's Dz), alpha-1 antitrypsin (r/o alpha-1 antitrypsin deficiency), antigliadin, and antiendomysial antibody (r/o celiac Dz). Patients who have chronic elevations in liver functions that remain asymptomatic and have a negative workup thus far may be considered for liver biopsy once a detailed discussion has been done regarding complications, benefits, risks, desire for prognostic information and intervention. *(Giboney, 2005, pp. 1105–1110)*

12. **(E)** Gastric lymphoma can occur as an isolated neoplasm confined to the stomach or it may be the manifestation of widespread infiltrative disease involving lymphatic and other organ systems. The stomach is the most common site of primary intestinal lymphoma. Anorexia and weight loss are the most common presenting complaints, whereas bleeding is relatively uncommon. Early satiety is a prominent symptom, as the gastric wall becomes thickened and the lumen is progressively compromised by the neoplastic infiltrate. Definitive diagnosis is made by endoscopy and biopsy. Radiation therapy provides a long-standing remission that may be equal to that of resection alone and has emerged as the treatment of choice. Patients who present with gastric outlet obstruction, however, are best treated by subtotal gastric resection and postoperative irradiation. A combined approach is associated with a 5-year survival rate of 85% when the malignant process is limited to the stomach. *(Schwartz et al., 1999, p. 1205)*

13. **(E)**

14. **(D)**

15. **(B)**

16. **(C)**

Explanations 13 through 16

The United States Preventative Services Task Force (USPSTF) has an A recommendation (strongly recommend) that clinicians routinely screen men aged ≥35 years and women aged ≥45 years for lipid disorders. The USPSTF has a D recommendation (against) routine screening with resting ECG. Colon cancer screening is recommended starting at the age of 50 for low-risk adults. The USPSTF has an I recommendation (insufficient evidence to recommend for or against routine screening) for prostate cancer using PSA testing or digital rectal examination (DRE). Most major U.S. medical organizations agree that the most appropriate candidates for prostate cancer screening include men older than 50 years and younger men at increased risk of prostate cancer, but that screening is unlikely to benefit men who have a life expectancy of less than 10 years. There is no recommendation for routine CBC screening of adults. (USPSTF: www.preventiveservices.ahrq.gov)

dT boosters are recommended every 10 years. HAV would be recommended for certain medical indications such as persons with clotting-factor disorders or chronic liver disease. It is also recommended for men who have sex with men, users of recreational drugs, persons working with hepatitis A-infected primates, or with HAV in a research laboratory setting. It should be considered by persons traveling to or working in countries that have high or intermediate endemicity of hepatitis A. (CDC 1999)

HBV is recommended for adults with certain indications. These include hemodialysis patients, patients who receive clotting-factor concentrates, health care and public safety workers who have exposure to blood in the workplace, persons in training for health professions. Behavioral indications for the HBV would include injecting drug users, persons with more than one sex partner in the previous 6 months, persons with a recently acquired sexually-transmitted disease (STD), all clients in STD clinics, and men who have sex with men. Household contacts and sex partners of persons with chronic HBV infection, clients and staff of institutions for the developmentally disabled, international travelers who will be in countries with high or intermediate prevalence of chronic HBV infection for more than 6 months, and inmates of correctional facilities should also be immunized. (CDC 1991)

The Centers for Disease Control (CDC) recommends that persons born after 1956 (like the patient in question) should have two doses of measles vaccine; additional doses should be given as MMR, but there is no need for MMR booster every 10 years. Pneumococcal vaccine should be given to patients with high-risk conditions, such as chronic obstructive pulmonary disease (COPD), chronic liver diseases, chronic renal failure, immunosuppressive conditions, and splenectomy.

This patient's LDL goal is less than 130 mg/dL as he has two coronary artery disease risk factors, a BMI of 30, and a low HDL. To achieve this goal you should recommend therapeutic lifestyle modification, including a low fat diet and regular exercises (30 min/day, most days of the week) to promote weight lose if overweight and stress management. He has normal triglycerides, so niacin is not indicated at this time. Lipid-lowering medication would not be indicated at this time. However, if he continues to have high LDL readings after trying the recommended lifestyle modifications, one could then consider the addition of lipid-lowering agents. (National Heart, Lung and Blood Institute of the National Institutes of Health, 2001)

17. (D)

18. (E)

Explanations 17 and 18

Body dysmorphic disorder involves the preoccupation with an imagined or exaggerated defect in appearance. Unlike the above case, the individual focuses on a perceived flaw rather than an internal symptom. Patients with conversion disorder display a neurologic deficit as a result of an unconscious conflict. The patient in the above case is anxious about having cancer, but she is not delusional regarding absolutely having the disease, as would be seen in delusional disorder. Somatization disorder requires the presence of multiple physical complaints covering several different body systems. The focus is on the somatic symptoms rather than having a specific disease. This individual displays features of hypochondriasis, a condition characterized by a preoccupation with fears of having a serious disease based on the misinterpretation of bodily sensations. In her case, it is her fearing having stomach cancer because of her gas pains. (*American Psychiatric Association, 2000*)

Confrontation is only necessary in cases of malingering. Confronting a patient with hypochondriasis would likely increase the individual's anxiety and anger, as well as damage the therapeutic alliance. An extensive evaluation in this case will not likely reassure the patient, will increase costs, and expose the person to possible side effects or complications from tests and procedures. Beginning an SSRI is indicated if there is a comorbid mental illness that will respond to the medication, such as major depressive disorder or panic disorder, neither of which appear to be present in this case. While referring the above patient to a psychiatrist may be useful for the same reasons, individuals with hypochondriasis are often resistant to psychiatric interventions. The best approach is to have regularly scheduled visits. These can both help provide the needed reassurance and enable time for limited physical examinations if indicated. (*Sadock and Sadock, 2003, p. 653*)

19. **(C)** Informed consent is a means by which the physician demonstrates respect for the patient's autonomy, so that the patient can make up his own mind to accept or refuse a proposed treatment or diagnostic test. The process of informed decision making involves two preconditions: that the patient is making the decision voluntarily (free of undue influence or coercion) and that the patient has the capacity to make the decision. Once these preconditions are met, the process of informed consent involves the disclosure of information, followed by the actual decision (either consent or refusal) made by the patient.

Disclosure of information must provide enough information on the patient's condition, the risks and benefits of the proposed treatment, and the alternatives available, so that the patient can make a rational decision. The standard that is used today for the amount of information to disclose is based on what would be expected by a reasonable person in order to make a decision. The subjective standard would be the amount of information that a particular individual requires, based on the physician's knowledge of that patient's characteristics and/or circumstances. The clinician should be aware of the possibility of framing effects when giving information, since framing (e.g., presenting only one side of pertinent statistics) may influence the patient's voluntariness.

In the case presented, it is important for the physician to explain why she is prescribing the statin, especially in light of the patient's cardiac risk factors. The physician should explain that there are other options for managing the patient's hypercholesterolemia, including other classes of medications or further lifestyle modification. Relevant side effects of the medication, including the need to monitor for liver toxicity with periodic blood tests, should be mentioned and the patient should be alerted as to what symptoms to report to the physician in this regard. Once the physician has disclosed the information, she should determine if the patient has any questions, both to check for comprehension and to fill in any gaps of knowledge, before the patient makes a decision about the medication.

20. **(D)** The average age of menarche is dependent on race but averages 12.8 years. For an adolescent female who has made no pubertal progression, an evaluation for primary amenorrhea (and delayed puberty) should be initiated by age 14. In the adolescent female who has met all of her other normal pubertal milestones (linear growth, breast development, and pubic and axillary hair growth), it is appropriate to delay the evaluation for primary amenorrhea until age 16. (*Beckmann et al., 2002, p. 463*)

21. **(C)**

22. **(B)**

Explanations 21 and 22

A cross-sectional study is the best study design to determine the prevalence of an event or characteristic at a single point in time. It is not useful in determining the etiology of the event in question. A randomized-controlled study is a prospective study design used to assess differences between two or more groups receiving different intervention or treatment. It is most often used to compare outcomes between different treatments or used in clinical decision analysis to compare outcomes. A case-control study is an observational study in which affected and unaffected subjects are identified after the fact and then compared regarding specific characteristics to determine possible associations or risks for the disease in question. A prospective cohort study is an observational study in which exposed and unexposed populations are identified and followed prospectively over time to determine the rate of a specific clinical event. A case-series study design is an objective report of clinical characteristic or outcomes from a group of clinical subjects. A case-series report can address almost any clinical issue, including screening test results, treatment outcomes, and natural history findings. It is most commonly used to describe clinical characteristics, such as signs and symptoms of disease or disease outcomes. *(Cassens, 1992)*

23. **(D)**

24. **(C)**

Explanations 23 and 24

Documentation of both affective and somatic symptoms by a menstrual calendar is critical to establish the diagnosis of PMS. The University of California at San Diego criteria for the diagnosis of PMS includes at least one of the following affective and somatic symptoms during the 5 days before menses in each of the three previous cycles:

- Affective symptoms: depression, angry outbursts, irritability, anxiety, confusion, social withdrawal
- Somatic symptoms: breast tenderness, abdominal bloating, headache, swelling of extremities
- Symptoms relieved from days 4 through 13 of the menstrual cycle

The National Institute of Mental Health diagnostic criteria include a 30% increase in the intensity of symptoms of PMS (measured by a standard instrument) from days 5–10 of the menstrual cycle as compared with the 6-day interval before the onset of menses and documentation of these changes in a daily symptom diary for at least two consecutive cycles. *(Dickerson et al., 2003, pp. 1743–1752)*

In clinical trials, SSRI therapy, particularly fluoxetine and sertraline, have been shown to be effective in treating PMS. While the other options listed, along with many others, are frequently tried, well-designed scientific studies have not consistently shown them to be helpful. *(Davis and Johnson, 2000)*

25. **(D)** This patient presents with the characteristic findings associated with undiagnosed ovarian cancer. The signs and symptoms in the early stages of the disease tend to be nonspecific, often gastrointestinal in nature. Patients with more advanced stage disease present with the classic constellation of abdominal distention, bloating, satiety, anorexia, dyspnea, and involuntary weight loss. The most appropriate diagnostic test to order in this situation would be a CT scan of the abdomen and pelvis to evaluate for extent of disease and potential respectability of disease. A CT scan can help to determine the presence or absence of liver metastases, hydronephrosis, and bowel obstruction.

Ultrasound is best reserved for the evaluation of the pelvic viscera, specifically the morphology and subtle detail associated with the uterus, ovaries, and fallopian tubes when abnormalities are suspected. It is not a good test to evaluate for abdominal extent of disease. Pelvic MRI, like ultrasound, does not provide any information relative to the abdominal extent of disease. Abdominal plain films are used primarily to assess bowel perforation or obstruction; it provides no fine detail about possible tumor burden of extent/location of disease. ERCP is used to evaluate the duct drainage of the gallbladder and pancreas. *(Togashi, 2003, pp. L87–L104)*

26. **(D)** The patient has nephrotic syndrome. The patient is also noted to have anemia and

leukopenia. HIV is one of the most common causes of nephrotic syndrome. While there are certainly many other conditions that can cause nephrotic syndrome, HIV is the most likely. A bone marrow examination would give important information to evaluate leukopenia and anemia but would be unlikely to yield a specific diagnosis. A chest x-ray is a poor way to rule out lung cancer. Other tests for systemic lupus erythematosus would be more useful than complement levels. The clinical history does not suggest mononucleosis. *(Mandell et al., 2000, pp. 1409–1410)*

27.   **(E)** There is a fundamental difference between human body metabolism in normal physiology and during starvation. A healthy 70-kg individual expends an average of 1800 kcal/day of energy obtained from lipid, carbohydrate, and protein sources. Obligate glycolytic cells include neurons, leukocytes, and erythrocytes. These cells require 180 g of glucose per day for basal energy needs.

During acute starvation, glucose is initially derived from the breakdown of hepatic glycogen. However, within 24 hours, hepatic glycogen storage is depleted. Thereafter, initiation of gluconeogenesis results in the production of glucose, mainly from the breakdown of amino acids and fatty acids. Ketones are derived from fatty acids during prolonged starvation. After 4 or 5 days, the rate of whole-body proteolysis diminishes significantly as the nervous system and other previous glucose-utilizing tissue begin to utilize ketones as the predominant energy source. Thus, ketones serve as the primary source of energy during prolonged starvation and have a protein sparing affect. *(Schwartz et al., 1999, pp. 26–28)*

28.   **(C)** Hydropic swelling among the placental tissues suggests the presence of a molar gestation. There are two types of molar pregnancies, each with distinctive clinical and cytogenetic features.

The partial mole has a triploid karyotype that results from dispermic fertilization of an egg with retention of the maternal haploid set. The placental tissue of the partial mole is characterized by focal, variable hydropic villi and usually by focal, slight trophoblastic hyperplasia. The embryo associated with partial molar pregnancies survives much longer than with complete moles, with embryonic deaths typically occurring at approximately 8 weeks estimated gestational age. Frequently, at the time of evacuation, there is macroscopic or microscopic evidence of a fetus. Fetal blood vessels are identified and usually contain nucleated fetal erythrocytes.

The complete mole has a diploid karyotype, resulting from paternal fertilization of an "empty egg" and subsequent replication of the paternal haploid karyotype within the empty egg, to produce 46 chromosomes, all paternal in origin. The placental tissue of the complete mole is remarkable for generalized edema of the chorionic villi, including central cistern formation, which results in a macroscopic appearance similar to a "bunch of grapes." The embryo associated with the complete mole undergoes resorption before the development of the cardiovascular system, when the embryo is less than 1 cm in length. Thus, fetal vessels generally degenerate soon after formation and no nucleated fetal erythrocytes are seen in the villous capillaries.

Partial moles account for 25–40% of all molar pregnancies and are typically diagnosed in the second trimester, when they present most commonly as a missed abortion. In contrast to the extremely high serum human chorionic gonadotropin (hCG) levels found in association with complete moles, partial moles typically have hCG levels in the low to normal range. The risk of subsequent gestational trophoblastic neoplasia associated with partial moles is 5–10%, compared to the increased risk of 10–30% associated with complete moles.

Complete moles typically present with vaginal bleeding in the first trimester. They can also be associated with hyperemesis gravidarum, toxemia, and hyperthyroidism in the first or second trimester. Complete moles are associated with an extremely high hCG value and a characteristic ultrasound "snowstorm" appearance.

Spontaneous miscarriage involves the loss of a nonmolar gestation, typically in the first trimester. The causes can include genetic defects, uterine anomalies, poorly controlled diabetes, or luteal phase defect. Cervical incompetence generally presents with painless cervical dilatation and spontaneous miscarriage at 18–22 weeks estimated gestational age. Intrauterine growth retardation generally refers to a viable intrauterine pregnancy in which fetal growth is inadequate for the gestational age. This causes a range from uteroplacental insufficiency to genetic abnormalities to in utero infection. *(Altieri, 2003, pp. 670–678)*

29. **(A)** The most common abdominal mass in a newborn infant is hydronephrosis. It is a common finding in prenatal ultrasounds. It will usually resolve without therapy. Neuroblastoma is the most common abdominal tumor of infancy. It is much less common than the relatively common hydronephrosis. Hepatomas and Wilms tumors are even rarer than neuroblastoma. Diaphragmatic hernia will usually present with respiratory embarrassment and feeding difficulties, not an abdominal mass. *(Rudolph et al., 2003, pp. 1375–1376)*

30. **(E)**

31. **(E)**

Explanations 30 and 31

This case is a typical description of a person with acute HIV infection. The duration of this patient's illness is against strep pharyngitis. The patient could have mononucleosis but a monospot would not be specific for this diagnosis. There is no history of oral sexual exposure, which would be necessary for *N. gonorrhea* pharyngitis. *N. gonorrhea* also does not cause meningitis in this setting. An HIV antibody test by ELISA is negative in a majority of cases of early acute HIV infection. The more sensitive polymerase chain reaction (PCR) test would be a better test to use.

After getting the results of the LP, the most appropriate next step is repeating LP in 2 days to see if there has been a change. The acute history is not indicative of tuberculosis. *H. influenzae* meningitis usually affects children less than 5 years of age. The only time opportunistic

infections or lymphoma occur in HIV is in the chronic setting of AIDS. Serum antibody tests for West Nile virus are indicated in patients with aseptic meningitis, but the clinical picture does not present with rash. Repeating an LP in 2 days to see if there is a change helps to exclude other infections that might cause a rash by identifying a change in the number and composition of cells. *(Mandell et al., 2000, pp. 1404–1405, 1432)*

32. **(C)** Any patient who develops bloody diarrhea following abdominal aortic surgery should be suspected of having ischemic colitis. It results from injury or ligation of the inferior mesenteric artery during the procedure. The estimated incidence is 1–6%. Patients may also present with abdominal distention, leukocytosis, and peritonitis as early as 24–48 hours following surgery. Immediate sigmoidoscopy is the diagnostic modality of choice, since it facilitates direct visualization of the colonic mucosa. In most instances the injury is mucosal, which appears as edematous, friable, and hemorrhagic mucosa with patchy ulceration. In these patients, the process is self-limited and treated with supportive measures including hydration, transfusion, and serial examination. In cases of full-thickness involvement, the mucosa will appear black or grey, indicating transmural ischemia and impending gangrene of the bowel. Surgical resection of the ischemic segment with proximal colostomy is indicated in these patients or patients with signs of sepsis or peritonitis. Arteriography and CT scan usually do not demonstrate specific vascular abnormalities. *(Schwartz et al., 1999, p. 948, 1284, 1285)*

33. **(D)** Down syndrome is caused by a trisomy of chromosome 21. Prominent epicanthic folds, mental retardation, congenital cardiovascular abnormalities, increased susceptibility to infections, hyperflexibility, muscle hypotonia, dysplastic ears, and infertility characterize the syndrome. Individuals with Down syndrome have a 20-fold risk in developing lymphoblastic leukemia during childhood. Infectious mononucleosis, although it can show lymphocytosis, would not be monomorphic of such high proportion. Infectious diseases will give an

increase in the myeloid series and leukemoid reaction. Reactive lymphocytosis is seen in viral infections and should not be considered in this case.

Down syndrome is the most common chromosome abnormality, occurring in 1 out of 800 live births. It is characterized by a trisomy 21 karyotype with an extra G group chromosome (chromosome 21), making a total of 47 chromosomes. The parents are phenotypically and genetically normal in the majority of cases and Down syndrome is secondary to a meiotic error in the ovum. The risk of having a Down syndrome child is proportional to increasing maternal age. The clinical features of Down syndrome include fat facies, epicanthic folds, oblique palpebral fissures, and mental retardation. The majority of affected individuals die early from cardiac or infectious complications. Thirty percent have a ventricular septal defect. Trisomy 13, also called Patau syndrome, causes microcephaly and severe mental retardation with absence of a portion of the forebrain. These children die soon after birth. Trisomy 18, or Edwards syndrome, is also a very severe genetic defect, and the average life span is 10 weeks. Affected children have severe mental retardation and cardiac anomalies, including ventricular septal defect. Persons with an XO karyotype have Turner syndrome and are phenotypically females. Only 3% of affected fetuses survive to birth; fetuses that do survive have severe edema of the hands, feet, and neck. Affected persons have a webbed neck, short stature, and congenital heart disease. At puberty, there is failure to develop normal secondary sex characteristics, so their genitals remain immature. Klinefelter syndrome, or testicular dysgenesis, is characterized by an XXY karyotype. It occurs in 1 out of 600 live births. Affected individuals usually are diagnosed after puberty and have eunuchoid habitus, long legs, small atrophic testes and penis and, often, low IQ. (Cotran et al., 1994, pp. 170–173)

34. (E)

35. (A)

Explanations 34 and 35

After the first 4–6 weeks of life, GBS begins to diminish as a cause of urinary tract infections (UTIs). The most common cause of UTIs then becomes E. coli. UTIs are more common in females. If infants develop fever and some degree of toxicity (vomiting, poor feeding, lethargy), they are commonly diagnosed clinically with pyelonephritis. The best clinical way to document pyelonephritis without any imaging would be seeing the presence of WBC casts in a urinary microscopic examination. (Rudolph et al., 2003, pp. 1667–1673)

While there are emerging data as to the short- and long-term management issues surrounding reflux nephropathy which may change the imaging recommendations, currently the American Academy of Pediatrics recommends a renal ultrasound and VCUG in all children with first time uncomplicated UTIs between 2 months and 2 years. IVPs are not studies performed in infants and children as part of evaluation of UTIs. Radionucleide cystography play a role in following children with abnormal collecting systems identified on prior studies, they are currently not the preferred modality in the initial evaluation regimen. (Downs, 1999, p. e54)

36. (C)

37. (D)

38. (D)

39. (C)

40. (E)

Explanations 36 through 40

Hyperglycemia results in "translocational hyponatremia." Increases in glucose concentration of 100 mg/dL will decrease the serum sodium by approximately 1.7 mmol/L. In this case, the sodium will correct to approximately 141.

This patient has an anion-gap metabolic acidosis from diabetic ketoacidosis, with an anion gap of 24. Using the formula to determine appropriate respiratory compensation [expected $pCO_2 = 1.5 \times (HCO_3) + 8 \pm 2$], we would expect the pCO_2 to be 26 ± 2. However, the pCO_2 here is less, indicating a concurrent respiratory alkalosis. The anion gap and bicarbonate levels show that the acidosis stems completely from the presence of unmeasured anions. Therefore, a concurrent nonanion-gap metabolic acidosis is not present.

Volume resuscitation is necessary, as patients with diabetic ketoacidosis are frequently volume depleted. Treatment of the ketosis with insulin is also necessary. This is typically done with a continuous infusion of intravenous insulin. The drip is maintained based on the presence of persistent ketoacidosis and should not be discontinued based on blood glucose values. Furthermore, dextrose should be added to the intravenous fluids when the blood glucose decreases, in order to avoid hypoglycemia from the insulin infusion. The administration of kayexalate is unnecessary, as the etiology of the hyperkalemia is due to the relative deficiency in insulin and will correct with the insulin drip.

Serum phosphate must be monitored closely during the treatment of diabetic ketoacidosis. The insulin drip can lead to intracellular uptake of phosphate, creating hypophosphatemia. This can result in muscle weakness and even respiratory paralysis. Hypokalemia is also a potential complication of the treatment of diabetic ketoacidosis, as insulin will increase the cellular uptake of potassium.

This patient has a combined anion-gap metabolic acidosis and respiratory alkalosis, which also can be seen in salicylate toxicity. Lithium toxicity can lead to diabetes insipidus and may create a low anion-gap picture. Ingestion of methanol and ethylene glycol can lead to an anion-gap metabolic acidosis but not necessarily a respiratory alkalosis. Isopropyl alcohol ingestions can lead to an osmolar gap, but usually will not lead to an anion-gap acidosis. (*Brenner, 2004, pp. 966–968*)

41. **(B)** Shock is defined as a state of inadequate supply of essential nutrients to the tissues. In the trauma setting, hypotension should be assumed to be secondary to hypovolemic

shock resulting from an acute loss of plasma volume, regardless of the patient presentation. Massive external or internal hemorrhage is the most common cause. Hypovolemic shock may also result from the loss of plasma into burned or injured tissues. Initial resuscitative efforts are therefore directed toward hypovolemic shock with a rapid intravenous infusion of crystalloid. (*Cameron, 2004, p. 909*)

42. **(D)**

43. **(D)**

Explanations 42 and 43

This patient displays criteria for bipolar disorder, manic with psychotic features. While alcohol can present with psychotic symptoms, it more commonly creates a depressed picture. Benzodiazepine intoxication rarely causes manic or psychotic symptoms. Although cannabis use is not infrequently associated with paranoia, it rarely displays frank psychosis. Opiate intoxication will appear more as a depressed syndrome. Individuals intoxicated with cocaine classically show signs similar to mania. Frank psychotic symptoms can occur in up to 50% of individuals. (*Sadock and Sadock, 2003, p. 433*)

While divalproex sodium (depakote) and lithium are both appropriate treatments for mania, it may take several days to weeks before significant therapeutic effects are achieved. Lamotrigine (lamictal) is efficacious in bipolar *depression* and in the maintenance phase, but it is not particularly effective in treating the manic phase. An antidepressant such as mirtazepine (remeron) may worsen mania in a bipolar patient. Lorazepam (ativan) or other high potency benzodiazepines are useful in the acute management of manic patients as the sedative effects are relatively rapid. (*American Psychiatric Association, 2000*)

44. **(D)** The triad of hypotension, elevated jugular venous pressure, and decreased or absent heart sounds in a patient with history of penetrating chest trauma should immediately raise the suspicion of either pericardial tamponade or tension pneumothorax. The distinction can readily

be made by chest x-ray, which will be normal in a patient with cardiac tamponade.

Cardiac tamponade develops when an injury causes blood to accumulate in the pericardial space between the heart and pericardium. Because the pericardium does not stretch, the heart is compressed and venous blood cannot enter the heart. The decreased diastolic filling results in a life-threatening decreased cardiac output.

Once the diagnosis of cardiac tamponade is established, immediate pericardiocentesis should be performed. Pericardiocentesis is successful in approximately 80% of cases and evacuation of as little of 15 cc may result in a dramatic response. Only if unsuccessful, and if the patient remains in severe hypotension, should an emergency room thoracotomy be performed. While the pericardiocentesis is being performed, the operating room should be prepared for emergent thoracotomy and definitive surgical repair. *(Schwartz et al., 1999, p. 150)*

45. (E)

46. (B)

Explanations 45 and 46

The initial management goals of caustic injuries are airway assessment, stabilization, and fluid resuscitation. The airway should be directly visualized with a fiberoptic nasopharyngoscope and, if edema or airway compromise is found, intubation is required. Induction of emesis re-exposes the upper esophagus to the corrosive agent. Well-intended measures to neutralize the corrosive agent with water, milk, or activated charcoal are contraindicated as they may elicit vomiting or obscure endoscopic visualization. Early endoscopy is essential to evaluate the extent and severity of injury and should be performed within 12–24 hours after injury. Recent controlled trials have shown no proven benefit of steroids.

The risk of developing a stricture is related to the degree of corrosive injury. Superficial mucosal injuries usually heal without complications, whereas deep or circumferential injuries usually result in a delayed stricture.

The risk of malignant degeneration in the strictured segment is 100–1000 times higher than the incidence in the general population. The other listed choices are not related to caustic injuries. *(Cameron, 2004, pp. 47–50)*

47. (D)

48. (D)

Explanations 47 and 48

The chest x-ray provided shows an infiltrate in the lingua of the left upper lobe. This is often confused with a left lower lobe infiltrate, but can be most readily distinguished by looking at the lateral image. On the lateral film, the left lower lobe—located posterior and inferior—is clear, documenting that the infiltrate is not in the lower lobe of the lung. The right lung is clear as well, ruling out bilateral interstitial infiltrates. Pulmonary abscesses, often associated with anaerobic infections, characteristically have air-fluid levels and are often located in dependent, poorly ventilated areas of the lung.

The most common cause of community-acquired pneumonia in adults is *S. pneumoniae*. Typical presentations would include a fairly sudden onset of a fever, productive cough, dyspnea, and pleuritic chest pain. *P. carinii* pneumonia is almost always associated with AIDS or other profound immunocompromised states. It is often seen as a diffuse, "ground-glass" appearing, interstitial infiltrate but may occur in the presence of a relatively normal chest x-ray. A pulmonary embolus can cause the sudden onset of dyspnea, pleuritic chest pain, hypoxia, dyspnea, and cough but is less likely to cause a fever or a typical appearing infiltrate on chest x-ray. While aspiration pneumonia cannot be definitively ruled out based on the presentation, it tends to be more common in lower lung fields and is, overall, much less common than pneumococcal pneumonia.

Approximately 20% of patients with community-acquired pneumonia are hospitalized. One frequently used scoring system for the determination of risk class, and need for hospitalization, comes from the Pneumonia

Patient Outcomes Research Team (PORT). They have created a system of assigning points based on the patient's age, comorbidities, symptoms and signs, from which a risk class can be determined (see Table 8-1). By applying this patient's age, lack of comorbidities, vital signs, and oxygen saturation, this patient falls into a risk class I and would be treated as an outpatient with oral antibiotics and close follow-up. *(Braunwald et al., 2001, pp. 1475–1480)*

TABLE 8-1

Source: Reproduced, with permission, from Kasper DL, Braunwald E, Fauci AS, et al. *Harrison's Principles of Internal Medicine,* 16th ed. New York, NY: McGraw-Hill, 2004, p. 1480.

BIBLIOGRAPHY

Altieri A. Epidemiology and etiology of gestational trophoblastic diseases. *Lancet Oncol* 2003;4(11): 670–678.

American Psychiatric Association. *Diagnostic and Statistical Manual of Mental Disorders*, 4th ed., Text Revision. Washington, DC: American Psychiatric Association, 2000.

Beckmann CRB, Ling FW, Laube DW, et al. *Obstetrics and Gynecology*, 4th ed. Baltimore, MD: Lippincot Williams & Wilkins, 2002.

Braunwald E, Hauser SL, Jameson JL, et al. *Harrison's Principles of Internal Medicine*, 15th ed. New York, NY: McGraw-Hill, 2001.

Brenner BM. *Brenner & Rectors's The Kidney*, 7th ed. Philadelphia, PA: W.B. Saunders, 2004.

Cameron JL, ed. *Current Surgical Therapy*, 8th ed. St. Louis, MO: C.V. Mosby, 2004.

Cassens BJ. NMS *Preventive Medicine and Public Health*, 2nd ed. Baltimore, MD: Lippincott Williams & Wilkins, 1992.

CDC. Prevention of Hepatitis A Through Active or Passive Immunization: Recommendations of the Immunization Practices Advisory Committee (ACIP). MMWR Recommendations and Reports. October 1, 1999;48(RR-12);1–37.

CDC. Hepatitis B Virus: A Comprehensive Strategy for Eliminating Transmission in the United States Through Universal Childhood Vaccination: Recommendations of the Immunization Practices Advisory Committee (ACIP). MMWR Recommendations and Reports. November 22, 1991;40(RR-13);1–19.

Committee on Genetics. Health supervision for children with neurofibromatosis. *Pediatrics* 1995; 96:368–372.

Cotran RS, Kumar V, Collins T. *Robbins Pathologic Basis of Disease*, 6th ed. Philadelphia, PA: W.B. Saunders, 1999.

Cotran RS, Kumar V, Robbins SL. *Robbins Pathologic Basis of Disease*, 5th ed. Philadelphia, PA: W.B. Saunders, 1994.

Davis AJ, Johnson SR. Premenstrual syndrome. *ACOG Pract Bull.* Number 15, April 2000; 95:1-9.

Dickerson LM, Mazyck PJ, Hunter MH. Premenstrual syndrome. *Am Fam Physician* 2003;67:1743–1752.

Downs SM. Technical report: UTIs in febrile infants and young children. The Urinary Tract Subcommittee of the American Academy of Pediatrics Committee on Quality Improvement. *Pediatrics* 1999;103(4):e54.

Giboney PT. Mildly elevated liver transaminases levels in the asymptomatic patient. *Am Fam Physician* 2005;71(6):1105–1110.

Greenfield LJ, Mulholland MW, Oldham KT, et al., eds. *Surgery: Scientific Principles and Practice*, 3rd ed. Philadelphia, PA: Lippincott Williams & Wilkins, 2001.

Jones KL, ed. *Smith's Recognizable Pattern of Human Malformations*, 5th ed. Philadelphia, PA: W.B. Saunders, 1997.

Mandell GL, Bennett JE, Mandell DR. *Mandell, Douglas and Bennett's Principles and Practice of Infectious Diseases*, 5th ed. Philadelphia, PA: Churchill Livingstone, 2000.

National Heart, Lung and Blood Institute of the National Institutes of Health. The Third Report of the National Cholesterol Education Program Expert Panel on the Detection, Evaluation and Treatment of High Blood Cholesterol in Adults (ATP III), 2001.

Rudolph CD, Rudolph AM, Hostetter MK, et al., eds. *Rudolph's Pediatrics*, 21st ed. New York, NY: McGraw-Hill, 2003.

Sadock BJ, Sadock VA. *Kaplan and Sadock's Synopsis of Psychiatry*, 9th ed. Philadelphia, PA: Lippincott Williams & Wilkins, 2003.

Schwartz SI, Shires GT, Spencer FC, et al., eds. *Principles of Surgery*, 7th ed. New York, NY: McGraw-Hill, 1999.

Togashi K. Ovarian cancer: the clinical role of US, CT, and MRI. *Eur Radiol* 2003;13(Suppl 4):L87–L104.

USPSTF: www.preventiveservices.ahrq.gov.

CHAPTER 9

Practice Test 2
Questions

Read each question carefully and in the order in which it is presented. Then select the one best response option of the choices offered. More than one option may be partially correct. You must select ONE BEST answer. You have 60 minutes to complete this test.

Setting I: Office/Health Center

You see patients in two locations: at your office suite, which is adjacent to a hospital, and at a community-based health center. Your office practice is a primary care generalist group. Most of the patients you see are from your own practice and are appearing for regularly scheduled return visits. Occasionally, you will encounter a patient whose primary care is managed by one of your associates. Reference may be made to the patient's medical records. Known patients may be managed by the telephone. You may have to respond to questions about information appearing in the public media, which will require interpretation of the medical literature. The laboratory and radiology departments have a full range of services available.

Questions 1 through 4

A 43-year-old African American female presents to your office for elevated blood pressure (BP). She has been having headaches for the last 3 weeks. She is a pharmacist and she checks her BP at her pharmacy. She presents with readings ranging between 160/104 and 155/95. After some research she did on her own, she has been exercising and following the "DASH (Dietary Approaches to Stop Hypertension)" diet for the past 3 months. Her BP in the office after more

than 10 minutes of resting was 153/89 in her left arm and 145/90 in her right. She tells you that both her mother and father have hypertension. She denies chest pain, shortness of breath, dizziness, or blurred vision. She denies tobacco use, drinks 2–4 beers on weekends, and uses no recreational drugs.

1. At this point you diagnose the patient with which of the following?

   (A) elevated BP without the diagnosis of hypertension
   (B) prehypertension
   (C) stage 1 hypertension
   (D) stage 2 hypertension
   (E) stage 3 hypertension

2. Your physical examination should include documentation of which of these?

   (A) cranial nerve examination
   (B) peripheral nerve examinations
   (C) auscultation for carotid, abdominal, and femoral bruits
   (D) palpation of the abdomen for hepatosplenomegaly
   (E) mental status examination

3. Which of the following tests would be recommended at this visit?

   (A) liver function tests
   (B) urine microalbumin
   (C) hemoglobin A1C
   (D) hematocrit
   (E) exercise stress test

4. Which of the following would be the most appropriate management recommendation at this time?

(A) No intervention at this time, but bring the patient back in 2 weeks for BP check.

(B) No pharmacologic treatment at this time, but advise her to continue lifestyle modifications such as the "DASH" diet plan and increase her physical activity.

(C) Continue lifestyle modifications and add a thiazide diuretic.

(D) Continue lifestyle modifications and add a beta-blocker.

(E) Continue lifestyle modifications and add an angiotensin-converting enzyme (ACE) inhibitor.

5. A 6-year-old is brought in by his mother. The mother noticed a cold sore on his lip 3 days ago. The mother now notices some spots on the upper lid of the left eye. The child seems comfortable but the eye is mildly inflamed with conjunctival hyperemia.

Which of the following is the most appropriate at this time?

(A) prescribe tears for the redness and irritation

(B) fluorescein stain of the cornea

(C) give ointment to prevent bacterial infection

(D) reassure the mother and ask her to check for fever

(E) give Benadryl for itching

6. A 32-year-old man was diagnosed with diabetes 2 years ago. The diagnosis was made at the time of an insurance examination, when he was incidentally found to have a fasting glucose of 150 mg/dL. He had no symptoms at that time. He has no family history of diabetes. At the time of diagnosis, his weight was 175 lbs and he is 5 ft 10 in. tall. He had no end-organ damage from diabetes detectable at the time of diagnosis. He was started on glyburide 5 mg daily, which controlled his glucose initially. One year ago, his average home blood glucose

readings were 120 mg/dL and his glycohemoglobin was 6.5% (normal 4–6%). However, over the past 2 months, he has become symptomatic with polyuria, polydipsia, and a 25-lb weight loss. His glyburide was increased to 10 mg twice daily without any improvement in his glucose readings. His current glycohemoglobin is 11%. Which of the following would be the most appropriate next step in his management?

(A) initiate a strict diet of 1000 cal/day

(B) switch glyburide to glipizide

(C) switch to insulin therapy

(D) add metformin 500 mg bid to his glyburide

(E) add rosiglitazone 8 mg daily to his glyburide

7. A 50-year-old male is evaluated for recurrent episodes of redness and swelling of the base of his great toe. He has also developed a small nodule overlying the joint. An aspiration biopsy of the nodule is performed and the result shown in Figure 9-1. What is the most likely cause of his recurrent symptoms?

FIG. 9-1

(A) rheumatoid arthritis

(B) suppurative arthritis

(C) gout

(D) osteoarthritis

(E) ankylosing spondylitis

Questions 8 and 9

A 21-year-old male is referred to the student health center because of unusual behavior in class for the past month. While discussing the reasons for the evaluation, the patient is noted to be glancing around the room nervously. When asked about this, he inquires whether there are any miniature listening devices present. He further explains that he is being followed by the CIA, which is tapping the phone line in his dormitory room. He claims to be an "inactive operative," but that he has nonetheless been receiving instructions from a transmitter implanted in his skull. These experiences have been occurring for the past 8 weeks. He is greatly distressed by what he considers to be harassment by the government. He is sleeping poorly due to the transmitting device, but his energy and appetite have been unchanged. He has been distracted and unable to study as a result, but he denies any suicidal ideation.

8. Which of the following is his most likely diagnosis?

   (A) brief psychotic disorder
   (B) delusional disorder
   (C) schizoaffective disorder
   (D) schizophrenia
   (E) schizophreniform disorder

9. After a full history and physical examination, medical conditions and substances are ruled out as causes of his symptoms. Treatment is initiated with olanzapine (Zyprexa). Which of the following laboratory values should be regularly monitored?

   (A) complete blood count (CBC)
   (B) kidney function tests
   (C) lipid panel
   (D) liver function tests
   (E) thyroid function tests

10. A 16-year-old female complains of worsening cyclic dysmenorrhea, lower back pain, and central pelvic pain. The pain with menses is no longer controlled with nonsteroidal anti-inflammatory agents. Her mother reports that she is missing 1 or 2 days of school each month due to the discomfort prior to her menstrual

bleeding. Oral contraceptives are prescribed but do not relieve the symptoms significantly.

Which diagnostic test would be most likely to confirm the diagnosis?

   (A) laparoscopy
   (B) computed tomography (CT) of the abdomen and pelvis
   (C) pelvic ultrasound
   (D) hysteroscopy
   (E) colonoscopy

Questions 11 through 14

A 24-year-old female presents to your office for the evaluation of 1 year of intermittent abdominal pain and diarrhea. The pain is most severe in the right lower quadrant, spastic, and often associated with fever. The patient intermittently manifests low-grade fevers, but often has asymptomatic periods as well. The pain does not seem to be related to her menses. The diarrhea is watery, nonbloody, and the patient states that she sometimes sees mucous in her stool. The patient smokes cigarettes but denies drug or alcohol use. Physical examination reveals a thin White female with unremarkable vital signs. She has one shallow oral ulcer that is mildly painful to her. Cardiopulmonary examination is normal. Her abdomen is flat, with normal bowel sounds and focal tenderness to palpation over the right lower quadrant. On rectal examination a perianal scar is noted. On questioning, the patient states that she once had an anal fissure that healed spontaneously.

11. An upper gastrointestinal (GI) series with small bowel follow through is performed. Which of the following would be the most likely finding?

   (A) gastric ulceration
   (B) duodenal ulceration
   (C) small bowel ulceration
   (D) small bowel volvulus
   (E) normal examination

A right upper quadrant ultrasound is obtained as part of the workup and gallstones are seen in the gallbladder, but the gallbladder wall is of normal thickness and there is no pericholecystic fluid.

12. What is the likely cause of the gallstones in this patient?

    (A) hypocholesterolemia
    (B) failure of enterohepatic bile salt circulation
    (C) chronic cholecystitis
    (D) primary sclerosing cholangitis (PSC)
    (E) tobacco use

13. This patient is at increased risk for developing which of the following malignancies?

    (A) esophageal cancer
    (B) gastric cancer
    (C) small bowel cancer
    (D) ovarian cancer
    (E) uterine cancer

14. Which of the following is the most likely diagnosis for this patient?

    (A) Crohn's disease
    (B) chronic pancreatitis
    (C) irritable bowel syndrome
    (D) endometriosis
    (E) ulcerative colitis

Questions 15 and 16

A 20-year-old G_1P_0 female at 20 weeks' gestation is seen for follow-up of an ultrasound (see Figure 9-2).

FIG. 9-2 (Courtesy of Christian A. Chisholm, MD.)

15. In the presence of this fetal anomaly, which of the following statements is true?

    (A) The likelihood of a chromosomal abnormality is increased.
    (B) The likelihood of additional structural abnormalities is increased.
    (C) The maternal serum alpha-fetoprotein (AFP) is likely to be elevated.
    (D) The likelihood that this fetal anomaly will recur in future pregnancies is increased.
    (E) It is likely that there is a family history of this fetal anomaly.

16. Which of the following should you explain in order to prepare the family and the labor and delivery team for her delivery?

    (A) In the presence of this anomaly, cesarean delivery is associated with fewer fetal/neonatal complications than is vaginal birth.
    (B) The surgical repair of this anomaly is typically accomplished within the first few hours after birth.
    (C) The herniated abdominal contents should be reduced into the abdomen immediately after birth to avoid damage.
    (D) Intrauterine repair of this anomaly is associated with improved outcomes when compared to postnatal repair.
    (E) It is anticipated that both solid and hollow abdominal organs will be in an extra-abdominal location at birth.

Questions 17 through 19

A woman brings her 15-year-old son to the office for an evaluation. She became concerned after she heard on the news that a student in the same school died suddenly while he was playing basketball. Her son is a talented and competitive basketball player who is being recruited by several Division 1 colleges.

17. You tell them that the most common cause of sudden death in athletic adolescents is which of the following?

(A) coronary artery abnormalities

(B) Marfan syndrome

(C) mitral valve prolapse

(D) aortic stenosis

(E) hypertrophic cardiomyopathy

18. What is the most appropriate cardiovascular screening method for average risk student athletes?

(A) history and physical examination

(B) history, physical examination, and screening echocardiogram

(C) history, physical examination, and screening electrocardiogram

(D) history, physical examination, and screening exercise stress test

(E) history, physical examination, CBC, and lipid panel

19. While examining this patient you hear a heart murmur. Which one of the following characteristics should prompt a referral to a cardiologist for further evaluation?

(A) any systolic murmur

(B) any diastolic murmur

(C) any murmur that gets softer with Valsalva maneuver

(D) any murmur that gets softer when the patient stands

(E) a late systolic murmur that is preceded by a midsystolic click

Questions 20 through 22

A 10-day-old infant is brought to your clinic for a checkup. The infant was born after an uncomplicated term gestation via an uncomplicated vaginal delivery. The mother's laboratory tests were negative. Both the mother and the baby have type O+ blood. The infant is breast-fed and has normal stool and urinary patterns. The mother noted that the child became jaundiced on day of life (DOL) 4 and that it peaked around DOL 6. She says that the jaundice seems to be slowly getting better. The infant is afebrile and, on initial examination, you note an otherwise healthy infant with moderate jaundice. The mother brings a discharge note from the newborn nursery

that indicates that on DOL 3 the total bilirubin was 8.7 with a conjugated bilirubin of 0.5.

20. What is the most likely diagnosis in this newborn?

(A) biliary atresia

(B) physiologic jaundice

(C) breast milk jaundice

(D) jaundice from isoimmune hemolysis

(E) jaundice from late-onset group B streptococcal sepsis

21. What is the most appropriate next step in management of this infant?

(A) Follow the clinical examination closely.

(B) Admit to the hospital for a sepsis workup and phototherapy.

(C) Draw total and direct serum bilirubin levels.

(D) Interrupt the breast-feeding for 24 hours and supplement with formula during that time.

(E) Draw a hematocrit and Coombs test on the infant.

22. On closer examination, you notice a crop of five clear vesicles with a mildly erythematous base on the infant's left shoulder. The mother denies seeing these in the past. She also denies having a history of herpes or having any symptoms. What should you do next?

(A) Begin the infant on topical mupirocin and oral cephalexin.

(B) Unroof one of the vesicles, send a swab from the base of the lesion for bacterial culture and herpes simplex virus (HSV) polymerase chain reaction (PCR), and treat only if positive.

(C) Follow the clinical examination closely for any changes.

(D) Admit to the hospital for a complete "sepsis workup" and empiric parenteral acyclovir.

(E) Unroof a vesicle, send for bacterial culture and HSV PCR, and begin oral acyclovir and cephalexin.

Questions 23 through 25

A 33-year-old nulligravid female presents to her internist complaining of vaginal and pelvic pain of 8 months' duration. The pain is diffuse, intermittent, 3/10 in severity, noncyclic, and does not radiate. It is exacerbated by bending and lifting and is not related to the timing of her menstrual cycle. She has internal vaginal pain with intercourse. The pain does not seem to be affected by urination or defecation. She has not noted any change in her vaginal discharge and is in a stable monogamous relationship. She has tried numerous over-the-counter medications, including acetaminophen and herbal remedies, without success. She has seen several other physicians for this problem, including a gynecologist, urologist, and gastroenterologist, none of whom "can find anything wrong with me."

23. An additional key element of her history today would include which of the following?

    (A) whether or not she has had a workup for systemic lupus erythematosus (SLE)
    (B) if she has had a history of recent travel outside the country
    (C) screening questions for depression, anxiety, and physical/sexual abuse
    (D) whether or not she has had a pelvic MRI
    (E) if she has a family history of colorectal cancer

24. On physical examination, the patient is afebrile with normal vital signs. Her urinalysis is unremarkable, she had a normal pap smear last month, her gonorrhea/chlamydia screen is negative, and her pregnancy test is negative. Her abdominal examination is normal with the exception of mild tenderness along the lower portion of her right abdomen which is exacerbated by raising her head from the table. Her cervix is normal appearing on speculum examination. On bimanual examination, she is tender along both lateral sidewalls of her vagina, and this tenderness increases with external rotation of her right hip. She had a pelvic ultrasound 1 week ago, which showed a 2-cm right ovarian cyst, normal uterus, and normal left adnexae.

What is your most plausible diagnosis?

    (A) ovarian cancer
    (B) endometriosis
    (C) musculoskeletal pain
    (D) somatization disorder
    (E) irritable bowel syndrome

25. The most appropriate management at this time is which of the following?

    (A) pelvic CT scan
    (B) laparoscopy
    (C) nonsteroidal anti-inflammatory drug (NSAID) and physical therapy
    (D) selective serotonin reuptake inhibitor (SSRI)
    (E) a high fiber diet and a prescription for dicyclomine (Bentyl)

26. A 42-year-old female patient with a history of diabetes develops necrolytic migratory erythema of her lower extremity. She most likely has which of the following?

    (A) gastrinoma
    (B) glucagonoma
    (C) insulinoma
    (D) VIPoma
    (E) somatostatinoma

27. What advice would you give to the parent of a teenager regarding adolescent immunization practices?

    (A) All adolescents should receive the hepatitis A vaccine prior to high school.
    (B) The meningococcal vaccine is recommended for first year college students who will be living in a college dorm.
    (C) All college students are required to be immunized against *Treponema pallidum* (syphilis).
    (D) After the initial series is completed, tetanus immunization is not required until college entry.
    (E) In adolescents, influenza immunization can be administered on alternate years.

Setting II: Emergency Department and Inpatient Facilities

You encounter patients in the emergency department and inpatient facilities, including the hospital, the adjacent nursing home/extended-care facility, and detoxification unit. Most patients in the emergency department are new to you and are seeking urgent care, but occasionally, you arrange to meet there with a known patient who has telephoned you. You have general admitting privileges to the hospital, including to the children's and women's services. On occasion you see patients in the critical care unit. Postoperative patients are usually seen in their rooms unless the recovery room is specified. You may also be called to see patients in the psychiatric unit. There is a short-stay unit where you may see patients undergoing same-day operations or being held for observation. Also available to you are a full range of social services, including rape crisis intervention, family support, and security assistance backed up by local police.

28. Tuboovarian abscess is one of the complications of acute pelvic inflammatory disease (PID), and occurs in up to 15–30% of women hospitalized with PID. The most cost-effective antibiotic regimen for treating inpatient women with tuboovarian abscess is which of the following?

    (A) ampicillin IV plus gentamycin IV plus clindamycin IV
    (B) cefotetan IV plus oral doxycycline
    (C) gentamycin IV
    (D) penicillin IM
    (E) ancef IV

29. A 62-year-old male smoker gradually develops dizziness, facial edema, and venous distention of the neck. An extensive workup including biopsy reveals the presence of a small cell carcinoma of the lung. Which of the following is the most appropriate management?

    (A) loop diuretics
    (B) radiation therapy
    (C) angioplasty
    (D) jugular vein bypass
    (E) thoracotomy with operative resection

Questions 30 and 31

A mother frantically brings in her 5-year-old son. She says that he was playing in the garage when she heard him cough and gag. The mother found him in the garage, his clothes stained with bright green liquid. The mother relates that the child has begun to "act drunk." The child denies drinking anything. You do not smell anything abnormal on his breath. His vital signs are normal. His examination reveals poor coordination with a stumbling gait. His lungs are clear. You suspect that he has had a toxic ingestion.

30. Which of the following is the most likely substance?

    (A) an alcoholic beverage
    (B) organophosphate pesticide
    (C) motor oil
    (D) ethylene glycol (antifreeze)
    (E) gasoline

31. Which of the following is the most appropriate course of action for this child?

    (A) gastric lavage with charcoal
    (B) administration of Fomepizole (4-methylpyrazole) followed by hemodialysis
    (C) administration of atropine in a controlled setting
    (D) careful observation at home until the effects wear off
    (E) serial chest x-rays (CXR)

32. A 42-year-old male, who has been on long-term oral steroid therapy, undergoes a partial small bowel resection for a near-obstructing Crohn's stricture. Which of the following vitamins is known to help counteract the ill effects of steroids on wound healing?

    (A) vitamin A
    (B) vitamin B_{12}
    (C) vitamin C
    (D) vitamin D
    (E) vitamin E

33. A 19-year-old nulliparous patient is being evaluated for a palpable abdominal mass and complaints of pelvic pain and pressure. A CT scan is obtained and suggests the presence of bilateral solid adnexal masses, each approximately 6 cm in diameter. As part of your preoperative assessment, you order appropriate tumor markers to assess the malignant potential of this pelvic mass. In this setting, what tumor markers would you order?

(A) ovarian cancer antigen 125 (CA-125)

(B) carcinoembryonic antigen (CEA), CA-125

(C) CA-19-9

(D) inhibin

(E) AFP, lactic dehydrogenase (LDH), beta-human chorionic gonadotropin (β-hCG)

34. A 45-year-old female, with a history of oral contraceptive use and right upper quadrant abdominal pain, has a 4 cm lesion in the right lobe of the liver seen on ultrasound. A CT scan reveals a hypodense lesion consistent with a hepatic adenoma. Which of the following is the most feared complication of the lesion?

(A) malignant transformation

(B) rupture and bleeding

(C) obstructive cholangitis

(D) anaphylactic shock

(E) peritoneal sepsis

35. A biopsy of a lateral neck mass in a 55-year-old man reveals normal thyroid tissue. Which of the following is the most appropriate management?

(A) suppression therapy with thioamides

(B) local excision of the neck mass

(C) excision of the neck mass and ipsilateral thyroid lobectomy

(D) excision of the neck mass and total thyroidectomy

(E) radioactive iodine ablation therapy

36. A 2-year-old female developed generalized edema and, on urine examination, revealed a heavy proteinuria of 5 g over the 24-hour period. Which of the following would be the diagnosis?

(A) acute diffuse proliferative glomerulonephritis

(B) membranoproliferative glomerulonephritis

(C) membranous glomerulonephritis

(D) minimal-change disease (lipoid nephrosis)

(E) rapidly progressive glomerulonephritis

Questions 37 and 38

A 58-year-old incoherent and agitated man wanders into the emergency room. He has no specific complaints, but he appears confused and mumbles about being homeless for a long time. His vitals are unremarkable except for a pulse of 110. His physical examination is remarkable for poor hygiene, body odor, a diffusely tender abdomen, nystagmus, and an unsteady gait.

37. Intravenous administration of what substance would be the most appropriate next step in the management of this patient?

(A) benzodiazepines

(B) naloxone (Narcan)

(C) thiamine

(D) glucose

(E) insulin

38. He is subsequently admitted to the medicine service for hepatitis. On day 3 of his admission, the nurses are concerned because he has mental status changes. On evaluation, he complains of extreme anxiety. He appears diaphoretic and tremulous. His vital signs demonstrate a temperature of 101.5°F, BP of 167/98, pulse of 120, and respirations of 24. Oral administration of which of the following benzodiazepines would be the most appropriate in the management of this patient?

(A) alprazolam (Xanax)

(B) clonazepam (Klonopin)

(C) diazepam (Valium)

(D) lorazepam (Ativan)

(E) triazolam (Halcion)

39. A 32-year-old female with anorexia nervosa complains of chronic epigastric pain, nausea, and bilious vomiting. Her symptoms are relieved when she assumes a knee to chest position. The etiology of the disorder is most likely which of the following?

(A) compression of the bowel by the inferior mesenteric artery

(B) kinking and obstruction of an afferent loop

(C) obstruction of the third portion of the duodenum

(D) obstruction from a cholangiocarcinoma

(E) obstructing gastric ulcer

Questions 40 through 42

While working in the emergency room, you see a patient with a cough, mild pleuritic chest pain, and a reduced oxygen saturation. Your differential diagnosis includes pulmonary embolus (PE). You order a D-dimer titer as a screening test, with a subsequent result of 6.2 (normal range 0–5.0). Your laboratory reports to you that this test has a sensitivity of 90% and a specificity of 50% for the diagnosis of pulmonary embolism.

40. If the occurrence of pulmonary embolism in persons with these symptoms and signs is 1 in 3, what is the predictive value of a positive test for the diagnosis of pulmonary embolism?

(A) 33%

(B) 47%

(C) 53%

(D) 67%

(E) 91%

41. What would be the predictive value of a negative D-dimer test?

(A) 99%

(B) 91%

(C) 85%

(D) 77%

(E) 67%

42. After a reanalysis of the test is performed, it is decided by the hospital laboratory director to change the reference range for the D-dimer test. Now, a normal D-dimer result will be 0–3.5. The laboratory director states that the new sensitivity will be 95% and the new specificity will be 30%. Based on this change, which of the following statements is true?

(A) The test now has a higher positive predictive value (PPV).

(B) The test now has a higher negative predictive value (NPV).

(C) Both the PPV and NPV are now higher.

(D) The test will now have more false negative results.

(E) The test will now have more true negative results.

43. A 14-month-old develops a fever in the middle of summer. His parents state that he has had mild upper respiratory symptoms. On examination, he is febrile and fussy, but otherwise is well appearing. A CBC reveals an elevated white blood cell count. A urinalysis is normal. A lumbar puncture is performed and the following cerebrospinal fluid (CSF) results are found: WBC 50/HPF (high-power field) (60% lymph, 40% PMN), RBC 3/HPF, protein 75, glucose 88. What is the most likely infectious agent?

(A) group B *Streptococcus* (GBS)

(B) HSV

(C) *Neisseria meningitidis*

(D) nonpolio enterovirus

(E) *Streptococcus pneumoniae*

Questions 44 through 48

A 48-year-old African American woman, with a history of hypertension, cocaine abuse, and medical noncompliance, arrives at the emergency room complaining of progressive dyspnea on exertion, fatigue, nausea, vomiting, and generalized malaise. She also has had generalized pruritis for the past 4 weeks. She was last seen by her primary care physician approximately 2-1/2 years ago but never followed-up. On questioning, she has not been taking her antihypertensive medication for the last 1 year because she "ran out of them." On physical examination, she has a BP of 185/98, with a heart rate of 85 bpm. She is somnolent but oriented and follows commands. Her examination is significant for pale conjunctiva and nail beds. The cardiac examination shows a regular heart rate and rhythm with a S$_4$ gallop. Her lungs have few bibasilar crackles and the abdominal examination is unremarkable. There is no audible abdominal bruit. Her extremities are significant for 1+ bilateral ankle edema and the neurologic examination was unremarkable. Rectal examination was negative for occult blood.

The laboratory values are:

Blood, serum value	
Sodium 138	Urinalysis:
Potassium 5.8	Specific gravity: 1.010
Chloride 107	Proteinuria: trace
CO$_2$ 15	Leukocytes (per HPF): 0–2
Blood urea nitrogen (BUN) 75	RBCs (per HPF): 1–3
Creatinine 8.4	Casts: 3–5 hyaline casts
Glucose 80	
Phosphate 9.5	Urine electrolytes
Calcium 7.7	Na$^+$: 80
LDH 235	K$^+$: 30
Total bilirubin 0.2	Cl$^-$: 50
WBC 10.5	
Hemoglobin 7.7	Toxicology: positive for cocaine
Hematocrit 22.3	
Platelets 194	

An ECG shows sinus rhythm at a rate of 75 with left ventricular hypertrophy (LVH). The CXR shows clear lung fields with an enlarged cardiac silhouette.

A kidney ultrasound shows bilateral 7.5 cm kidneys (normal >11–12 cm) with increased echogenicity.

44. Which statement regarding the etiology of this patient's kidney failure is correct?

   (A) This patient has chronic kidney disease most likely from renal artery stenosis.

   (B) She has chronic kidney disease most likely secondary to hypertensive nephrosclerosis.

   (C) Her ultrasound findings are suggestive of HIV-associated nephropathy.

   (D) This patient has acute renal failure resulting from hypertensive emergency due to cocaine.

   (E) She has chronic kidney disease most likely from chronic glomerulonephritis.

45. What diagnostic test would it be necessary to perform next?

   (A) cardiac catheterization to evaluate patient for coronary artery disease

   (B) a renal artery angiogram to evaluate for renal artery stenosis

   (C) a kidney biopsy

   (D) HIV serology to evaluate for HIV-associated nephropathy

   (E) no further diagnostic testing is indicated

46. Which statement best describes the mechanism explaining this patient's anemia?

   (A) development of polyclonal antibodies against erythropoietin

   (B) diminished production of erythropoietin by bone marrow

   (C) decreased production of erythropoietin by kidney cells

   (D) increased erythropoietin production by red blood cells

   (E) decreased production of bone marrow erythropoietin receptors due to uremic toxins

47. Which of the following would be the next best step?

   (A) placement of an arteriovenous (AV) fistula and initiation of hemodialysis
   (B) intravenous infusion of sodium bicarbonate and furosemide
   (C) placement of a temporary hemodialysis catheter and initiate hemodialysis immediately
   (D) intravenous infusion of calcium gluconate, insulin, and dextrose to treat hyperkalemia
   (E) placement of an AV graft and initiate hemodialysis as soon as possible

48. Which of the following is an indication for emergent hemodialysis?

   (A) BUN of 110 and creatinine of 10.0
   (B) urine output of <5 cc/h for the past 24 hours
   (C) pericardial friction rub on physical examination
   (D) ingestion of toxic levels of acetaminophen
   (E) asymptomatic, but profound, hyponatremia (Na <115)

Answers and Explanations

1. **(C)**

2. **(C)**

3. **(D)**

4. **(C)**

Explanations 1 through 4

The seventh report of the Joint National Committee on the prevention, detection, evaluation, and treatment of high blood pressure (JNC 7) key recommendations classify this patient in hypertension stage 1, as most of her BP readings are systolic blood pressure (SBP) in the 140–159 range and diastolic blood pressure (DBP) between 90 and 99.

Category	SBP and/or DBP
Normal	<120 and <80
Prehypertension	120–139 or 80–90
Hypertension stage 1	140–159 or 90–99
Hypertension stage 2	≥160 or ≥100

The primary purpose of the initial physical examination is to look for causes of secondary hypertension and for early organ damage due to untreated hypertension. In your physical examination for a newly diagnosed patient with hypertension, you should include BP measurement in both arms, examination of the optic fundi, BMI calculation, auscultation for carotid, abdominal and femoral bruits, palpation of the thyroid gland, examination of the heart and lungs, and examination of the abdomen for enlarged kidneys, masses, and abnormal aortic pulsation. Cranial/peripheral nerve examination, mental status examination, and palpation of the abdomen for hepatosplenomegaly are not an essential part of this physical examination.

Initial laboratory tests should include urinalysis (not urine microalbumin), blood glucose (not hemoglobin A1C), hematocrit, lipid panel and serum potassium, creatinine and calcium, which is part of a basic metabolic panel (not liver function tests). There is no indication for exercise stress testing at this time.

The JNC 7 recommends that the most appropriate initial management for this patient is lifestyle modification and a thiazide-type diuretic. Lifestyle modification includes weight reduction (goal BMI 18.5–24.9), adopting the DASH diet plan, dietary sodium reduction, regular aerobic physical activity such as brisk walking at least 30 min/day most days of the week, and no more than two alcoholic drinks per day in most men and no more than one alcoholic drink per day in women.

Beta-blockers should be the initial pharmacologic agents in postmyocardial infarction patients. ACE inhibitors should be the initial pharmacologic agents in patients with chronic kidney diseases. (*National Heart, Lung and Blood Institute, 2003*)

5. **(B)** The presence of a red eye in a patient with signs of a herpes viral infection (cold sore) raises the possibility of herpetic infection of the eye. This can be in the form of eyelid involvement only, conjunctivitis, or corneal disease, with corneal disease being the most serious and potentially vision threatening. The most appropriate and important intervention at this time would be flourescein staining of the cornea with a slit-lamp examination to look for the presence of corneal epithelial ulcers, particularly dendritic ulcers characteristic of HSV, or abnormalities of the deeper corneal stroma. Most cases of herpes simplex can be diagnosed clinically, but corneal scrapings or viral cultures may be taken. Patients with corneal herpes infections require antiviral therapy—either topical or systemic—and

frequent ophthalmologic follow-up. *(Kunimoto et al., 2004, Sect. 4.14)*

6. **(C)** The patient appears to be insulin deficient with uncontrolled hyperglycemia and weight loss. He now weighs 150 lbs, which is about 15 lbs below his ideal body weight. Type 1 diabetes can occur at any age. Although there is a genetic component to type 1 diabetes, it is less consistent than type 2 diabetes, so his negative family history tends to favor this entity. Each of the oral medications, even if effective, would only reduce glycohemoglobin by 1–2%. Therefore, there is no single agent that will correct his glucose level into a target range. As he is underweight and losing weight, it is unlikely that insulin resistance is playing a major role. Thus, rosiglitazone or metformin would not be advisable. Glyburide and glipizide are similar sulfonylureas, so there is no advantage of switching from one to another. Only insulin will immediately correct the hyperglycemia and the weight loss. *(Larsen et al., 2003, pp. 1460–1466)*

7. **(C)** The pathognomonic lesion of gout is the tophus, a collection of crystalline or amorphous urates surrounded by an inflammatory response consisting of macrophages, lymphocytes, fibroblasts, and foreign body giant cells. In the photomicrograph that accompanies the question, the darker stellate deposits denote the center of the tophus. These urate deposits would appear golden brown, in contrast to the pink-staining tissue about them on hematoxylin-eosin staining. Gout is a systemic disorder of uric acid metabolism resulting in hyperuricemia. Urates precipitate out of the supersaturated blood and deposit in the joints and soft tissue. Rheumatoid arthritis and ankylosing spondylitis are characterized by a diffuse proliferative synovitis; suppurative arthritis, by a prominent neutrophilic inflammation; and osteoarthritis, by cartilaginous and subchondral bone changes. *(Cotran et al., 1994, pp. 1253–1257)*

8. **(E)**

9. **(C)**

Explanations 8 and 9

This individual is experiencing a psychotic illness, manifested by paranoia, delusions, and hallucinations, lasting for several months. Brief psychotic disorder is characterized by psychotic symptoms similar to those above but only lasting for 1 day up to 1 month, with a subsequent return to premorbid functioning. Delusional disorder typically affects patients in midlife and involves the presence of a nonbizarre delusion without prominent hallucinations or significant impairment in functioning, as seen in the above case. A diagnosis of schizoaffective disorder requires both 1 month of psychotic symptoms and an additional mood disorder; this patient does not display evidence of a significant affective component. The diagnosis of schizophrenia similarly necessitates at least 1 month of active psychosis, but some indication of the disorder must be present for at least 6 months. While this patient may actually have and be eventually diagnosed with schizophrenia, his above presentation is consistent with schizophreniform disorder, the criteria of which require prominent psychotic symptoms to be present for at least 1 month but less than 6 months. *(American Psychiatric Association, 2000)*

The introduction of second-generation, so-called atypical, antipsychotics have markedly improved the armamentarium in the treatment of psychotic disorders such as schizophrenia. They are at least as effective as older medications in decreasing the positive symptoms, such as delusions, hallucinations, or disorganized speech/behavior. Their advantage over neuroleptics such as haloperidol comes with the presumed superior management of negative symptoms, including apathy, anhedonia, and poor attention. As a class, second-generation antipsychotics do have disadvantages. They can cause a significant amount of weight gain as well as metabolic effects, such as elevated blood sugar (including new-onset diabetes) and lipid indices. Therefore, regular monitoring of weight (such as BMI), fasting glucose, and lipids are recommended. Frequent monitoring of the CBC is only recommended for clozapine given the risk of agranulocytosis. Kidney function should be monitored for all patients treated with lithium. Anticonvulsants such as valproic acid and carbamazepine may cause hepatotoxicity, so liver function tests such as alanine aminotransferase (ALT) and aspartate aminotransferase (AST) should be routinely checked. *(Sadock and Sadock, 2003, p. 498)*

10. **(A)** Direct visualization of the pelvic organs during laparoscopy is required to definitively diagnose endometriosis. In some cases, biopsy of one or more of the lesions for pathologic confirmation may also be useful. Cystic collections of endometriosis in the ovaries, termed endometriomas, can often be visualized by CT, MRI, or ultrasonography. However, intraoperative confirmation is still required to exclude other common causes of cystic ovarian masses. *(Stenchever et al., 2001, p. 532)*

11. **(C)**

12. **(B)**

13. **(C)**

14. **(A)**

Explanations 11 through 14

The history and physical examination are all highly suspicious for Crohn's disease, an inflammatory bowel disorder that can affect the entire gut from the mouth to the anus. Gastric and duodenal ulcers would likely present with bleeding and not diarrhea. A small bowel volvulus would be more acute and would have signs of an obstruction. A normal examination would be unlikely.

Patients with Crohn's disease often have ileal inflammation, which leads to the loss of bile acid receptors in the terminal ileum. This results in net bile salt loss with a decreased overall bile acid pool and, thus, bile in the biliary tree that is more lithogenic. Hypercholesterolemia, not hypocholesterolemia, is associated with gallstones. PSC is associated with ulcerative colitis, not Crohn's disease. The ultrasound findings are not compatible with chronic cholecystitis, as the gallbladder

wall is normal and there is not pericholecystic fluid. Tobacco use is not associated with gallstones.

Patients with Crohn's disease are at increased risk of developing cancer in areas of chronic inflammation. In this patient, as she has primarily small bowel disease, she is at risk for small bowel adenocarcinoma. Adenocarcinoma of the ileum, where this patient likely has the most inflammation, can be seen 100 times more frequently in Crohn's patients than in age and sex matched controls. The other malignancies listed are not strongly associated with Crohn's disease, although patients with Crohn's disease are also at increased risk for squamous cell cancers of the anus and vulva, as well as certain hematologic malignancies such as lymphomas. Patients with Crohn's colitis are at increased risk for colorectal cancer.

The history and physical are most consistent with Crohn's disease. The patient is young, a smoker, and has right lower quadrant pain associated with diarrhea. The presence of oral ulcers and a history of an anal fissure are all strongly associated with Crohn's disease. Irritable bowel syndrome is not associated with fevers, but can produce diarrhea and abdominal pain. Ulcerative colitis would likely produce bloody diarrhea. Endometriosis would be expected to flare during menses. Chronic pancreatitis could present with diarrhea but would be very unusual in a young female who does not consume alcohol. *(Braunwald et al., 2001, pp. 1683–1692)*

15. **(C)**

16. **(B)**

Explanations 15 and 16

Gastroschisis is one of the two common fetal ventral wall defects, omphalocele being the other. Any open fetal defect, including open neural tube defects, increases the amniotic fluid AFP, and thus the maternal serum AFP by transudation across the fetal membranes. Both gastroschisis and omphalocele are 10-fold less common than open neural tube defects, with an incidence of approximately 1–2/10,000 births. While omphalocele is associated with a significant risk of chromosomal aneuploidy (trisomy 13 and 18 occur in 33–50%) and associated structural malformations in up to 70%, these associations are not seen in gastroschisis. Gastroschisis is thought to occur secondary to a fetal vascular accident in early gestation, resulting in full-thickness necrosis of the abdominal wall and extrusion of fetal bowel through the defect. The risk of recurrence is not increased in future pregnancies, and there is not thought to be a hereditary component.

When gastroschisis is present, delivery should occur at a tertiary care center with a neonatal intensive care unit and pediatric surgery capabilities. Intrauterine repair has not been reported and is not likely to be attempted. The maternal risk involved in such a procedure would be excessive in light of the typically good outcomes of neonatal care. The only special care required in the delivery room is to gently wrap the bowel in saline-moistened sterile gauze to avoid dessication, and to avoid excessive manipulation of the bowel, which could result in volvulus. The abdominal defect in gastroschisis is small and to the right of the umbilical cord insertion, thus only allows herniation of intestine. If liver is in an extracorporeal location, the entity is more likely a ruptured omphalocele. (*Cunningham et al., 2001, p. 1127*)

17. (E)

18. (A)

19. (B)

Explanations 17 through 19

Sudden cardiac death is defined as a nontraumatic, nonviolent, and unexpected event resulting from sudden cardiac arrest within 6 hours of a previously witnessed state of normal health. It occurs in about 1 per 200,000 high school athletes per academic year. The most common cause of sudden death in athletic adolescents is hypertrophic cardiomyopathy (36%), followed by coronary artery abnormalities

(19%). Marfan syndrome, aortic stenosis, and mitral valve prolapse are rare causes of sudden death in athletic adolescents.

Detection of cardiovascular abnormalities that may cause sudden death is difficult, as congenital cardiac abnormalities relevant to athletic screening account for a combined prevalence of only about 0.2% in athletic populations. Currently, there is no cost-effective battery of tests to identify all, or even most, dangerous cardiovascular conditions. A complete and careful personal and family history and physical examination are recommended to identify, or raise suspicion of, cardiovascular lesions known to cause sudden cardiac death or disease progression in young athletes.

During the physical examination, auscultation of the heart should be performed with the patient in standing and supine positions. The following murmurs should be referred to a cardiologist for further evaluation: any systolic murmur grade 3/6 or higher, any diastolic murmur, and any murmur that gets louder with Valsalva maneuver. Murmurs that get softer when a patient stands include tricuspid stenosis (most commonly rheumatic in origin), and atrial or ventricular septal defects. A late systolic murmur that is preceded by a midsystolic click is characteristic of mitral valve prolapse. (*Lyznicki et al., 2000, pp. 765–784*)

20. (B)

21. (A)

22. (D)

Explanations 20 through 22

Approximately one-third of newborn infants will have some degree of recognizable jaundice. This is termed physiologic jaundice. This physiologic jaundice is usually present after the first 2 days of life and will usually peak by day 5. This jaundice usually lasts no longer than 10–14 days and has no conjugated portion. Breast milk jaundice is seen when the jaundice in a newborn is prolonged, typically longer than 2 weeks. GBS infection is a cause of jaundice in the newborn infant, but it is very rare compared to physiologic jaundice. Biliary atresia causes a cholestatic (or conjugated) jaundice. Isoimmune hemolysis is a cause of a rapid increase in the bilirubin level and is usually seen in the first 1–3 days of life. Jaundice from hemolysis is much less common than physiologic jaundice.

Physiologic jaundice is usually a benign, self-limited condition. It usually does not require therapy once it begins to resolve. Breast milk jaundice may improve with interruption of breast-feeding, but that is not recommended by the American Academy of Pediatrics. If this infant's bilirubin level were increasing, it could be anticipated that hemolysis were present. If that were the case, the amount of hemolysis can be judged by a hematocrit and reticulocyte count. *(Rudolph et al., 2003, pp. 164–169)*

What is described in the vignette is cutaneous herpes simplex infection (HSV). A negative maternal history for HSV is seen in approximately 50% of infants with perinatally acquired HSV disease. The absence of a maternal history of HSV should not dissuade one from entertaining the diagnosis. Neonatal HSV occurs in one of three common presentations: skin-eye-mucous membrane (SEM), disseminated, and central nervous system (CNS) disease. What is described is the SEM manifestation. Approximately one-third of infants with SEM HSV will develop CNS or disseminated disease. All infants with SEM HSV in the newborn period should be treated aggressively with a full evaluation and parenteral acyclovir. Oral acyclovir has no role in the management of perinatal HSV disease. SEM manifestation of HSV needs to be distinguished from a simple impetigo, which may present with cloudy blisters, most commonly in the diaper region. This entity could potentially be treated with topical or oral antimicrobials. If HSV cannot be adequately ruled out, aggressive intervention is warranted. *(American Academy of Pediatrics, 2003, pp. 344–353)*

23. **(C)**

24. **(C)**

25. **(C)**

Explanations 23 through 25

Physical and sexual abuses are associated with various chronic pain disorders. Studies have found that up to 50% of women with chronic pelvic pain have a history of past or current abuse. *(Jamieson and Steege, 1997, pp. 1408–1412)*

Primary or secondary myofascial pelvic pain is an underrecognized and undertreated aspect of pelvic pain. Common findings include exacerbation of symptoms with movement, lifting, and/or vaginal penetration, along with localization to the abdominal wall and/or vaginal sidewalls. NSAIDs and physical therapy can be helpful for these patients. *(King et al., 1991, pp. 87–98; Weiss, 2001, pp. 2226–2231)*

26. **(B)** Glucagonoma is a tumor that arises from α_2 cells in the islets of Langerhans of the pancreas. They produce a distinctive syndrome consisting of migratory necrolytic dermatitis of the legs and perineum, weight loss, stomatitis, hypoaminoacidemia, anemia, and diabetes mellitus. Patients also have a risk of venous thrombosis and pulmonary emboli. The diagnosis is confirmed by demonstrating elevated plasma glucagon levels. Workup should include an abdominal CT scan and, if necessary, arteriography to localize the lesion. The majority of glucagonomas are malignant and have metastasized by the time of diagnosis. The most common sites of metastases include the liver, lymph nodes, adrenal gland, and vertebrae. Treatment includes surgical excision of the primary tumor and debulking of metastases. Oral zinc supplement may improve the dermatitis. Somatostatin has been reported to return serum glucagon and amino acid levels to normal, clear the rash, and promote weight gain. Streptozotocin and dacarbazine are the most effective chemotherapeutic agents. *(Schwartz et al., 1999, p. 1496)*

27. **(B)** With the advancing of immunizations, more and more opportunities for disease prevention in adolescents arise. Hepatitis A vaccine is recommended to all children between 12 and 23 months of age. There are no specific recommendations with regard to hepatitis A vaccine

and adolescents. Meningococcal vaccine (MCV4) is to be administered to all 11- to 12-year-old children and, if unimmunized, to any student entering high school. While the MCV4 may be appropriate for all college students, specific recommendations currently apply only to those students living in college dorms. A tetanus booster is recommended for all children at their 11- to 12-year visit who have completed their primary series. Influenza vaccination should be given each year in all adolescents. There is currently no vaccine available against syphilis. *(Pediatrics 117; No. 1, January 2006, pp. 239–240)*

28. **(A)** A tuboovarian abscess is more likely to respond to triple antibiotic therapy. Lack of response within 48 hours usually requires surgical intervention. *(McNeely et al., 1998, pp. 1272–1278)*

29. **(B)** Superior vena cava (SVC) obstruction is caused by a bronchogenic carcinoma in over 85% of cases. The majority of these carcinomas are small cell tumors. Obstruction is caused by compression or direct invasion and results in impairment of the venous return from the head, neck, and upper extremities. Patients present with venous distention, facial edema, and plethora. Less common symptoms include headache, respiratory symptoms, and life-threatening laryngeal edema with airway compression.

The presence of SVC obstruction in a patient with a bronchogenic carcinoma portends a grave prognosis, with survival measured in weeks to months. Radical surgical resection in these patients is contraindicated and treatment is aimed at palliation. Palliative radiation, with or without chemotherapy, has proven effective to help downsize the tumor and ameliorate many of the accompanying symptoms. It is therefore the preferred treatment modality. *(Schwartz et al., 1999, p. 784)*

30. **(D)**

31. **(B)**

Explanations 30 and 31

This child likely has ethylene glycol ingestion. The absence of a smell along with the bright green color is indicative of ethylene glycol. The most common use of ethylene glycol is in antifreeze for automobiles. The sweet taste associated with ethylene glycol makes it a common target for curious children. The initial clinical findings are neurobehavioral and have the appearance of being "drunk." Serum ethylene glycol levels are an important diagnostic and therapeutic adjunct. Ethylene glycol metabolism produces a number of toxic organic acid metabolites and can result is death (from cardiac dysfunction) or long-term morbidity (from renal insult). Fomepizole is an inhibitor of alcohol dehydrogenase and limits the accumulation of toxic metabolites. Hemodialysis has also been shown to limit the long-term sequellae. *(Brent, 2001, pp. 979–988)*

32. **(A)** Vitamin A plays an important role in wound healing. It is involved in the stimulation of fibroblasts, collagen cross-linking, and epithelialization. In addition, it has been shown to help reverse many of the inhibitory effects of glucocorticoids on the inflammatory phase of wound healing. Vitamin A may be indicated in steroid-dependent patients undergoing extensive surgery or for those with problematic wounds. *(Greenfield et al., 2001, p. 78)*

33. **(E)** Epithelial ovarian tumors arise from the surface epithelium of the ovary and comprise approximately 75–80% of all ovarian neoplasms; the mean age of onset is 60 years of age. Germ cell neoplasms arise from the germ cell, or eggs of the ovary, and comprise 10–15% of ovarian tumors; the mean age of onset is 19 years of age. Sex cord stromal neoplasms arise from the connective tissue of the ovary and comprise approximately 5% of ovarian neoplasms. Their occurrence is rather evenly spread over the childhood and adult years, with a minimal propensity toward bilateralism.

Ovarian tumors are capable of producing peptides that can be detected in the peripheral circulation and, if present, that can suggest the presence of these tumors preoperatively.

For example, CA-125 will be elevated in the presence of epithelial ovarian cancers in approximately 80% of all cases. Unfortunately, elevations in CA-125 are found most commonly in association with advanced stage, incurable disease. CA-125 will be elevated in less than 50% of curable stage 1 disease. The usefulness of CA-125 as a screening tumor marker for epithelial ovarian cancer is also limited by the fact that CA-125 can be elevated in association with a number of benign gynecologic conditions including endometrioisis, PID, menstruation, adenomyosis, leiomyomata, and pregnancy.

Germ cell neoplasms comprise the second largest category of ovarian neoplasm. Characteristic germ cell neoplasms include dysgerminoma, immature teratoma, endodermal sinus tumor, embryonal tumor, gonadoblastoma, and mixed germ cell neoplasms. Dysgerminomas comprise 50% of all germ cell neoplasms and have a propensity toward bilateralism. Dysgerminomas are associated with elevated levels of LDH, endodermal sinus tumors with elevated levels of AFP, and embryonal tumors with elevated levels of AFP and β-hCG. Immature teratomas can be associated with elevated levels of LDH and AFP.

CEA is a nonspecific tumor antigen that can be elevated in the setting of GI tumors, breast cancer, and mucinous ovarian neoplasms. Inhibin is a tumor marker that can be elevated in association with granulosa cell tumors, a specific type of ovarian sex cord stromal neoplasm.

Given the age of the patient in this case, the most likely category of ovarian tumor present would be a germ cell tumor. Thus, the appropriate panel of tumor markers to order would be AFP, LDH, and β-hCG. (*Schwartz, 1991, pp. 423–432*)

34. **(B)** Hepatic adenoma is a benign tumor of the liver that is strongly associated with oral contraceptive use. Ninety percent of patients with hepatic adenomas have a history of oral contraceptive use. The diagnosis is typically made in women of childbearing age who present with right upper quadrant pain or mass effect. Liver function tests are usually normal. The hepatic lesion is identified on ultrasound, CT, and MRI. Characteristic findings include a hypodense lesion on CT scan and early enhancement on MRI with contrast. Percutaneous biopsy is contraindicated because it is associated with a high risk of bleeding.

Hepatic adenomas are associated with up to a 30% risk of spontaneous rupture with life-threatening massive hemorrhage. Although much less common, malignant transformation has also been described.

Although regression and disappearance of hepatic adenomas have been reported after the discontinuation of contraceptives, the potential for bleeding and malignant transformation warrants routine surgical resection. They often can be removed by enucleation with a narrow rim of normal hepatic parenchyma. (*Cameron, 2004, p. 318*)

35. **(D)** The finding of normal thyroid tissue in the lateral side of the neck, previously known as lateral aberrant thyroid, is, in fact, a metastasis from an occult papillary type thyroid carcinoma. Therefore, definitive treatment mandates total thyroidectomy with excision of the metastatic neck lesion. Medical therapy and radioactive iodine ablation are treatment modalities for benign disease, such as a toxic goiter. (*Charles et al., 1995*)

36. **(D)** In minimal-change disease (lipoid nephrosis), the classic clinical findings secondary to glomerular injury are massive proteinuria, hypoalbuminemia, peripheral edema, and hyperlipidemia. Lipoid nephrosis is of unknown etiology and pathogenesis. Epidemiologically it is seen in children, usually between the ages of 1 and 4. The clinical picture gives the pure nephrotic syndrome, which is selective proteinuria in over 90% of the cases (only albumin is lost in the urine). The BP generally remains normal and the urine sediment is free of RBCs or WBCs. Of the other selections listed, membranous glomerulonephritis occurs in adults, while rapidly progressive glomerulonephritis and acute diffuse proliferative glomerulonephritis have different symptomatology and clinical presentation. (*Cotran et al., 1999, pp. 954–956*)

37. (C)

38. (D)

Explanations 37 and 38

This case is demonstrative of Wernicke's encephalopathy, caused by acute thiamine deficiency. Intravenous benzodiazepines would be an appropriate treatment for delirium caused by either alcohol or benzodiazepine withdrawal, which might present with confusion and agitation. However, the patient would likely display an elevated BP, as well as flushing, diaphoresis, and tremor. Intravenous naloxone is the treatment of choice for acute opiate overdose. This would more likely present with a diminished level of consciousness, a decreased pulse, BP, and respirations, as well as constricted and unresponsive pupils. Intravenous insulin would be essential for treating diabetic ketoacidosis. The classic triad of Wernicke's encephalopathy includes confusion, oculomotor disturbances, and ataxia. The treatment of choice is parenteral thiamine given prior to glucose, as administering glucose prior to thiamine can cause a worsening of symptoms or even permanent damage. *(Sadock and Sadock, 2003, p. 908)*

This presentation is consistent with acute alcohol withdrawal. While the primary treatment for alcohol withdrawal is benzodiazepines, alprazolam is a shorter-acting but high potency drug, which would require more frequent dosing and may potentially build up in the patient's system given his hepatic disease. Clonazepam is longer acting but also higher potency, and could cause over-sedation given its active metabolites. Diazepam can be an appropriate treatment for alcohol withdrawal; however caution should be used in patients with questionable hepatic function given the long half-life of the medication and its metabolite. It is also poorly absorbed when given intramuscularly. Triazolam is a very short-acting benzodiazepine, used only for insomnia, and as such can cause rebound anxiety in individuals. Lorazepam has the advantage of having an intermediate half-life and not being dependent on liver function for its breakdown. It is also well absorbed when

given orally and parenterally. *(Sadock and Sadock, 2003, pp. 908, 404–405)*

39. (C) The superior mesenteric artery arises directly from the aorta and crosses in front of the third portion of the duodenum to enter the root of the mesentery. Superior mesenteric artery compression syndrome occurs when the acute angle between the aorta and superior mesenteric artery results in compression of the third portion of the duodenum. This syndrome usually occurs in young, thin women who have a loss of the retroperitoneal fat cushion. The syndrome is also known as "cast syndrome" because of its association with patients in body casts. Symptoms include bilious vomiting and postprandial pain. Medical treatment consists of eliminating all contributing factors (such as casts), lying in the supine position, and increasing weight. Surgery is reserved for those who fail conservative measures. Surgical interventions include releasing the ligament of Treitz, which moves the duodenum out from beneath the superior mesenteric artery, or bypassing the obstruction. *(Schwartz et al., 1999, p. 1560)*

40. (B)

41. (B)

42. (B)

Explanations 40 through 42

In order to determine the answers to questions 40 and 41, we must first take the information provided and place it into 2×2 table form. With the given prevalence of the disease being 1 in 3, we will assume a population of 300 people, as this makes the mathematical calculations as easy as possible—100 people will have a PE and 200 will be free of this disease.

With the sensitivity of the test being 90%, then the number of true positive test results is calculated as: $0.9 \times 100 = 90$. The number of false negative test results would then be: $100 - 90 = 10$.

With the specificity of the test being 50%, then the number of true negative test results is calculated as: $0.5 \times 200 = 100$. The number of false positive test results would then be: 200 – 100 = 100.

A 2 × 2 table with this information would appear as follows:

Disease: pulmonary embolism

		+	−
D-dimer	+	True positives 90	False positives 100
	−	False negatives 10	True negatives 100

The calculation of predictive values is then:

$$PPV = true\ positives/(true\ positive + false\ positive)$$

$$PPV = 90/(90 + 100) = 0.47 = 47\%$$

$$NPV = true\ negatives/(true\ negative + false\ negative)$$

$$NPV = 100/(100 + 10) = 0.91 = 91\%$$

The answer to question 42 requires the understanding of the concepts of sensitivity and specificity as characteristics of a test. By lowering the threshold for a test to be abnormal, in this case lowering the upper limit of the normal D-dimer range from 5.0 to 3.5, one can reasonably expect to have more test results that are abnormal (i.e., all of the test results from 3.6 to 4.9 that used to be considered normal will now be considered abnormal). Some of these results will be true positives and some of them will be false positives. The net effect of this will be to increase the sensitivity of the test and to lower its specificity. However, the prevalence of the disease in the population will remain the same, because changing a test characteristic does not change the occurrence of the disease. Putting the new numbers into a 2 × 2 table results in:

Disease: pulmonary embolism

		+	−
D-dimer	+	True positives 95	False positives 140
	−	False negatives 5	True negatives 60

The PPV now equals $95/(95 + 140) = 0.40 = 40\%$

The NPV now equals $60/(60 + 5) = 0.92 = 92\%$

Conceptually, this can be remembered by using the following mnemonics: SpPIn and SnNOut. In the first, when a test is highly **Sp**ecific, a **P**ositive test helps to rule **In** a disease (SpPIn). In the second, when a test is highly **Sen**sitive, a **N**egative helps to rule **Out** a disease. (*Slawson and Shaughnessy, 2003*)

43. **(D)** The "summer flu" is commonly a nonpolio enterovirus infection. In children this may manifest itself in a range from simply fever to shock and encephalitis. Most infant and children with enteroviral infection have fever, fussiness, and a nominal amount of upper respiratory infection (URI) symptoms. The CSF findings described are most consistent with aseptic meningitis. The lymphocytic predominant CSF pleocytosis, with a normal glucose and protein level, would speak against this being bacterial meningitis. The CSF findings may also be consistent with HSV meningoencephalitis, but the child would not typically be well appearing clinically. Enterovirus infections usually warrant supportive care only. (*American Academy of Pediatrics, 2003, pp. 269–270*)

44. **(B)**

45. **(E)**

46. **(C)**

47. **(C)**

48. **(C)**

Explanations 44 through 48

This patient most likely has hypertensive nephrosclerosis. Furthermore, the findings in her history suggest that she has chronic kidney disease. The presence of LVH and an S_4 gallop suggest long-standing hypertension with end-organ damage. Small, echogenic kidneys are consistent with a chronic process; therefore, this is unlikely to be a presentation of acute renal failure. HIV-associated nephropathy is usually associated with large kidneys on ultrasound. There is no evidence, by urinalysis, of glomerulonephritis.

At this time, there is no indication for any invasive evaluation of coronary artery disease. Moreover, there is nothing on physical examination (such as abdominal bruit) to suggest renal artery stenosis. Given the small, echogenic kidneys, any intervention at this point would not likely make a difference in her kidney function. HIV-associated nephropathy usually is associated with significant proteinuria and large kidneys on ultrasound—neither of which is presented in this case. Lastly, a kidney biopsy would not likely yield any information that could improve the renal outcome in this case. Moreover, biopsy of small, scarred kidneys is not recommended, as this poses a significant risk of bleeding.

Erythropoietin is a glycoprotein that is synthesized in kidney cells adjacent to the proximal tubule. Erythropoietin then stimulates erythropoiesis in the bone marrow. In chronic kidney disease, the synthesis of erythropoietin is diminished, resulting in anemia. This anemia can be treated by administering recombinant human erythropoietin.

This patient requires urgent hemodialysis as she is presenting with uremic symptoms, that is, nausea, vomiting, and malaise. An AV fistula is the best form of permanent hemodialysis access (owing to its less frequent rate of infections), followed by AV graft. However, an AV fistula takes weeks to mature. Similarly, an AV graft cannot be used immediately. As this patient has chronic kidney disease with symptoms of uremia, she will need dialysis much sooner. Placement of a temporary dialysis catheter, which can be used immediately, would be the best choice at the present time. An alternative access would be the placement of a tunneled permanent hemodialysis catheter, if this could be done in quick fashion. The acid-base and electrolyte abnormalities will be managed with hemodialysis and, at this time, there is no emergency stemming from the hyperkalemia and metabolic acidosis.

Emergent hemodialysis is indicated for hyperkalemia, metabolic acidosis, or pulmonary edema that are refractory to medical management. The presence of symptomatic uremia, including uremic encephalopathy or uremic pericarditis (characterized by the presence of a pericardial friction rub), would also be an indication for emergency dialysis. Ingestions or overdoses of certain toxic substances, such as ethylene glycol, lithium, or salicylates, are an indication for emergent hemodialysis. Acetaminophen overdose is treated with acetylcysteine, not dialysis. High levels of BUN and creatinine and low urine output are not strict indications for emergent hemodialysis. (Brenner, 2004, pp. 1085–1095, 2567)

BIBLIOGRAPHY

American Academy of Pediatrics. *The Red Book, 2003 Report of the Committee on Infectious Diseases*, 26th ed. Elk Grove Village, IL: American Academy of Pediatrics, 2003.

American Psychiatric Association. *Diagnostic and Statistical Manual of Mental Disorders*, 4th ed., Text Revision. Washington, DC: American Psychiatric Association, 2000.

Braunwald E, Hauser SL, Jameson JL, et al. *Harrison's Principles of Internal Medicine*, 15th ed. New York, NY: McGraw-Hill, 2001.

Brenner BM. *Brenner & Rectors's The Kidney*, 7th ed. Philadelphia, PA: W.B. Saunders, 2004.

Brent J. Current management of ethylene glycol poisoning. Therapy in practice. *Drugs 2001;61(7):979–988.*

Cameron JL, ed. *Current Surgical Therapy*, 8th ed. St. Louis, MO: C.V. Mosby, 2004.

Charles VM, Russell RCG, Williams NS. *Bailey & Love's Short Practice of Surgery*, 22nd ed. London: Chapman & Hall, 1995.

Committee on Infectious Diseases, "*Recommended Childhood and Adolescent Immunization Schedule—United States*, 2006." Pediatrics 117; No. 1, January 2006, pp. 239–240.

Cotran RS, Kumar V, Collins T. *Robbins Pathologic Basis of Disease*, 6th ed. Philadelphia, PA: W.B. Saunders, 1999.

Cotran RS, Kumar V, Robbins SL. *Robbins Pathologic Basis of Disease*, 5th ed. Philadelphia, PA: W.B. Saunders, 1994.

Cunningham FG, Gant NF, Leveno KJ, et al. *Williams Obstetrics*, 21st ed. New York, NY: McGraw-Hill, 2001.

Greenfield LJ, Mulholland MW, Oldham KT, et al., eds. *Surgery: Scientific Principles and Practice*, 3rd ed. Philadelphia, PA: Lippincott Williams & Wilkins, 2001.

Hoffman R, Benz EJ Jr, Shattil SJ, et al. *Hematology: Basic Principles and Practice*, 3rd ed. New York, NY: Churchill Livingstone, 2000.

Jamieson EF, Steege JF. The association of sexual abuse with pelvic pain complaints in a primary care population. *Am J Obstet Gynecol* 1997;177: 1408–1412.

King PM, Myers CA, Ling FW, et al. Musculoskeletal factors in chronic pelvic pain. *J Psychosom Obstet Gynaecol* 1991;12(Suppl):87–98.

Kunimoto DY, Rapuano CJ, Friedberg MA, et al. *The Wills Eye Manual: Office and Emergency Room Diagnosis and Treatment of Eye Disease*, 4th ed. Philadelphia, PA: Lippincott Williams & Wilkins, 2004.

Larsen PR, Kronenberg HM, Melmed S, et al. *Williams Textbook of Endocrinology*, 10th ed. Philadelphia, PA: W.B. Saunders, 2003.

Lyznicki JM, Nielsen NH, Schneider JF. Cardiovascular screening of student athletes. *Am Fam Physician* 2000;62:765–784.

McNeely S, Hendrix S, Mazzoni M, et al. Medically sound, cost-effective treatment for pelvic inflammatory disease and tubo-ovarian abscess. *Am J Obstet Gynecol* 1998;178(6):1272–1278.

National Heart, Lung and Blood Institute. The 7th Report of the Joint National Committee on Prevention, Detection, Evaluation and Treatment of High Blood Pressure, 2003.

Rudolph CD, Rudolph AM, Hostetter MK, et al., eds. *Rudolph's Pediatrics*, 21st ed. New York, NY: McGraw-Hill, 2003.

Sadock BJ, Sadock VA. *Kaplan and Sadock's Synopsis of Psychiatry*, 9th ed. Philadelphia, PA: Lippincott Williams & Wilkins, 2003.

Schwartz PE. Ovarian masses: serologic markers. *Clin Obstet Gynecol* 1991;34:423–432.

Schwartz SI, Shires GT, Spencer FC, et al., eds. *Principles of Surgery*, 7th ed. New York, NY: McGraw-Hill, 1999.

Slawson D, Shaughnessy A. *Becoming an Information Master*. Course materials, 2003.

Stenchever M, Droegemueller W, Herbst A, et al. *Comprehensive Gynecology*, 4th ed. St. Louis, MO: Mosby, 2001.

Weiss JM. Pelvic floor myofascial trigger points: manual therapy for interstitial cystitis and the urgency-frequency syndrome. *J Urol* 2001;166: 2226–2231.

CHAPTER 10

Practice Test 3
Questions

Read each question carefully and in the order in which it is presented. Then select the one best response option of the choices offered. More than one option may be partially correct. You must select ONE BEST answer. You have 60 minutes to complete this test.

Setting I: Office/Health Center

You see patients in two locations: at your office suite, which is adjacent to a hospital, and at a community-based health center. Your office practice is a primary care generalist group. Most of the patients you see are from your own practice and are appearing for regularly scheduled return visits. Occasionally, you will encounter a patient whose primary care is managed by one of your associates. Reference may be made to the patient's medical records. Known patients may be managed by the telephone. You may have to respond to questions about information appearing in the public media, which will require interpretation of the medical literature. The laboratory and radiology departments have a full range of services available.

Questions 1 and 2

You see a 6-year-old girl in your office for leg aches. The mother relates that she has been complaining that her knees and ankles have been bothering her for the past 3 months. The pain is worse in the morning. She has not noticed any swelling, redness, or warmth in her joints. The mother says that she seems to have a fever once a day. She has never taken her temperature, but she seems flushed and has a lacy rash in the evening. She has not lost any weight. Her examination is essentially normal, with the exception of mild fluid notable in both of her knees. The knees have full range of motion and do not seem to bother her when you move them. You perform some blood tests which reveal the following: white blood cell (WBC) 28,000 (polymorphonuclear [PMN] 88%, lymph 10%, and no blasts on the smear), hematocrit 10.2 mg/dL, platelets 765,000, and erythrocyte sedimentation rate (ESR) 112.

1. What is the most likely diagnosis?

   (A) juvenile rheumatoid arthritis (JRA) (Still's disease)
   (B) growing pains
   (C) osteogenic sarcoma
   (D) infectious arthritis
   (E) acute toxic synovitis (ATS)

2. What is the most appropriate next step?

   (A) diagnostic arthrocentesis
   (B) bilateral hip, knee, and ankle x-rays
   (C) a trial of oral corticosteroids
   (D) a trial of nonsteroidal anti-inflammatory medication (NSAID)
   (E) MRI of both knees

3. A 74-year-old woman presents for routine physical examination. She is accompanied by her daughter, who reports that her mother has become increasingly forgetful. The patient has been misplacing objects and forgetting the names of her children and grandchildren. On examination, the patient demonstrates some paucity of speech, frequently nodding and smiling in response to questions posed. A Mini-Mental Status Examination reveals her score to be 21/30. The physician suspects she has dementia and may benefit from initiation of donepazil. Before doing so, the physician wants to order some tests to rule out treatable causes of dementia. In getting the patient's consent for both the tests and the treatment, what statement is correct when determining whether the patient has the ability to make her own decisions?

    (A) Since the patient has dementia, she automatically does not have decision-making capacity.

    (B) If the patient's condition were life threatening, the physician would not have to worry about whether the patient had decision-making capacity.

    (C) If the patient agrees with the recommendations of the physician, it does not matter whether she has decision-making capacity.

    (D) The patient may have the capacity to make a decision about whether or not to have the tests but not have the capacity to accept or refuse the proposed treatment.

    (E) The determination of capacity need not factor in whether there is any concomitant depression.

Questions 4 and 5

The patient is a 16-year-old girl attending a primary care clinic appointment with her mother. The mother is worried that her daughter is "too skinny." She apparently picks at her food, skips meals altogether, and exercises several hours per day. When asked about her behavior, she claims to be "fat" and expresses the need to lose more weight. She appears pale and cachectic, and her weight is markedly below that expected for her height.

4. Which of the following would be the most likely associated finding in this patient?

    (A) absence of menstrual cycles

    (B) abuse of diuretics or laxatives

    (C) eating large amounts of food

    (D) self-induced vomiting

    (E) sense of loss of control over behavior

5. Which of the following laboratory results would most likely be present in this individual?

    (A) decreased corticotropin-releasing hormone level

    (B) elevated fasting glucose level

    (C) high serum cholesterol level

    (D) hyperthyroidism

    (E) leukocytosis

Questions 6 and 7

A 38-year-old manager of a construction company presents to your office for the first time for evaluation of diffuse joint pain and swelling that has persisted for the past 4 weeks. His symptoms began with gradual pain and swelling in his knees which subsequently involved the joints of his hands and wrists. He reports some improvement with over-the-counter nonsteroidal anti-inflammatory agents but "the symptoms keep coming back." He denies any genitourinary symptoms. His physical examination demonstrates symmetrical swelling and warmth of his proximal interphalangeal joints (PIP), metacarpophalangeal joints (MCP), and knees bilaterally.

6. At this time, what would be the best test to order to confirm your diagnosis and affect the management of this patient?

    (A) HLA-B27

    (B) urinalysis

    (C) plain radiographs of the sacroiliac joints

    (D) antinuclear antibodies (ANA)

    (E) plain radiographs of the hands and knees

7. You suspect that your patient may have rheumatoid arthritis. In addition to the test you ordered above, you also order rheumatoid factor (RF) testing. Imaging studies demonstrate bony decalcification that is most marked adjacent to the PIP, MCP, and knee joints. Laboratory testing demonstrates mild leukocytosis, an elevated ESR, and a negative RF test.

How will the result of RF testing affect your management of this patient?

(A) Since the RF test is negative, he does not have rheumatoid arthritis and should not be exposed to the side effects of medications such as methotrexate and prednisone, but instead should receive anti-inflammatory medications.

(B) Test the patient for ANA, as the negative RF suggests that your diagnosis of rheumatoid arthritis is incorrect.

(C) Make the diagnosis of "general" arthritis NOS (not otherwise specified) and treat the patient with 10 mg of daily prednisone as sole therapy, as this will control his inflammation and has relatively few side effects.

(D) Diagnose the patient with rheumatoid arthritis and refer the patient to a rheumatologist for management with methotrexate.

(E) Verify your suspicion that this is indeed rheumatoid arthritis by ordering a C-reactive protein (CRP).

Questions 8 through 10

A 67-year-old Hispanic female is seen in the clinic for a well-woman examination. The patient has a history of type II diabetes mellitus (DM) and hypertension. Her medications include hydrochlothiazide 50 mg qd and metformin (Glucophage) 500 mg bid. She does not check her blood pressure (BP) at home and she told you that her fasting blood sugar is ranging 110–140 mg/dL. In reviewing some health maintenance issues, she tells you that her last dT (diphtheria-tetanus) was 5 years ago, she had a normal mammogram 1 year ago, she had an undilated eye examination at "a place in the mall" 1 year ago that was normal and she had a screening colonoscopy 8 years ago that was normal. She has had normal pap smears throughout her life, including annually for the last 5 years. She is widowed and not sexually active. Today she has no complaints. Her vital signs are: BP 140/85, heart rate 84, respiration rate 18, and temperature 98.7°F.

8. At this office visit, you should order which of the following?

(A) CA-125 for ovarian cancer screening

(B) pap smear

(C) chest x-ray (CXR) for lung cancer screening

(D) referral to an ophthalmologist

(E) colonoscopy for colon cancer screening

9. After the patient rested for more than 10 minutes, you rechecked her BP and it was 144/88. Her goal BP should be less than which of the following?

(A) 120/80

(B) 130/80

(C) 135/85

(D) 140/85

(E) 140/90

10. At this time, what would be the most appropriate management?

(A) add a low dose of atenolol

(B) increase the hydrochlothiazide dose

(C) add a low dose of amlodipine

(D) add a low dose of lisinopril

(E) add a low dose of clonidine

11. A 15-year-old male presented with fever, sore throat, generalized lymph node enlargement, and lymphocytosis with atypical lymphocytes on the peripheral smear. These findings are characteristic of which of the following?

(A) chronic lymphocytic leukemia

(B) infection with Epstein-Barr virus (EBV)

(C) streptococcal pharyngitis

(D) allergic drug reaction

(E) pulmonary tuberculosis

Questions 12 and 13

A 23-year-old mother brings her 5-month-old child to your office for nasal congestion, runny nose, mild wheezing, red watery eyes, and vomiting that started suddenly 45 minutes ago. The mother took her child's temperature and it was 98.5(F. The child had not had a cough or diarrhea. There have been no known ill contacts. This is the first time that her baby has had these symptoms. Further history reveals that this happened after the child was breast-fed and given a small part of a boiled egg. On examination, the infant's pulse is 140, respiratory rate is 24, and temperature is 98.6°F. The patient has nasal and conjunctival congestion, bilateral wheezing and flushing of the skin over the trunk.

12. At this time, what should you do?

   (A) Tell the mother that this is a self-limited viral illness and ask her to return to your office in 3 days if symptoms persist.

   (B) Give a prescription for Tylenol as needed and advise mother to give the child plenty of water.

   (C) Order a CXR in your office to rule out pneumonia.

   (D) Ask the mother to take her child to the emergency room (ER), which is a 10-minute drive from your office.

   (E) Call 911 and closely monitor the patient until they arrive to transport the patient to the ER.

13. One month later, the mother brings her child for a well-child examination. Which of the following vaccinations would be contraindicated?

   (A) diphtheria, tetanus, acellular pertussis (DTaP)

   (B) *Haemophilus influenzae,* type B (HIB)

   (C) hepatitis B

   (D) injectable polio vaccine (IPV)

   (E) influenza

14. The major method of action of combined oral contraceptives (containing both an estrogen and a progestin) is due to which of the following?

   (A) cervical mucus thickening

   (B) decreased Fallopian tube transport of the fertilized egg

   (C) suppression of endogenous follicle-stimulating hormone (FSH)

   (D) changes in the uterine endometrium

   (E) suppression of endogenous luteinizing hormone (LH)

15. A 22-year-old woman presents with depression, hypertension, 20-lb weight gain over 6 months, and amenorrhea. She is currently on fluoxetine and oral contraceptives. She admits to drinking four to six beers per day on weekends. On examination, she weights 160 lbs, her height is 5 ft, and she has supraclavicular fullness, abdominal striae, ecchymoses on her arms, and facial acne.

   Which of the following would be the most appropriate next step?

   (A) morning adrenocorticotropic hormone (ACTH) level

   (B) morning cortisol level

   (C) MRI of pituitary

   (D) 24-hour free urinary cortisol

   (E) 1 µg cosyntropin stimulation test

Questions 16 through 18

A 46-year-old man presents with a 2-year history of dysphagia. Initially the dysphagia was for solid foods only, especially meats, but has progressed over time to the point where he mostly consumes liquids or soft foods such as pudding and ice cream. He occasionally awakens with regurgitated food on his pillow in the morning. He has lost 10 lbs over the past year. His physical examination is unremarkable. He has no other medical problems. He drinks one to two alcoholic beverages per day and smoked one pack of cigarettes per day for 10 years, stopping 15 years ago.

16. The most appropriate test to evaluate the patient would be which of the following?

(A) upper endoscopic examination (esophagogastroduodenoscopy)

(B) barium swallow

(C) computed tomography (CT) scan of the chest and abdomen

(D) esophageal pH testing

(E) esophageal manometry (motility testing)

17. Further studies reveal the following: the esophageal mucosa is normal, as is the proximal stomach. The esophagus is dilated and contains residual food despite an overnight fast. The lower esophageal sphincter (LES) is tight.

Which condition is the patient most likely to have?

(A) Barrett esophagus

(B) diffuse esophageal spasm (DES)

(C) achalasia

(D) nutcracker esophagus

(E) scleroderma

18. The patient is at increased risk for which of the following disorders?

(A) esophageal squamous cell carcinoma

(B) esophageal adenocarcinoma

(C) gastroesophageal reflux disease (GERD)

(D) gastric adenocarcinoma of the proximal stomach

(E) Barrett esophagus

19. A family with a newborn infant comes to your office for a 2-week checkup. The parents are first-time parents and they have significant concern about "sudden death." Which of the following would be the most important counseling regarding SIDS (sudden infant death syndrome) prevention?

(A) ensure that the crib has plenty of pillows in it to prevent the baby from rolling

(B) ensure that all pets are restricted from the baby's room

(C) delay immunizations until 6 months of age

(D) encourage the family to always place the baby on her back to sleep

(E) offer the use of a home apnea and bradycardia monitor

Questions 20 and 21

20. A 21-year-old college student calls your answering service requesting a prescription for emergency contraception. During intercourse 6 hours ago her partner's condom broke. You advise her of the nonprescription availability of *Plan B*, which contains which of the following?

(A) misiprostol 300 µg

(B) gonadotropin releasing hormone (GnRH) agonist

(C) ethinyl estradiol and norgestimate

(D) levonorgestrel 0.75 mg

(E) conjugated equine estrogens (Premarin) 0.625 mg

21. While she does not want to become pregnant, your patient also says that she would not want to cause an abortion if she were already pregnant. You advise her that this type of emergency contraception works by which mechanism?

(A) inhibiting ovulation and works for up to 1 week after the last unprotected intercourse

(B) causing insufficient corpus luteum function, altering the histology of the endometrium, and must be taken within 72 hours of unprotected intercourse

(C) interrupting an implanted pregnancy within 18 hours of ingestion

(D) causing an imbalance between testosterone and estrogen if taken within 24 hours

(E) evoking a surge in inhibin and decrease in FSH which diminishes ovarian follicular production if taken within 5 days of unprotected intercourse

Questions 22 through 24

A 36-year-old White female comes to your office complaining of an unintentional 15-lb weight loss in the last 3 months. Her review of systems is notable for fatigue, a skin rash over her face and upper chest, hair loss, mild bilateral knee swelling, and shortness of breath with exertion. On physical examination, there is an erythematosus macular rash on her face and upper chest. She has a pericardial friction rub and a normal pulmonary examination. She has mild bilateral knee swelling and tenderness.

22. Which of the following laboratory tests would be most likely to help in diagnosing this patient's condition?

   (A) complete blood count
   (B) comprehensive metabolic panel
   (C) CRP
   (D) antinuclear antibody
   (E) RF

23. A CXR would be most likely to show which of the following?

   (A) cardiomegaly
   (B) bilateral pulmonary congestion
   (C) bilateral pleural effusion
   (D) pulmonary fibrosis
   (E) diffuse bilateral infiltrates

24. You institute appropriate therapy and 2 months later the patient returns for follow-up. She is feeling much better, has regained some of her weight, her skin rash has resolved, and her knee pain has improved. She would like to get pregnant in the next few months. Regarding pregnancy, you advise her of which of the following?

   (A) She can get pregnant at any time as she is much better now.
   (B) She should wait until her symptoms resolve completely and she regains her initial weight.
   (C) She can get pregnant, but she needs to stop her medications now.

   (D) She should wait until the disease has been quiescent for at least 6 months.
   (E) This is a life-long disease that needs chronic treatment; therefore, she should not attempt to become pregnant.

Setting II: Emergency Department and Inpatient Facilities

You encounter patients in the emergency department and inpatient facilities, including the hospital, the adjacent nursing home/extended-care facility, and detoxification unit. Most patients in the emergency department are new to you and are seeking urgent care, but occasionally, you arrange to meet there with a known patient who has telephoned you. You have general admitting privileges to the hospital, including to the children's and women's services. On occasion you see patients in the critical care unit. Postoperative patients are usually seen in their rooms unless the recovery room is specified. You may also be called to see patients in the psychiatric unit. There is a short-stay unit where you may see patients undergoing same-day operations or being held for observation. Also available to you are a full range of social services, including rape crisis intervention, family support, and security assistance backed up by local police.

25. Eight hours following an uneventful kidney transplant, a 57-year-old patient develops fever and renal failure. What is the most likely cause?

   (A) preformed antibodies
   (B) immunosuppressive drug reaction
   (C) T-cell-mediated immune response
   (D) wound infection
   (E) graft versus host disease

26. An 18-year-old G_1 White woman who has received no prenatal care is brought in to Labor and Delivery by rescue squad. She called for an ambulance when she noted the sudden onset of heavy vaginal bleeding. Earlier the same day she noted the onset of painful hardening of her abdomen every 5–7 minutes. She reports that she believes she is about "7 months" pregnant. She has no significant medical or surgical

history. She denies use of alcohol, tobacco, or illicit drugs. You confirm fetal heart tones in the range of 140–150 beats per minute (bpm) and place the patient on a fetal heart rate monitor and tocometer. The next step in this patient's management should be which of the following?

(A) sterile speculum examination of vagina and cervix
(B) digital examination for cervical dilation
(C) emergency caesarian delivery
(D) ultrasound
(E) amniocentesis

Questions 27 and 28

A 60-year-old female is treated with trimethoprim/sulfamethoxazole (Bactrim) for a urinary tract infection. One week after completing the course, she develops blisters on her abdomen and thighs. After another 2 weeks, the patient presents for evaluation and has multiple flaccid bullae and superficial erosions on the chest, abdomen, back, and thighs. She also has painful erosions of the oral mucosa. A skin biopsy reveals an intraepidermal split.

27. What is the most likely diagnosis?

(A) toxic epidermal necrolysis
(B) bullous pemphigoid
(C) primary varicella
(D) pemphigus vulgaris (PV)
(E) disseminated herpes simplex

28. The most appropriate initial therapy for this patient would be which of the following?

(A) oral valacyclovir
(B) inpatient admission to the Burn Unit
(C) oral prednisone
(D) oral dicloxacillin
(E) watchful observation

29. An 82-year-old female returns to the intensive care unit (ICU) after a partial colectomy with a diverting colostomy for an acute large bowel obstruction. The following morning, the nurse records a total of 100 cc of urine over the past 6 hours. Which of the following criteria suggest prerenal failure?

(A) urine osmolarity of 300 mOsm/kg
(B) urine sodium level of 50 meq/L
(C) urine/plasma creatinine ratio of 15
(D) fractional excretion of sodium (FeNa) <1
(E) central venous pressure greater than 15 cmH$_2$O

30. A 69-year-old male with history of coronary artery disease and high lipids is admitted to the coronary care unit (CCU) with an acute inferior myocardial infarction. He is placed on a continuous infusion of unfractionated heparin and undergoes a cardiac catheterization with stent placement. On day 7, he complains of a swollen left leg. A Doppler ultrasound confirms a deep vein thrombosis of the femoral vein. The intern notices that his platelet count has dropped to 70,000 from 300,000 at admission.

What is the next step in the management of this patient?

(A) continue heparin at the same dose
(B) increase the dose of heparin since it seems not to be working
(C) stop heparin
(D) start warfarin and continue heparin
(E) stop heparin and start a low molecular weight heparin

31. A 3 cm lesion in the right lobe of the liver is found in a 65-year-old male suspected of having cholethiasis. A CT scan is obtained which reveals the lesion to have an enhancing rim with centripetal filling (see Figure 10-1). The most appropriate management is which of the following?

FIG. 10-1

(A) observation

(B) estrogen therapy

(C) percutaneous CT-guided biopsy

(D) laparotomy with wide excision with 1 cm margins

(E) laparotomy with right hepatic lobectomy

Questions 32 and 33

You are called to the newborn nursery to see a baby with a birthmark on his face. You note a port-wine stain on the right forehead and cheek. The port-wine stain is only on the right side.

32. What is the most likely condition?

(A) Sturge-Weber syndrome

(B) neurofibromatosis, type 1 (von Recklinghausen's disease)

(C) tuberous sclerosis

(D) CHARGE Association

(E) Beckwith-Wiedemann syndrome

33. What is the most common complication of the above disorder?

(A) cardiac abnormalities

(B) seizures and mental retardation

(C) polycystic kidney disease

(D) cystic or fibrous pulmonary changes

(E) hypoglycemia

34. A patient who sustained extensive burns developed shock and acute renal failure. Which would be the most accurate description of pathologic changes seen in the kidney?

(A) crescents in the glomeruli

(B) fibrinoid necrosis of the arterioles and hyperplastic atherosclerosis

(C) patchy necrosis of the proximal tubular epithelium

(D) multiple infarctions

(E) pus within the tubules and abscess in the interstitium

35. Which of the following is the most appropriate treatment for a 32-year-old male with a toxic nodular goiter and compressive airway symptoms?

(A) radioactive iodine therapy

(B) propranolol

(C) propylthiouracil

(D) Lugol solution

(E) total lobectomy

Questions 36 and 37

36. A 3-year-old child is seen in the ER with a history of a recent acute respiratory infection. The mother reports that the child has been complaining of bilateral knee pain and abdominal discomfort. On examination, you notice a palpable purpuric rash on the buttocks extending to both lower extremities. What is the most likely diagnosis?

(A) immune thrombocytopenic purpura (ITP)

(B) Henoch-Schönlein purpura (HSP)

(C) Evans syndrome

(D) meningococcemia

(E) hemolytic uremic syndrome (HUS)

37. Treatment of the above condition should include which of the following?

(A) course of antibiotics

(B) no specific treatment is required at this time

(C) blood transfusion

(D) corticosteroids

(E) intravenous immunoglobulin (IVIG)

Questions 38 through 40

A 23-year-old male checks into the ER with his girlfriend. His chief complaint is, "I can't look to my side." The patient was released from a local community hospital 5 days ago, after a 3-week hospitalization. While there, he was diagnosed with schizophreniform disorder and treated with risperidone (Risperdal), which was just increased to 2 mg orally two times per day. His mental status examination is notable for significant anxiety without overt psychotic symptoms. He is afebrile, and his vital signs are normal. His physical examination is remarkable for rotation of his head toward the left with tender neck musculature in spasm.

38. What is the most likely etiology of his presentation?

(A) acute dystonic reaction

(B) akathisia

(C) conversion disorder

(D) parkinsonism

(E) tardive dyskinesia

39. What is the most appropriate next step in the management of his condition?

(A) discontinue the risperidone

(B) intramuscular injection of benztropine (Cogentin)

(C) intramuscular injection of haloperidol (Haldol)

(D) intramuscular injection of lorazepam (Ativan)

(E) reassurance and suggestion that it will improve

40. The patient returns to the ER 1 week later complaining of "feeling more agitated." He states he has felt "edgy" over the past several days. His girlfriend confirms that he has been pacing around the apartment during the day and night. On mental status examination, he demonstrates good hygiene and is cooperative. He displays some psychomotor agitation with

moving in his chair and standing up frequently. His thought processes are logical without looseness of association. His thought content is without suicidal or homicidal ideation. He denies paranoia, ideas of reference, or delusions. He denies perceptual disturbances and does not appear to respond to internal stimuli.

What is the most appropriate next step in the management of this patient?

(A) add a mood stabilizer to the regimen

(B) add propranolol (Inderal) to the regimen

(C) decrease the dose of risperidone

(D) increase the dose of risperidone

(E) switch to another antipsychotic

Questions 41 through 44

A 68-year-old woman, with a history of hypertension, type 2 diabetes, and a previous myocardial infarction, presents to the ER with dyspnea. She gives a history of progressively worsening dyspnea on exertion and lower extremity edema. She sleeps on three pillows and will get short of breath if she tries to lay flat for any period of time. She came to the ER because she feels "like I'm not getting any air." On examination, her pulse is 110 bpm, BP is 160/100, and her respiratory rate is 28. Her oxygen saturation is 91% by pulse oximetry at room air.

41. Which of the following physical examination findings is she most likely to have?

(A) tracheal deviation

(B) pericardial rub

(C) diastolic murmur along the left sternal border

(D) perioral cyanosis

(E) S_3 gallop

42. Which of the following should be administered first?

(A) furosemide 80 mg IV

(B) continuous infusion of IV nitroglycerin

(C) aspirin 650 mg PO

(D) enalapril 1.25 mg IV

(E) oxygen

43. A subsequent echocardiogram reveals an ejection fraction of 35%. Which of the following medications has been shown to reduce mortality in this setting?

   (A) angiotensin-converting enzyme (ACE) inhibitors
   (B) digoxin
   (C) dihydropyridine calcium channel blockers
   (D) alpha-adrenergic antagonists
   (E) warfarin

44. Which of the following medications would be contraindicated in this patient?

   (A) insulin
   (B) metformin (Glucophage)
   (C) glyburide (DiaBeta, Micronase)
   (D) acarbose (Precose)
   (E) glimepiride (Amaryl)

Questions 45 and 46

A 52-year-old male, with past medical history of gallbladder stones and hypertension, presents to the emergency department with midabdominal pain radiating to the back and nausea and vomiting for 2 days. Initial laboratory tests showed a WBC count of 19,000, hemoglobin of 14 g/dL, total bilirubin of 1.1, aspartate transaminase (AST) of 430 mg, alanine transaminase (ALT) of 420, amylase of 860, lipase of 620, lactate dehydrogenase (LDH) of 590, glucose of 364, creatinine of 0.8, and blood urea nitrogen (BUN) of 19. Abdominal x-ray was negative and CT scan is consistent with acute pancreatitis.

45. Which of the following is the most appropriate management of this patient?

   (A) outpatient management with oral pain medications and antiemetics, with follow-up in a week
   (B) 23-hour observation
   (C) admission to the general medical floor, NPO (nothing by mouth), pain medications, and antiemetics

   (D) ICU admission, NPO, nasogastric (NG) tube, IV fluid, antibiotics
   (E) immediate surgery for debridement of pancreatic debris

46. The estimated mortality of this patient is what percentage?

   (A) 2%
   (B) 15%
   (C) 40%
   (D) 80%
   (E) 100%

47. A 65-year-old gentleman suddenly notices he can't see from one eye but he is not having any pain or redness. Which of the following is the most likely diagnosis?

   (A) cataract
   (B) angle closure glaucoma
   (C) corneal abrasion
   (D) retinal detachment
   (E) primary open angle glaucoma

48. A 32-year-old male is seen in the ER with a nondisplaced fracture of the ulna after a fall. Incidentally, you notice that the patient is jaundiced and has a palpable spleen. You order a CBC which shows hemoglobin of 10.2 g/dL. The patient reveals a history of having chronic anemia and that he has intermittently been prescribed iron pills to take. He says that at age 23 he had a cholecystectomy. He has several family members with similar symptoms. You review the peripheral smear and find spherocytes. The best way to confirm this man's diagnosis would be which of the following?

   (A) splenectomy
   (B) hemoglobin electrophoresis
   (C) osmotic fragility
   (D) glucose-6-phosphate dehydrogenase (G-6PD) level
   (E) indirect Coombs test

Answers and Explanations

1. **(A)**

2. **(D)**

Explanations 1 and 2

Leg aches are a common complaint and are usually nonspecific in nature. The presence of a lacy rash with arthralgias and daily fever spikes, in an otherwise healthy child, is a common presentation of systemic-onset JRA (Still's disease). "Growing Pains" is a term used for a common, yet nonspecific, constellation of complaints. The typical compliant associated with growing pains is in a 7- to 12-year-old who has vague pain in the midthigh or calf (but not the joints) which is at its worst in the evening. The pain is usually symmetric and the therapy is usually massage and analgesia. Osteogenic sarcomas are rare bone tumors. Their most common location is around the knee, but the bilateral nature of this child's presentation makes a tumor unlikely. Infectious arthritis (or septic arthritis) is usually a single joint which is very tender and warm. A septic joint has an acute course with limp, fever, and some degree of toxicity. In septic arthritis, the ESR and WBC counts will usually be markedly elevated, but the 3-month history would exclude this diagnosis. ATS is a postinfectious arthralgia. The screening tests of a CBC and ESR are typically normal in ATS.

The best first-line therapy in the treatment of JRA is a trial of NSAIDs. If this trial fails then a course of prednisone is usually undertaken. Given the "classic" nature of this child's presentation, and the nominal fluid in the joint, an arthrocentesis is uncalled-for. Plain films of the entire lower extremity would be unrevealing and expose the child to excessive radiation. Close follow-up of this child is a necessity until the diagnosis is made and the disease under control. Some children

with JRA can have other systemic findings, the most concerning of which is uveitis. *(Rudolph et al., 2003, pp. 836–839)*

3. **(D)** Decision-making capacity can be determined by the patient's attending physician and need not involve consultation with a psychiatrist, although this may provide helpful information when there is cognitive impairment or mental illness. Cognitive impairments, such as mental illness, mental retardation, or dementia, do not automatically entail decisional incapacity. Decision-making capacity is not to be confused with competency, which is a legal determination made by a court of law to decide whether the patient can handle her own affairs. Determination of decision-making capacity is dependent on the decision to be made, wherein complex or riskier decisions require a higher threshold in assessing capacity. This sliding scale notion of capacity may entail that a patient is capable of making some medical decisions but not others.

There are seven requirements for decision-making capacity: (1) ability to communicate a choice and preference; (2) ability to understand medical condition; (3) ability to understand risks and benefits of condition and treatment options; (4) intact judgment (e.g., not impaired through depression or substance abuse); (5) consistency with previously expressed wishes or values; (6) ability to reason through issues at hand; (7) some fixity in the decision made (although this does not exclude the possibility of a patient changing her mind for compelling reasons).

In the case presented, the patient may be able to weigh the risks, benefits, and options of testing but may not have this capacity for the proposed treatment. Just because the patient may agree with the recommendations made by the physician does not imply that she has the capacity or that it is not necessary to assess decisional capacity. Were the patient found to lack decision-making capacity, the physician is obligated to obtain consent from the patient's appropriate surrogate decision maker, whether it is an appointed health care agent or a decision maker chosen from a hierarchy of relationships (spouse, adult child, parent, other relative, close personal friend).

4. **(A)**

5. **(C)**

Explanations 4 and 5

This patient likely has anorexia nervosa. Abuse of diuretics, laxatives or enemas, and self-induced emesis are all considered to be purging behaviors. While there is a purging subtype of anorexia, these symptoms are also commonly seen in bulimia nervosa. Eating excessively large amounts of food, or binging, can also be present during an episode of anorexia, but, like purging, binging is not specific for anorexia nervosa. Binging is necessary for the diagnosis of bulimia nervosa. Feeling a loss of control is part of the clinical picture of bulimia, but in anorexia the patients display a dramatic sense of denial regarding their weight loss and physical appearance. Amenorrhea, or the absence of three consecutive menstrual cycles, is not only characteristic of, but also necessary, for the diagnosis of anorexia nervosa. (*American Psychiatric Association, 2000*)

Because of the recurrent vomiting, the purging type of anorexia nervosa can demonstrate electrolyte disturbances such as a hypokalemic, hypochloremic alkalosis and elevated serum amylase levels. The prolonged state of starvation seen in anorexia can also cause various laboratory abnormalities including hypersecretion of corticotrophin-releasing hormone, low fasting glucose concentrations, mild hypothyroidism, leukopenia, and elevated serum cholesterol levels. These irregularities normalize with the regaining of sufficient weight. (*Sadock and Sadock, 2003, p. 743*)

6. **(E)**

7. **(D)**

Explanations 6 and 7

This patient presents with symptoms typical for rheumatoid arthritis but has not met diagnostic criteria. He has had arthritis of three different joint areas simultaneously, involvement (swelling) of the MCP and PIP joints, and a symmetrical arthritis. These three symptoms plus one of the following would make the diagnosis of rheumatoid arthritis: morning stiffness greater than 1 hour, rheumatoid nodules, serum RF or radiographs demonstrating erosions or unequivocal bony decalcification. In the event that the patient does have erosions on plain radiographs, your management of his rheumatoid arthritis would be more aggressive and referral to a rheumatologist would be indicated. HLA-B27 is associated with spondyloarthropathy but should never be ordered when there is no clinical suspicion for spondyloarthropathy (due to the presence of this antigen in the normal population). The diagnosis of spondyloarthropathy requires inflammatory spinal pain or asymmetric synovitis and either family history, psoriasis, inflammatory bowel disease, urethritis, buttock pain, or sacroiliitis, which this patient does not have. A urinalysis would not confirm a diagnosis. Plain radiographs of the sacroiliac joints, in the absence of symptoms of spondyloarthropathy, are not indicated. Similar to HLA-B27 testing, ANA testing, in the absence of clinical history and examination suggesting a connective tissue disease, is not indicated, due to the false positive results occurring in the normal population.

This patient has clinical criteria suggestive of rheumatoid arthritis and the radiographic changes fulfill criteria for rheumatoid arthritis (as there can be erosions OR bony decalcification). The absence of RF does not contradict the diagnosis of rheumatoid arthritis. However, once rheumatoid arthritis has been diagnosed, patients who are RF-positive tend to have more severe disease. Joint inflammation is more severe and there is more joint destruction in RF-positive compared to RF-negative rheumatoid arthritis patients. However, RF-negative patients are still at risk for joint damage and warrant therapy with a disease modifying antirheumatic drugs (DMARD), such as methotrexate, under the supervision of a rheumatologist. ANA testing is a "fishing expedition" in the absence of clinical suspicion for a connective tissue disease and, therefore, should not be ordered. Arthritis NOS is a vague diagnosis, but the side effects of 10 mg of prednisone, as sole therapy, are very clear and very real. Although prednisone will control his inflammation, steroid-induced osteoporosis, avascular necrosis, or other steroid-associated morbidities may ensue. This is the reason that DMARD therapy is used in rheumatoid arthritis. DMARD therapy will enable the physician to either lower the dosage of or discontinue prednisone and effectively treat the rheumatoid arthritis. CRP is an acute-phase reactant produced by the liver. It can be elevated as early as 4 hours after tissue injury and peaks within 1–3 days. It is elevated in many diseases associated with inflammation. Even if this test was positive in this patient, systemic inflammation was already indicated by the mild leukocytosis and the elevated ESR. *(Ruddy et al., 2001, pp. 970–980, 1001–1003)*

8. (D)

9. (B)

10. (D)

Explanations 8 through 10

The basic guidelines for diabetic care recommend that patients with type 2 DM should have a dilated eye examination by a trained expert shortly after diagnosis and then every year afterward. The United States Preventive Services Task Force (USPSTF) has a D recommendation (against) checking CA-125 levels for ovarian cancer screening. They also have a D recommendation (against) routinely screening women older than 65 for cervical cancer if they have had adequate recent screening with normal pap smear and are not otherwise at high risk for cervical cancer. The USPSTF has an I recommendation (insufficient evidence for recommending for or against screening asymptomatic persons) for lung cancer with CXR, low-dose CT, sputum cytology, or a combination of these tests. The USPSTF has an A

recommendation (found fair to good evidence that several screening methods are effective in reducing mortality) for screening for colorectal cancer in men and women 50 years of age or older with colonoscopy every 10 years. There are other equally effective methods for screening for colorectal cancer, such as sigmoidoscopy every 5 years, double-contrast barium enema every 5 years, or fecal occult blood testing (FOBT) yearly, or the combination of sigmoidoscopy and FOBT every 5 years. There are insufficient data to determine which strategy is best in terms of the balance of benefits and potential harms or cost-effectiveness.

In this patient with a history of hypertension and DM, her BP goal is 130/80, as recommended by the JNC 7. To achieve this goal for patients with DM or chronic renal disease, the best management is to add a low dose of an ACE inhibitor, such as lisinopril. The American Diabetes Association (ADA) recommends an ACE inhibitor for all patients over the age of 55 years with hypertension or without hypertension but with another cardiovascular risk factor (history of cardiovascular disease, dyslipidemia, microalbuminuria, smoking). *(American Diabetes Association, 2004, pp. S15–S35; USPSTF: www.preventiveservices.ahrq.gov)*

11. (B) Infection with EBV is transmitted by close human contact. The clinical picture of infectious mononucleosis is typically fever, generalized lymphadenopathy, sore throat, and splenomegaly. On examination of the peripheral blood, there is a lymphocytosis with atypical lymphocytes. These cells are proved to be activated T cells. The virus attacks the epithelial cells as well as the B lymphocytes. On examination of the peripheral blood, the atypical lymphocytes represent suppressor T lymphocytes characteristic of this disease. Lymphoid organs, such as spleen and lymph nodes, are enlarged, although the architecture is usually preserved. The final diagnosis of this disease includes specific findings such as lymphocytosis, atypical lymphoid cells previously described, a positive heterophile reaction (monospot test), and specific antibodies for EBV antigens. *(Cotran et al., 1999, pp. 371–373)*

12.   (E)

13.   (E)

Explanations 12 and 13

This child is showing the symptoms of an anaphylactic reaction, most likely to egg protein. Cutaneous manifestations, with or without angioedema, are characteristic of systemic anaphylactic reactions. Upper or lower airway obstruction may occur, which can cause hoarseness, stridor, or wheezing. Gastrointestinal symptoms may include nausea, vomiting, diarrhea, or abdominal pain. Vascular collapse or shock may occur. In this patient, vascular collapse or respiratory compromise due to bronchospasm or laryngeal edema could occur quickly. Therefore, the child should be closely monitored while emergency medical technicians are called for safe transport. As the child's condition could quickly deteriorate, allowing the parent to drive the child to the ER would be unsafe.

Eggs, milk, seafood, and nuts are common food causes of anaphylaxis. The influenza vaccine is contraindicated in persons who have a history of anaphylaxis to egg proteins, as the virus is grown in chicken eggs and small amounts of egg protein may be present in the vaccine. Vaccines to measles, mumps, and yellow fever are also prepared in eggs and would be similarly contraindicated. *(Braunwald et al., 2001, pp. 785, 1915–1916)*

14.   **(E)** Combination oral contraceptives have both an estrogen and a progestin component. The overall effect of oral contraceptives is progestational. Although progestins can affect Fallopian tube function, endometrial maturation, and cause thickened cervical mucus, the major contraceptive effect of progestins is to suppress LH release thereby preventing ovulation. Estrogen in the oral contraceptive primarily acts to suppress FSH release. *(Beckmann et al., 2002, pp. 331–333)*

15.   **(D)** The patient has the clinical features of Cushings syndrome. Initial screening tests for determining if she has hypercortisolism include dexamethasone suppression testing,

midnight cortisol measurement, and urinary free cortisol. Of these tests, the urinary free cortisol is best in this patient as depression, obesity, and oral contraceptives all interfere with the 1 mg dexamethasone suppression test. Depression is known to be associated with abnormal glucocorticoid metabolism and oral contraceptives increase cortisol-binding globulin, thus increasing total serum cortisol levels. The other tests listed are not useful in the initial evaluation of hypercortisolism. *(Larsen et al., 2003, pp. 509–511, 516)*

16.   (A)

17.   (C)

18.   (A)

Explanations 16 through 18

The next best test would be an upper endoscopy. The patient has some alarm symptoms in his history, including progression of his dysphagia and weight loss. His history of smoking also puts him at increased risk for squamous cell esophageal cancer. Endoscopy would allow direct inspection of the esophagus, stomach, and duodenum. An obstructing malignancy, if present, could be identified and biopsies could be obtained. A barium swallow or a CT scan would be helpful, but would not allow tissue samples to be obtained were a mass identified. Esophageal pH testing and esophageal manometry are not yet indicated at this time.

The patient has achalasia, manifesting as failure of relaxation of the LES despite the initiation of a swallow. His esophagus has dilated over time in response to swallowing against a chronic obstruction, although the LES does still occasionally relax. DES and nutcracker esophagus would have a normal appearing esophagus endoscopically but would have manometric abnormalities on formal testing. Scleroderma esophagus is associated with chronic relaxation of the LES, esophagitis, and strictures. Barrett esophagus would not manifest as dysphagia, but represents a mucosal change seen at the gastroesophageal junction in patients with GERD.

Patients with achalasia are at increased risk for esophageal squamous cell carcinoma, possibly secondary to chronic esophageal inflammation from retained food. The tumors often arise in the dilated portion of the esophagus. Other complications in patients with achalasia include aspiration pneumonia and chronic cough. GERD and its complication, Barrett esophagus, are less common in patients with achalasia as gastric contents usually cannot reflux through the chronically closed LES. *(Braunwald et al., 2001, pp. 233–236, 1644–1645)*

19. **(D)** The rates of SIDS in the United States have decreased over the past 15 years from 1.2 per 1000 births to .56 per 1000 births. This 53% decrease is attributed partly to the "Back To Sleep" campaign. While the cause (or causes) of SIDS is (are) unknown, there are some well-recognized risk factors. These include: prone sleeping, cigarette smoke exposure (both pre- and postnatally), overheating, thick bedding and pillows and stuffed animals in the sleep environment. Additionally, the use of pacifiers has been shown to decrease the rates of SIDS in infants. The home use of monitors has not been shown to decrease the rates of SIDS and should be discouraged. Likewise, there has been no relationship demonstrated between immunizations and SIDS. *(AAP Task Force on Sudden Infant Death Syndrome, 2005, pp. 1245–1255)*

20. **(D)**

21. **(B)**

Explanations 20 and 21

Plan B is comprised of two tablets, each containing 0.75 mg of the progesterone agent levonorgestrel. The second pill is ingested 12 hours after the first.

Although a single mechanism of action for emergency contraception has not been clearly established, it is generally thought to work by inhibiting ovulation, causing insufficient corpus luteum formation, and alteration of the histology and biochemistry of the endometrium. The method does not interrupt an implanted pregnancy. Effectiveness ranges from 75 to 90%

and is more likely to be successful in preventing pregnancy if taken within 72 hours of unprotected intercourse. *(Chez, 2001, pp. 1–6)*

22. **(D)**

23. **(A)**

24. **(D)**

Explanations 22 through 24

Systemic lupus erythematosus (SLE) is diagnosed by the presence of 4 of the following 11 signs or symptoms: malar rash; discoid rash; photosensitivity; oral ulcers; arthritis; serositis; renal disorder; neurologic disorder; hematologic disorder; immunologic disorder; ANA. In this case, the patient has the presence of a characteristic rash, arthritis, and serositis (pericardial friction rub suggestive of a pericardial effusion). The presence of ANA on blood testing would, therefore, be diagnostic for SLE. The other tests listed may be helpful but are nonspecific.

All of the CXR findings listed can occur in the presence of SLE. Pericarditis is the most common manifestation of cardiac lupus and effusions can occur. Pleurisy and pleural effusions are also common. Lupus pneumonitis can cause fleeting infiltrates on x-ray, but the most common cause of pulmonary infiltrates in patients with SLE is infection. *(Braunwald et al., 2001, pp. 1924–1925)*

SLE can lead to recurrent pregnancy loss. Reports have indicated that during pregnancy, approximately one-third of women reported that their lupus improved, one-third stayed the same, and one-third worsened. In general, pregnancy outcomes are better if the disease has been quiescent for at least 6 months, there is no active renal involvement, superimposed preeclampsia does not develop, and there is no evidence of antiphospholipid antibody. *(Cunningham et al., 2001, pp. 1386–1387)*

25. **(A)** Transplant rejection is classified as hyperacute, acute, and chronic. Hyperacute rejection is a B-cell-mediated process and occurs when the serum of the recipient has preformed anti-donor antibodies. These antibodies adhere to

and kill endothelium, which results in rapid graft infarction. The rejection characteristically occurs within the first 24 hours. The presence of preformed antibodies can be predicted by a positive cross-match and is an absolute contraindication to transplant. The rejection does not respond to medical treatment and the transplanted organ must be removed.

Acute rejection is a cell-medicated immune response initiated by helper T cells. It occurs 1 week to 3 months following the transplant and rarely occurs after 1 year. The diagnosis is made by detection and workup of graft dysfunction, culminating in a biopsy. It can be treated medically by a course of high-dose immunosuppressive drugs.

Chronic rejection usually occurs more than 1 year posttransplant. It has an insidious onset and is multifactorial, with both the cell-mediated and humoral arms of the immune system involved. Chronic rejection is usually not reversible.

Graft versus host disease occurs with transplant of tissues that contain immunocompetent cells, such as during a bone marrow transplant. Surgical wound infection typically takes place 3–5 days after surgery and does not result in organ failure. *(Jarrell et al., 2000, p. 464)*

26. **(D)** In a patient with no prenatal care who presents with vaginal bleeding, ultrasound should be the first diagnostic test. It is needed to rule-out placenta previa or vasa previa. It would be dangerous to proceed with a digital or speculum examination when the placenta or its vessels might be located at or near the cervical os. *(Marx et al., 2002, Chap. 172)*

27. **(D)**

28. **(C)**

Explanations 27 and 28

PV is an autoimmune blistering skin disease that occurs mainly in elderly patients. Affected patients have circulating autoantibodies against keratinocyte adhesion molecules (desmogleins). The typical skin lesion of pemphigus is a flaccid blister that ruptures to leave large erosions,

especially on the head, neck, axillae, and trunk. Mortality in untreated patients is often due to bacteremia (or fungemia) that occurs in the setting of a severely compromised cutaneous barrier. Most patients with PV have oral mucosal erosions; other mucosae may be affected as well.

Skin biopsy of a pemphigus blister shows an intraepidermal split. Biopsy for direct immunofluorescence reveals intercellular deposits of IgG in the epidermis. By contrast, the skin biopsy of a patient with Stevens-Johnson syndrome shows a subepidermal split. In addition, the cutaneous manifestations of Stevens-Johnson syndrome are unlikely to continue to progress 3 weeks after the causative drug has been discontinued.

Standard therapy for PV is oral prednisone at an initial dose of about 1 mg/kg/day. Patients may also be treated with a steroid-sparing agent such as azathioprine. *(Braunwald et al., 2001, pp. 311–312)*

29. **(D)** Oliguria is defined as urine output less than 400 cc/day and results from prerenal, renal, or postrenal failure. Prerenal failure is the most common type following surgery and usually results from a relative state of hypovolemia. Renal causes include intrinsic renal pathology, such as acute tubular necrosis (ATN). Postrenal causes are obstructive in nature, as in those with benign prostate hyperplasia or ureteral stone. The distinction between prerenal and renal oliguria can be made based on laboratory data. In prerenal oliguria, the kidneys function to preserve water and sodium, which results in a highly concentrated urine with Na sparing. FeNa is characteristically less than one in prerenal failure, as in the chart *(Schwartz et al., 1999, p. 503)*:

	Prerenal	Renal
Urine osmolarity	>500	<350
U/P osmolarity	>1.25	<1.1
U/P creatinine	>40	<20
Urine Na	<20	>40
FeNa	<1%	>1%

30. **(C)** This patient has heparin-induced thrombocytopenia with thrombosis (HITT). Heparin-induced thrombocytopenia (HIT) is estimated

to occur in about 1% of individuals exposed to heparin. The diagnosis should be considered in any individual who develops thrombocytopenia (platelet count less than 100,000/µL) or a fall in platelet count greater than 50% after the initiation of heparin. Thromboembolic complications (arterial and/or venous) can occur in 10–70% of patient with HIT. HIT seem to be caused by the development of heparin-dependent antibodies that recognize platelet factor 4 and heparin complexes. The mainstay of treatment is the cessation of heparin. The use of low molecular heparin is not recommended because in vitro cross-reactivity surpasses 90%. *(Hoffman et al., 2000, p. 2052)*

31. **(A)** Hemangioma is the most common benign lesion of the liver. Unlike hepatic adenomas, malignant degeneration does not occur and spontaneous rupture is rare. Most patients are asymptomatic and the lesion is found incidentally. Large lesions, however, can result in a palpable right upper quadrant mass and abdominal pain. In addition, platelet trapping in giant hemangiomas may result in thrombocytopenia.

The diagnosis of hepatic hemangiomas can usually be made on CT scan with the classic findings of a rim-enhancing lesion with central filling. If needed, additional studies including a T2-weighted MRI, technetium-labeled red blood cell scan, and arteriogram can be helpful to confirm the diagnosis. Percutaneous biopsy often provides the histologic diagnosis but is rarely indicated and is associated with the complication of bleeding.

Most hepatic hemangiomas should not be excised. Even large lesions followed for long periods of time show no notable increase in size or clinical manifestations. The potential for rupture is minimal and should not constitute an indication for excision. Pain, mass effect, significant growth, platelets trapping, and early rupture are indications for surgical excision. In these patients, large lesions may necessitate anatomic resection, but enucleation is often feasible. *(Schwartz et al., 1999, pp. 1407–1409)*

32. **(A)**

33. **(B)**

Explanations 32 and 33

Sturge-Weber syndrome is a neurocutaneous syndrome which involves port-wine stains, typically in V_1 or V_2 (trigeminal nerve) distribution. The port-wine stain usually is unilateral and respects the midline. There is a concomitant leptomeningeal vascular anomaly and underlying cerebral cortical atrophy. Seizures develop in most patients during the first year of life. Typically, they are tonic-clonic in nature and may involve the contralateral side of the facial nevus. In at least 50% of children, mental retardation or severe learning disabilities will be present. *(Behrman, p. 2018; Jones, 1997, p. 495)*

34. **(C)** ATN is a clinico-pathologic entity characterized pathologically by destruction of tubular epithelium and clinically by acute renal failure. ATN is the most common cause of acute renal failure. ATN can be divided into ischemic, in which the causes are shock, burns, and crush injury, and toxic tubular necrosis, caused by heavy metals, drugs, and organic solvents. The clinical course has an initial phase followed by a maintenance phase in which there is a decrease in urine output (oliguria), elevated BUN, hyperkalemia, and metabolic acidosis. All of this is followed by a recovery phase. *(Cotran et al., 1999, pp. 969–971)*

35. **(E)** Toxic nodular goiter, also known as Plummer's disease, is a consequence of one or more thyroid nodules secreting inappropriately high levels of thyroid hormone independently of thyroid-stimulating hormone (TSH) control. Hyperthyroidism in patients with toxic nodular goiter is milder than in those with Graves' disease and the condition is not accompanied by extrathyroidal manifestations such as ophthalmopathy, pretibial myxedema, vitiligo, or thyroid acropathy.

Patients with toxic multinodular goiter are older at presentation than those with Graves' disease. The thyroid gland goiter characteristically has one or more nodules on palpation. Local symptoms of compression, such as dysphasia and dyspnea, may occur. The diagnosis is suggested by a thorough history and physical examination and confirmed by documenting suppressed serum TSH level and raised serum thyroid hormone level.

Therapy with antithyroid medications or beta-blockers may help alleviate symptoms but is not definitive treatment, especially if the patient possesses local symptoms of compression. Radioiodine therapy is not as effective as in Graves' disease because of lower uptake. I^{131} ablation may be used in patients who are unsuitable for surgery but, because of the high failure rate, local resection is considered the treatment of choice. For solitary nodules, nodulectomy or thyroid lobectomy is the treatment of choice. (Schwartz et al., 1999, p. 1674)

36. (B)

37. (B)

Explanations 36 and 37

HSP is also commonly referred to as anaphyllactoid purpura. HSP is a small vessel vasculitis. The rash of HSP is very characteristic and is commonly located on the lower extremities and buttocks. Abdominal pain, joint pain, and nephritis are common features of the disease as well. These complaints are usually self-limiting. Symptomatic treatment including hydration and pain control with acetaminophen may be given. Avoidance of competitive activities and elevation of the lower extremities may help reduce any local edema. (Behrman, p. 827; Rudolph et al., 2003, pp. 842–844)

38. (A)

39. (B)

40. (B)

Explanations 38 through 40

This individual is being treated with an antipsychotic medication. The presumed mechanism of action involves the blockade of dopamine receptors in the mesolimbic and mesocortical regions of the brain. Dopamine blockade in other areas, such as the nigrostriatal pathways, accounts for many of the side effects

seen with this class of medications. Akathisia is described as an inner feeling of restlessness, which usually appears after several weeks of treatment with antipsychotics. Conversion disorder is the unconscious production of neurologic deficits due to unconscious conflict. Antipsychotic-induced parkinsonism also appears after several weeks of treatment and is characterized by the triad of a resting (pill-rolling) tremor, bradykinesia, and rigidity (either lead-pipe or cogwheel). Tardive dyskinesia is a long-term consequence of chronic antipsychotic use. It involves involuntary choreoathetoid movements, especially of the face, mouth, tongue, and hands. It occurs in up to 25% of patients medicated over 4 years and often progresses over time. Acute dystonic reactions, as in this case, occur within hours to days of initiating or increasing an antipsychotic medication and are categorized by the painful contraction of muscles.

Although consideration should always be given to either lowering the dose of or switching to another medication if intolerable side effects occur, discontinuing the risperidone will not immediately treat the dystonic reaction and will increase the risk for a relapse of psychotic symptoms. Injection of haloperidol or lorazepam may be indicated in the management of an acutely agitated patient. In this example, the individual is without current psychotic symptomatology and is anxious due to his painful muscle spasms. Injection of haloperidol may also worsen his dystonia. Reassurance and suggestion are often effective in managing conversion symptoms, but acute dystonia requires immediate treatment with an anticholinergic agent such as benztropine or an antihistaminic agent such as diphenhydramine.

This patient is exhibiting symptoms and signs of akathisia. Adding a mood stabilizer or increasing the dose of antipsychotic might be appropriate if he were showing indications of manic excitement or psychotic agitation, but his psychotic symptoms appear to be in remission. Increasing the risperidone may actually worsen his akathisia. Decreasing the current dose or switching to another antipsychotic would be indicated if he were experiencing intolerable side effects. Both of these options could also result in a relapse of his psychosis. Given the apparent remission of his symptoms on risperidone, the most reasonable approach would be to add a beta-adrenergic blocker such as propranolol which has been shown to be beneficial in treating akathisia. *(Sadock and Sadock, 2003, pp. 992–995, 1058)*

41. (E)

42. (E)

43. (A)

44. (B)

Explanations 41 through 44

This patient is presenting with symptoms and signs of congestive heart failure. She has evidence of both left and right ventricular failure, with orthopnea, hypoxia, and peripheral edema. Along with peripheral edema, signs that one would be expected to find on physical examination would include pulmonary rales, elevated jugular venous pressure, hepatojugular reflux, and an S_3 gallop. This is a "protodiastolic" sound that would be expected to occur 0.13–0.16 seconds after the second heart sound. These sounds may occur in healthy children and young adults, but are rare in healthy adults over the age of 40 and are common in persons of any age in heart failure. Tracheal deviation may be expected to occur in a person with a tension pneumothorax. A pericardial friction rub, while possible in the setting of heart failure, is less likely to occur than an S_3 gallop and may lead toward a consideration of the diagnosis of pericarditis. A diastolic murmur along the left sternal border may be associated with, among other valvular abnormalities, aortic insufficiency. This may be a specific cause of heart failure but, again, is much less likely to be heard than an S_3 gallop in this setting. Perioral cyanosis is unlikely to occur at an oxygen saturation of 91%. In a hypoxic patient presenting with dyspnea, the first drug to be administered should be oxygen. In the primary survey of emergency patients, the mnemonic "ABC"—

for airway, breathing, and circulation—should always come first. The other medications listed, which all may play a role in the management of this patient in the acute or long-term settings, would be appropriate after assuring airway, breathing, and circulation.

Alpha-adrenergic antagonists have been shown to be no better than placebo in their reduction in mortality in heart failure. Dihydropyridine class calcium channel blockers have not been shown to produce improvement in congestive heart failure. Some agents in this class may worsen symptoms and actually increase mortality. Newer dihydropyridines—felodipine and amlodipine—do not appear to worsen mortality, so they may be safe to use in this setting. In patients with sinus rhythm and reduced ejection fraction, digoxin is often used. Study results have been conflicting; however mortality does not seem to be affected by the use of digoxin in this setting. The use of warfarin in systolic dysfunction is controversial. While many patients with moderate-to-severe left ventricular dysfunction are given warfarin in order to reduce the risk of thromboembolic events, evidence of improved outcomes is, at present, lacking. Warfarin would be indicated in those with atrial fibrillation, visualized thrombus, or previous thromboembolic disease. Multiple studies have consistently shown an improvement in the natural history of congestive heart failure, along with reductions in mortality, with the use of ACE inhibitors. Their use should be considered first-line in all patients with congestive heart failure due to systolic dysfunction. *(Braunwald et al., 2001, pp. 503–543, 570–582, 645)*

The use of metformin is contraindicated in the setting of congestive heart failure that requires drug treatment. The thiazolidinediones are also contraindicated for New York Heart Association (NYHA) class III and IV heart failure and must be used with caution in class I and II heart failure. The other diabetic medications listed may be used in the clinical setting of congestive heart failure. Caution may be required, however, in the setting of renal or hepatic insufficiencies that may be associated with congestive heart failure.

45. (D)

46. (B)

Explanations 45 and 46

Several scales and criteria have been devised to assess the prognosis of patients with pancreatitis. The most widely used is Ranson's criteria. Ranson's criteria are not diagnostic; however, they help estimate the severity of the disease, the prognosis, and serve as a guide to management decisions. Ranson's criteria are divided into two groups. The first group contains five criteria that are used to assess the severity in the first 24 hours of admission. This group includes: age above 55 years, WBC count higher than 16,000/mm^3, serum glucose higher than 200 mg/dL, serum AST higher than 250 IU/L, serum LDH higher than 350 IU/L. The second group is the 48-hour criteria (the second day of admission) and includes: hematocrit decrease more than 10%, increase in BUN level of more than 5 mg/dL, serum calcium level lower than 8 mg/dL, partial pressure of oxygen in arterial blood lower than 60 mmHg, base deficit higher than 4 meq/L, and fluid sequestration of more than 6 L.

If a patient meets 0–2 of the criteria, the mortality rate is only 2%, whereas the presence of 3–4 criteria bears a mortality rate of 15%. If a patient meets 5–6 criteria, the mortality rate is 40%, and if patient meets 7 criteria, the mortality rate is nearly 100%. Patients presenting with three or more of the Ranson's criteria should be admitted to the ICU for aggressive resuscitation, bowel rest, NG tube decompression, and serial laboratory and physical examination. Surgery is reserved for complications of pancreatitis, including pancreatic abscess formation, hemorrhagic pancreatitis, infected pancreatic necrosis, or recalcitrant disease with deterioration of the patient's general status. (*Schwartz et al., 1999, pp. 1476–1478*)

47. (D) Common causes of sudden, painless vision loss lasting more than 24 hours would include retinal detachment, retinal artery or vein occlusion, and ischemic optic neuritis. Cataracts and open angle glaucoma would be among the most common causes of painless vision loss that is gradual over the course of months or years. Acute angle closure glaucoma is a cause of acute, painful vision loss. Corneal abrasions are usually painful and associated with eye redness. (*Kunimoto et al., 2004, Chap. 1*)

48. (C) Hereditary spherocytosis (HS) is a hemolytic anemia characterized by abnormal flexibility and shape of red cells, due to a deficiency or dysfunction of multiple membrane proteins. Clinically, patients with HS can vary from having an asymptomatic condition with almost normal hemoglobin levels to severe hemolysis and anemia, leading to life-threatening jaundice and congestive heart failure in neonates. Patients who maintain mild anemia are usually diagnosed later in life during evaluation for unrelated conditions. Some patients may develop bilirubin gallstones at early age that require cholecystectomy. The hallmark for the diagnosis of HS is the presence of sphrerocytes in the peripheral smear. In addition to the indices of hemolysis (reticulocytosis, elevated LDH, and elevated unconjugated bilirubin), the red cell osmotic fragility is characteristically increased. Splenectomy in these individuals is the main treatment producing improvement in red cell survival and a rise in hemoglobin levels. (*Hoffman et al., 2000, pp. 584–585*)

BIBLIOGRAPHY

AAP Task Force on Sudden Infant Death Syndrome. The changing concept of sudden infant death syndrome: diagnostic coding shifts, controversies regarding the sleeping environment, and new variables to consider in reducing risk. *Pediatrics* 2005;116(5):1245–1255.

American Diabetes Association. Standards of medical care in diabetes. *Diabetes Care* 2004;27:S15–S35.

American Psychiatric Association. *Diagnostic and Statistical Manual of Mental Disorders*, 4th ed., Text Revision. Washington, DC: American Psychiatric Association, 2000.

Beckmann CRB, Ling FW, Laube DW, et al. *Obstetrics and Gynecology*, 4th ed. Baltimore, MD: Lippincot Williams & Wilkins, 2002.

Behrman RE, Kliegman RM, Jensen HD. *Nelson Textbook of Pediatrics*, 17th ed. Philadelphia, PA: W.B. Saunders, 2004.

Braunwald E, Hauser SL, Jameson JL, et al. *Harrison's Principles of Internal Medicine*, 15th ed. New York, NY: McGraw-Hill, 2001.

Braunwald E. *Heart Disease: A Textbook of Cardiovascular Medicine,* 6th ed. Philadelphia, PA: W.B. Saunders, 2001.

Cameron JL, ed. *Current Surgical Therapy*, 8th ed. St. Louis, MO: C.V. Mosby, 2004.

Chez R. Emergency oral contraception. *ACOG Pract Bull* 2001;(25).

Cotran RS, Kumar V, Collins T. *Robbins Pathologic Basis of Disease*, 6th ed. Philadelphia, PA: W.B. Saunders, 1999.

Cunningham FG, Gant NF, Leveno KJ, et al. *Williams Obstetrics*, 21st ed. New York, NY: McGraw-Hill, 2001.

Hoffman R, Benz EJ Jr, Shattil SJ, et al. *Hematology: Basic Principles and Practice*, 3rd ed. New York, NY: Churchill Livingstone, 2000.

Jarrell BE, Carabasi RA III, Radomski JS. *National Medical Series for Independent Study, Surgery,* 4th ed. Philadelphia, PA: Lippincott Williams & Wilkins, 2000, p. 464.

Jones KL, ed. *Smith's Recognizable Pattern of Human Malformations*, 5th ed. Philadelphia, PA: W.B. Saunders, 1997.

Kunimoto DY, Rapuano CJ, Friedberg MA, et al. *The Wills Eye Manual: Office and Emergency Room Diagnosis and Treatment of Eye Disease*, 4th ed. Philadelphia, PA: Lippincott Williams & Wilkins, 2004.

Larsen PR, Kronenberg HM, Melmed S, et al. *Williams Textbook of Endocrinology*, 10th ed. Philadelphia, PA: W.B. Saunders, 2003.

Marx J, Hockenberger R, Walls R. *Rosen's Emergency Medicine: Concepts and Clinical Practice*, 5th ed. St. Louis, MO: Mosby, Chap. 172, 2002.

Ruddy S, Harris ED Jr, Sledge CB, et al. *Kelley's Textbook of Rheumatology*, 6th ed. Philadelphia, PA: W.B. Saunders, 2001.

Rudolph CD, Rudolph AM, Hostetter MK, et al., eds. *Rudolph's Pediatrics*, 21st ed. New York, NY: McGraw-Hill, 2003.

Sadock BJ, Sadock VA. *Kaplan and Sadock's Synopsis of Psychiatry*, 9th ed. Philadelphia, PA: Lippincott Williams & Wilkins, 2003.

Schwartz SI, Shires GT, Spencer FC, et al., eds. *Principles of Surgery*, 7th ed. New York, NY: McGraw-Hill, 1999.

Townsend CM, Beauchamp RD, Evers BM, et al., eds. *Sabiston Textbook of Surgery: The Biological Basis of Modern Surgical Practice*, 17th ed. Philadelphia, PA: W.B. Saunders, 2004.

USPSTF: www.preventiveservices.ahrq.gov.

CHAPTER 11

Practice Test 4
Questions

Read each question carefully and in the order in which it is presented. Then select the one best response option of the choices offered. More than one option may be partially correct. You must select ONE BEST answer.

Setting I: Office/Health Center

You see patients in two locations: at your office suite, which is adjacent to a hospital, and at a community-based health center. Your office practice is a primary care generalist group. Most of the patients you see are from your own practice and are appearing for regularly scheduled return visits. Occasionally, you will encounter a patient whose primary care is managed by one of your associates. Reference may be made to the patient's medical records. Known patients may be managed by the telephone. You may have to respond to questions about information appearing in the public media, which will require interpretation of the medical literature. The laboratory and radiology departments have a full range of services available.

Questions 1 through 3

A 19-year-old African American male presents to your office for a precollege sports examination. He is planning to be on the college basketball team. He is playing basketball 5 days per week for 1–2 hours each day. He has been healthy. He complains today of mild right flank discomfort which comes and goes. He denies any fever, chills, dysuria, or polyuria. He has no history of significant trauma or previous hematuria. He smokes one pack of cigarettes every 2–3 days, drinks 4–6 beers on weekends, and denies recreational drug abuse. His last diphtheria-tetanus (dT) shot was at age 14. His examination is normal. You order a urinalysis which shows 8 red blood cells (RBCs) per high-power field (HPF). Review of his chart shows that he had 6 RBCs/HPF in a urinalysis 6 months ago but he never returned for the requested follow-up examination.

 1. What is the appropriate next step at this point?

(A) observation
(B) repeat urinalysis in 3 months
(C) empiric antibiotic treatment of urinary tract infection (UTI)
(D) intravenous pyelogram
(E) plain abdominal x-ray

2. During this visit, what should you do?

(A) counsel patient regarding low back pain prevention
(B) counsel patient regarding skin cancer prevention
(C) provide alcohol abuse counseling
(D) give dT booster
(E) advise patient to do frequent testicular examination for testicular cancer screening

3. The number one cause of death in this patient's age group is which of the following?

(A) acquired immune deficiency syndrome (AIDS)
(B) homicide
(C) suicide
(D) motor vehicle accident
(E) cardiovascular disease

Questions 4 and 5

A 42-year-old woman is referred to the clinic after recently moving to the area. She presents with numerous chief complaints including severe headaches since childhood, arthritis pain, atypical chest pain, and chronic lower back pain. She also describes a history of intermittent diarrhea and unusual food intolerances. She has had irregular menstrual periods since menarche, and she often becomes dizzy and unsteady on her feet. Her large medical chart documents frequent outpatient appointments, a number of hospitalizations, abundant tests and procedures, and multiple surgeries. Despite her extensive evaluations, there have not been definitive diagnoses or sufficient treatments to adequately address all of her difficulties. She clearly appears in significant distress regarding the amount of her suffering and perceived lack of attention she has received.

4. Which of the following is her most likely diagnosis?

   (A) conversion disorder
   (B) hypochondriasis
   (C) pain disorder
   (D) somatization disorder
   (E) undifferentiated somatoform disorder

5. Which of the following is the most useful approach in her management?

   (A) admission to the hospital for extensive workup
   (B) confrontation about the psychological nature of her symptoms
   (C) reassurance that a diagnosis will eventually be found
   (D) referral to various outpatient specialists
   (E) regularly scheduled follow-up appointments

Questions 6 through 8

A 60-year-old White female presents to your office with the complaints of aching shoulders and sides of her hips. These symptoms have persisted for the past 4 weeks and have prompted her to avoid her water aerobics class at her local YMCA. She has lost 15 lbs in the past 4 weeks but denies any joint symptoms.

Her physical examination demonstrates no loss of joint range or mobility, no synovitis in any joint, and tenderness of the neck and shoulders. Her motor strength in the upper and lower extremities is normal. Laboratory testing is significant only for an erythrocyte sedimentation rate (ESR) of 99 mm/h, a negative antinuclear antibody (ANA), and a normal creatine phosphokinase (CPK).

6. Her clinical history and examination suggest which of the following diagnoses?

   (A) polymyositis
   (B) hypothyrodism
   (C) polymyalgia rheumatica
   (D) osteoarthritis of the neck and shoulders
   (E) fibromyalgia

7. What would be the most appropriate medical management for this patient?

   (A) thyroid hormone replacement
   (B) analgesic such as acetaminophen
   (C) prednisone in a dose of 20 mg daily
   (D) antidepressant medication (Amitryptiline 50 mg daily)
   (E) muscle relaxant (cyclobenzaprine 10 mg daily)

8. The patient returns to your clinic 5 days later saying that the symptoms are still present. In addition, the patient reports that she has been having headaches and blurriness of her vision. Laboratory studies demonstrate an ESR of 100 mm/h. These additional symptoms suggest which of the following diagnoses?

   (A) rheumatoid arthritis
   (B) giant cell arteritis
   (C) systemic lupus erythematosus
   (D) hypothyroidism
   (E) the patient is depressed and is amplifying her symptoms

9. A 6-month-old female is brought to your clinic for a well-child examination. Her height and weight are below the 50th percentile. The child has otherwise been healthy. On examination, the child has good color and is in no acute distress. During auscultation, you hear a loud, harsh, and

blowing holosystolic murmur over the left sternal border. Which of the following would be the most likely cause of your clinical findings?

(A) ventricular septal defect (VSD)
(B) tetralogy of Fallot
(C) transposition of the great vessels
(D) truncus arteriosis
(E) pulmonic atresia

Questions 10 through 12

A previously healthy 27-year-old female comes to your office with complaints of recurrent headaches over the past few days. She became alarmed when she recently visited a health fair and was told that she had elevated blood pressure (BP). She was started on oral contraceptives (OCPs) after the birth of her last child 1 year ago. In that year, she has gained 20 lbs and has developed bilateral ankle edema that worsens at night. She missed her last two menstrual periods and, this morning, she woke up with some vaginal bleeding. She wants to know what to do because at this point of her life "she just can't afford to get pregnant."

10. Which of the following would be the most appropriate next step?

(A) Advise that she stop the OCPs and get a urine pregnancy test.
(B) Obtain a urine pregnancy test but continue the OCPs.
(C) Reassure her that all of her symptoms are likely caused by the onset of menses.
(D) Emphasize to her that the headaches are likely due to social stressors and that her weight will likely stabilize in time.
(E) Recommend that she be started on diuretic medication to control her BP and reduce her edema.

11. Which of the following is an absolute contraindication to taking OCPs?

(A) a diagnosis of major depression
(B) a history of migraine headaches
(C) a history of oligomenorrhea
(D) smoking after the age of 35
(E) a history of any hemolytic anemia

12. Which of the following is considered an adverse effect of OCPs?

(A) thrombocytopenia
(B) ovarian cancer
(C) cholelithiasis
(D) irreversible infertility
(E) endometrial cancer

13. A 19-year-old college student is found to have an elevated serum calcium on routine physical examination. She has a family history of hypercalcemia that has not resulted in any known symptoms. Further workup reveals a slightly elevated serum parathyroid hormone with depressed levels of serum phosphate. A 24-hour urine calcium excretion is obtained and is low. Which of the following is the correct diagnosis?

(A) familial hypocalciuric hypercalcemia (FHH)
(B) primary hyperparathyroidism
(C) secondary hyperparathyroidism
(D) tertiary hyperparathyroidism
(E) metastatic bone cancer

Questions 14 through 16

A 44-year-old divorced male is referred to the clinic for ongoing management of his hypertension and hypercholesterolemia. He begins the evaluation by remarking, "I came here because I heard you are the best. Those other doctors didn't like me very much. Besides, they don't know what they are doing." He subsequently admits to poor compliance with taking his medications or maintaining a low salt, low fat diet. He blames this on his boss, whom he calls a "task master . . . he works me to the bone, and I don't have time to eat properly." He denies pervasive depressive symptoms but claims to be "lonely and bored." He admits to "mood swings," where he will be "happy," but within minutes to hours can become depressed and feel hopeless. He describes lifelong difficulties with his temper, and he has frequently broken items of value when angry. He is not in a stable relationship but does admit to repeated promiscuity with women, where he will impulsively purchase expensive jewelry to curry favor with them in order to have sexual intercourse.

14. Which of the following is his most likely diagnosis?

(A) avoidant personality disorder
(B) borderline personality disorder
(C) dependent personality disorder
(D) paranoid personality disorder
(E) schizoid personality disorder

15. The above patient's comments demonstrate which prominent defense mechanism?

(A) denial
(B) displacement
(C) intellectualization
(D) splitting
(E) sublimation

16. Which of the following medications would be the most appropriate first-line treatment for his symptoms?

(A) clonazepam (Klonopin)
(B) haloperidol (Haldol)
(C) lithium
(D) sertraline (Zoloft)
(E) valproic acid (Depakene)

17. Which of the following patients with thyroid cancer has the best prognosis?

(A) a 16-year-old child with papillary carcinoma metastatic to three cervical lymph nodes
(B) a 42-year-old male with papillary carcinoma
(C) a 52-year-old female with follicular carcinoma confined to the thyroid capsule
(D) a 44-year-male with an occult focus of medullary carcinoma found incidentally after a subtotal thyroidectomy
(E) a 53-year-old female with a Hurthle cell carcinoma

18. A 36-year-old patient presents to her physician for a prescription for OCP. What medical history elicited from this patient would be an absolute contraindication to prescribing her OCP?

(A) hypertension
(B) type II diabetes mellitus
(C) epilepsy
(D) cigarette smoker
(E) menstrual migraines (without aura)

Questions 19 and 20

You are evaluating a 4-month-old girl for persistently poor weight gain. The mother relates that the child is "a very good eater" but cannot seem to keep weight on and that she has seemed to have an increase in her "spitting up." She was born at term with an uneventful perinatal history. On examination, she appears as a vigorous but wasted infant with decreased adiposity. Her weight and height are both below the 3rd percentile. Her examination is otherwise essentially normal. Laboratory studies include the following:

Na 135	K 5.2	Cl 111	Bicarbonate 16
BUN 15	Creatinine 0.9	Glucose 79	
Urinalysis:	Specific gravity 1.010	pH 6.0	Blood and protein (–)

19. What is the most likely explanation for this child's poor weight gain?

(A) pyloric stenosis
(B) formula intolerance
(C) duodenal stenosis
(D) gastroesophageal reflux
(E) renal tubular acidosis (RTA)

20. Which of the following would help confirm the diagnosis?

(A) an upper gastrointestinal (GI) contrast study
(B) an upper GI endoscopy
(C) a trial of sodium bicarbonate to assess urinary pH
(D) a trial of metoclopramide (Reglan)
(E) a trial of an elemental formula

21. A 55-year-old woman presents to her internist complaining of urinary frequency and irritation for the past 2 months. Last weekend your partner called her in a prescription for trimethoprim/sulfamethoxazole (Bactrim DS) for a presumed UTI. Her symptoms have persisted. In addition, she has noted increasing vaginal dryness and irritation during intercourse. These problems have been exacerbated since she discontinued her oral hormone replacement therapy last year. On examination, you would expect to find which of the following?

(A) white, curdy vaginal discharge
(B) thin, pale vulvar skin and vaginal mucosa
(C) a fungating, friable lesion on her cervix
(D) a retained tampon
(E) a vesicovaginal fistula

22. Which of the following is true regarding parental refusal for vaccination administration?

(A) As some vaccines are unsafe, parents may "opt out" of immunizations due to personal preference.
(B) If the parents decline immunizations, then all care to the child should be curtailed.
(C) If parents refuse immunizations, and this refusal is deemed to harm the child, state authorities may need to be involved.
(D) If the parents refuse immunizations, they should be administered to the child while the parent is unaware.
(E) Immunization refusal, in and of itself, is considered medical neglect.

23. A 25-year-old woman presents with bilateral galactorrhea, fatigue, and weight gain. She had menarche at age 12, had normal monthly periods until age 20, and then was placed on birth control pills for contraception until 18 months ago. She subsequently had a normal pregnancy with vaginal delivery 6 months ago. She nursed the child for 3 months and restarted her birth control pills. She also started a vigorous exercise program to lose weight. However, over the past 3 months, she has felt fatigued and has gained about 15 lbs. She has noticed muscle cramps while exercising, dry skin, and persistent hair loss. She also has felt depressed. On examination, her BP is 130/90, heart rate 60 bpm. There is a rough texture to her skin and her deep tendon reflexes are slow to relax.

Labs:	Total T4	4.5 (5–12 µg/dL)
	T3-resin uptake	20% (25–35%)
	Free thyroid index	0.9 (1.2–4.2)
	Thyroid-stimulating hormone (TSH)	35 (0.4–5 µU/mL)
	Prolactin	40 (5–15 ng/mL)

Which of the following would be the most appropriate next step?

(A) MRI of pituitary
(B) nuclear thyroid scan
(C) stop OCP and repeat studies in 6 weeks
(D) initiate levothyroxine therapy
(E) thyroid replacement hormone (TRH) stimulation test

24. An 18-year-old primigravid woman had a complete hydatidiform mole evacuated by suction curettage. Her preevacuation serum human chorionic gonadotropin (hCG) level was 125,000 mIU/mL and her uterus was 22 weeks' gestational size. Postevacuation serum quantitative hCG levels were obtained every 2 weeks. Her hCG level decreased to 25,000 mIU/mL at 2 weeks, but then began to climb and is currently 32,000 mIU/mL after 4 weeks. Physical examination suggests a boggy uterus only. What is the most appropriate step in management at this point?

(A) repeat dilatation and curettage
(B) weekly hCG testing
(C) computed tomography (CT) scan of the head, chest, abdomen, and pelvis
(D) hysterectomy
(E) pelvic ultrasound

Setting II: Emergency Department and Inpatient Facilities

You encounter patients in the emergency department and inpatient facilities, including the hospital, the adjacent nursing home/extended-care facility, and detoxification unit. Most patients in the emergency department are new to you and are seeking urgent care, but occasionally, you arrange to meet there with a known patient who has telephoned you. You have general admitting privileges to the hospital, including to the children's and women's services. On occasion you see patients in the critical care unit. Postoperative patients are usually seen in their rooms unless the recovery room is specified. You may also be called to see patients in the psychiatric unit. There is a short-stay unit where you may see patients undergoing same-day operations or being held for observation. Also available to you are a full range of social services, including rape crisis intervention, family support, and security assistance backed up by local police.

25. A 74-year-old female, with a history of hypertension and hypothyroidism, is admitted with easy bruising, guaiac positive stools, and anemia (hemoglobin 8.1 g/dL). Screening coagulation tests reveal a prolonged activated partial thromboplastin time (aPTT) with a normal prothrombin time (PT) and platelet count. What is the next step in the diagnosis of this woman's problem?

    (A) perform upper and lower endoscopy with biopsies
    (B) check factors II, VII, IX, and X levels
    (C) check factor VII level
    (D) check factors XI, VII, IX, and VIII levels
    (E) check an aPTT 1:1 mix with normal plasma

26. A 42-year-old male with extensive Crohn's disease undergoes a near complete resection of the ileum. A deficiency of which of the following vitamin is likely to result?

    (A) niacin
    (B) thiamine

    (C) vitamin B_{12}
    (D) vitamin C
    (E) vitamin B_6

Questions 27 through 29

A 55-year-old female presented with a 3-week history of feeling a lump in her breast on self-examination. The mass was painless and she did not notice skin changes, nipple discharge, or retraction. There was no family history of breast or ovarian cancer. The patient was otherwise healthy. On physical examination, a hard mass was found on the left upper quadrant of the breast measuring approximately 2 cm in diameter. After a mammography and clinical testing she underwent an excisional biopsy. The photomicrograph shown in Figure 11-1 is a representative histologic section representing the tumor mass.

FIG. 11-1 (*Courtesy of Edison Catalano, MD.*)

27. What would be the diagnosis on the palpable tumor seen on the microphotograph?

    (A) infiltrating ductal carcinoma, poorly differentiated (grade III)
    (B) infiltrating ductal carcinoma low grade
    (C) microinvasive ductal carcinoma, papillary variant

(D)   atypical ductal hyperplasia

(E)   colloid carcinoma (mucinous secreting)

28.   What is the most important prognostic finding in carcinoma of the breast?

(A)   presence of estrogen receptors

(B)   lymphatic invasion

(C)   cellular anaplasia

(D)   metastasis to the regional lymph nodes

(E)   nipple retraction

29.   With which of the following breast tumors will you find axillary metastasis?

(A)   atypical lobular hyperplasia

(B)   lobular carcinoma in situ

(C)   atypical ductal hyperplasia

(D)   tubular adenoma

(E)   infiltrating ductal carcinoma

30.   A patient with uncontrolled diabetes and chronic renal failure undergoes an uneventful debridement of a necrotic venous ulcer. On the second postoperative night, she is noted to have persistent bleeding and a prolonged bleeding time. Which of the following is the best intervention at this time?

(A)   compression dressing and subcutaneous injection of vitamin K

(B)   platelet transfusion

(C)   intravenous desmopressin (DDAVP)

(D)   transfuse fresh frozen plasma

(E)   correct hyperglycemic state

31.   With pregnancy, physiologic alterations occur in nearly all organ systems. Regarding the hematologic system, which of the following is true?

(A)   The blood volume increases by 100% by the end of pregnancy.

(B)   The maternal red cell mass increases by 50% by the end of pregnancy.

(C)   The total iron demands for a term pregnancy to meet both maternal and fetal needs are 2500 mg.

(D)   Supplementation with 30 mg of elemental iron per day during pregnancy effectively prevents iron depletion.

(E)   Mean platelet counts in pregnant and nonpregnant women are the same.

32.   Which of the following is an indication to resect a Meckel's diverticulum found incidentally during a laparoscopic appendectomy in a 52-year-old male?

(A)   any Meckel's diverticulum found incidentally should be removed

(B)   location within 12 in. of the ileocecal valve

(C)   history of rectal bleeding

(D)   presence of a wide neck

(E)   presence of firm tissue at the base of the diverticulum

Questions 33 and 34

33.   A 34-year-old male undergoes an uneventful excision of a parathyroid adenoma. The following postoperative day, he complains of numbness around his lips. Which of the following is the most likely cause of this symptom?

(A)   hypocalcemia secondary to hypomagnesemia

(B)   hypocalcemia due to acute renal failure

(C)   hypocalcemia due to hungry bone syndrome

(D)   hypocalcemia due to inadvertent injury to the recurrent laryngeal nerve

(E)   postoperative hematoma of the neck

34.   Which of the following is the most appropriate intervention?

(A)   oral calcium gluconate

(B)   intravenous rehydration with normal saline

(C)   intravenous magnesium sulfate infusion

(D)   blood transfusion

(E)   reassurance and close observation

35. A 7-year-old girl presents to the emergency room (ER) with complaints of fatigue and pallor. She was treated by her primary care physician (PCP) earlier in the week for an upper respiratory infection. Your examination reveals splenomegaly and bruising on her upper extremities. You order laboratory work that shows a WBC of 11,000, hemoglobin of 6 g/dL, and a platelet count of 40,000. A Coombs' test is also positive. What is the most likely cause?

(A) immune thrombocytopenic purpura (ITP)

(B) Henoch-Schönlein purpura

(C) Evans syndrome

(D) meningococcemia

(E) hemolytic uremic syndrome

Questions 36 through 48

A 78-year-old female is transferred from the nursing home with nausea, vomiting, abdominal distention, and obstipation for the last 3 days. On examination, she is somnolent and tachycardic. Her abdomen is distended, tympanic, and diffusely tender. An abdominal x-ray is obtained and is shown in Figure 11-2.

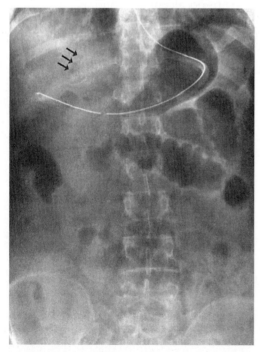

FIG. 11-2 (*Reproduced, with permission, from Chen MYM, Pope TL Jr, Ott DJ.* Basic Radiology. *New York, NY: McGraw-Hill, 2004, p. 220.*)

36. These findings are most consistent with which of the following?

(A) gallstone ileus

(B) pancreatitis

(C) cholangitis

(D) small bowel neoplasm

(E) perforated appendicitis

37. The patient is at risk for which of the following?

(A) ascending cholangitis

(B) small bowel perforation

(C) colonic perforation

(D) Ogilvie syndrome

(E) massive lower GI bleed

38. What is the most appropriate intervention?

(A) IV fluids, gastric decompression, antibiotics, and close observation

(B) endoscopic retrograde cholangiopancreatography (ERCP) with decompression of the biliary tree

(C) cholecystectomy

(D) surgical exploration with enterotomy to relieve the obstruction

(E) surgical exploration with enterotomy to relieve the obstruction and concomitant cholecystectomy

39. Which of the following conditions is the leading cause of death in the United States of infants between the ages of 1 and 12 months?

(A) bacterial meningitis

(B) congenital heart disease

(C) congenital malformation syndromes

(D) accidental poisonings

(E) sudden infant death syndrome (SIDS)

Questions 40 and 41

An 84-year-old White female presents with acute vision loss that occurred several hours ago. She has a past history of hypertension and atrial fibrillation which are both controlled. She has been generally tired lately and is not eating well.

40. Which of the following tests should be ordered first?

(A) MRI of brain and orbits with contrast

(B) carotid Doppler

(C) ESR

(D) cardiac echo

(E) complete blood count with differential and platelet count

41. Which of the following would you most likely find on fundoscopic examination?

(A) retinal hemorrhages

(B) lipid exudation

(C) cherry red spot

(D) arteriovenous (AV) nicking

(E) cotton wool spots

42. A 62-year-old male presents to the ER with severe substernal pain following a prolonged episode of retching and vomiting. Workup, including a chest x-ray (CXR), reveals minimal air in the mediastinum. Which of the following is the most appropriate intervention at this time?

(A) upper endoscopy

(B) gastrografin swallow

(C) place nasogastric and chest tubes, make NPO (nothing by mouth), and begin broad-spectrum antibiotics

(D) emergent left thoracotomy

(E) emergent right thoracotomy

43. What is the most likely infectious agent in a 4-month-old with copious nasal secretions, wheezing, and cough in the winter?

(A) group B *Streptococcus*

(B) group A *Streptococcus*

(C) respiratory syncytial virus

(D) nonpolio enterovirus

(E) *Haemophilus influenzae*

44. A 35-year-old man presents to the ER with a third-degree flame burn of his right upper extremity, anterior trunk, and right lower extremity, sparing the genitalia. What is his estimated burn percentage?

(A) 15%

(B) 25%

(C) 35%

(D) 45%

(E) 55%

Questions 45 through 48

A 50-year-old man presents to the ER following three episodes of massive hematemesis. The patient has never had prior similar episodes and is not currently bleeding. His vital signs are: temperature 98.8°F, BP 98/72 supine, 75/50 sitting up, pulse 110, respirations 17, oxygen saturation of 100% on room air. On examination, he is pale, dizzy, and weak. He has scleral icterus, spider angiomata on his chest, splenomegaly, and shifting dullness in his abdomen. His initial hematocrit is 30%. His PT is 31 seconds with an international normalized ratio (INR) of 3.1. The patient denies taking any anticoagulant medications. A GI consultation is requested.

45. Prior to upper endoscopy, what is the best initial step in the patient's management?

(A) obtain hepatitis serologies

(B) gastric lavage with nasogastric tube

(C) CT scan to rule out hepatic disease

(D) IV fluid resuscitation

(E) correction of the patient's coagulopathy

46. Upper endoscopy reveals multiple grade 3 (out of 4) varices in the esophagus. One of the larger varices has a fibrin plug over what appears to be a break in the mucosa and is oozing fresh blood. What is the next best step in the patient's management?

(A) endoscopic esophageal banding to treat the varices

(B) endoscopic esophageal sclerotherapy to treat the varices

(C) surgical therapy for definitive ligation of varices

(D) institution of high-dose proton pump inhibitor (PPI) therapy

(E) placement of a transjugular intrahepatic portosystemic shunt (TIPS) via interventional radiology

47. The patient does well and does not rebleed while in hospital. Which additional therapy that can help prevent rebleeding in this patient should be provided as an outpatient management strategy?

   (A) endoscopic esophageal banding to treat the varices

   (B) endoscopic esophageal sclerotherapy to treat the varices

   (C) surgical therapy for definitive ligation of varices

   (D) institution of high-dose PPI therapy

   (E) placement of a TIPS via interventional radiology

48. Six months later the patient returns to the ER following another episode of massive hematemesis. Upper endoscopy performed in the hospital reveals actively bleeding gastric varices below the esophagogastric junction. The bleeding is torrential and the patient is hemodynamically unstable.

What is the next best step in the patient's management?

   (A) endoscopic esophageal banding to treat the varices

   (B) endoscopic esophageal sclerotherapy to treat the varices

   (C) surgical therapy for definitive ligation of varices

   (D) institution of high-dose PPI therapy

   (E) placement of a TIPS via interventional radiology

Answers and Explanations

1. **(D)**

2. **(C)**

3. **(D)**

Explanations 1 through 3

Microscopic hematuria is defined as >3 RBCs/ HPF on microscopic evaluation of the urinary sediment from two of three properly collected urinalysis specimens. Because the degree of hematuria bears no relation to the seriousness of the underling cause, hematuria should be considered a symptom of serious disease until proved otherwise (observation is incorrect). The initial step in evaluating microscopic hematuria is a thorough medical history and physical examination. Evaluation of the upper urinary tract is the next recommended step. Options for this include intravenous pyelography, ultrasonography, and CT scanning. *(Grossfeld et al., 2001, pp. 1145–1154)*

During this visit you should provide alcohol abuse counseling. The United States Preventive Services Task Force (USPSTF) has a B recommendation (recommend routinely) for screening and behavioral counseling interventions to reduce alcohol misuse by adults in primary care settings. The USPSTF has an I recommendation (insufficient evidence) for skin cancer and low back pain prevention counseling and D recommendation (against) routine screening for testicular cancer in asymptomatic adolescent and adult males. The patient's last dT booster was at age 14, 5 years ago, so he does not need a dT booster at this time. *(USPSTF: www.preventiveservices.ahrq.gov)*

The number one cause of death in this patient's age group is motor vehicle-related injuries. The mortality rate for the 15- to 24-year age range due to unintentional injury is 38.7/100.000, most of it due to motor vehicle accidents. The next most common causes of death are other traumas, including homicide, suicide, and drowning. *(Last et al., 1992)*

4. **(D)**

5. **(E)**

Explanations 4 and 5

Conversion disorder is diagnosed by the presence of neurologic symptoms or deficits associated with largely unconscious psychological factors or conflicts, without the myriad of different symptoms seen in this case. Hypochondriasis is characterized by a preoccupation with fears of having a serious illness based on a misinterpretation of bodily sensations. Pain disorder involves significant distress or impairment in functioning as a result of pain. Psychological factors are felt to play a role in the onset, severity, exacerbation, and maintenance of the pain. Non-pain-related symptomatology, as demonstrated in this patient, is not a feature. Undifferentiated somatoform disorder is diagnosed when there are unexplained physical complaints which do not meet full criteria for somatization disorder. This case represents somatization disorder, characterized by a pattern of recurring, multiple somatic complaints, beginning before the age of 30, which are not fully explained by any known medical condition. *(American Psychiatric Association, 2000)*

If a patient is diagnosed with somatization disorder, admission to the hospital for an extensive workup and multiple referrals may reinforce the process of somatization and worsen symptoms. Confronting the individual will likely anger the patient and lead to an increase in somatic complaints. Reassurance that a diagnosis will be discovered is inaccurate, misleading, and can eventually result in a lawsuit. The most appropriate management for these individuals is to schedule regular, brief appointments addressing any new physical complaints. Laboratory tests, studies, and procedures should be limited in nature. An abbreviated physical examination will reassure the patient that he/she is cared for and taken seriously. After a therapeutic alliance is better established, eventual referral to a psychiatrist may help to decrease health care utilization and to treat any comorbid psychopathology. *(Sadock and Sadock, 2003, p. 647)*

6. **(C)**

7. **(C)**

8. **(B)**

Explanations 6 through 8

Polymyalgia rheumatica is an inflammatory syndrome of older individuals characterized by pain and stiffness in the shoulder and pelvic girdles. Patients are typically >50 years old, have bilateral symptoms, and the ESR is frequently elevated above 40 mm/h. The absence of muscle weakness and normal CPK argue against polymyositis. Although hypothyroidism can cause musculoskeletal pain, it is not associated with an ESR of 99 or weight loss (typically weight gain). Osteoarthritis of the neck and shoulders would demonstrate abnormalities in the range of motion associated with pain—this patient has muscle tenderness only. Fibromyalgia is a chronic noninflammatory and nonautoimmune diffuse pain syndrome of unknown etiology, with an average age of onset of between 35 and 40 years of age and characteristic tender points (11 of the 18 tender points need to be present for at least 3 months and exist both above and below the waist). Given the advanced age of this patient (60-year-old), the presence of symptoms for only 1 month and evidence for systemic inflammation (ESR = 99), the diagnosis of fibromyalgia is highly unlikely.

Prednisone in a dose of 10–20 mg daily usually results in a dramatic and rapid response in polymyalgia rheumatica. Most patients are significantly better in 1–2 days and the ESR

should steadily decline. The use of TRH would be appropriate if this patient's symptoms were due to hypothyroidism. Analgesics will not help the inflammation (indicated by the elevated ESR) in polymyalgia rheumatica. Although this patient could have depression, the elevated ESR argues against this and the use of a muscle relaxant for a systemic inflammatory disease is unlikely to be helpful.

Giant cell (or temporal) arteritis occurs synchronously or sequentially in patients with polymyalgia rheumatica (PMR). Symptoms include headache, jaw claudication, visual disturbance, and scalp tenderness. The failure of prednisone to significantly improve symptoms (at doses of 20 mg daily) or normalize the ESR should suggest the presence of temporal arteritis and prompt temporal artery biopsy. Rheumatoid arthritis is unlikely, as there is no evidence of synovitis of any of the joints. Systemic lupus erythematosus is possible, but highly unlikely, in a patient of this age who is ANA negative. This patient's symptoms are not typical for hypothyroidism (absence of muscle weakness, weight loss instead of weight gain, and an elevated ESR ~100 mm/h). To assume that the patient is depressed and is amplifying her symptoms despite laboratory evidence of systemic inflammation (ESR ~100 mm/h) would not be prudent. *(Ruddy et al., 2001, pp. 1155–1162)*

9. **(A)** Cyanotic congenital heart lesions are usually the result of right-to-left shunting. This results in the shunting of blood past the pulmonary system and the absence of gas exchange. Tetralogy of Fallot, transposition of the great vessels, truncus arteriosus, and pulmonic atresia are all causes of cyanotic congenital heart disease. The child in the case presented, however, does not have a cyanotic lesion. Of the listed heart lesions, only the VSD results in left-to-right shunting. *(Fleisher and Ludwig, 2000, pp. 187–191)*

10. **(A)**

11. **(D)**

12. **(C)**

Explanations 10 through 12

The patient likely has elevated BP secondary to OCP medication. This is the most common cause of secondary hypertension in the patient and, at its onset, the medication should be stopped. In addition, she has developed other side effects from OCPs, including weight gain and edema. Given her current symptoms, it is reasonable to assume that her BP may be elevated and hence should be checked during this visit. The vaginal bleeding and missed menses may signify that she is currently pregnant. Therefore, a urine pregnancy test should be obtained and the OCP stopped immediately until pregnancy is ruled out.

The only absolute contraindication listed is smoking after the age of 35, although heavy smoking at any age is also considered a relative contraindication. With the exception of hemolytic anemia, the rest of the choices are all considered relative contraindications to prescribing OCPs. The only hemolytic anemia which is considered an absolute contraindication is sickle cell disease, due to an increased risk of thrombosis.

Cholelithiasis is a well-established potential side effect of OCPs. Others include thromboembolic disease, hypertension, weight gain, fluid retention, edema, glucose intolerance, headaches, melasma, and nausea. The risk of developing endometrial cancer and ovarian cancer may, in fact, be reduced with the use of OCPs. The temporary infertility induced by OCPs should be reversible on discontinuation. Prolonged infertility following the cessation of OCPs should prompt a workup for other causes. Thrombocytopenia is not considered to be an expected side effect of OCPs. *(Larsen et al., 2003, pp. 672–691)*

13. **(A)** FHH, or familial benign hypercalcemia, is a rare condition characterized by asymptomatic or mildly symptomatic hypercalcemia. It is inherited as an autosomal dominant trait and the parathyroid glands are usually normal in size. The basis for the development of FHH appears to be mutations in the calcium-sensing receptor gene which regulates the parathyroid gland set point and modulates the extracellular calcium concentration. The condition may be mistaken for primary hyperparathyroidism because, in both conditions, the serum calcium and parathyroid hormone levels are elevated with a concomitant low serum phosphate. The distinction is made by obtaining a 24-hour urine calcium excretion level. In patients with FHH, the urine calcium level is low, whereas in primary hyperparathyroidism the level is high. The distinction is important, as patients with primary hyperparathyroidism benefit from surgery and those with FHH do not. *(Cameron, 2004, p. 602)*

14. **(B)**

15. **(D)**

16. **(D)**

Explanations 14 through 16

Avoidant personality disorder is characterized by a pattern of inhibition in social situations and feelings of inadequacy. These individuals are more likely to blame themselves for their difficulties rather than criticize others, as illustrated in the above case. Patients with dependent personality disorder display a pervasive need to be taken care of that leads to submissive behavior. They are not likely to be hostile or as labile as in the above example. Paranoid individuals maintain chronic mistrust and suspiciousness of others. They assume that others will or have harmed them. They are not liable to enter into numerous relationships or admit to feelings of loneliness in the way that the above patient demonstrates. Schizoid personality disorder is diagnosed in patients with a pervasive pattern of detachment and restricted range of expression in interpersonal relationships. Schizoid individuals do not seek out relationships, preferring solitary activities. They are not as explosive as the patient in this case. The above example represents a man with borderline personality disorder, characterized by instability of relationships, affects and sense of self, as well as impulsivity, anger control problems, and chronic feelings of emptiness. *(American Psychiatric Association, 2000)*

Denial is classified as a primitive or psychotic defense mechanism, where an individual avoids awareness of an external reality by negating sensory data. Displacement is considered a neurotic defense, characterized by shifting feeling from one person or situation to another that will evoke less distress. Intellectualization is another neurotic defense, utilizing intellectual processes in order to avoid affective experience. Sublimation is classified as a mature defense, where a person will direct an impulse toward a socially acceptable goal. The above patient demonstrates the defense mechanism of splitting. Splitting is considered a primitive defense and is commonly seen in severe personality disorders, especially borderline personality disorder. In splitting, patients divide feelings, people, and behavior into separate good and bad categories rather than deal with their ambivalence. (Sadock and Sadock, 2003, pp. 207–208, 802)

While benzodiazepines such as clonazepam may help with anxiety and agitation in individuals with borderline personality disorder, they are not considered first-line medications due to the paucity of data, the risk of abuse, and the possibility of worsening behavioral dyscontrol. Antipsychotics such as haloperidol may be beneficial for control of anger and self-mutilation, but the effects are nonspecific. Given the significant side effects, especially the risk of tardive dyskinesia, they are not considered appropriate for use as solo agents. Mood stabilizers, such as lithium and valproic acid, are sometimes used to treat the impulsive aggression and mood lability common in borderline patients. However, there is legitimate concern in using lithium in these impulsive, often suicidal patients, given its toxicity in overdose. While valproate is safer in overdose, there are less data to support its efficacy in this patient population. Antidepressants in general, especially serotonin-specific reuptake inhibitors (SSRIs) such as sertraline, have been shown to be efficacious in treating the symptoms of mood lability, impulsivity, aggression, hostility, and self-mutilation seen in borderline personality disorder. SSRIs have been the most widely studied medications and are very safe in the event of an overdose.

These factors favor their use as a first-line pharmacotherapy in these patients, although no agents are currently Food and Drug Administration (FDA) approved for this illness. (American Psychiatric Association, 2001)

17. **(A)** Thyroid cancer is classified as papillary, follicular, Hurthle cell, medullarly, or anaplastic. Of all subtypes, papillary carries the best overall prognosis. In addition to the subtype of cancer, there are several important prognostic indicators, referred to as the AGES scale. The AGES scale includes the **A**ge of the patient, pathologic tumor **G**rade, **E**xtent of disease, and **S**ize of tumor. Other important factors include the presence of distant metastases, the extent of original surgical resection, and the presence of extrathyroidal invasion. Of all factors, age is the most important (age <40). For instance, a 16-year-old male with thyroid cancer and metastasis to regional lymph nodes has a 90% chance of survival. (Schwartz et al., 1999, pp. 1682–1683)

18. **(D)** Absolute contraindications to the use of combined OCPs include history of thrombotic disorders, vascular disease (e.g., cerebral, coronary), impaired liver function (or liver tumor), history of hormone-dependent cancer (e.g., breast), smoker over the age of 35, known or suspected pregnancy, undiagnosed vaginal bleeding, and congenital hyperlipidemia. (Beckmann et al., 2002, p. 335)

19. **(E)**

20. **(C)**

Explanations 19 and 20

This child has a "narrow-gap" metabolic acidosis. Given her history, this would be most consistent with RTA. In her case, this represents the presence of a proximal renal bicarbonate threshold (proximal RTA). She is unable to retain bicarbonate enough to raise her serum level. Persistent vomiting (pyloric stenosis, duodenal stenosis, or gastroesophageal reflux) would result in the loss of bicarbonate and thus a serum alkalosis, not acidosis.

In proximal RTA (type II RTA), there is a failure to reabsorb bicarbonate. There is a "threshold" level of serum bicarbonate above which the kidney will "spill" the bicarbonate into the urine. For example, if the "threshold" is a serum level of 15, the addition of bicarbonate to the serum will result in the bicarbonate spilling into the urine, with a resulting increase in the urinary pH. The addition of bicarbonate into the serum would result in a transient increase in the serum level, with a gradual decrease back to the "threshold" level. When the serum bicarbonate level reaches 15, the threshold level, the urinary pH will return to normal (slightly acidic, pH of approximately 5–7). In distal RTA (type I RTA), there is an inability to maintain a proton "gradient." This results in an abnormally high urinary pH in the face of acidemia (the inability to lower urinary pH). Distal RTA will also have hypokalemia, as a result of maintaining electroneutrality. In evaluation of a proximal RTA, the diagnostic workup includes a trial of bicarbonate. This trial will demonstrate the transient rising of the urinary pH and serum bicarbonate. *(Rudolph et al., 2003, pp. 1710–1712)*

21. **(B)** This patient has symptoms and physical findings of vulvovaginal atrophy due to the hypoestrogenic state of menopause. Irritative bladder symptoms are common with this condition as the lower genitourinary (GU) tract has estrogen receptors like the vagina and vulva. A white, curdy discharge of a yeast infection is possible, and would be more common following a course of antibiotic. It would not be consistent with the time course of her symptoms, however. A retained tampon would tend to cause a malodorous vaginal discharge. The likelihood of this woman using a tampon would also be low, as she is postmenopausal. A vesicovaginal fistula would tend to cause a leakage of urine from the vagina rather than irritative bladder symptoms. A fungating cervical mass (i.e., advanced cervical carcinoma) would be a rare occurrence. *(Hendrix, 2003, pp. 1029–1037)*

22. **(C)** There are few situations in which a state's medical or legal authorities should be involved in the care of a child. Refusal of vaccinations during an epidemic may be one of those situations. Parents may have personal preferences regarding immunizations but these preferences do not reach the threshold of a true religious exemption. If a parent declines an immunization, routine care, including any "nonobjectionable" vaccinations should be continued. All opportunities should be afforded to engage the parents during future visits to readdress an incomplete immunization status. At no time should immunizations be administered against a parent's expressed wishes (without appropriate legal and judicial intervention). While immunization delinquency may be part of a medical neglect picture, it would be unlikely that declining immunization alone would be considered true medical neglect. *(Diekema, 2005, pp. 1428–1431)*

23. **(D)** The diagnosis is primary hypothyroidism, most likely due to postpartum thyroiditis. The essential laboratory finding is the elevated TSH and low free thyroid hormone levels in the setting of weight gain and fatigue. The low T3-resin uptake indicates increased thyroid-binding globulin (TBG) from either hypothyroidism or estrogen effect. The free thyroid index is derived by multiplying T3-uptake times the total T4. As both levels are low, the free thyroid index will also be low. The galactorrhea and the elevated prolactin are not uncommon in patients with hypothyroidism and relate to the increased levels of TRH, a potent stimulant for prolactin. The prolactin should no longer be elevated from nursing, but OCPs also increase prolactin levels. As the baseline TSH is elevated, there is no indication for a TRH stimulation test. Nuclear thyroid scans give useful information in the differential diagnosis of hyperthyroidism but are not helpful in the diagnosis of hypothyroidism. *(Larsen et al., 2003, pp. 423–428, 440)*

24. **(C)** Follow-up of patients with hydatidiform mole indicates evacuation is curative in 80% of cases. In roughly 20% of cases, however, trophoblastic tissue will persist and the diagnosis of gestational trophoblastic neoplasia (GTN) will be made. This diagnosis includes a

spectrum of disease including invasive mole, choriocarcinoma, and placental site trophoblastic tumor.

Following evacuation of a molar gestation, appropriate surveillance follow-up should include serial hCG values obtained for 1–2 weeks until normal times three and then monthly thereafter, to complete 1 year of surveillance. Birth control is recommended during this period, preferably with OCPs. In the setting of stable or rising hCG levels, as in the case noted above, metastatic workup is indicated with a CT scan of the head, chest, abdomen, and pelvis.

Patients at risk for the development of postevacuation GTN include those with (1) preevacuation uterus >16 weeks' size; (2) preevacuation bilateral ovarian enlargement (theca-lutein cysts); (3) age greater than 40; (4) preevacuation hCG levels greater than 100,000 mIU/mL; (5) prior hydatidiform mole; (6) medical complications of molar pregnancy including toxemia, hyperthyroidism, and trophoblastic embolization.

Indications for treatment of postmolar trophoblastic tumor include: (1) plateauing hCG levels for three consecutive determinations; (2) rising hCG levels for two consecutive determinations; (3) hCG levels greater than 20,000 mIU/mL 4 or more weeks postevacuation; (4) detection of metastases; or (5) histopathologic diagnosis of choriocarcinoma.

A repeat D&C (dilation & curettage) is rarely indicated following evacuation of a molar gestation; it is not curative in the setting of GTN and may be associated with an increased risk of uterine perforation. (Ng and Wong, 2003, pp. 893–903)

25. **(E)** The initial step in identification of the cause of a prolonged PT or aPTT is to establish if the addition of normal plasma can correct the deficit. Failure to correct the prolonged PT or aPTT by addition of 50% normal plasma is indicative of the presence of a specific (against one of the coagulation factors) or nonspecific inhibitor (e.g., lupus anticoagulant). If, after the 1:1 mix, the PT or aPTT tests correct, a plasma factor(s) deficiency is the most likely cause. The most common inhibitor in a nonhemophilia

individual is against factor VIII, as is this woman's case. (Hoffman et al., 2000, p. 1843)

26. **(C)** The distal small bowel (ileum) is the site of absorption of fat-soluble vitamins (vitamins A, D, E, and K) as well as vitamin B_{12}. Vitamin B_{12} binds with intrinsic factor, a glycoprotein secreted from parietal cells of the gastric fundus and body. Specific receptors in the terminal ileum take up the B_{12} intrinsic factor complex. Vitamin B_{12} deficiency leads to megaloblastic anemia. The patient will require monthly vitamin B_{12} injections. (Schwartz et al., 1999, p. 1255)

27. **(A)**

28. **(D)**

29. **(E)**

Explanations 27 through 29

The photomicrograph shows malignant tumor cells infiltrating between the collagen bundles and in some focal areas, growing as a solid nest. The tumor shows high degree of anaplasia with prominent nucleoli and scant cytoplasm. Formation of ductal structures is minimal and, for all of these reasons, it is a poorly differentiated tumor (grade III). Carcinoma of the breast affects one out of nine women in the United States and one-third of these patients will die of the disease. Cancer of the breast is rarely found before the age of 25, except when there is a familial predisposition. Family history is a risk factor for the development of breast cancer in 5–10% of the cases. Two genes have been implicated in the genetic inheritance of cancer of the breast those are, BRCA-1 and BRCA-2; however, less than 20% of women with a family history of breast cancer carry these genes. A proliferative breast disease (atypical ductal hyperplasia) is also associated with an increase in risk for developing breast cancer. Also associated with the increased risk of developing carcinoma of the breast is increasing age, carcinoma of the contralateral breast or endometrium, radiation exposure, length of reproductive life, parity, obesity, and estrogen (although questionable).

Invasive or infiltrating ductal carcinomas are the major variety of the carcinomas (70–80%). Most of these cancers exhibit a marked increase in fibrous tissue stroma, which gives the stony hard consistency. On histologic examination, the tumor consists of malignant cells forming cords, solid nests, and tubules. The cytologic appearance of these tumor cells varies from low to high grade. *(Cotran et al., 1999, pp. 1104–1111)*

The prognosis of breast cancer is directly related to its staging using the TNM system. In the absence of distant metastasis, the stage of the tumor is determined by the size of the primary tumor and the presence or absence of regional lymphadenopathy. Other prognostic factors, such as the presence of lymphatic invasion or hormone receptor status, may influence survival, but it is not clear whether they add to the information from pathologic staging.

Atypical lobular hyperplasia, atypical ductal hyperplasia, and tubular adenoma are benign breast diseases and would not cause adenopathy. Lobular carcinoma in situ, by definition, is not an invasive cancer and, therefore, would not cause the presence of axillary adenopathy. However, approximately 30% of patients who undergo excision of lobular neoplasia may develop invasive carcinoma in the following 15–20 years, usually infiltrating ductal carcinoma. Of the options listed, only infiltrating ductal carcinoma would be expected to cause axillary metastasis. *(Braunwald et al., 2001, pp. 574–577)*

30. **(C)** Prolonged bleeding time is the hallmark of platelet pathology. Impaired platelet adhesion is seen in both acute and chronic renal insufficiency. The mechanism is unclear, although data imply that uremic toxins in plasma result in disaggregation of factor VIII, which is required for proper platelet function. DDAVP (1-desamino-8-D-arginine vasopressin) is a synthetic derivative of vasopressin and administration results in a dose-dependent increase of factor VIII from endothelial cells. It is therefore used to help control postoperative bleeding in uremic patients. Alternatively, transfusion with cryoprecipitate is useful because it contains high levels of factor VIII. Ultimately, correction of the uremic state with dialysis may be indicated. Transfused platelets will not correct the condition, as they will be deactivated by the circulating toxins. Vitamin K is used to correct bleeding caused by a defective extrinsic pathway of the coagulation cascade. Fresh frozen plasma does not contain high levels of factor VIII. Hyperglycemia is not related to bleeding tendency. *(Jarrell et al., 2000, pp. 130–131; Schwartz et al., 1999, p. 82)*

31. **(D)** Physiologic changes in the cardiovascular and circulatory systems are significant and may affect underlying maternal illness. Blood volume increases by 40–50% by term pregnancy, with red cell mass lagging behind and increasing by only 20–25%; this differential has been referred to as the physiologic anemia of pregnancy. The total requirement for term pregnancy to meet maternal, fetal, and placental needs is 1000 mg of iron. This need can be met by preexisting iron stores in iron-replete women, but at the risk of depleting their iron stores, resulting in postpartum anemia. Iron depletion can be prevented by the administration of 30 mg of elemental iron per day, which can be obtained by taking one ferrous gluconate 325 mg tablet per day. *(Romslo et al., 1983, pp. 101–107)*

32. **(E)** Meckel's diverticulum, the most common true diverticulum of the GI tract, is a congenital diverticulum that results from incomplete closure of the omphalomesenteric, or vitelline, duct. It is characteristically found within 2 ft of the ileocecal junction and along the antimesenteric border of the ileum. A Meckel's diverticulum may be asymptomatic and found incidentally during surgical exploration. In this scenario, resection is indicated only if there are signs of potential complications. Such findings include the presence of palpable firm tissue at the base. This represents heterotrophic gastric or pancreatic tissue, which may result in an adjacent ulcer and bleeding. If a connection or adhesion from the Meckel's diverticulum to the umbilicus is present, resection would be indicated to prevent the risk of future intestinal rotation, volvulus, and obstruction around the adhesion. Finally, resection should

be contemplated if the neck of the Meckel's diverticulum is narrow, as this may result in future obstruction by a fecalith with resulting diverticulitis and perforation. The morbidity from incidental removal can be as high as 12% and is therefore limited to these indications. *(Schwartz et al., 1999, p. 1249)*

33.   (C)

34.   (A)

Explanations 34 and 35

Hungry bone syndrome refers to hypocalcemia following surgical correction of hyperparathyroidism in patients with severe, prolonged disease, as serum calcium is rapidly taken from the circulation and deposited into the bone. Symptoms usually occur within 24–48 hours following parathyroidectomy, when calcium levels reach a nadir. Early symptoms include numbness and tingling in the perioral area, fingers, or toes. Advanced symptoms include nervousness, anxiety, and increased neuromuscular transmission evidenced by positive Chvostek's and Trousseau's signs, carpal pedal spasm, and hyperactive tendon reflexes. In severe cases, one may develop a prolonged QT interval on ECG.

Patients who manifest any signs or symptoms of hypocalcemia always require intervention. In severely symptomatic patients, treatment should begin with intravenous calcium gluconate. Mildly symptomatic patients may be given oral calcium in the form of calcium lactate, calcium carbonate, or calcium gluconate. If hypocalcemia remains despite calcium supplementation, additional therapy with vitamin D may be needed. Supplemental calcium and vitamin D therapy should be continued until serum calcium levels return to normal. *(Schwartz et al., 1999, p. 1701)*

35.   (C) Evans syndrome is the combination of ITP and autoimmune hemolytic anemia. The triggers of these events remain speculative. Children with Evans syndrome will have a Coombs' positive anemia with various levels of thrombocytopenia. Corticosteroids may be

warranted to control acute hemolysis or thrombocytopenia. *(Rudolph et al., 2003, p. 1546)*

36.   (A)

37.   (B)

38.   (D)

Explanations 36 through 38

Gallstone ileus causes 1–2% of mechanical small-intestine obstructions. It results from erosion of an impacted gallstone through the wall of the gallbladder into the wall of the adjacent duodenum. The gallstone then passes through the small intestine. The size of the stone is important, since stones smaller than 2 cm usually pass, while larger stones may cause an obstruction. When obstruction occurs, the site is usually at the terminal ileum, which is the narrowest portion of the small intestine. The resulting obstruction results in large fluid losses and electrolyte abnormalities. Edema, ulceration and, ultimately, necrosis of the bowel may occur, resulting in perforation.

The correct preoperative diagnosis is infrequently made. However, radiographic examination is diagnostic if gas is demonstrated within the biliary tree in the presence of a small intestine obstruction. In 20% of cases a radiopaque stone is also visualized.

Definitive therapy requires urgent surgical intervention. The patient is explored and the small bowel is opened (enterotomy) just proximal to the lodged stone. The stone is extracted and the small bowel is primarily closed. Prolonging the operation to perform a cholecystectomy in an ill, elderly patient adds to potential operative morbidity and is generally not warranted. *(Schwartz et al., 1999, pp. 1450–1452)*

39.   (E) SIDS is the most common cause of death in children between 1 and 12 months of age. In the first month of life, perinatal complications (i.e., prematurity) are the most common cause of death. The diagnosis of SIDS requires a review of the medical history, a death scene investigation, as well as a full postmortem examination.

The rate of SIDS has decreased dramatically with the onset of the "Back to Sleep" campaign, which recommends placing infants on their back or side—not abdomen—to sleep. While bacterial meningitis can be a devastating disease, it is rarely fatal when treated. Death from congenital malformations will usually occur within the first month of a neonate's life. (*Rudolph et al., 2003, pp. 1935–1936*)

40. **(C)**

41. **(C)**

Explanations 40 and 41

This patient is presenting with symptoms most consistent with central retinal artery occlusion. This typically causes painless, acute, unilateral vision loss. Sometimes there will be an associated history of amaurosis fugax. Characteristic diagnostic signs of this are a cherry red spot in the center of the macula and superficial opacification or whitening of the retina in the posterior pole. Common etiologies of this include embolus from the heart or carotid artery, thrombosis, giant cell arteritis, other collagen vascular disease, and hypercoagulable states.

For this patient, who has atrial fibrillation, which would put her at an increased risk of embolic disease, the most important test to order emergently would be an ESR. This would help to determine whether the etiology of the event is more likely embolic or related to giant cell arteritis. If the ESR were markedly elevated then high-dose steroids should be immediately started. The other tests listed may be part of the later workup but would not be as important immediately to determine the urgent treatment required. (*Kunimoto et al., 2004, Sect. 11.5*)

42. **(B)** Esophageal perforation has a poor survival rate, especially if the diagnosis is delayed. When suspected, urgent posterior-to-anterior (PA) and lateral CXRs should be obtained. Positive findings include mediastinal emphysema, mediastinal-widening secondary to edema, pneumothorax, and pleural effusion; however, these findings may take over an hour

to appear. The diagnosis is confirmed with a water-soluble contrast (gastrografin) esophagogram. If the gastrografin study is negative, a thin-barium swallow should be performed. Barium extravasation may result in a severe mediastinitis. (*Cameron, 2004, p. 8*)

43. **(C)** In the wintertime, greater than 90% of children younger than 3 years of age will become infected with respiratory syncytial virus (RSV). It can cause a bronchiolitis in infants which occasionally results in hypoxia. Most otherwise healthy infants will not require hospitalization. Risk factors for complications from RSV bronchiolitis include bronchopulmonary dysplasia, congenital heart disease, and prematurity. (*American Academy of Pediatrics, 2003, pp. 523–528*)

44. **(D)** There are two methods commonly utilized to estimate the total burn surface area: the palm method and the rule of nine. The palm method is based on the fact that patient's palm approximates 1% of his/her total body surface area. This method is particularly useful in those with a patchy pattern of burn injury. Rule of nine divides the body surface into several areas, each of which represents 9% or an interval of 9%. The head and neck represents 9% and each of the upper extremeties equals 9% of the total body surface area. The anterior and posterior trunk each accounts for 18% as does each lower extremity. The genital area is 1%. In the above scenario, the patient has a burn involving his right upper extremity (9%), anterior trunk (18%), and right lower extremity (18%), a total of 45%. (*Schwartz et al., 1999, p. 228*)

45. **(D)**

46. **(A)**

47. **(A)**

48. **(E)**

Explanations 45 through 48

The patient is symptomatically orthostatic when switching from a supine to sitting position following massive hematemesis and needs urgent IV volume repletion to help prevent end-organ damage from hypovolemia. Hepatitis serology data, gastric lavage, correction of coagulopathy, and radiologic studies, while all important, should be deferred until after the patient has been hemodynamically stabilized.

Endoscopic esophageal banding would be the procedure of choice for this patient. Banding is superior to sclerotherapy in terms of efficacy for stopping variceal bleeding, although sclerotherapy might be a second option if banding fails or causes more bleeding. Surgery in patients with bleeding esophageal varices involves a very high risk due to portal hypertension and concomitant coagulopathy. PPI therapy would do little to help this patient as his illness is not due to acid reflux. A TIPS is not first-line therapy for acute variceal bleeding.

The patient had bleeding esophageal varices that have been successfully treated via banding. Banding rarely completely ablates varices in a single session. Multiple sessions are often required to completely thrombose and scar the varices to the point where they cannot rebleed. Sclerotherapy is not usually performed in patients who have responded to banding. High-dose PPI therapy would not help to prevent rebleeding from esophageal varices. A TIPS is not required in patients who have had bleeding controlled endoscopically and are doing well. Endoscopic therapy is preferable to surgery as an outpatient management strategy in patients with portal hypertension.

Gastric varices, often seen in patients with portal hypertension, respond poorly to endoscopic banding or sclerotherapy. A PPI would not help to stop the bleeding. Surgery in this patient is possible but highly risky given his hemodynamic instability. A TIPS could be performed in an emergent fashion and would decompress his portal system and would have the best chance of stopping the bleeding from the gastric varices. (Braunwald et al., 2001, pp. 252–253, 1760–1761)

American Academy of Pediatrics. *The Red Book, 2003 Report of the Committee on Infectious Diseases,* 26th ed. Elk Grove Village, IL: American Academy of Pediatrics, 2003.

American Psychiatric Association. *Diagnostic and Statistical Manual of Mental Disorders,* 4th ed., Text Revision. Washington, DC: American Psychiatric Association, 2000.

American Psychiatric Association. *Practice Guideline for the Treatment of Patients with Borderline Personality Disorder.* Washington, DC: American Psychiatric Association, 2001.

Beckmann CRB, Ling FW, Laube DW, et al. *Obstetrics and Gynecology,* 4th ed. Baltimore, MD: Lippincot Williams & Wilkins, 2002.

Braunwald E, Hauser SL, Jameson JL, et al. *Harrison's Principles of Internal Medicine,* 15th ed. New York, NY: McGraw-Hill, 2001.

Cameron JL, ed. *Current Surgical Therapy,* 8th ed. St. Louis, MO: C.V. Mosby, 2004.

Cotran RS, Kumar V, Collins T. *Robbins Pathologic Basis of Disease,* 6th ed. Philadelphia, PA: W.B. Saunders, 1999.

Diekema DS. Responding to parental refusals of immunizations of children. *Pediatrics* 2005;115(5): 1428–1431.

Fleisher GR, Ludwig S, eds. *Textbook of Pediatric Emergency Medicine,* 4th ed. Baltimore, MD: Lippincott Williams & Wilkins, 2000.

Grossfeld GD, Wolf JS, Litwin MS, et al. Asymptomatic microscopic hematuria in adults: summary of the AUA best practice policy recommendations. *Am Fam Physician* 2001;63:1145–1154.

Hendrix SL. Long-term use of hormone therapy for urogenital complaints. *Med Clin North Am* 2003;87(5):1029–1037.

Hoffman R, Benz EJ, Shattil SJ, et al. *Hematology: Basic Principles and Practice,* 3rd ed. New York, NY: Churchill Livingstone, 2000.

Jarrell BE, Carabasi RA. *National Medical Series for Independent Study, Surgery,* 4th ed. Philadelphia, PA: Lippincott Williams & Wilkins, 2000, pp. 130–131.

Kunimoto DY, Kanitkar KD, Makar MS, et al. *The Wills Eye Manual: Office and Emergency Room Diagnosis and Treatment of Eye Disease,* 4th ed. Philadelphia, PA: Lippincott Williams & Wilkins, 2004.

Larsen PR, Davies TF, Hay ID, et al. *Williams Textbook of Endocrinology,* 10th ed. Philadelphia, PA: W.B. Saunders, 2003.

Last JM, Wallace RB. *Maxcy-Rosenau-Last Public Health and Preventive Medicine,* 14th ed. Norwalk, CT: Appleton and Lange, 1992.

Ng TY, Wong LC. Diagnosis and management of gestational trophoblastic neoplasia. *Best Pract Res Clin Obstet Gynaecol* 2003;17(6):893–903.

Romslo I, Haram K, Sagan N, et al. Iron requirement in normal pregnancy is assessed by serum ferritin, serum transfer and saturation and erythrocyte protoporphyrin determinations. *Br J Obstet Gynecol* 1983;90:101–107.

Ruddy S, Harris J, Sledge CM, et al. *Kelley's Textbook of Rheumatology,* 6th ed. Philadelphia, PA: W.B. Saunders, 2001.

Rudolph CD, Rudolph AM, Hostetter MK, et al., eds. *Rudolph's Pediatrics,* 21st ed. New York, NY: McGraw-Hill, 2003.

Sadock BJ, Sadock VA. *Kaplan and Sadock's Synopsis of Psychiatry,* 9th ed. Philadelphia, PA: Lippincott Williams & Wilkins, 2003.

Schwartz SI, Shires GT, Spencer FC, et al., eds. *Principles of Surgery,* 7th ed. New York, NY: McGraw-Hill, 1999.

USPSTF: www.preventiveservices.ahrq.gov.

Index